Essentials of
Applied Microbiology
for NURSES
Including Infection Control and Safety

Essentials of
Applied Microbiology for NURSES
Including Infection Control and Safety

As per the Revised INC Syllabus for BSc Nursing

Apurba S Sastry MD (JIPMER) DNB MNAMS PDCR
Officer In-charge, Hospital Infection Control and Prevention Unit (HICP)
Antimicrobial Stewardship Lead
Additional Professor
Department of Microbiology
Jawaharlal Institute of Postgraduate Medical Education and Research (JIPMER)
Puducherry, India

Sandhya Bhat (Gold medalist) MD DNB MNAMS PDCR
Professor
Department of Microbiology
Pondicherry Institute of Medical Sciences (PIMS)
(A Unit of Madras Medical Mission)
Puducherry, India

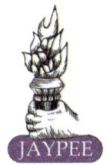

JAYPEE BROTHERS MEDICAL PUBLISHERS
The Health Sciences Publisher
New Delhi | London

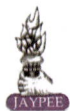 **Jaypee Brothers Medical Publishers (P) Ltd**

Headquarters

Jaypee Brothers Medical Publishers (P) Ltd
EMCA House, 23/23-B
Ansari Road, Daryaganj
New Delhi 110 002, India
Landline: +91-11-23272143, +91-11-23272703
+91-11-23282021, +91-11-23245672
Email: jaypee@jaypeebrothers.com

Corporate Office

Jaypee Brothers Medical Publishers (P) Ltd
4838/24, Ansari Road, Daryaganj
New Delhi 110 002, India
Phone: +91-11-43574357
Fax: +91-11-43574314
Email: jaypee@jaypeebrothers.com

Overseas Office

J.P. Medical Ltd
83 Victoria Street, London
SW1H 0HW (UK)
Phone: +44 20 3170 8910
Fax: +44 (0)20 3008 6180
Email: info@jpmedpub.com

Website: www.jaypeebrothers.com
Website: www.jaypeedigital.com

© 2022, Jaypee Brothers Medical Publishers

The views and opinions expressed in this book are solely those of the original contributor(s)/author(s) and do not necessarily represent those of editor(s) and Publisher of the book.

All rights reserved. No part of this publication may be reproduced, stored or transmitted in any form or by any means, electronic, mechanical, photocopying, recording or otherwise, without the prior permission in writing of the publishers.

All brand names and product names used in this book are trade names, service marks, trademarks or registered trademarks of their respective owners. The publisher is not associated with any product or vendor mentioned in this book.

Medical knowledge and practice change constantly. This book is designed to provide accurate, authoritative information about the subject matter in question. However, readers are advised to check the most current information available on procedures included and check information from the manufacturer of each product to be administered, to verify the recommended dose, formula, method and duration of administration, adverse effects and contraindications. It is the responsibility of the practitioner to take all appropriate safety precautions. Neither the publisher nor the author(s)/editor(s) assume any liability for any injury and/or damage to persons or property arising from or related to use of material in this book.

This book is sold on the understanding that the publisher is not engaged in providing professional medical services. If such advice or services are required, the services of a competent medical professional should be sought.

Every effort has been made where necessary to contact holders of copyright to obtain permission to reproduce copyright material. If any have been inadvertently overlooked, the publisher will be pleased to make the necessary arrangements at the first opportunity.

Inquiries for bulk sales may be solicited at: jaypee@jaypeebrothers.com

Essentials of Applied Microbiology for Nurses Including Infection Control and Safety

First Edition: 2022

Reprint: 2023, **2024**

ISBN: 978-93-5465-938-6

Printed at Rajkamal Electric Press, Kundli, Haryana.

Dedicated to

Our Beloved Parents, Family Members
And, above all, the Almighty

Become an Infection Control Nurse

- Pursue a career as an infection control nurse—a highly demanding and specialized area.
- Infection control nurses are the pillar behind the implementation of infection control activities in healthcare facilities.
- Have in-depth knowledge of Microbiology and infection control to prevent cross-transmission of organisms in hospital.

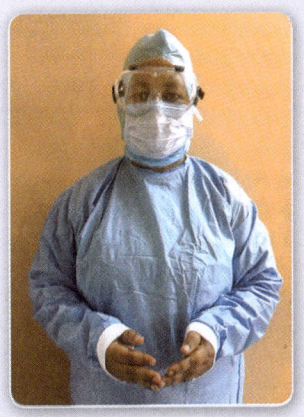

Golden Rules of Goal Setting

Dear Students

Here are some important tips which will help you in setting your goals in studies:
1. Set Goals That Motivate You: This means making sure that they are important to you, and that there is value in achieving them
2. Set SMART Goals
    - Specific: Your goal must be clear and well defined, not vague or generalized
    - Measurable: Goals must have measurable objectives
    - Attainable: Make sure that your goals are achievable and within your limit
    - Relevant: Will take you to the direction you want your life and career to go
    - Time Bound: You must know when you have the deadline and can celebrate success
3. Set Goals in Writing: Written commitment in presence of your close people (parents, close friends) will always push and remind you whenever you tend to deviate from your goal
4. Make an Action Plan: Do not focus only on the outcome, but make planning of all small steps that collectively take to the outcome. This is especially important if your goal is big and demanding, or long-term
5. Monitor Yourself: Compliance to the action plan should be monitored at least weekly (for one month goal) or monthly (for a yearly goal), depending upon your goal size.

Remember,

"Success is not final; failure is not fatal: It is the courage to continue that counts."
—Winston S Churchill

"There are two types of people who will tell you that you cannot make a difference in this world: those who are afraid to try and those who are afraid you will succeed."
—Ray Goforth

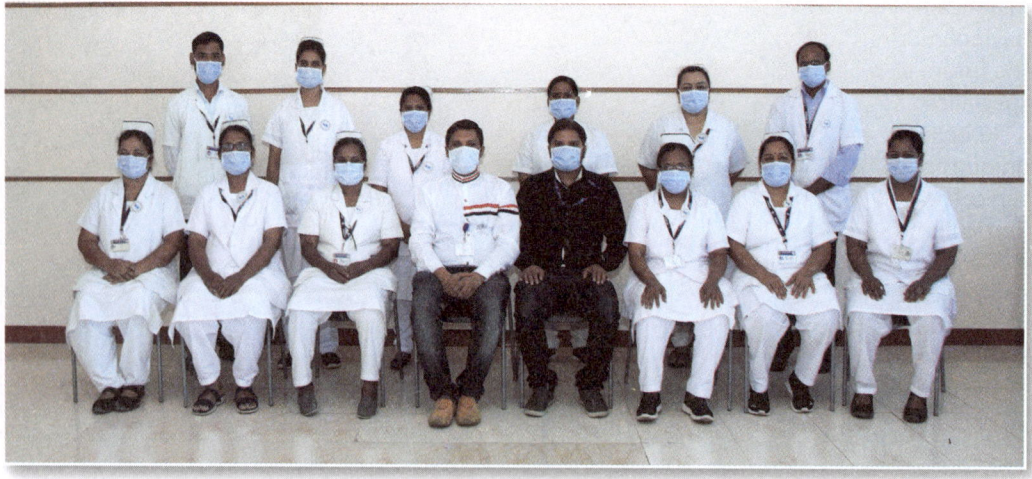

Hospital Infection Control and Prevention (HICP) Unit, JIPMER, Puducherry, India

PREFACE

It gives us immense pleasure to announce the release of *Essentials of Applied Microbiology for Nurses*. The excitement reaches its pinnacle as our sleepless nights of the last three months have come to an end.

The idea of scripting a Nursing book on Microbiology came to our mind as we received numerous requests from the Microbiology and Nursing faculties across the country to write a Microbiology book with a different approach exclusively catering to the nurses. The existing nursing books on this subject are discouraging with suboptimal matter and do not cover the infection control part, which is the most important area of Microbiology for Nurses.

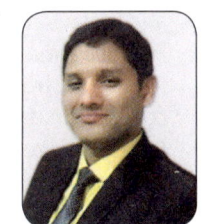

Apurba S Sastry

Nurses are the pillar behind the success of any hospital. Their motherly care gives great relief to the patients. Proper training in Microbiology and infection control can produce competent nurses who will deliver better patient care.

- **Infection control activities:** The thorough knowledge of Nurses on various aspects of infection control such as contact precautions, e.g. hand hygiene with correct indications and steps, appropriate use of PPE is of immense help to prevent cross-transmission of infection in hospital.
- **Antimicrobial stewardship activities:** Nurses play a crucial role in several key activities of antimicrobial stewardship such as—(1) appropriate specimen collection by correct technique and at right time, (2) apposite administration of antimicrobials in the correct dose, frequency, etc.

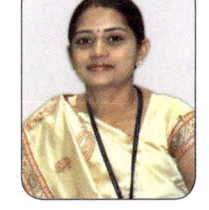

Sandhya Bhat

- Comprehensive knowledge of **sterilization and disinfection** would help the Nurses to adhere to the disinfection policy and monitor environmental cleaning protocols in the healthcare facility.

Infection Control Nurses are the functional unit of the hospital infection control and prevention (HICP) unit and are pillars behind the implementation of infection control activities in healthcare facilities. Unfortunately, there is a paucity of infection control nurses in India. Therefore having in-depth knowledge of Microbiology and infection control can help nursing students in the future to pursue their careers as infection control nurses, which is a highly demanding and specialized area.

Keeping all the above-mentioned aspects in mind, we have drafted this textbook with a very unique approach to suit the need of nursing students of India—both in their examination and in clinical practice. The book has been thoroughly framed as per the revised Indian Nursing Council Curriculum for BSc Nursing 2021.

- Divided into two parts: Applied Microbiology and Infection Control Including Safety
- Applied Microbiology Part comprises of sections: General Microbiology, Immunology, Bacterial Infections, Viral Infections, Parasitic Infections, and Fungal Infections
- **Section 1:** *General Microbiology* section is meticulously structured with the inclusion of general bacteriology, general virology, general parasitology, and general mycology chapters. General bacteriology is reorganized into a single chapter with several sub-chapters
- **Section 2:** *Immunology* section covers topics such as immunity, components of the immune system, immune response, antigen, antibody and complement, antigen-antibody reaction, hypersensitivity reactions and immunoprophylaxis, and national immunization schedule

- **Section 3:** *Systematic Bacteriology* section covers topics such as gram-positive cocci (*Staphylococcus, Streptococcus,* Pneumococcus, *Enterococcus*), and gram-negative cocci infections (meningococcus and gonococcus), gram-positive bacilli infections (*Corynebacterium* and *Bacillus*), anaerobic infections, mycobacteria infections, gram-negative bacilli infections (Enterobacterales, *Vibrio,* non-fermenters, fastidious bacteria) and others
- **Section 4:** *Virology* section covers topics such as DNA viral infections like Herpes and others, and RNA viral infections such as Myxoviruses, rubella, coronaviruses, arboviruses, rabies, polio, HIV, hepatitis viruses, Ebola, viral gastroenteritis, oncogenic viruses, and others. COVID-19, the most catastrophic disease of today's date has been addressed as a completely new chapter covering in detail.
- **Section 5:** *Parasitology* section covers topics such as Amoebae, flagellates (*Giardia, Trichomonas, Leishmania,* and *Trypanosoma*), malaria parasite (*Plasmodium*), coccidian parasites infections, cestode, trematode and nematode (intestinal and tissue) infections
- **Section 6:** *Mycology* section covers topics such as superficial mycoses, subcutaneous mycoses, systemic (deep) mycoses, and opportunistic fungal infections
- **Section 7:** *Infection control* section comprises of topics such as healthcare-associated infections (HAI), standard precautions including hand hygiene and PPE, transmission-based precautions, major HAI types, HAI surveillance, and infection control committee, sterilization and disinfection (Including CSSD), biomedical waste management, needle stick injury, environmental surveillance, laundry management, immunization program for healthcare workers and antimicrobial stewardship
- **Section 8:** *Applied Microbiology* section comprises of topics on various infective syndromes such as bloodstream infection, meningitis, UTI, diarrhea, respiratory infection, and others.
- A separate chapter on *Specimen Collection* has been incorporated covering in-depth various aspects of appropriate specimen collection—correct technique, adequate volume, and at the correct time (before the start of antimicrobials),
- The chapter on Practical Microbiology has been incorporated covering the various practical aspects of Microbiology and Infection Control relevant to Nurses including several problem-solving exercises
- Patient Safety and Safety Protocol for Healthcare Personnel have been added as separate chapters, which is as per the new curriculum for BSc Nurses
- Most features of the author's popular MBBS book have been maintained in this book
  - More content, less pages—saves student's time
  - Concise, bulleted format, and to-the-point text—easy to read during the examination
  - Simple and lucid language—makes the understanding easy
  - Separate highlight boxes—for important topics and treatment boxes for quick review.

We hope that the nursing students will relish reading this book and find it useful. We also hope that we have made a good start in addressing the varied needs of nursing students and faculties teaching microbiology for nurses with a single comprehensive book. We will feel glad to receive your valuable feedback, which will enable us to improve further.

Apurba S Sastry
apurbasastrymicrobiology@gmail.com

Sandhya Bhat
sandhyabhatk@gmail.com

ACKNOWLEDGMENTS

The release of *Essentials of Applied Microbiology for Nurses* would not have been possible without our close association with many people. We take this opportunity to extend our sincere gratitude and appreciation to all those who made this book possible.

Hearty acknowledgments to our teachers, departmental staff, family members, and others, for their blessings and support.

1. We are extremely thankful to Director, JIPMER, Puducherry, and Director-Principal, Pondicherry Institute of Medical Sciences (PIMS), Puducherry for giving permission to write this textbook.
2. We would like to sincerely thank **Dr Deepashree R**, Assistant Professor of Microbiology, JSS Medical College, Mysuru, Karnataka, for her input during the manuscript preparation.
3. We would like to sincerely thank **Dr Ketan Priyadarshi**, Senior Resident and Fellow in Hospital Infection Control, JIPMER for his inputs during the manuscript preparation.
4. **Faculty of Department of Microbiology, JIPMER** for their constant support, inputs and help during preparation—Dr Sujatha S (Professor), Dr Rakesh Singh (Professor and Head), Dr Jharna Mandal (Professor), Dr Rahul Dhodapkar (Professor), Dr Noyal M Joseph (Additional Professor), Dr Rakhi Biswas (Additional Professor), Dr Nonika Rajkumari (Additional Professor) and Dr Maanasa Bhaskar (Assistant Professor).
5. **Faculty of Department of Microbiology, PIMS** for their constant support, inputs, and help during preparation—Dr Shashikala, (Professor and Head), Dr Sheela Devi (Professor), Dr Johny Asir (Professor), Dr Vivian Joseph P (Professor), Dr Sujitha E (Associate Professor), Dr Arthi E (Associate Professor), Dr Patricia Anita (Associate Professor), Dr Meghna (Assistant Professor), Mrs Desdemona Rasitha (Tutor) and Mr Gnanavelu E (Tutor).
6. **Residents and postgraduates,** Department of Microbiology, JIPMER and Pondicherry Institute of Medical Sciences (PIMS), Puducherry.
7. **HICP, JIPMER**—infection control nurses and support office staff such as Ms Ilaveni, Ms Ramya, and Mr Venkat.
8. **Infection control nurses,** HICC, Pondicherry Institute of Medical Sciences, Puducherry.
9. **Microbiology faculty from various institutes**—for their inputs during manuscript preparation
    - **Dr Anand B Janagond**, Professor of Microbiology, S Nijalingappa Medical College, Bagalkot, Karnataka
    - **Dr Tessa Antony,** Faculty of Microbiology, Ramachandra Medical College, Chennai
    - **Dr Sribal Selvarajan,** Faculty of Microbiology, Ramachandra Medical College, Chennai
    - **Dr MJ Kumari,** Professor cum Principal (Ag.) and Vice Principal, College of Nursing, JIPMER, Puducherry
    - **Sr Dr Mony K,** Principal, College of Nursing, PIMS, Puducherry
    - **Mrs Jessica Shushma D'Souza and Dr Mridula M,** Faculty of Microbiology, Kasturba Medical College, Manipal, Karnataka.
10. **Special thanks to our teachers**—Dr Reba Kanungo (PIMS, retired), Dr SC Parija (JIPMER, retired), Dr BN Harish (JIPMER, retired), Dr ER Nagaraj (SSMC Tumkur, retired), Dr Sharadadevi Mannur (CDSIMER, Bengaluru) and Dr Renushree (SSMC, Tumkur).
11. **For providing photographs**—We are extremely thankful to all people/institutes/companies who have agreed to provide valuable photographs.

Acknowledgments

As you know, human errors are inevitable; and no book is immune to them. We would request all the readers to provide any errata found and also valuable inputs.

If any reader wishes to share feedback, suggestions, updates, and errata, please feel free to mail us at *apurbasastrymicrobiology@gmail.com*. As a token of gratitude, the reader will be acknowledged in the subsequent edition of the book.

Special Acknowledgments to My Publishers

Jaypee Brothers Medical Publishers (P) Ltd, New Delhi, India

- Shri Jitendar P Vij (Group Chairman)
- Mr Ankit Vij (Managing Director)
- Mr MS Mani (Group President)
- Dr Madhu Choudhary (Director–Educational Publishing): She has been a great support throughout the manuscript preparation
- Ms Pooja Bhandari (Production Head)
- Ms Seema Dogra (Cover Visualizer)
- Dr Astha Sawhney (Assistant Manager): Extremely dynamic, have lot of patience and available 24x7 to address to our queries
- **The Development Team:** Mr Deepak Saxena (Typesetters), Mr Nitin Bhardwaj (Graphic Designer), Mr Binay Kumar (Proofreader). These guys are simply outstanding in their work. A special mention for Mr Deepak Saxena, we must say that he is the best operator of India in medical publishing. The way Nitin Bhardwaj does the designing of photographs is extraordinary. It is a treat for us to work with all of them. These guys are extremely workaholic and have a very good team spirit. We salute them, for their professionalism.
- **Marketing heads from various zones:** Mr Narendra Shekhawat (Vice President–Sales), Mr Venugopal V (South Head), Mr Rishi Sharma (North Region Head), CS Gawde (Western Head) and Sandip Gupta (Eastern Head).
- **Branch managers and Sales manager from various branches:** Bengaluru branch (Ravi Kumar, A Palani, E Venkatesh), Chennai branch (Maran A [Adoption Head for South], Dharani Kumar P, RK Dharani, Dharanidaran), Kochi branch (Sujeesh VS, Diffin Robin, Arun Kumar), Hyderabad branch (Parimal Guha Neogy, Marthanda Sarma, Rajesh Malothu, Hamza Ali), Mumbai branch (Sameer S Mulla), Nagpur branch (Rajesh Shrivas), Ahmedabad branch (Ms Priyanka Kansara, Dinesh Waghade), Delhi branch (Sujatha Puri), Kolkata branch (Sanjoy Chakraborthy).

Lastly, we would like to keep in record that without the support of our son, parents (of both Dr Sandhya and Dr Apurba) and other family members, it would have been impossible to continue the spirit on, during the journey of the current edition. A special mention to our son (Master Adarsh), who really helped us being very much cooperative. In fact, he was encouraging us to work for the book. We deeply apologize to you as well as our parents (Mr Anooj Sastry and Ms Tarini Purohit), as we could not give enough time and care during the manuscript preparation.

Apurba S Sastry
Sandhya Bhat

CONTENTS

Section 1: General Microbiology

1. Introduction, History and Microscopy — 3
2. General Bacteriology:
   - 2.1. Morphology and Physiology of Bacteria — 9
   - 2.2. General Bacteriology: Laboratory Diagnosis of Bacterial Infections — 18
   - 2.3. General Bacteriology: Bacterial Genetics — 31
   - 2.4. General Bacteriology: Antimicrobial Agents and Antimicrobial Resistance — 34
   - 2.5. General Bacteriology: Normal Flora and Bacterial Pathogenesis — 39
3. General Virology — 43
4. General Parasitology — 51
5. General Mycology — 55
6. Epidemiology of Infectious Disease — 59

Section 2: Immunology

7. Immunity, Components of Immune System, Immune Response — 67
8. Antigen, Antibody and Complement — 74
9. Antigen–Antibody Reaction — 80
10. Hypersensitivity Reactions — 89
11. Immunoprophylaxis and Immunization Schedule — 93

Section 3: Bacterial Infections

12. Gram-positive and Gram-negative Cocci Infections — 103
13. Gram-positive Bacilli Infections — 112
14. Anaerobic Infections — 116
15. Mycobacteria Infections — 120
16. Gram-negative Bacilli Infections-I — 126
17. Gram-negative Bacilli Infections-II — 135
18. Miscellaneous Bacterial Infections — 141

Section 4: Viral Infections

19. Herpes and Other DNA Virus Infections — 149
20. Myxoviruses and Rubella Virus Infections — 155
21. Coronavirus Infections including COVID-19 — 161
22. Arbovirus Infections — 165
23. Rabies and Polio — 170
24. HIV/AIDS — 176
25. Viral Hepatitis — 183
26. Miscellaneous RNA Virus Infections — 191

Section 5: Parasitic Infections

27. Amoeba, *Giardia* and *Trichomonas* Infections — 197
28. Hemoflagellates: Leishmania and Trypanosoma — 204
29. *Plasmodium* (Malaria Parasite) — 208
30. Opportunistic Coccidian Parasites and Others — 215
31. Cestode Infections — 219
32. Trematode Infections — 226
33. Intestinal Nematode Infections — 229
34. Tissue Nematode Infections — 237

Section 6: Fungal Infections

35. Medical Mycology — 245

Section 7: Hospital Infection Control

36. Healthcare-associated Infections — 259
37. Standard Precautions: Hand Hygiene and PPE — 262
38. Transmission-based Precautions — 274
39. Major Healthcare-associated Infection Types — 280
40. HAI Surveillance and HICC — 292
41. Sterilization and Disinfection — 297
42. Biomedical Waste Management — 313
43. Needle Stick Injury — 321
44. Environmental Surveillance — 326
45. Laundry Management — 331
46. Immunization of Healthcare Workers — 333
47. Antimicrobial Stewardship — 335

Section 8: Applied Microbiology and Miscellaneous

48. Bloodstream Infections — 345
49. Meningitis — 349
50. Urinary Tract Infection (UTI) — 353
51. Diarrheal Diseases — 357
52. Respiratory Tract Infections — 361
53. Miscellaneous Infectious Syndromes — 366
54. Specimen Collection and Transport — 372
55. Practical Microbiology — 380
56. Patient Safety — 388
57. Safety Protocol for Healthcare Personnel — 394

Index — *399*

INC SYLLABUS

APPLIED MICROBIOLOGY AND HOSPITAL INFECTION CONTROL INCLUDING SAFETY

Placement: III SEMESTER
Theory: 2 Credits (40 hours)
Practical: 1 Credit (40 hours) (Lab/Experiential Learning – L/E)

SECTION A: APPLIED MICROBIOLOGY

Theory: 20 hours
Practical: 20 hours (Lab/Experiential Learning – L/E)

Description: This course is designed to enable students to acquire understanding of fundamentals of Microbiology, compare and contrast different microbes and comprehend the means of transmission and control of spread by various microorganisms. It also provides opportunities for practicing infection control measures in hospital and community settings.

Competencies: On completion of the course, the students will be able to:
1. Identify the ubiquity and diversity of microorganisms in the human body and the environment.
2. Classify and explain the morphology and growth of microbes.
3. Identify various types of microorganisms.
4. Explore mechanisms by which microorganisms cause disease.
5. Develop understanding of how the human immune system counteracts infection by specific and non-specific mechanisms.
6. Apply the principles of preparation and use of vaccines in immunization.
7. Identify the contribution of the microbiologist and the microbiology laboratory to the diagnosis of infection.

COURSE OUTLINE

T – Theory, L/E – Lab/Experiential Learning

Unit	Time (Hrs) T	Time (Hrs) P	Learning Outcomes	Content	Teaching/ Learning Activities	Assessment Methods
I	3		Explain concepts and principles of microbiology and its importance in nursing	**Introduction:** • Importance and relevance to nursing • Historical perspective • Concepts and terminology • Principles of microbiology	• Lecture cum Discussion	• Short answer • Objective type
II	10	10 (L/E)	Describe structure, classification morphology and growth of bacteria	**General characteristics of Microbes:** • Structure and classification of Microbes • Morphological types • Size and form of bacteria	• Lecture cum Discussion • Demonstration • Experiential Learning through visual	• Short answer • Objective type

Contd...

INC Syllabus

Contd...

Unit	Time (Hrs) T	Time (Hrs) P	Learning Outcomes	Content	Teaching/ Learning Activities	Assessment Methods
			Identify Microorganisms	• Motility • Colonization • Growth and nutrition of microbes • Temperature • Moisture • Blood and body fluids • Laboratory methods for identification of microorganisms • Types of staining—simple, differential (Gram's, AFB), special—capsular staining (negative), spore, LPCB, KOH mount • Culture and media preparation—solid and liquid. Types of media—semi-synthetic, synthetic, enriched, enrichment, selective and differential media. Pure culture techniques—tube dilution, pour, spread, streak plate. Anaerobic cultivation of bacteria		
III	4	6 (L/E)	Describe the different disease producing organisms	**Pathogenic organisms** • Micro-organisms: Cocci—gram-positive and gram-negative; Bacilli—gram-positive and gram-negative • Viruses • Fungi: Superficial and deep mycoses • Parasites • Rodents and Vectors ➢ Characteristics, source, portal of entry, transmission of infection, identification of disease producing micro-organisms	• Lecture cum Discussion • Demonstration • Experiential learning through visual	• Short answer • Objective type
IV	3	4 (L/E)	Explain the concepts of immunity, hyper sensitivity and immunization	**Immunity** • Immunity: Types, classification • Antigen and antibody reaction • Hypersensitivity reactions • Serological tests • Immunoglobulins: Structure, types and properties • Vaccines: Types and classification, storage and handling, cold chain, immunization for various diseases • Immunization schedule	• Lecture • Discussion • Demonstration • Visit to observe vaccine storage • Clinical practice	• Short answer • Objective type • Visit report

SECTION B: INFECTION CONTROL AND SAFETY

Theory: 20 hours

Practical/Lab: 20 hours (Lab/Experiential Learning – L/E)

Description: This course is designed to help students to acquire knowledge and develop competencies required for fundamental patient safety and infection control in delivering patient care. It also focuses on identifying patient safety indicators, preventing and managing hospital acquired infections, and in following universal precautions.

Competencies: The students will be able to:
1. Develop knowledge and understanding of Hospital Acquired Infections (HAIs) and effective practices for prevention.
2. Integrate the knowledge of isolation (Barrier and reverse barrier) techniques in implementing various precautions.
3. Demonstrate and practice steps in Handwashing and appropriate use of different types of PPE.
4. Illustrate various disinfection and sterilization methods and techniques.
5. Demonstrate knowledge and skill in specimen collection, handling and transport to optimize the diagnosis for treatment.
6. Incorporate the principles and guidelines of Biomedical waste management.
7. Apply the principles of antibiotic stewardship in performing the nurses' role.
8. Identify patient safety indicators and perform the role of nurse in the patient safety audit process.
9. Apply the knowledge of International Patient Safety Goals (IPSG) in the patient care settings.
10. Identify employee safety indicators and risk of occupational hazards.
11. Develop understanding of the various safety protocols and adhere to those protocols.

COURSE OUTLINE

T – Theory, L/E – Lab/Experiential Learning

Unit	Time (Hrs) T	P	Learning Outcomes	Content	Teaching/ Learning Activities	Assessment Methods

I	2	2 (E)	Summarize the evidence based and effective patient care practices for the prevention of common healthcare associated infections in the healthcare setting	**HAI (Hospital Acquired Infection)**
				• Hospital acquired infection
				• Bundle approach
				  ➤ Prevention of Urinary Tract Infection (UTI)
				  ➤ Prevention of Surgical Site Infection (SSI)
				  ➤ Prevention of Ventilator Associated Events (VAE)
				  ➤ Prevention of Central Line Associated Blood Stream Infection (CLABSI)
				• Surveillance of HAI—Infection control team and Infection control committee
					• Lecture and Discussion
					• Experiential Learning
						• Knowledge assessment
						• MCQ
						• Short answer

Contd...

Contd...

Unit	Time (Hrs) T	Time (Hrs) P	Learning Outcomes	Content	Teaching/ Learning Activities	Assessment Methods
II	3	4 (L)	Demonstrate appropriate use of different types of PPEs and the critical use of risk assessment	**Isolation Precautions and use of Personal Protective Equipment (PPE)** • Types of isolation system, standard precaution and transmission-based precautions (direct contact, droplet, indirect) • Epidemiology and infection prevention—CDC guidelines • Effective use of PPE	• Lecture • Demonstration and Re-demonstration	• Performance assessment • OSCE
III	1	2 (L)	Demonstrate the hand hygiene practice and its effectiveness on infection control	**Hand Hygiene** • Types of hand hygiene • Hand washing and use of alcohol hand rub • Moments of hand hygiene • WHO hand hygiene promotion	• Lecture • Demonstration and Re-demonstration	• Performance assessment
IV	1	2 (E)	Illustrates disinfection and sterilization in the healthcare setting	**Disinfection and sterilization** • Definitions • Types of disinfection and sterilization • Environment cleaning • Equipment cleaning • Guides on use of disinfectants • Spaulding's principle	• Lecture • Discussion • Experiential learning through visit	• Short answer • Objective type
V	1		Illustrate on what, when, how, why specimens are collected to optimize the diagnosis for treatment and management	**Specimen Collection (Review)** • Principle of specimen collection • Types of specimens • Collection techniques and special considerations • Appropriate containers • Transportation of the sample • Staff precautions in handling specimens	• Discussion	• Knowledge evaluation • Quiz • Performance assessment • Checklist
VI	2	2 (E)	Explain on Biomedical waste management and laundry management	**BMW (Biomedical Waste Management)** *Laundry management process and infection control and prevention* • Waste management process and infection prevention • Staff precautions • Laundry management • Country ordinance and BMW National Guidelines 2017: Segregation of wastes, color coded waste containers, waste collection and storage, packaging and labeling, transportation	• Discussion • Demonstration • Experiential learning through visit	• Knowledge assessment by short answers, objective type • Performance assessment

Contd...

Contd...

Unit	Time (Hrs) T	Time (Hrs) P	Learning Outcomes	Content	Teaching/ Learning Activities	Assessment Methods
VII	2		Explain in detail about antibiotic stewardship, AMR Describe MRSA/ MDRO and its prevention	**Antibiotic stewardship** • Importance of antibiotic stewardship • Anti-microbial resistance • Prevention of MRSA, MDRO in healthcare setting	• Lecture • Discussion • Written assignment– Recent AMR (Antimicrobial resistance) guidelines	• Short answer • Objective type • Assessment of assignment
VIII	3	5 (L/E)	Enlist the patient safety indicators followed in a health care organization and the role of nurse in the patient safety audit process	**Patient Safety Indicators** • Care of vulnerable patients • Prevention of latrogenic injury • Care of lines, drains and tubing's • Restrain policy and care – Physical and chemical • Blood and blood transfusion policy • Prevention of IV complication • Prevention of fall • Prevention of DVT • Shifting and transporting of patients • Surgical safety • Care coordination event related to medication reconciliation and administration • Prevention of communication errors • Prevention of HAI • Documentation	• Lecture • Demonstration • Experiential learning	• Knowledge assessment • Performance assessment • Checklist/ OSCE
			Captures and analyzes incidents and events for quality improvement	**Incidents and Adverse Events** • Capturing of incidents • RCA (Root cause analysis) • CAPA (Corrective and preventive action) • Report writing	• Lecture • Role play • Inquiry based learning	• Knowledge assessment • Short answer • Objective type
IX	1		Enumerate IPSG and application of the goals in the patient care settings	**IPSG (International Patient Safety Goals)** • Identify patient correctly • Improve effective communication • Improve safety of high alert medication • Ensure safe surgery • Reduce the risk of health care associated infection • Reduce the risk of patient harm resulting from falls • Reduce the harm associated with clinical alarm system	• Lecture • Role play	• Objective type

Contd...

Contd...

Unit	Time (Hrs) T	Time (Hrs) P	Learning Outcomes	Content	Teaching/ Learning Activities	Assessment Methods

X	2	3 (L/E)	Enumerate the various safety protocols and its applications	**Safety protocol**
				• 5S (Sort, Set in order, Shine, Standardize, Sustain)
				• Radiation safety
				• Laser safety
				• Fire safety
				  ➢ Types and classification of fire
				  ➢ Fire alarms
				  ➢ Firefighting equipment
				• HAZMAT (Hazardous Materials) safety
				  ➢ Types of spill
				  ➢ Spillage management
				  ➢ MSDS (Material Safety Data Sheets)
				• Environmental safety
				  ➢ Risk assessment
				  ➢ Aspect impact analysis
				  ➢ Maintenance of temp and humidity (Department wise)
				  ➢ Audits
				• Emergency codes
				• Role of nurse in times of disaster
					• Lecture
					• Demonstration/ Experiential learning
						• Mock drills
						• Post tests
						• Checklist

XI	2		Explain importance of employee safety indicators	**Employee Safety Indicators** • Vaccination • Needle stick injuries (NSI) prevention • Fall prevention • Radiation safety • Annual health check **Healthcare Worker Immunization Program and management of occupational exposure**	• Lecture • Discussion • Lecture method • Journal review	• Knowledge assessment by short answers, objective type • Short answer
			Identify risk of occupational hazards, prevention and post exposure prophylaxis.	• Occupational health ordinance • Vaccination program for healthcare staff • Needle stick injuries and prevention and post exposure prophylaxis		

*Experiential Learning:

Experiential learning is the process by which knowledge is created through the process of experience in the clinical field.

SECTION 1: General Microbiology

SECTION OUTLINE

1. Introduction, History and Microscopy
2. General Bacteriology
   - 2.1. Morphology and Physiology of Bacteria
   - 2.2. Laboratory Diagnosis of Bacterial Infections
   - 2.3. Bacterial Genetics
   - 2.4. Antimicrobial Agents and Antimicrobial Resistance
   - 2.5. Normal Flora and Bacterial Pathogenesis
3. General Virology
4. General Parasitology
5. General Mycology
6. Epidemiology of Infectious Disease

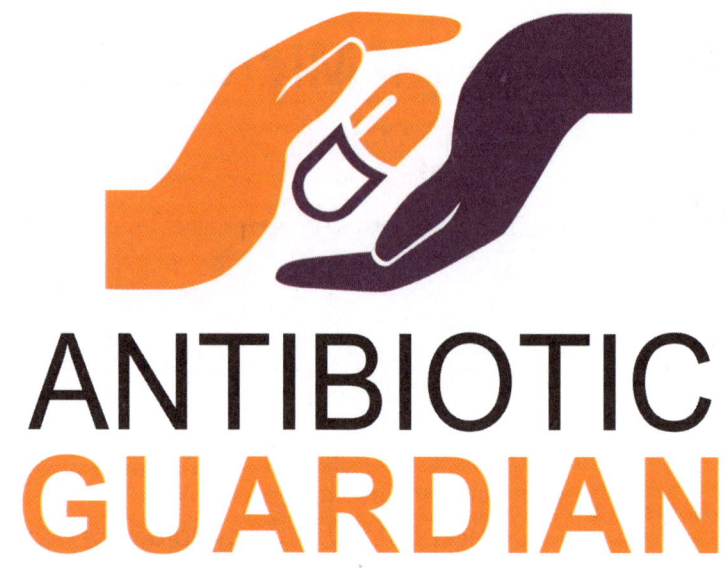

ANTIBIOTIC
GUARDIAN

*If we use antibiotics when not needed,
we may not have them when they are most needed*

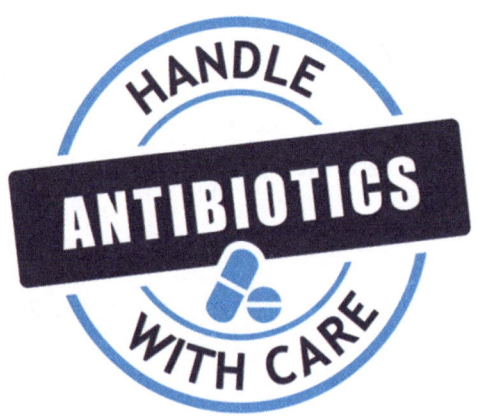

CHAPTER 1

Introduction, History and Microscopy

CHAPTER PREVIEW

- Classification of Microorganisms
- History
- Microscopy

Medical microbiology is a branch of medicine that deals with the study of microorganisms and their role in human health and disease. It also concerns with the diagnosis, treatment and prevention of various infectious diseases.

The branches of medical microbiology are as follows:

- ❖ **General microbiology:** It deals with the study of general properties of microorganisms—taxonomy, morphology, pathogenesis, laboratory diagnosis, and treatment for their effective killing
- ❖ **Immunology**: It deals with the study of the immune system and various immunological methods for the diagnosis of infectious diseases
- ❖ **Systemic microbiology:** Microorganisms infect various organ systems of our body. There are four kinds of microorganisms that cause infectious disease: bacteria, fungi, parasites, and viruses
    - *Bacteriology:* The study of bacteria
    - *Virology:* The study of viruses
    - *Mycology:* The study of fungi
    - *Parasitology:* The study of parasites; has two arms:
        - ♦ Protozoology: The study of protozoa
        - ♦ Helminthology: The study of helminths.
- ❖ **Hospital infection control:** It deals with the study of various control measures to prevent the transmission of healthcare-associated infections.

CLASSIFICATION OF MICROORGANISMS

Microorganisms are grouped under both prokaryotes and eukaryotes.
- ❖ Bacteria are placed under prokaryotes. They have a primitive nucleus and other properties of a prokaryotic cell **(Table 1.1)**
- ❖ Whereas fungi and parasites (protozoa and helminths) belong to eukaryotes;

Table 1.1: Characteristics of prokaryotes and eukaryotes.

Characteristics	Prokaryotes	Eukaryotes
Major groups	Bacteria	Fungi, parasites, plants, animals
Nucleus	Diffuse	Well-defined
Nuclear membrane	Absent	Present
Nucleolus	Absent	Present
Cell division	Binary fission	Mitosis, meiosis
Plasmid	Present	Absent
Cell membrane	No sterols	Contains sterols
Cellular organelles	Absent (except ribosome)	Present
Ribosome	70S	80S

Abbreviation: S, Svedberg unit.

having a well-defined nucleus and various eukaryotic cellular organelles
❖ Viruses are neither considered prokaryotes nor eukaryotes because they lack the characteristics of living things, except the ability to replicate.

HISTORY

There were several eminent personalities in the field of Microbiology, whose important contributions have been described below.

Louis Pasteur

Louis Pasteur (1822–1895), also known as '**father of microbiology**' has made several remarkable contributions **(Fig. 1.1A)**.
❖ He had proposed the **principles of fermentation** for the preservation of food
❖ He introduced the **sterilization techniques** and developed steam sterilizer, hot air oven, and autoclave
❖ He described the method of **pasteurization of milk**
❖ He contributed to the vaccine development against anthrax, fowl cholera, and rabies
❖ He postulated the '**germ theory of disease**', which states that disease cannot be caused by bad air, but it is produced by the organisms present in the air
❖ **Liquid media concept:** He used nutrient broth to grow microorganisms
❖ He was the founder of the Pasteur Institute, Paris.

Joseph Lister

Joseph Lister (1867) is considered to be the '**father of antiseptic surgery**'. He postulated that postoperative infections can greatly be reduced by using disinfectants to sterilize the surgical instruments and to clean the wounds.

Robert Koch

Robert Koch (1843–1910), made notable contributions to the field of microbiology **(Fig. 1.1B)**. His contributions were as follows:
❖ He introduced **solid media** for the culture of bacteria
❖ He introduced methods for isolation of bacteria in pure culture
❖ He described **hanging drop** method for testing motility
❖ He **discovered bacteria** such as the anthrax bacilli, tubercle bacilli and cholera bacilli
❖ **Koch's postulates:** Robert Koch had postulated that a microorganism can be accepted as the causative agent of an infectious disease only if four criteria are fulfilled. These criteria are as follows:
  1. The microorganism should be constantly associated with the lesions of the disease
  2. It should be possible to isolate the organism in pure culture from the lesions of the disease
  3. The same disease must result when the isolated microorganism is inoculated into a suitable laboratory animal
  4. It should be possible to re-isolate the organism in pure culture from the lesions produced in the experimental animals.

Exceptions to Koch's postulates: There are some bacteria that do not satisfy one or more of the four criteria of Koch's postulates. *Mycobacterium leprae* and *Treponema pallidum* cannot be grown in culture; whereas *Neisseria gonorrhoeae* has no animal model.

Other Important Contributors

❖ **Antonie van Leeuwenhoek** (1676): He was the first scientist who observed bacteria

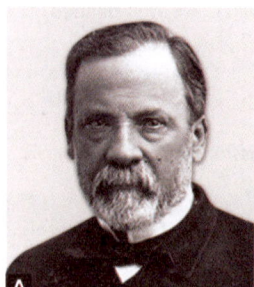
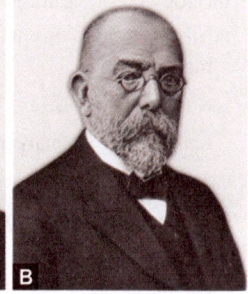

Figs. 1.1A and B: Eminent microbiologists: **A.** Louis Pasteur; **B.** Robert Koch.
Source: Wikipedia (*with permission*).

and other microorganisms, using a single-lens microscope constructed by him and he named those small organisms as *'Little animalcules'*
- **Edward Jenner** (1796): He, developed the first vaccine of the world, the smallpox vaccine. He used the cowpox virus (*Variolae vaccinae*) to immunize children against smallpox from which the term **'vaccine'** has been derived. The same principles are even used today for developing vaccines
- **Paul Ehrlich** (1854–1915): He is known as *'father of chemotherapy'.* He was also the first to report the *acid-fast nature* of tubercle bacillus
- **Hans Christian Gram (in 1884):** He developed a method of staining bacteria which was named as 'Gram stain' to make them more visible and differentiable under a microscope
- **Ernst Ruska:** He was the *founder of electron microscope* (1931)
- **Alexander Fleming (in 1929):** He discovered the most commonly used antibiotic substance of the last century, i.e., penicillin
- **Karry B Mullis:** Discovered polymerase chain reaction (PCR) and was awarded Noble Prize in 1993
- **Ignaz Semmelweis (1846):** He introduced the importance of hand hygiene in healthcare facilities. He proposed that improper hand hygiene practice during delivery led to the transmission of infection causing outbreak of puerperal fever.

Nobel Laureates

A number of scientists in the field of medicine or physiology have been awarded Nobel Prizes for their contributions in microbiology (Table 1.2).

MICROSCOPY

Microorganisms are extremely small. The size of the bacteria, fungi and parasites is expressed in micrometers (1 µm = 10^{-3} mm); whereas viruses are measured in nanometers (1 nm = 10^{-3} µm). Therefore organisms require

Table 1.2: Nobel laureates in medicine or physiology for their contributions in microbiology.

Nobel laureate	Year	Research done
Sir Ronald Ross	1902	Life cycle of malarial parasite in mosquitoes
Robert Koch	1905	Discovery of the causative agent of tuberculosis
Charles LA Laveran	1907	Discovery of malarial parasite in unstained preparation of blood
Sir Alexander Fleming	1945	Discovery of penicillin
J Lederberg and EL Tatum	1958	Discovery of conjugation in bacteria
Watson and Crick	1962	Discovered double helix structure of DNA
Holley, Khurana and Nirenberg	1968	Discovered genetic code
BS Blumberg	1976	Discovered Australia antigen (HBsAg)
Barbara McClintoch	1983	Discovered mobile genetic elements (transposon)
Georges Kohler	1984	Developed hybridoma technology for monoclonal antibodies
Kary B Mullis	1993	Invented polymerase chain reaction
Stanley B Prusiner	1997	Described Prions
Luc Montagnier and Barre-Sinoussi	2008	Discovery of human immunodeficiency virus (HIV)
William C Campbell and S. Omura	2015	For discovering ivermectin for the treatment of roundworm infections
Youyou Tu	2015	For discovering artemisinin, a novel drug used for malaria

specialized instrument— called 'microscope' to view objects and areas of objects that cannot be seen with the naked eye.

There are various types of microscopes that are used in diagnostic microbiology.
* Bright-field or light microscope
* Dark-field (or dark ground) microscope
* Phase contrast microscope
* Fluorescence microscope
* Electron microscope.

Bright-field or Light Microscope

The bright-field or light microscope forms a dark image against a brighter background.

Structure

The parts of a bright-field microscope are divided into three groups **(Fig. 1.2)**:
1. **Mechanical parts:**
   - *Base*: It holds various parts of the microscope, such as the light source, the fine and coarse adjustment knobs
   - *C-shaped arm*: It holds the microscope, and it connects the ocular lens to the objective lens
   - *Mechanical stage:* The arm bears a stage with stage clips to hold the slides and the stage control knobs to move the slide during viewing. It has an aperture at the center that permits light to reach the object from the bottom.
2. **Magnifying parts:**
   - *Ocular lens:* The arm contains an eyepiece that bears an ocular lens of 10x magnification power
   - *Objective lens*: The arm also contains a revolving nose piece that bears three to four objectives with lenses of differing magnifying power (4x, 10x, 40x and 100x).
3. **Illuminating parts:**
   - *Condenser:* It is mounted beneath the stage which focuses a cone of light on the slide
   - *Iris diaphragm*: It controls the light that passes through the condenser
   - *Light source:* It may be a mirror or an electric bulb
   - *Adjustment knobs:* Fine and coarse adjustment knobs help to sharpen the image.

Working Principle

The rays emitted from the light source pass through the iris diaphragm and fall on the specimen. The light rays passing through the specimen are gathered by the objective and a magnified image is formed. This image is further magnified by the ocular lens to produce the final magnified virtual image **(Fig. 1.3)**.

Dark-field Microscope

In dark-field (or dark ground) microscope, the object appears bright against a dark background.
* This is made possible by use of a special dark-field condenser
* *Applications:* It is used to identify the living, unstained cells and thin bacteria like spirochetes which cannot be visualized by light microscopy **(Fig. 1.4)**.

Phase Contrast Microscope

In this type of microscope, the contrast is enhanced. This microscope visualizes the

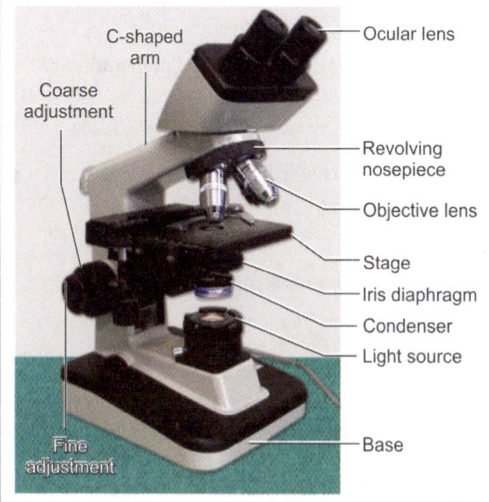

Fig. 1.2: Bright-field microscope.
Source: Nikon Alphaphot (*with permission*).

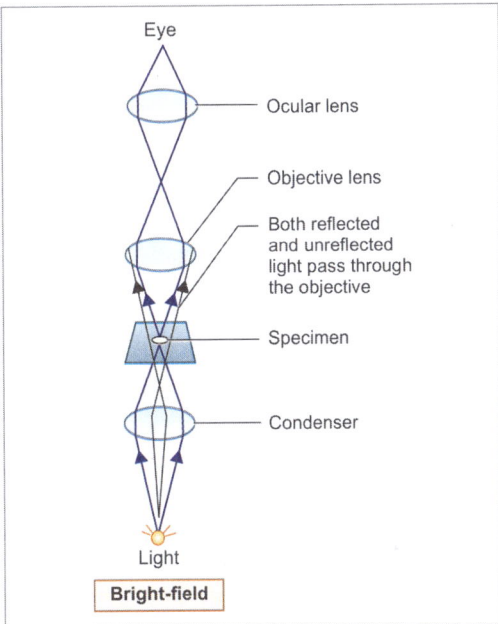

Fig. 1.3: Light pathways of bright-field microscope.

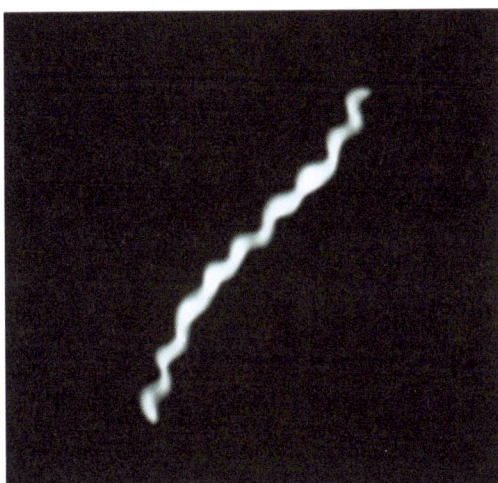

Fig. 1.4: Dark ground microscopic picture demonstrating spirally coiled bacteria (spirochete).
Source: Public Health Image Library, ID# 2043; Centers for Disease Control and Prevention (CDC), Atlanta (with permission).

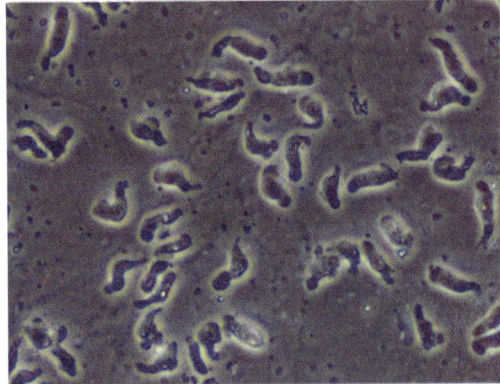

Fig. 1.5: Phase-contrast microscopic picture demonstrating *Naegleria fowleri* trophozoites (free-living amoeba)
Source: Centers for Disease Control and Prevention (CDC), Atlanta (with permission).

unstained living cells by creating a difference in contrast between the cells and water.
❖ This is made possible by the use of a special condenser, similar to the dark-field condenser, and a special optical disc located in the objective called a phase plate
❖ **Applications:** A phase-contrast microscope is useful for studying **(Fig. 1.5):**
  ■ Microbial motility
  ■ Determining the shape of living cells
  ■ Detecting microbial internal cellular components, such as the cell membrane, nuclei, mitochondria, chromosomes, Golgi apparatus, inclusion bodies, etc.

Fluorescence Microscope

The "fluorescence microscope" refers to any microscope that uses fluorescence property to generate an image.
❖ The source of light may be a mercury lamp that emits UV light rays
❖ The specimen should be stained with fluorescent dyes for visualization
❖ **Applications:** Certain microbes fluoresce when they are stained nonspecifically by fluorochrome dyes
  ■ Acridine orange dye is used for the detection of parasites such as *Plasmodium* and filarial nematodes
  ■ Auramine phenol is used for the detection of tubercle bacilli **(Fig. 1.6).**

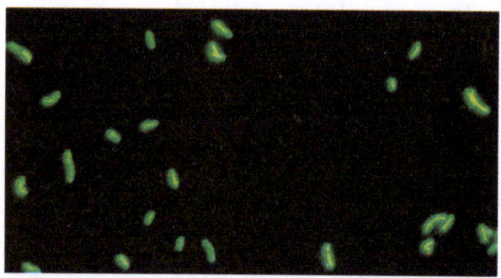

Fig. 1.6: Tubercle bacilli seen under fluorescence microscope.
Source: Department of Microbiology, JIPMER, Puducherry (*with permission*).

Electron Microscope

An electron microscope (EM) uses accelerated electrons as a source of illumination. EM has a much better resolving power than a light microscope; hence, it can reveal the details of flagella, fimbriae and intracellular structures of a cell. It was invented by German physicist **Ernst Ruska** in 1931. Electron microscopes are of two types:
1. Transmission electron microscope (TEM, the most common type)
2. Scanning electron microscope (SEM).

EXPECTED QUESTIONS

I. Write short notes on:
1. Contributions of Louis Pasteur to Microbiology.
2. Koch's postulates.
3. Principle and uses of bright-field microscope.

II. Multiple Choice Questions (MCQs):
1. Who has described the germ theory of life?
    a. Antonie van Leeuwenhoek
    b. Louis Pasteur
    c. Robert Koch
    d. Paul Ehrlich
2. Who has introduced the sterilization techniques?
    a. Louis Pasteur
    b. Edward Jenner
    c. Robert Koch
    d. Paul Ehrlich
3. Who discovered tubercle bacilli?
    a. Edward Jenner
    b. Alexander Fleming
    c. Robert Koch
    d. Joseph Lister
4. Which of the following microscope, the object appears bright against a dark background?
    a. Light microscope
    b. Phase-contrast microscope
    c. Dark ground microscope
    d. Electron microscope
5. Which of the following organism follows Koch's postulates?
    a. *Mycobacterium leprae*
    b. *Treponema pallidum*
    c. *Neisseria gonorrhoeae*
    d. *Bacillus anthracis*
6. Electrons are used as a source of illumination in:
    a. Light microscope
    b. Dark field microscope
    c. Phase contrast microscope
    d. Electron microscope
7. Who developed smallpox vaccine?
    a. Louis Pasteur
    b. Edward Jenner
    c. Robert Koch
    d. Paul Ehrlich

Answers
1. b   2. a   3. c   4. c   5. d   6. d   7. b

CHAPTER 2.1

General Bacteriology: Morphology and Physiology of Bacteria

CHAPTER PREVIEW

- Medically Important Bacteria
- Morphology of Bacteria
- Physiology of Bacteria

MEDICALLY IMPORTANT BACTERIA

Based on Gram stain, the bacteria can be grouped into gram-positive cocci, gram-negative cocci, and gram-positive bacilli, gram-negative bacilli and miscellaneous bacteria (that do not take up/poorly take up Gram stain) **(Table 2.1.1)**.

MORPHOLOGY OF BACTERIA

Shape of Bacteria

Depending on their shape, bacteria are classified into:
- Cocci (singular coccus, from; kokkos, meaning berry) are oval or spherical cells, and
- Bacilli or rods (singular bacillus, meaning rod-shaped).

Cocci are arranged in groups (clusters), pairs, or chains. Similarly, bacilli can be arranged in chains, pairs, and some bacilli are curved, comma-shaped, or cuneiform-shaped **(Table 2.1.2 and Fig. 2.1.1)**.

Based on Gram staining property, both cocci and bacilli are further classified into **(Table 2.1.2 and Fig. 2.1.1)**:
- Gram-positive cocci
- Gram-negative cocci
- Gram-positive bacilli
- Gram-negative bacilli.

Table 2.1.1: Medically important bacteria.

Gram-positive cocci
- Staphylococcus—e.g. *S. aureus*
- Streptococcus—e.g. β-hemolytic streptococci, and pneumococcus
- Enterococcus—e.g. *E. faecalis, E. faecium*

Gram-negative cocci

Neisseria—e.g. meningococcus and gonococcus

Gram-positive bacilli
- Corynebacterium—e.g. *C. diphtheriae*
- Bacillus—e.g. *B. anthracis*
- Mycobacterium—e.g. *M. tuberculosis, M. leprae*
- Miscellaneous gram-positive bacilli—*Listeria, Actinomycetes* and *Nocardia*

Gram-negative bacilli
- Enterobacterales—e.g. *Escherichia coli, Klebsiella, Proteus, Shigella, Salmonella, Yersinia*
- Non-fermenting gram-negative bacilli—e.g. *Pseudomonas, Acinetobacter, Burkholderia*
- Vibrio—e.g. *Vibrio cholerae*
- Fastidious gram-negative bacilli—*Haemophilus, Bordetella, Brucella*
- Miscellaneous gram-negative bacilli—*Campylobacter, Helicobacter, Legionella*, etc.

Anaerobic bacterial infections
- Sporing anaerobes—*Clostridium*
- Non-sporing anaerobes—*Bacteroides*

Miscellaneous bacteria
- Spirochetes—*Treponema, Borrelia, Leptospira*
- Rickettsiae, Chlamydiae and *Mycoplasma*

Table 2.1.2: Classification of bacteria depending on their morphology and Gram staining property.	
Bacteria	**Example**
Gram-positive cocci arranged in	
Cluster	Staphylococcus
Short chain	Streptococcus
Long chain	Viridans streptococci
Pairs, lanceolate shaped	Pneumococcus
Pairs or in short chain	Enterococcus
Gram-negative cocci arranged in	
Pairs, lens-shaped	Meningococcus
Pairs, kidney-shaped	Gonococcus
Gram-positive bacilli arranged in	
Chain (bamboo stick appearance)	Bacillus anthracis
Chinese letter or cuneiform pattern	Corynebacterium diphtheriae
Branched and filamentous form	Actinomyces, Nocardia
Gram-negative bacilli arranged in	
Pleomorphic (various shapes—cocci, coccobacilli, bacilli, etc.)	Haemophilus, Proteus
Coccobacilli	Acinetobacter
Comma shaped	Vibrio cholerae
Others	
Spirally coiled, flexible	Spirochetes
Bacteria that lack cell wall	Mycoplasma

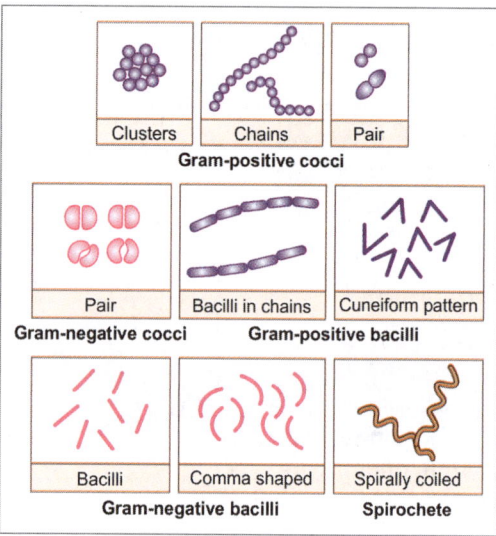

Fig. 2.1.1: Different morphology of bacteria and Gram staining property.

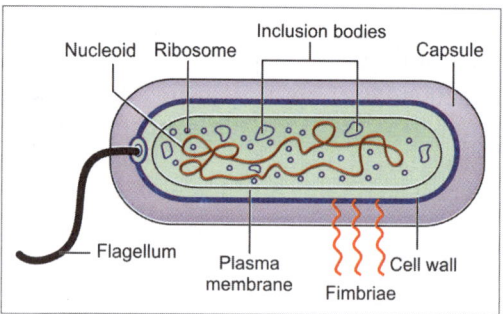

Fig. 2.1.2: Structure of bacterial cell.

Miscellaneous group: However, some bacteria are weakly Gram stained and hence need special stains for their demonstration, such as:
* Spirochetes (*Treponema* and *Leptospira*)—thin spirally coiled bacilli
* *Mycoplasma* (cell wall deficient free-living bacteria)
* Rickettsiae and chlamydiae are obligate intracellular bacteria.

Bacterial Cell Anatomy

Bacterial cell anatomy comprises the following structures **(Fig. 2.1.2)**:
* The **outer layer** or the envelope of a bacterial cell consists of—(1) a rigid cell wall, and (2) an underlying plasma membrane
* The **cytoplasm** contains cytoplasmic inclusions (mesosomes, ribosomes, inclusion granules, vacuoles) and a diffuse nucleoid containing a single circular chromosome
* Some bacteria may possess additional **cell wall appendages** such as capsule, flagella and fimbriae.

Bacterial Cell Wall

The cell wall is a tough and rigid structure, surrounding the bacterium. It is 10–25 nm in thickness.

The cell wall has the following functions:
* It protects the cell against osmotic lysis
* It confers rigidity upon bacteria due to the presence of a peptidoglycan layer in the cell wall

CHAPTER 2.1 ♦ General Bacteriology: Morphology and Physiology of Bacteria

- It is the site of action of several antibiotics
- **Virulence factors:** Bacterial cell wall contains certain virulence factors (e.g. endotoxin), which contribute to their pathogenicity
- **Immunity:** Antibody raised against specific cell wall antigens (e.g. antibody to LPS) may provide immunity against some bacterial infections.

Gram-positive Cell wall

The cell wall of gram-positive bacteria is simpler than that of gram-negative bacteria **(Table 2.1.3)**, made up of the following structure.

- **Peptidoglycan:** It is made up of layers of mucopeptide chains. It is much thicker (50–100 layers thick, 16–80 nm) than the gram-negative cell wall **(Fig. 2.1.3)**
- **Teichoic acid:** Gram-positive cell wall contains a significant amount of teichoic acid; which is absent in gram-negative bacteria. It constitutes major surface antigens of gram-positive bacteria.

Gram-negative Cell wall

The gram-negative cell wall is thinner and more complex than the gram-positive cell wall, comprising of the following components **(Fig. 2.1.4 and Table 2.1.3)**.

- **Peptidoglycan layer:** It is very thin (2 nm) compared to that of the gram-positive cell wall, made up of 1–2 layers of mucopeptide chain
- **Outer membrane:** This is a phospholipid layer that lies outside the thin peptidoglycan layer. It serves as a protective barrier to the cell. Outer membrane proteins (OMP) or porin proteins help in the transport of smaller molecules and also they are target sites for many antibiotics

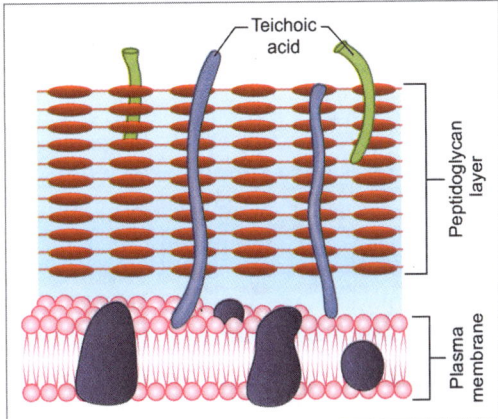

Fig. 2.1.3: Structure of gram-positive cell wall.

- **Lipopolysaccharide (LPS):** This layer is unique to gram-negative bacteria, which is absent in gram-positives. It consists of three parts as:
  1. *Lipid A or the endotoxin*: It is an important virulence factor for gram-negative bacteria
  2. *Core polysaccharide*: It projects from lipid A region
  3. *O side chain*: O antigens are used for serotyping for bacteria and they also induce antibody formation.
- **Periplasmic space:** It is the space between the inner cell membrane and outer membrane. It encompasses the peptidoglycan layer.

Cell Membrane

The plasma membrane is essential for the survival of the bacteria. It is 5–10 nm thick, and composed of bilayered phospholipid in which several proteins are embedded **(Figs. 2.1.2 to 2.1.4)**. The plasma membrane serves important functions in the bacterial cell such as:

- It is a **semipermeable membrane** that acts as an osmotic barrier; selectively allows particular ions, nutrients into the cell, and also helps in waste excretion

Table 2.1.3: Differences between gram-positive and gram-negative cell wall.

Characters	Gram-positive cell wall	Gram-negative cell wall
Peptidoglycan layer	Thicker (16–80 nm)	Thinner (2 nm)
Lipid content	Nil or scanty (2–5%)	Present (15–20%)
Lipopolysaccharide	Absent	Present (endotoxin)
Teichoic acid	Present	Absent

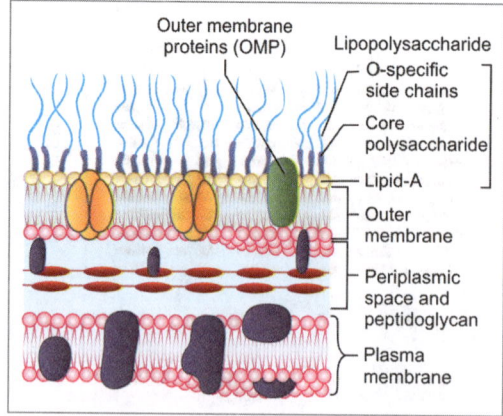

Fig. 2.1.4: Gram-negative cell wall.

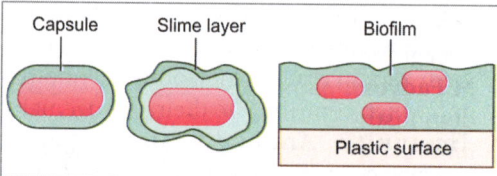

Fig. 2.1.5: Capsule, slime layer and biofilm.

❖ It acts as the site for a variety of crucial metabolic processes such as respiration, synthesis of lipids and cell wall, etc.

Cytoplasmic Matrix

Bacterial cytoplasm is mainly composed of water and is packed with the following structures.
- ❖ **Ribosomes:** They are the sites for protein synthesis; composed of rRNA and ribosomal proteins. Ribosomes are integrated with the mRNA and at this site, the genetic codons of the mRNA are translated into peptide sequences
- ❖ **Intracytoplasmic inclusions:** They are the storage sites of nutrients/energy present in some bacteria. They are formed by the bacteria under nutritional deficiency conditions. For examples, include glycogen granules and metachromatic granules
- ❖ **Mesosomes:** They are invaginations of the plasma membrane. They possess respiratory enzymes and are involved in bacterial respiration; are analogous to the mitochondria of eukaryotes
- ❖ **Nucleoid:** Bacteria do not have a true nucleus, but the genetic material is located in an irregularly shaped region called the nucleoid. There is no nuclear membrane or nucleolus
  - ▪ Bacteria possess a single haploid chromosome, comprising circular double-stranded DNA
  - ▪ Bacterial DNA divides by simple binary fission.

▪ Bacteria also possess extrachromosomal DNA called **plasmids**.

Cell Wall Appendages

Capsule and Slime Layer

Some bacteria possess a layer of amorphous viscid material lying outside the cell wall called **capsule**. When the capsule is in the form of unorganized loose material, it is called a **slime layer (Fig. 2.1.5)**.

Function/Uses

Most of the bacterial capsules are polysaccharide in nature—e.g. pneumococcus, meningococcus, *Haemophilus influenzae*, *Klebsiella pneumoniae*. In *Bacillus anthracis*, the capsule is polypeptide in nature.

The capsule has various functions as follows:
- ❖ **Bacterial virulence:** (i) Capsule protects the bacterium from phagocytosis and from the action of host cell lysozymes. (ii) It also helps in biofilm formation. Biofilm is an extracellular polysaccharide layer, which helps in bacterial adhesion to foreign body surfaces and thereby promotes diseases such as prosthetic valve endocarditis and catheter-associated urinary tract infections, etc.
- ❖ **Identification:** Capsular antigens can be used for the identification and typing of bacteria
- ❖ **Used as vaccine:** Capsular antigens of a few bacteria are used for vaccine preparation; e.g. pneumococcus, meningococcus, and *Haemophilus influenzae* serotype-b.

Demonstration of Capsule

Capsule can be detected by various methods as follows:
- ❖ **Negative staining** by India ink and nigrosin stain: Capsule appears as a clear refractile

halo around the bacteria against a black background
- **M'Fadyean capsule stain:** It is used for demonstration of the capsule of *Bacillus anthracis* by using polychrome methylene blue stain
- **Quellung reaction** for demonstrating capsule in *Streptococcus pneumoniae* by adding capsular antisera mixed with methylene blue
- **Latex agglutination test:** Capsular antigens can be detected in the sample (e.g. CSF) by latex agglutination test by using specific anticapsular antibodies coated on latex particles. This is available for pneumococcus, *Haemophilus influenzae* and meningococcus.

Flagella

Flagella are thread-like appendages, protruding from the cell wall. They measure 5–20 μm in length and 0.01–0.02 μm in thickness.
- **Arrangement:** There are various patterns of arrangement of flagella with respect to the bacterial surface **(Figs. 2.1.6A to D)**:
  - Peritrichous (flagella distributed over the entire cell surface), e.g. *Escherichia coli*
  - Monotrichous (single polar flagellum), e.g. *Vibrio cholerae*
  - Lophotrichous (multiple polar flagella)
  - Amphitrichous (single flagellum at both the ends).
- **Ultrastructure of flagella:** Flagellum is composed of three parts—(i) filament, (ii) basal body, and (iii) hook
- **Bacterial motility:** Flagella confer motility to the bacteria (organ of locomotion). Bacteria can produce characteristic type of

Table 2.1.4: Types of motility shown by different bacteria.

Types of motility	Bacteria
Tumbling motility	*Listeria*
Gliding motility	*Mycoplasma*
Stately motility	*Clostridium*
Darting motility	*Vibrio cholerae*
Swarming on agar plate	*Proteus*
Corkscrew motility	*Spirochetes*

motility which helps in their identification **(Table 2.1.4)**
- **Detection of flagella:** Flagella can be demonstrated by:
  - Direct demonstration by electron microscopy
  - Indirect means by demonstrating the motility by hanging drop method, dark ground or phase contrast microscopy.

Fimbriae or Pili

Fimbriae or pili are short, fine, hair-like appendages, smaller to flagella, but numerous in number. According to the functions, pili are of two types **(Fig. 2.1.7A)**.
1. **Common pili or fimbriae:** They help in **bacterial adhesion** to epithelial surfaces helping in colonization. They are present in gram-negative and some gram-positive bacteria
2. **Sex pili:** They help in bacterial conjugation by forming a conjugation tube through which the bacterial gene transfer takes

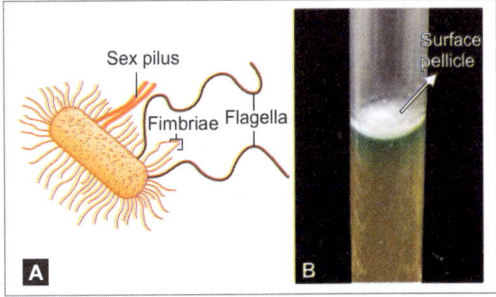

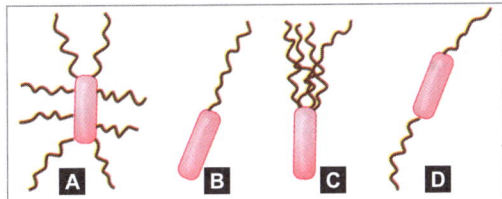

Figs. 2.1.6A to D: Types of bacterial flagellar arrangement: **A.** Peritrichous; **B.** Monotrichous; **C.** Lophotrichous; **D.** Amphitrichous.

Figs. 2.1.7A and B: A. Differentiation between fimbriae, sex pilus and flagella; **B.** Surface pellicle (arrow showing).
Source: Department of Microbiology, JIPMER *(with permission).*

place. They are only found in gram-negative bacteria.

Detection of fimbriae: Fimbriae can be detected either directly by electron microscope, or indirectly through the formation of the **surface pellicle**. It is a thin layer formed at the surface of liquid culture **(Fig. 2.1.7B)**.

L Form (Cell Wall Deficient Forms)

They are the cell wall deficient bacteria, discovered by E Klieneberger. She named it as L form after its place of discovery, i.e. Lister Institute, London (1935).
- When bacteria lose cell wall, they become spherical irrespective of their original shape. This may occur spontaneously or after exposure to lysozyme or cell wall-acting antibiotics such as penicillin
- L forms play a role in the persistence of pyelonephritis and other chronic infections
- Some bacteria like *Mycoplasma* lack cell wall permanently and has been suggested that they may represent stable L form.

Bacterial Spores

Spores are highly resistant resting stage of the bacteria formed in unfavorable environmental conditions as a result of the depletion of exogenous nutrients.

Structure

The bacterial spore comprises several layers. From the innermost to the outermost, the layers are—core, cortex, coat, and exosporium **(Fig. 2.1.8)**.

- The core is the innermost part containing the DNA material and is walled off from the cortex by an inner membrane and the germ cell wall
- Cortex and the coat layers lie external to the core and are separated from each other by an outer membrane
- The outermost layer is called the exosporium.

Sporulation

Sporulation refers to the process of formation of spores from the vegetative stage of bacteria. Sporulation commences when growth ceases due to a lack of nutrients. The mature spore formed is extremely resistant to heat and disinfectant.

Germination

It is the transformation of dormant spores into active vegetative cells when grown in a nutrient-rich medium.

Shape and Position of Spores

For a given species, the position, shape, and relative size of the spore are constant.
- **Position:** Spores may be central, sub-terminal, or terminal **(Figs. 2.1.9 A to F)**
- **Shape:** They may be oval or spherical
- **Width:** The diameter of the spore may be the same or less than the width of bacteria (non-bulging spore—e.g. as in *Bacillus*), or may be wider than the bacillary body producing a bulge in the cell (bulging spore, e.g. as in *Clostridium*).

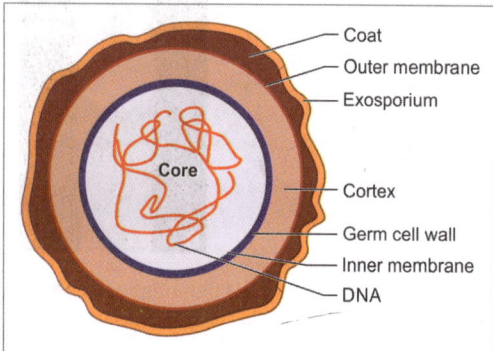

Fig. 2.1.8: Structure of bacterial spore.

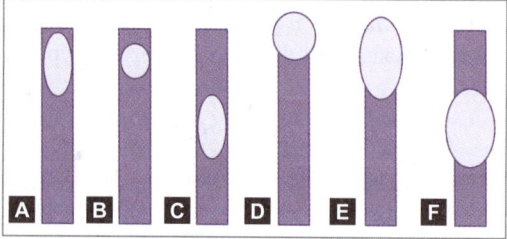

Figs. 2.1.9A to F: Position and shape of spores: **A.** Non-bulging, oval and terminal; **B.** Non-bulging, round, and subterminal; **C.** Non-bulging, oval and central; **D.** Bulging, round and terminal; **E.** Bulging, oval and terminal; **F.** Bulging, oval, and central.

Sporicidal Agents

Spores are resistant to most of the routinely used disinfectants. Only limited agents called sterilants are capable of killing the spores, e.g. autoclave, ethylene oxide sterilizer, etc. (refer to Chapter 41).

Demonstration of Spores

- **Gram staining:** Spores appear as unstained refractile bodies within the cells
- **Modified Ziehl–Neelsen staining:** Spores are weakly acid-fast and appear red color when ZN staining is performed using 0.25–0.5% sulfuric acid as a decolorizer
- **Schaeffer–Fulton stain:** It is a special staining technique to demonstrate spores.

Applications

Spores of certain bacteria are employed as indicators of proper sterilization. Absence of the spores (inability to grow) after autoclaving or processing in hot air oven indicates proper sterilization.
- Spores of *Geobacillus stearothermophilus* are used as sterilization control for autoclave and plasma sterilizer
- Spores of *Bacillus atrophaeus* are used as sterilization control for hot air oven and ethylene oxide sterilizer.

PHYSIOLOGY OF BACTERIA

Bacterial Growth and Nutrition

Water constitutes about 80% of the total bacterial cell. The minimum nutritional requirements essential for the growth of bacteria include sources of carbon, nitrogen, hydrogen, oxygen, and small amounts of inorganic salts such as sulfur, phosphorus, and sodium, etc.

Some fastidious bacteria require additional growth factors called **bacterial vitamins**, which need to be added to the culture medium for their growth; e.g.—*Haemophilus influenzae* requires niacin.

Bacterial Cell Division

Bacteria divide by **binary fission**. The nuclear division precedes cytoplasmic division and then the two daughter cells get separated. In a few bacteria, the daughter cells may remain partially attached even after cell division; so that the bacterial cells are arranged in pairs or chains (e.g. streptococci) or clusters (e.g. staphylococci).

Rate of Multiplication in Bacteria

Generation time is the time required for a bacterium to give rise to two daughter cells under optimum conditions. The generation time for most of the important pathogenic bacteria (e.g. *Escherichia coli*) is 20 minutes. In *Mycobacterium tuberculosis,* it is about 10–15 hours and for *Mycobacterium leprae,* it is about 12–13 days.

Bacterial Count

The bacterial count may be expressed in terms of the total count and viable count. **The total count** indicates the total number of bacteria (live or dead) in the specimen. **Viable count** measures the number of living (viable) cells in the given specimen.

Bacterial Growth Curve

When a bacterium is inoculated into a suitable liquid culture medium and incubated, its growth follows a definite course. When the bacterial count of such culture is determined at different intervals and plotted in relation to time, a **bacterial growth curve** is obtained comprising of four phases **(Table 2.1.5 and Fig. 2.1.10)**.

1. **Lag phase:** It is the period between inoculation and the beginning of the multiplication of bacteria. After inoculating into a culture medium, bacteria do not start multiplying immediately but take some time to build up enzymes and metabolites
   - Bacteria increase in size due to the accumulation of enzymes and metabolites
   - Bacteria reach their maximum size at the end of the lag phase.
2. **Log phase:** In this phase bacteria divide exponentially so that the growth curve takes

Table 2.1.5: Various phases of bacterial growth curve.

	Lag	Log	Stationary	Decline
Bacteria divide	No	Yes	Yes	No
Bacterial death	No	No	Yes	Yes
Total count	Flat	Raises	Raises	Flat
Viable count	Flat	Raises	Flat	Falls
Special features	Accumulation of enzymes and metabolites Attains a maximum size	Uniformly stained Metabolically active Small size	Gram variable **Produce:** Granules, spores, exotoxin, bacteriocin	**Produce:** Involution forms

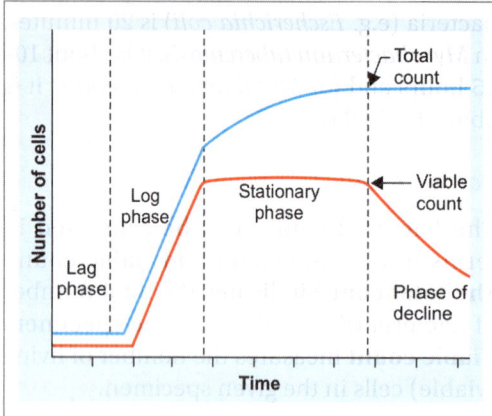

Fig. 2.1.10: Bacterial growth curve.

a shape of a straight line. At this stage, the bacterium is:
- Smaller in size and biochemically active
- Uniformly stained: It is the best time to perform the Gram stain.

3. **Stationary phase:** After the log phase, the bacterial growth ceases almost completely due to exhaustion of nutrients, accumulation of toxic products, and autolytic enzymes
   - The number of progeny cells formed is just enough to replace the number of cells that die
   - Hence, the number of viable cells remains stationary as there is almost a balance between the dying cells and the newly formed cells. But the total count keeps rising. In this phase:
     ♦ Bacterium becomes gram-variable
     ♦ More storage granules are formed
     ♦ Sporulation occurs in this phase
     ♦ Bacteria produce exotoxins, antibiotics, and bacteriocins.

4. **Decline phase:** Gradually, the bacteria stop dividing completely; while the cell death continues due to exhaustion of nutrients, and accumulation of toxic products. Involution forms are seen in this phase. There is a decline in the viable count but not in total count.

Factors Affecting Growth of Bacteria

Several environmental factors affect the growth of the bacteria.

Oxygen

Based on their oxygen requirements bacteria are classified as:
- **Obligate aerobes:** They can grow only in the presence of oxygen (e.g. *Pseudomonas, Mycobacterium tuberculosis, Bacillus*)
- **Facultative anaerobes:** They are aerobes that can also grow anaerobically (e.g. most of the pathogenic bacteria, e.g. *Escherichia coli, Staphylococcus aureus*, etc.)
- **Microaerophilic bacteria:** They can grow in the presence of low oxygen tension, i.e. 5–10% of oxygen (e.g. *Campylobacter* and *Helicobacter*)
- **Obligate anaerobes:** These bacteria can grow only in absence of oxygen, as oxygen is lethal to them (e.g. *Clostridium tetani*).

Temperature

Most of the pathogenic bacteria grow optimally at 37°C (i.e. human body temperature). However, the optimal temperature range varies with different bacterial species.
- **Psychrophiles**—grow best at temperatures below 20°C, e.g. *Pseudomonas*

- **Mesophiles**—grow within a temperature range 25°C and 40°C, e.g. most of the pathogenic bacteria
- **Thermophiles**—these bacteria grow at a high-temperature range of 55°C–80°C, e.g. *Geobacillus stearothermophilus*.

Other Important Factors Affecting Growth of Bacteria

- **Carbon dioxide:** Organisms that require higher amounts of carbon dioxide (5–10%) for growth are called *capnophilic bacteria*. Examples include *Brucella abortus*, *Streptococcus pneumoniae*, etc.
- **pH:** Most pathogenic bacteria grow between pH 7.2-and pH 7.6. Very few bacteria (e.g. lactobacilli) can grow at acidic pH and *Vibrio cholerae* are capable of growing at alkaline pH
- **Light:** Bacteria (except phototrophs) grow well in darkness. Photochromogenic mycobacteria produce pigments only on exposure to light
- **Moisture and desiccation:** Moisture is an essential requirement for the growth of bacteria because 80% of the bacterial cell consists of water. Some organisms like *Treponema pallidum* and *N. gonorrhoeae* die quickly after drying, while *M. tuberculosis* and *S. aureus* may survive drying for several weeks.

EXPECTED QUESTIONS

I. **Write an essay on:**
   Describe in detail the structure and function of the cell wall and cell membrane of gram-negative bacilli with the help of a diagram.

II. **Write short notes on:**
   1. Bacterial capsule.
   2. Bacterial growth curve.

III. **Multiple Choice Questions (MCQs):**
   1. The cuneiform arrangement is characteristic of:
      a. *Staphylococcus*
      b. *Streptococcus*
      c. *Corynebacterium diphtheriae*
      d. *Bacillus anthracis*
   2. A bacterial capsule can be best demonstrated by:
      a. Gram staining
      b. Acid-fast staining
      c. Negative staining
      d. Albert staining
   3. The bacterial structure involved in motility is:
      a. Ribosome   b. Pili
      c. Mesosome   d. Flagella
   4. Which of the following cocci–arrangement is wrong?
      a. Chain-*Streptococcus*
      b. Pair-Pneumococcus
      c. Chain-Gonococcus
      d. Cluster-*Staphylococcus*
   5. Lipopolysaccharide is a component of cell wall of:
      a. Gram-positive bacteria
      b. Gram-negative bacteria
      c. Virus
      d. Fungi
   6. Bacterial structure involved in respiration is:
      a. Ribosome   b. Pili
      c. Mesosome   d. Flagella

Answers
1. c   2. c   3. d   4. c   5. b   6. c

CHAPTER 2.2

General Bacteriology: Laboratory Diagnosis of Bacterial Infections

CHAPTER PREVIEW
- Specimen Collection
- Direct Detection
- Culture, Identification and AST
- Serology
- Molecular Methods

Laboratory diagnosis of bacterial infections comprises of several steps—as discussed in the highlight box.

Laboratory diagnosis of bacterial infections
1. **Specimen collection**
2. **Direct detection**
   - Microscopy: Gram stain, acid-fast stain, Albert stain, histopathological staining, dark ground, phase-contrast, and fluorescence microscopy
   - Antigen detection from a clinical specimen (Chapter 9)
   - Molecular diagnosis: Detecting bacterial DNA or RNA from a clinical specimen
3. **Culture**
   - Culture media
   - Culture methods
   - Colony morphology, smear, and motility testing
4. **Identification**
   - Biochemical identification
   - Automated identification methods
5. **Antimicrobial susceptibility testing**
6. **Serology**—Antigen and antibody detection (Chapter 9)
7. **Molecular methods**—PCR, real-time PCR

SPECIMEN COLLECTION

Specimen collection depends upon the type of underlying infections **(Table 2.2.1)**. The proper collection of the specimen is of paramount importance for the isolation of the bacteria in culture.

General Principles
The following general principles should be followed while collecting the specimen:
- **Standard precautions** should be followed for collecting and handling all specimens (Chapter 37 for details)
- **Before the start of antibiotics** specimens for culture should be collected
- **Contamination** with normal flora should be avoided, especially when collecting urine and blood culture specimens
- **Swabs** are though convenient but considered inferior to tissue, aspirate, and body fluids
- **Container:** Specimens should be collected in sterile, tightly sealed, leak-proof, wide-mouthed, screw-capped containers **(Fig. 2.2.1A)**
- **Labeling:** All specimens must be appropriately labeled with name, age, gender, treating physician, diagnosis, antibiotic history, type of specimen, and desired investigation name
- **Rejection:** Specimens grossly contaminated or compromised or improperly labeled may be rejected

CHAPTER 2.2 ♦ General Bacteriology: Laboratory Diagnosis of Bacterial Infections

Table 2.2.1: Types of infections and various specimens collected.

Type of infections	Specimens collected
Bloodstream infection, sepsis, endocarditis	Paired blood culture specimens • Collected aseptically by two-step disinfection of skin; first with alcohol followed by chlorhexidine • 8–10 mL of blood (for adults) collected in blood culture bottles **(Fig. 2.2.7B)**
Infectious diseases requiring serology	• Blood (2 mL/investigation) • Collected by minimal asepsis • Collected in vacutainer **(Fig. 2.2.1B)**
Diarrheal diseases	Stool (mucus flakes), rectal swab
Meningitis	Cerebrospinal fluid (CSF)
Infections of other sterile body areas	Sterile body fluids; e.g. pleural fluid, synovial fluid, peritoneal fluid
Skin and soft tissue infections	Pus or exudate, wound swabs, aspirates from abscess and tissue bits
Anaerobic infections	Aspirates, tissue specimens, blood and sterile body fluids, bone marrow (swabs, sputum not satisfactory)
Upper respiratory tract infections	Throat swab with a membrane over the tonsil, nasopharyngeal swab, per-nasal swab
Lower respiratory tract infections	Sputum, endotracheal aspirate, bronchoalveolar lavage (BAL), protected specimen brush (PSB), and lung biopsy
Pulmonary tuberculosis	• Sputum—early morning and spot • Collected in a well-ventilated area • Gastric aspirate for infants
Urinary tract infections	• Midstream urine • Suprapubic aspirated urine • Catheterized patient—collected from the catheter tube, after clamping distally and disinfecting; not from urobag
Genital infections	• Urethral swab, cervical swab—for urethritis • Exudate from genital ulcers
Eye infections	• Conjunctival swabs • Corneal scrapings • Aqueous or vitreous fluid
Ear infections	• Swabs from the outer ear • Aspirate from the inner ear

❖ If **anaerobic culture** is requested, proper anaerobic collection containers with media should be used
❖ The specimen should not be sent in a container containing **formalin** for microbiological analysis.

Specimen Transport

The specimens should reach the laboratory for further processing as soon as possible after the collection. If required appropriate transport media should be used. For most of the specimens, transport time should not exceed **two hours**. However, there are some exceptions.

❖ CSF and body fluids, ocular specimens, tissue specimens, suprapubic aspirate and bone specimen require an **immediate transport** (<15 minutes)
❖ **Urine (midstream)** added with preservative (boric acid) is acceptable up to 24 hours, otherwise should be transported within 2 hours

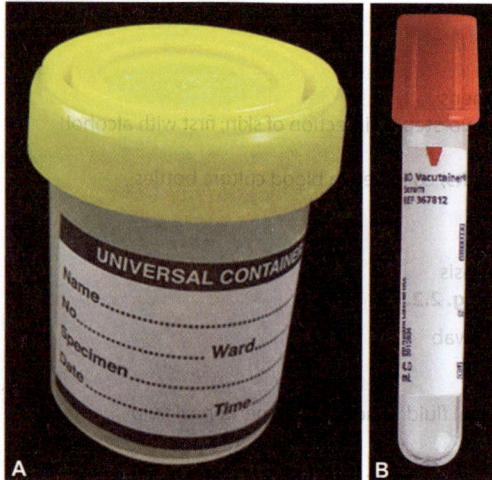

Figs. 2.2.1A and B: A. Sterile universal container; **B.** Blood collection Vacutainer tube.

- **Stool culture:** Stool specimen should be transported within 1 hour, but with transport medium (Cary-Blair medium) up to 24 hours is acceptable
- **For anaerobic culture:** Specimens should be put into Robertson's cooked meat broth or any specialized anaerobic transport system and transported immediately to the laboratory.

Specimen Storage before Processing

Most specimens can be stored **at room temperature** immediately after receipt, for **up to 24 hours**. However, there are some exceptions.
- **Blood cultures**—should be incubated at 37°C immediately upon receipt
- **Sterile body fluids**, bone, vitreous fluid, suprapubic aspirate—should be immediately plated upon receipt and incubated at 37°C
- **Corneal scraping**—should be immediately plated at *bed-side* on to blood agar and chocolate agar
- **Stool culture**—can be stored up to 72 hours at 4°C
- **Urine** and **lower respiratory** tract specimens can be stored up to 24 hours at 4°C.

For details on specimen collection, refer Chapter 54.

DIRECT DETECTION

Specimens upon receipt to the laboratory are subjected to various direct detection methods, which help in the early institution of antimicrobial therapy and also guide the microbiologist for further culture processing. The most important direct detection method includes the microscopic demonstration of bacteria by various staining techniques. The other methods are the detection of antigen (discussed in Chapter 9) and nucleic acid detection methods (discussed subsequently in this chapter).

STAINING TECHNIQUES

Common staining techniques used in diagnostic bacteriology include:
- **Simple stain:** Basic dyes, such as methylene blue or basic fuchsin is used as simple stains. They provide color contrast for visualization
- **Differential stain:** Here, two stains are used which impart different colors and help in differentiating bacteria. The most commonly employed differential stains are Gram stain and acid-fast stain
- **Special stains:** These staining techniques are useful to identify various bacterial structures of importance. Examples include—(1) Albert staining (to demonstrate metachromatic granules), (2) Spore staining (e.g. Schaeffer–Fulton stain) and (3) Flagellar staining (e.g. Leifson's method)
- **Negative staining:** A drop of bacterial suspension is mixed with dyes, such as India ink or nigrosin. The background gets stained black whereas the unstained bacterial capsule stands out in contrast.

Gram Stain

This staining technique was originally developed by Hans Christian Gram (1884). Gram stain is the most widely used test in diagnostic bacteriology.

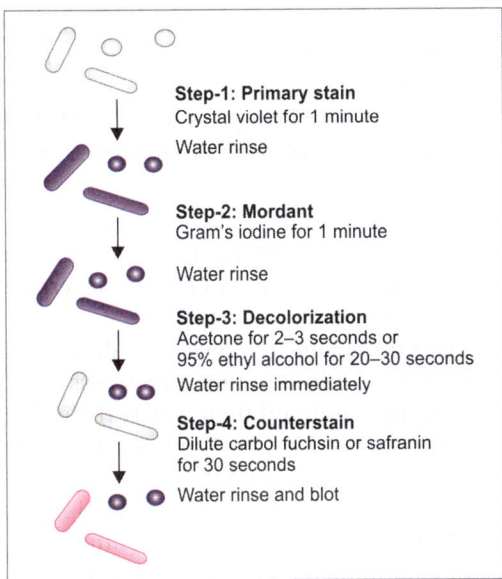

Fig. 2.2.2: Principle and procedure of Gram staining.

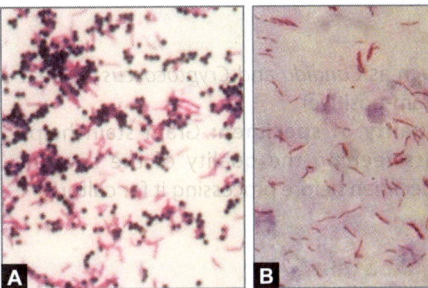

Figs. 2.2.3A and B: A. Gram staining demonstrating violet-colored gram-positive cocci in clusters and pink-colored gram-negative bacilli; **B.** Acid-fast stained smear showing long slender slightly curved beaded red acid-fast bacilli.

Source: Department of Microbiology, JIPMER, Puducherry (*with permission*).

Procedure (Fig. 2.2.2)

❖ **Step 1 (Primary stain):** Heat-fixed smear is stained with crystal violet (or gentian violet or methyl violet) for one minute. Then the slide is rinsed with water. Crystal violet stains all the bacteria violet in color

❖ **Step 2 (Mordant):** Gram's iodine is poured over the slide for one minute. Then the slide is rinsed with water. Gram's iodine acts as a mordant, binds to the dye to form bigger dye-iodine complexes in the cytoplasm

❖ **Step 3 (Decolorization):** Next step is pouring of few drops of decolorizer to the smear, e.g. acetone (for 2–3 sec) or ethyl alcohol (20–30 sec). The slide is immediately rinsed with water. Decolorizer removes the primary stain from gram-negative bacteria while the gram-positive bacteria retain the primary stain

❖ **Step 4 (Counterstain):** Secondary stains such as safranin or dilute carbol fuchsin is added for 30 seconds. It imparts pink or red color to the gram-negative bacteria.

Interpretation of Gram Stain

Smear is examined under oil immersion objective (**Fig. 2.2.3A**).

❖ Gram-positive bacteria appear violet colored
❖ Gram-negative bacteria are decolorized and, therefore, take counterstain and appear pink.

Principle of Gram Staining

The gram-positive cell wall has a thick peptidoglycan layer, which acts as a permeability barrier preventing loss of the primary stain. Whereas a gram-negative cell wall is more permeable due to the thin peptidoglycan layer and lipopolysaccharide layer, which gets easily disrupted by the decolorizer; thus allowing the outflow of the primary stain easily.

> **Uses of Gram Stain**
> The various uses of Gram stain include:
> - To **differentiate bacteria** into gram-positive and gram-negative
> - **To start empirical treatment:** Gram stain from the specimen gives a preliminary clue about the bacteria present so that the empirical treatment with broad-spectrum antibiotics can be started early, before the culture report is available
> - **Anaerobic organisms** if detected in the Gram stain of the clinical specimen, gives a preliminary clue to perform an anaerobic culture of the specimen
> - **Yeasts:** In addition to staining the bacteria, Gram stain is useful for staining certain fungi
>
> *Contd...*

Contd...

- such as *Candida* and *Cryptococcus* (appear gram-positive)
- **Quality of specimen:** Gram stain helps in screening the quality of the sputum specimen before processing it for culture.

Acid-fast Stain

The acid-fast stain was discovered by Paul Ehrlich and subsequently modified by Ziehl-Neelsen. This staining is done to identify acid-fast organisms, such as *Mycobacterium tuberculosis* and others. Acid-fastness is due to the presence of mycolic acid in the cell wall.

Ziehl-Neelsen Technique (Hot Method)

Smear is air-dried and heat-fixed before staining.

Procedure

- **Step 1 (primary stain):** Smear is poured with strong carbol fuchsin for 5 minutes. Intermittent heating is done for better penetration of the stain. Rinse the slide with tap water
- **Step 2 (Decolorization):** It is done by pouring 25% sulfuric acid over the slide for 2–4 minutes. The slide is gently rinsed with tap water and tilted to drain off the water
- **Step 3 (Counterstaining):** Methylene blue is poured onto the slide for 30 seconds. Then the slide is rinsed gently with tap water and allowed to dry
- The slide is examined under the bright-field microscope under an oil immersion field (100x).

Interpretation

Mycobacterium tuberculosis appears as long slender, straight, or slightly curved and beaded, red colored acid-fast bacillus and background take up the counterstain and appear blue **(Fig. 2.2.3B)**.

Modifications of Acid-fast Staining

Modifications of acid-fast staining include:
- **Cold method (Kinyoun's method):** In this technique heating is not required, phenol concentration in carbol fuchsin is increased and duration of carbol fuchsin staining is more
- **Decolorization using acid-alcohol** (3 mL of HCl and 97 mL of ethanol) can also be used.

Albert Stain

Albert stain is used to demonstrate the metachromatic granules of *Corynebacterium diphtheriae*.
- **Procedure:** Smear is covered with Albert I stain for 5 minutes, then the excess stain is drained out and then Albert II (iodine solution) is added for 1 minute. The slide is washed with water, blotted dry, and examined under oil immersion field
- **Interpretation:** *Corynebacterium diphtheriae* appears as green-colored bacilli arranged in a cuneiform pattern, with bluish-black metachromatic granules at polar ends (Refer to **Fig. 13.1B** of Chapter 13).

Other Microscopic Techniques

Other microscopic techniques include:
- **Dark-ground microscopy**—for demonstration of spirochetes in genital specimens (Refer **Fig. 1.4** of Chapter 1)
- **Hanging drop preparation** for stool specimen—for demonstration of darting motility; gives a clue about *V. cholerae*.

CULTURE, IDENTIFICATION AND AST

Culture is the most common diagnostic method used for the detection of bacterial infections. Specimens are inoculated onto various culture media and incubated. The colonies grown are subjected to identification and antimicrobial susceptibility test (AST).

CULTURE MEDIA

A microbiological culture medium is a liquid or solid substance that contains nutrients to support the growth, and survival of microorganisms.
- **Constituents of culture media:** The important constituents of culture media

are water, electrolytes, peptone, agar (solidifying agent), meat extract, and yeast extract. In addition, blood or serum may be added to provide extra-nutrition to fastidious bacteria

- **Types of culture media:** Based on consistency, culture media are grouped into—liquid (or broth), semisolid and solid media
- **Based on the method of growth detection**, culture media are classified as—conventional or automated culture media
  - *Conventional culture media:* They are of various types such as—simple/basal media, enriched media, enrichment broth, selective media, differential media, transport media, and anaerobic media
  - *Automated culture media*: They are mainly available for blood and sterile body fluid culture. The growth is detected automatically by the equipment.

Conventional Culture Media

Simple/Basal Media

They contain minimum ingredients that support the growth of non-fastidious bacteria.
- Examples include—Peptone water, nutrient broth, and nutrient agar **(Figs. 2.2.4A and B)**
- Basal media support the growth of non-fastidious bacteria, helpful in studying the bacterial growth curve
- They are the preferred media for performing the biochemical tests and to describe colony morphology.

Enriched Media

When a basal medium is added with additional nutrients, such as blood, serum or egg, it is called an enriched medium. They support the growth of fastidious nutritionally exacting bacteria. Examples include:
- **Blood agar:** It is useful to test the hemolytic property of the bacteria, which may be either: Partial or α (green) hemolysis and complete or β-hemolysis **(Fig. 2.2.4C)**
- **Chocolate agar:** It is more nutritious than blood agar, and even supports the growth of *Haemophilus influenzae* that does not grow on blood agar **(Fig. 2.2.4D)**
- **Blood culture media:** They are also enriched media, used for isolating organisms from blood (discussed later in this chapter).

Enrichment Broth

They are the liquid media added with some inhibitory agents which selectively allow certain organism to grow and inhibit others.
- Useful for isolation of the pathogens from stool specimen, which also contain normal flora
- Examples include—selenite F broth for isolation of *Shigella* and alkaline peptone water (APW) for *Vibrio cholerae*.

Selective Media

They are solid media containing inhibitory substances that inhibit the normal flora present in the specimen and allow the pathogens to grow. Examples include—
- Lowenstein–Jensen (LJ) medium **(Fig. 2.2.5A)** for isolation of *Mycobacterium tuberculosis*

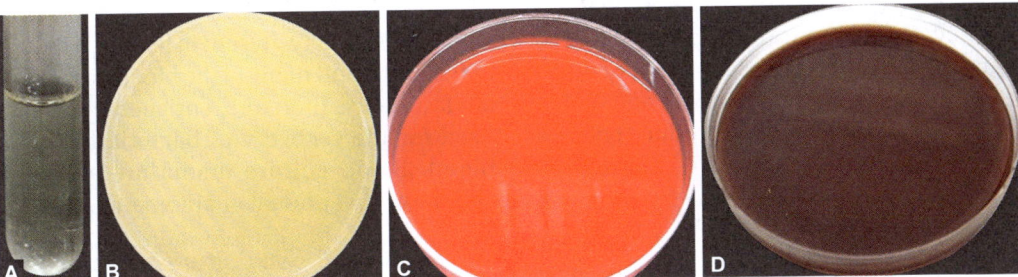

Figs. 2.2.4A to D: A. Peptone water; **B.** Nutrient agar; **C.** Blood agar; **D.** Chocolate agar.
Source: **A to D.** Department of Microbiology, JIPMER, Puducherry (*with permission*).

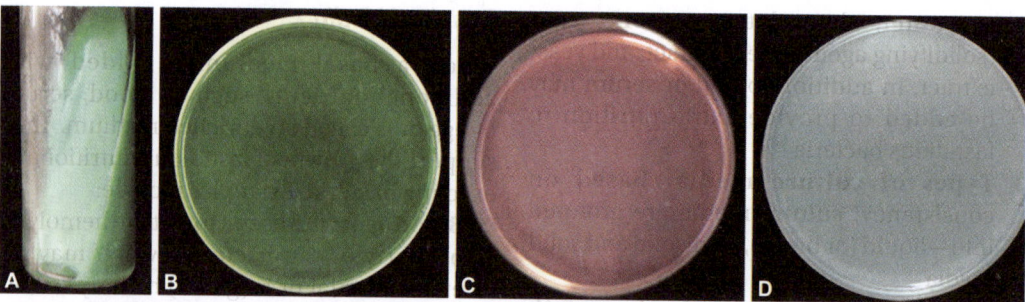

Figs. 2.2.5A to D: A. Lowenstein–Jensen medium; **B.** TCBS agar; **C.** MacConkey agar; **D.** CLED agar.
Source: Department of Microbiology, JIPMER, Puducherry (*with permission*).

* Thiosulfate-citrate-bile salt-sucrose (TCBS) agar (**Fig. 2.2.5B**) for isolation of *Vibrio* species.

Transport Media

They are used for the transport of the clinical specimens suspected to contain delicate organisms or if a delay is expected for specimen transport.
* Bacteria only remain viable; do not multiply in this media
* Examples include—(1) Cary-Blair medium for *Salmonella*, and *Shigella*, (2) Venkatraman-Ramakrishnan medium for *Vibrio cholerae* and (3) Amies medium for gonococcus.

Differential Media

These media differentiate between two groups of bacteria by changes in the color of the colonies produced.
* Examples include— (1) **MacConkey agar** (most commonly used medium for all specimens), and (2) **CLED agar** (cysteine lactose electrolyte-deficient agar, used for urine specimen) (**Figs. 2.2.5C and D**)
* They differentiate organisms into LF or lactose fermenters (produce pink-colored colonies, e.g. *Escherichia coli*) and NLF or non-lactose fermenters (produce colorless colonies, e.g. *Shigella*).

Anaerobic Culture Media

Anaerobic media contain reducing substances that take-up oxygen and create lower redox potential and thus permit the growth of obligate anaerobes, such as *Clostridium*. Examples include—**Robertson's cooked meat (RCM) broth** and thioglycollate broth (**Fig. 2.2.6A**).

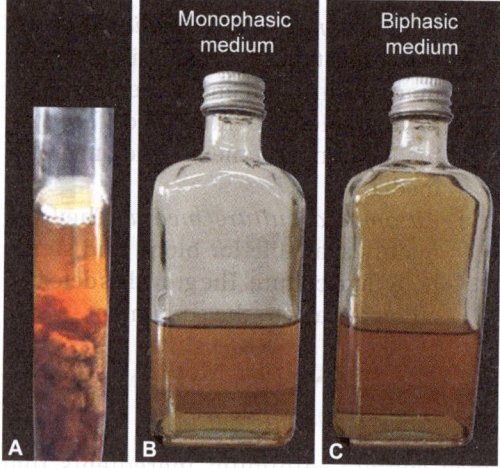

Figs. 2.2.6A to C: A. Robertson's cooked meat medium; **B.** Brain-heart infusion broth; **C.** Biphasic medium (Brain-heart infusion broth/agar).
Source: **A to C.** Department of Microbiology, JIPMER, Puducherry (*with permission*).

Blood Culture Media

Organisms usually present in lesser quantities in the blood and many of the blood pathogens are fastidious. Therefore, enriched media are used for the recovery of bacteria from the blood. Blood culture media are available either as conventional or automated media.

Conventional Blood Culture Media

The conventional blood culture media are of two types.

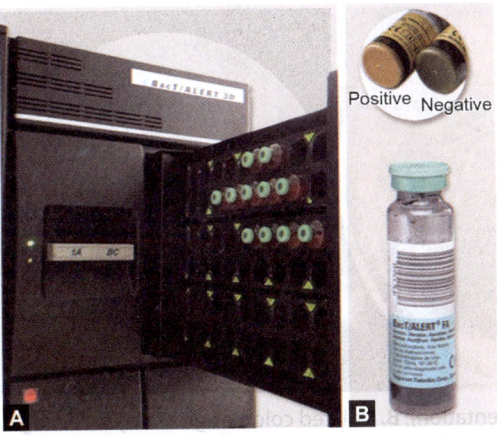

Figs. 2.2.7A and B: A. BacT/ALERT automated blood culture system; **B.** BacT/ALERT blood culture bottle.
Source: Department of Microbiology, JIPMER, Puducherry (with permission).

1. **Monophasic medium:** It contains brain-heart infusion (BHI) broth **(Fig. 2.2.6B)**
2. **Biphasic medium:** It has a liquid phase containing BHI broth and a solid agar slope made up of BHI agar **(Fig. 2.2.6C)**.

Automated Blood Culture Systems

Automated blood culture techniques are revolutionary and offer several advantages over conventional blood cultures, such as—(i) continuous automated monitoring, (ii) faster recovery of organisms, and (iii) lesser contamination risk.
- ❖ **Medium:** They contain tryptic soy broth and/or brain heart infusion broth
- ❖ **Other specimens:** In addition to blood, they can also be used for culture of bone marrow, sterile body fluids such as CSF, peritoneal, pleural fluids, etc.
- ❖ **Examples** of automated blood culture systems are BacT/ALERT 3D and BACTEC systems **(Fig. 2.2.7A)**
- ❖ **Principle:** When bacteria multiply, they produce CO_2 by metabolism, which decreases the pH of the medium, which in turn triggers the sensor resulting in:
  - Color change at the bottom of the bottle (BacT/ALERT)
  - Production of fluorescence (BACTEC).
- ❖ **Growth signal:** The instrument gives a signal (producing beep or color change on the screen) once the growth is detected **(Fig. 2.2.7B)**.

CULTURE METHODS

Culture methods involve inoculating the specimen onto appropriate culture media, followed by incubating the culture plates in appropriate conditions.
- ❖ **Selection of media:** A combination of blood agar and MacConkey agar is commonly used for the processing of most specimens
- ❖ **Inoculation of the specimens** onto the culture media is done with the help of bacteriological loops made up of platinum or nichrome wire
- ❖ **Inoculation methods:** Common inoculation methods are streak culture, liquid culture, and lawn culture
  - *Streak culture* method is used for the inoculation of the specimens onto the solid media. Here, a loopful of the specimen is smeared onto the solid media to form round-shaped primary inoculum, which is then spread over the culture plate by streaking parallel lines. This technique is followed to get isolated colonies **(Figs. 2.2.8A and B)**
  - *Lawn* or *carpet culture:* It is useful to carry out antimicrobial susceptibility testing (AST) by disk diffusion method **(Fig. 2.2.8C)**
  - *Liquid culture:* It is used for the culture of blood and body fluids and also for water analysis. Bacterial growth is observed by turbidity in the medium
  - *Pour plate technique:* Used for quantifying the bacterial load present in the specimens such as urine or blood. Here, serial dilutions of the specimen are added on to the molten agar. After being cooled and solidified, the Petri dishes are incubated and then the colony count is estimated.

Incubatory Conditions

Most of the pathogenic bacteria are aerobes or facultative anaerobes; grow best when incubated at 37°C in the bacteriological

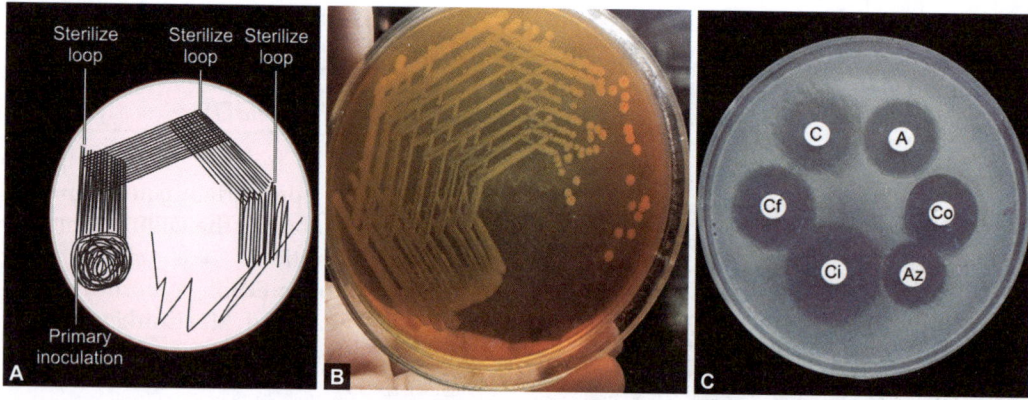

Figs. 2.2.8A to C: A. Streak culture (schematic representation); **B.** Isolated colonies grown by following streak culture; **C.** Lawn culture of a bacterial isolate to perform the antimicrobial susceptibility testing.
Source: Department of Microbiology, JIPMER, Puducherry *(with permission)*.

incubator. For capnophilic bacteria (e.g. *Brucella*, *Streptococcus*, pneumococcus) candle jar is used to provide 5% CO_2. For obligate anaerobes, anaerobic culture methods are used (see below).

Anaerobic Culture Methods

Obligate anaerobic bacteria can grow only in the absence of oxygen. The following are the methods used to create anaerobiosis.

* **Evacuation and replacement method** by using:
  ■ **McIntosh and Filde's anaerobic jar (Fig. 2.2.9A):** It was the most popular method in the past
  ■ *Anoxomat:* It automatically evacuates air and replaces it with hydrogen gas from a cylinder. It is easier to use and highly effective for creating anaerobiosis **(Fig. 2.2.9B)**.
* **Absorption of oxygen by chemical methods**: *GasPak system* works on this principle. It is the most commonly used method for anaerobiosis. Here, the oxygen is removed by chemical reactions **(Fig. 2.2.9C)**
* **Anaerobic glove box** and **anaerobic work station** for easy processing, incubation and examination of the specimens
* **Reducing agents** such as glucose, thioglycollate, and cooked meat pieces can

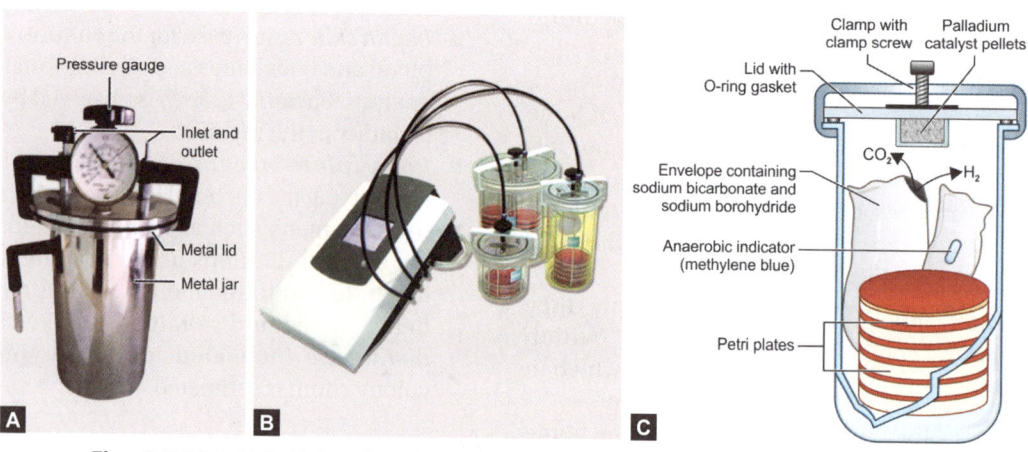

Figs. 2.2.9A to C: A. McIntosh and Filde's anaerobic jar; **B.** Anoxomat anaerobic system; **C.** GasPak anaerobic system.
Source: **A.** Department of Microbiology, Pondicherry Institute of Medical Sciences, Puducherry; **B.** Department of Microbiology, JIPMER, Puducherry *(with permission)*.

be used to reduce oxygen in culture media. Robertson cooked meat broth (**RCM**) is commonly used; which uses chopped meat particles as reducing agent (**Fig. 2.2.6A**).

Colony Morphology

After overnight incubation, the culture media are removed from the incubator and examined under bright illumination.
- ❖ The appearance of the bacterial colony on the culture medium helps in their preliminary identification
- ❖ The colony characteristics that help in the preliminary identification are—
  - Size, shape, consistency (e.g. dry, moist or mucoid)
  - Color (pink or pale on MacConkey agar)
  - Pigment production (e.g. blue-green pigments by *Pseudomonas*)
  - Hemolysis on blood agar: e.g. (i) α or partial hemolysis, (ii) β or complete hemolysis.

Culture Smear and Motility Testing

The colonies grown on the culture media are subjected to Gram staining and motility testing by hanging drop method. **Hanging drop preparation** is one of the most common and easiest method to demonstrate bacterial motility.
- ❖ A drop of bacterial broth is prepared on a coverslip and kept over a cavity slide
- ❖ Then the edge of the drop is focused under the microscope for demonstration of motile bacteria
- ❖ Hanging drop may give some clue about the identification, especially for gram-negative bacilli.

CULTURE IDENTIFICATION

Identification of bacteria from culture is made either by conventional biochemical tests or automated identification systems.

Conventional Biochemical Identification

Based on the type of colony morphology and Gram staining appearance observed in culture smear, the appropriate biochemical tests are employed.
1. **Initially,** catalase and oxidase tests are done on all types of colonies grown on the media
2. **For gram-negative bacilli:** The following are the common biochemical tests done routinely, abbreviated as 'ICUT':
   - Indole test
   - Citrate utilization test
   - Urea hydrolysis test
   - Triple sugar iron test (TSI).
3. **For gram-positive cocci:** The useful biochemical tests are as follows:
   - Coagulase test (for *Staphylococcus aureus*)
   - CAMP (Christie-Atkins-Munch-Petersen) test for group B *Streptococcus*
   - Bile esculin hydrolysis test (for *Enterococcus*)
   - Inulin fermentation and bile solubility test (for pneumococcus).

Automated Systems for Bacterial Identification

Automated identification systems are revolutionary in diagnostic microbiology.
- ❖ They have several advantages—(i) produce faster results, (ii) can identify a wide range of organisms with accuracy, which are otherwise difficult to identify (e.g. anaerobes) through conventional biochemical tests
- ❖ Examples of automated systems used for bacterial identification are—
  - MALDI-TOF: Matrix-assisted laser desorption ionization time-of-flight
  - VITEK 2 automated ID and AST system.

ANTIMICROBIAL SUSCEPTIBILITY TEST

Antimicrobial susceptibility test (AST) is the most important investigation carried out by a microbiology laboratory. Bacteria exhibit great variations in susceptibility to antimicrobial agents. Therefore, AST plays a vital role to guide the clinician in tailoring the empirical antibiotic therapy to pathogen-directed therapy.

AST Methods

Antimicrobial susceptibility testing methods are:
- Disk diffusion method, e.g. Kirby–Bauer's disk diffusion (DD) test
- Dilution tests: Broth dilution and agar dilution methods
- Epsilometer or E-test
- Automated AST: e.g. VITEK and Phoenix systems.

Disk Diffusion Method

Kirby–Bauer's disk diffusion (DD) test is the most widely used AST method. They are suitable for rapidly growing pathogenic bacteria.
- **Procedure:** Mueller–Hinton agar (MHA) is the medium used for DD test
  - Bacterial suspension is inoculated onto this medium by spreading (lawn culture) with sterile swabs
  - Antimicrobial disks are then placed on the surface of MHA plate. Then the plates are incubated at 37°C for 16–18 hours and then interpreted.
- **Interpretation:** Susceptibility to the drug is determined by the zone of inhibition of bacterial growth around the disk. The interpretation of zone size into sensitive, intermediate or resistant is based on the standard zone size interpretation chart, provided by standard guidelines (e.g. CLSI) (Fig. 2.2.10).

Dilution Tests

Here, the inoculum of the test organism is added to serial dilutions of antimicrobial agent in presence of a suitable medium. After overnight incubation, it is examined to determine the MIC.
- **MIC (minimum inhibitory concentration):** It is the lowest concentration of the drug that will inhibit the visible growth of an organism
- **Types:** Based on the platform where the test is performed, there are various types of dilution methods
  - *Broth dilution:* It uses Mueller-Hinton broth. It can be performed using tube (broth macrodilution) or microtiter plate (broth microdilution)
  - *Agar dilution:* It is performed on Mueller-Hinton agar.

Epsilometer or E-test

E-test is an absorbent strip that contains predefined gradient of antibiotic concentrations along its length. It is a MIC-based method, that uses the principles of both dilution and diffusion of the drug into the medium.

Automated Antimicrobial Susceptibility Tests

Several automated systems are available now, such as: VITEK 2 and Phoenix system for bacterial identification and AST. They are MIC-based methods, that work on the principle of broth microdilution. They provide more rapid results compared with traditional methods.

Interpretation of AST

The result of AST is always expressed in the following interpretative categories.
- **Susceptible (S):** Indicates that the antimicrobial agent is clinically effective when used in a standard therapeutic dose
- **Intermediate (I):** Indicates that the antimicrobial agent is not clinically effective when used in standard dose, but may be active when used in increased dose
- **Resistant (R):** Indicates that the antimicrobial agent is NOT clinically effective when used in either standard dose or increased dose, and therefore should not be included in the treatment regimen.

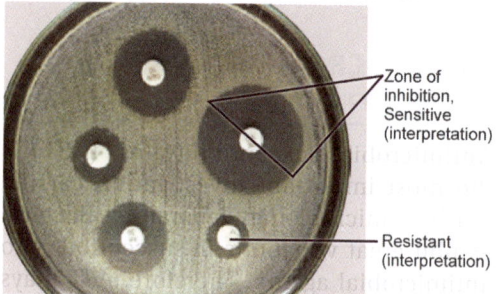

Fig. 2.2.10: Kirby–Bauer disk diffusion method.
Source: Department of Microbiology, PIMS Puducherry (with permission).

SEROLOGY

The serological tests play an important role in the diagnosis of various bacterial infections. These include detection of either antigen or antibody in the serum of the patient, by various immunological assays—precipitation, agglutination, ELISA, rapid tests, etc. The detail of these methods is discussed in Chapter 9.

MOLECULAR METHODS

Molecular methods are broadly grouped into amplification-based and non-amplification-based methods.
- *Nucleic acid amplification techniques (NAATs)* have been increasingly used in diagnostic microbiology. Various NAATs used are:
  - Polymerase chain reaction (PCR)
  - Real-time polymerase chain reaction (rt-PCR)
  - Automated real-time PCR such as cartridge-based nucleic acid amplification test (CBNAAT).
- *Non-amplification molecular methods* include DNA hybridization method, e.g. line probe assay.

Polymerase Chain Reaction

Polymerase chain reaction (PCR) is a technology in molecular biology used to amplify a single or few copies of a piece of DNA to generate millions of copies of DNA. It was developed by Kary B Mullis (1983) for which he and Michael Smith were awarded the Nobel Prize in Chemistry in 1993.

Principle of PCR
PCR involves three basic steps:
1. **DNA extraction from the organism:** This involves lysis of the organisms and release of the DNA by—boiling or adding enzymes (e.g. proteinase K).
2. **Amplification of extracted DNA:** This is carried out in a special PCR machine called thermocycler **(Fig. 2.2.11A)**. The extracted DNA is subjected to repeated cycles (30–35 numbers) of amplification which takes about

Contd...

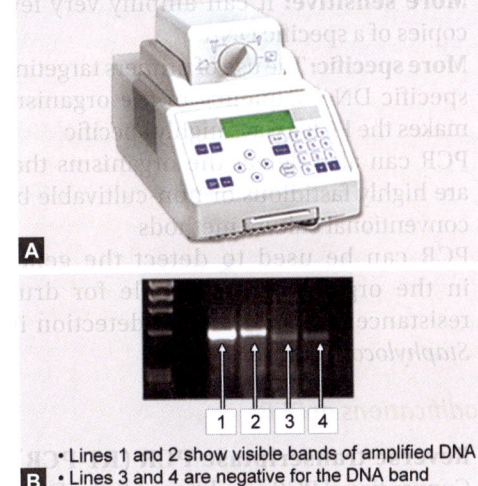

- Lines 1 and 2 show visible bands of amplified DNA
- Lines 3 and 4 are negative for the DNA band

Figs. 2.2.11A and B: A. Thermocycler machine; **B.** Visualization of amplified DNA under UV light.
Source: Department of Microbiology, JIPMER, Puducherry *(with permission).*

Contd...

3–4 hours. Each amplification cycle has three steps:
  - **Denaturation at 95°C:** This involves separation of the dsDNA into two separate single strands
  - **Primer annealing (55°C):** Primer is a short oligonucleotide complementary to a small sequence of the target DNA. It anneals to the complementary site on the target ssDNA
  - **Extension of the primer (72°C):** This step is catalyzed by Taq Polymerase enzyme which keeps on adding the free nucleotides to the growing end of the primer.
3. **Gel electrophoresis of amplified product:** The amplified DNA is electrophoretically migrated according to its molecular size by performing agarose gel electrophoresis. The amplified DNA forms clear band, which can be visualized under ultraviolet (UV) light **(Fig. 2.2.11B)**.

Applications of PCR

Polymerase chain reaction is now a common and often indispensable technique used in medical diagnostics for a variety of applications. It has the following advantages compared to the conventional culture methods:

- **More sensitive:** It can amplify very few copies of a specific DNA
- **More specific:** The use of primers targeting specific DNA sequence of the organism makes the PCR assays highly specific
- PCR can also detect the organisms that are highly fastidious or non-cultivable by conventional culture methods
- PCR can be used to detect the genes in the organism responsible for drug resistance (e.g. *mec* A gene detection in *Staphylococcus aureus*).

Modifications of PCR

1. **Reverse transcriptase PCR (RT-PCR):** Conventional PCR amplifies only the DNA. For detection of RNA, reverse transcription step is done prior to PCR which converts RNA into DNA
2. **Nested PCR:** It uses two sets of primers that are targeted against two different DNA sequences of same organism. It is more sensitive and specific. Nested PCR is used for detection of *Mycobacterium tuberculosis* (targeting *IS6110* gene) in samples
3. **Multiplex PCR:** It uses more than one primer that is targeted against DNA sequences of several organisms in one reaction
   - It is useful for the syndromic diagnosis of infectious diseases that are caused by more than one organism
   - For example, for the diagnosis of pyogenic meningitis, PCR can be performed using different primers targeting common agents of meningitis such as pneumococcus, meningococcus and *H. influenzae*.

Real-time PCR (rt-PCR)

It is an advanced PCR technology, which is used to amplify and simultaneously detect or quantify a DNA sequence on a real-time basis.
- **Advantages:** It is quantitative, takes lesser time, higher rate of sensitivity and specificity as compared to conventional PCR
- **RT rt-PCR:** Reverse transcriptase rt-PCR formats can detect and quantify RNA of the test organism in the sample on a real-time basis—e.g. for COVID-19.

EXPECTED QUESTIONS

I. Write short notes on:
1. Gram staining.
2. Selective media.
3. Transport media.
4. Anaerobic culture methods.
5. Polymerase chain reaction.

II. Multiple Choice Questions (MCQs):
1. Recommended transport medium for stool specimen suspected to contain *Vibrio cholerae* is:
   a. Buffered glycerol saline medium
   b. Venkatraman-Ramakrishnan medium
   c. Nutrient broth
   d. Blood agar
2. Which is an enriched medium?
   a. Selenite F broth
   b. Peptone water
   c. MacConkey agar
   d. Chocolate agar
3. Robertson cooked meat broth is an example of:
   a. Enriched media
   b. Enrichment media
   c. Anaerobic media
   d. Nutrient media
4. The blood culture bottle contains:
   a. Enriched media
   b. Enrichment media
   c. Anaerobic media
   d. Nutrient media
5. The three components of PCR involve all, *except*:
   a. DNA extraction
   b. Amplification
   c. Gel documentation
   d. Blotting

Answers
1. b   2. d   3. c   4. a   5. d

CHAPTER 2.3

General Bacteriology: Bacterial Genetics

CHAPTER PREVIEW

- Mutation
- Gene Transfer
  - Transformation
- Transduction
- Lysogenic Conversion
- Conjugation

PRINCIPLES OF BACTERIAL GENETICS

Bacterial DNA is present in the chromosome as well as in extrachromosomal genetic material as a plasmid.

- **Chromosome:** Bacteria possess a single haploid chromosome, comprising of coiled circular double-stranded DNA. Bacteria do not have a true nucleus; but the genetic material is located in an irregularly-shaped region called the nucleoid
- **Plasmids:** They are the extrachromosomal ds circular DNA molecules that exist in a free state in the cytoplasm of bacteria. They are capable of replicating independently. They may contain genes that code for resistance to various antimicrobial agents.

Bacteria acquire new genes including those that code for drug resistance either by—(i) mutation or (ii) gene transfer from other bacteria.

MUTATION

A mutation is a random, undirected heritable variation caused by a change in the nucleotide sequence of the genome of the cell. Mutations can be spontaneous or induced by physical or chemical agents.

Impact: Mutation can affect any gene and hence may modify any characteristic of the bacterium, for example—
- Loss of ability to produce capsule or flagella
- Loss of virulence
- Alteration in colony morphology
- Alteration in drug susceptibility.

Detection: Mutation can be detected by gene sequencing. Other less commonly used phenotypic methods include—(i) fluctuation test, (ii) replica plating method, (iii) Ames test.

GENE TRANSFER

Gene transfer occurs between bacteria by four distinct methods, such as:
1. Transformation (uptake of naked DNA)
2. Transduction (through bacteriophage)
3. Lysogenic conversion
4. Conjugation (plasmid mediated via conjugation tube).

Transformation

When bacteria die, the cell wall gets lysed and the DNA fragmented are released to the surrounding environment.
- Transformation is a natural process of random uptake of free DNA fragment from the surrounding medium by a bacterial cell

and incorporation of this DNA fragment into its chromosome in a heritable form
- **Griffith experiment:** It was an experiment performed by Griffith (1928) on mice using pneumococci and provided direct evidence of transformation
- Transformation has been studied in certain bacteria—*Streptococcus, Bacillus, Haemophilus,* and *Pseudomonas,* etc.

Transduction

Transduction is defined as the transfer of a portion of DNA from one bacterium to another by a bacteriophage.

Mechanism of transduction: Bacteriophage (or phage) is a virus that infects and multiplies inside the bacterium
- During the transfer of phage from one bacterium to other, a part of the host DNA may accidentally get incorporated into the phage and then gets transferred to the recipient bacterium
- This leads to acquisition of new characters by the recipient bacterium coded by the donor DNA.

Life cycles of phage: After entering into a new bacterium, the phage can perform two types of life cycle.
1. *Lytic or virulent cycle:* The phage multiplies in host cytoplasm, produces a large number of progeny phages, which subsequently are released causing lysis and death of the host cell. In this cycle, inserting a new gene to the bacterium is difficult
2. *Lysogenic or temperate cycle:* Here, the phage DNA remains integrated with the bacterial chromosome and multiplies synchronously with bacterial DNA
    - The phage DNA when transferring to a new bacterium gets disintegrated from the parent bacterial chromosome and in the process, may take up a few bacterial genes
    - These bacterial genes along with the phage DNA get transferred to a new bacterium
    - The donor bacterial genes can provide several properties to the new bacterium such as coding for drug resistance (e.g. plasmid coded penicillin resistance in staphylococci).

Lysogenic Conversion

Here, the phage DNA which is integrated into the host bacterial chromosome (during the lysogenic cycle), itself codes for several virulence factors such as diphtheria toxin, cholera toxin, etc. When the bacteriophage infects a new host, the virulence genes also get transferred.

Conjugation

Conjugation refers to the transfer of genetic material from one bacterium (donor) to another bacterium (recipient) through a conjugation tube **(Fig. 2.3.1)**.
- **F factor:** The donor bacterium contains a special type of plasmid called, the F factor or fertility factor; which encodes a type of pilus called sex pilus
- **Conjugation tube:** The sex pilus forms the conjugation tube when a donor bacterium comes in contact with the recipient bacterium
- **Transfer of F factor:** The donor F factor gets replicated and a copy moves to the recipient bacterium through the conjugation tube. As a result, the recipient bacterium becomes a donor bacterium (as it acquires the F factor) and the process continues
- **Transfer of other genes:** In some cases, along with the F factor, few other donor genes coding for virulence or drug resistance, etc. may also get transferred
- **Role in drug resistance:** Conjugation is the most common mechanism of the transfer of drug resistance genes in bacteria. Several drug resistance genes can be transferred together along with the F factor, which is the main reason for the emergence of **multidrug resistance** in bacteria.

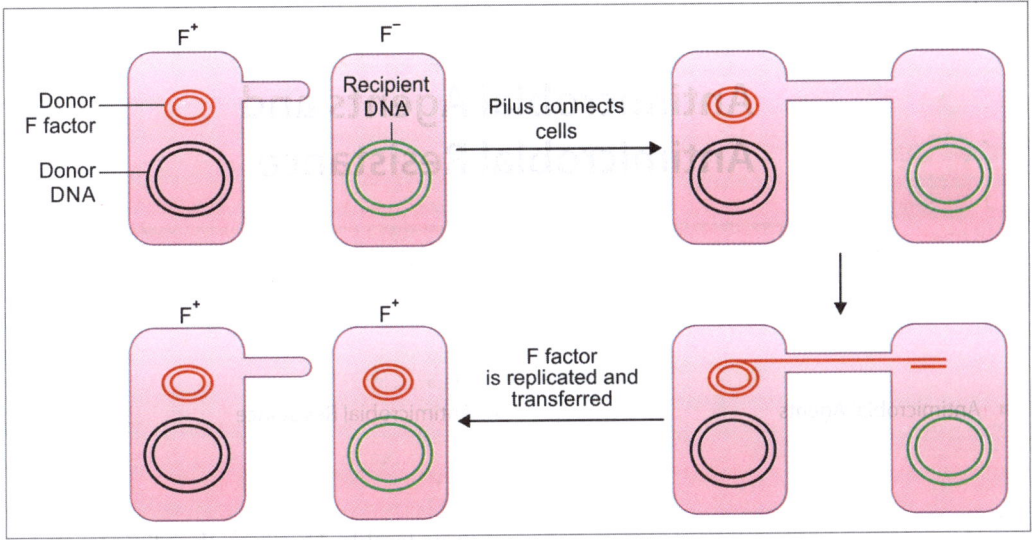

Fig. 2.3.1: Bacterial conjugation.

EXPECTED QUESTIONS

I. Write short notes on:
1. Transformation.
2. Transduction.
3. Conjugation.

II. Multiple Choice Questions (MCQs):
1. The most common method to transfer drug-resistant genes is ____.
    a. Transformation
    b. Transduction
    c. Lysogenic conversion
    d. Conjugation
2. Diphtheria toxin is transferred between bacteria by which of the following method?
    a. Transformation
    b. Transduction
    c. Lysogenic conversion
    d. Conjugation
3. The transfer of bacterial genes through bacteriophage is called as ____.
    a. Transformation
    b. Transduction
    c. Lysogenic conversion
    d. Conjugation
4. Plasmid coded penicillin resistance in staphylococci is transferred between bacteria by which of the following method?
    a. Transformation
    b. Transduction
    c. Lysogenic conversion
    d. Conjugation

Answers
1. d   2. c   3. b   4. b

CHAPTER 2.4

General Bacteriology: Antimicrobial Agents and Antimicrobial Resistance

CHAPTER PREVIEW

- Antimicrobial Agents
- Antimicrobial Resistance

ANTIMICROBIAL AGENTS

Antimicrobials are the agents that kill or inhibit the growth of microorganisms. They can be classified in various ways:

1. According to microorganisms against which they are used—antibacterial, antifungal, antiparasitic, antiviral agents. Only antibacterial agents are discussed in this chapter
2. According to their ability to kill (ends with suffix cidal) or inhibit (ends with suffix static) the microorganism, e.g. bactericidal and bacteriostatic
3. According to the chemical structure and mechanism of action—the antimicrobial agents can be further divided into many classes, as described in **Table 2.4.1**.

ANTIMICROBIAL RESISTANCE

Antimicrobial resistance refers to the development of resistance to an antimicrobial agent by a microorganism. It can be of two types—intrinsic and acquired resistance.

Intrinsic Resistance

It refers to the innate ability of a bacterium to resist a class of antimicrobial agents due to its inherent structural or functional characteristics.

❖ This imposes negligible threat as it is a defined pattern of resistance and is non-transferable. However, the clinicians must be aware to exclude these antibiotics from therapy
❖ Some of the important examples include—
  - Gram-negative bacteria are resistant to vancomycin
  - Gram-positive bacteria are resistant to colistin
  - Aerobic bacteria are resistant to metronidazole
  - *Klebsiella pneumoniae* are resistant to ampicillin and ticarcillin
  - *Proteus* species are resistant to ampicillin, first and second-generation cephalosporins, tetracyclines, nitrofurantoin, and polymyxins
  - *Pseudomonas aeruginosa* is resistant to ampicillin, ceftriaxone, amoxicillin-clavulanate, ampicillin-sulbactam, ertapenem, tetracyclines, tigecycline, co-trimoxazole, and chloramphenicol
  - *Acinetobacter baumannii* is resistant to ampicillin, amoxicillin, amoxicillin-clavulanate, ertapenem, aztreonam, chloramphenicol, and fosfomycin

Acquired Resistance

This refers to the emergence of resistance in bacteria that are ordinarily susceptible to antimicrobial agents, by acquiring the genes coding for resistance. Most of the antimicrobial resistance shown by bacteria belongs to this category.

CHAPTER 2.4 ♦ General Bacteriology: Antimicrobial Agents and Antimicrobial Resistance

Table 2.4.1: Antimicrobial agents—classification and indication.

Class/mechanism		Drugs	Spectrum of activity
A. Inhibit Cell wall Synthesis			
β-lactam antibiotics: Binds to penicillin-binding protein, thereby blocking peptidoglycan cross-linking			
Penicillins	Penicillin	Penicillin G Procaine penicillin G Benzathine penicillin G	*Streptococcus,* pneumococcus, meningococcus, gonococcus, *Corynebacterium diphtheriae, Clostridium perfringens,* and *Treponema pallidum*
	Penicillinase-resistant- penicillins	Cloxacillin, dicloxacillin, nafcillin, oxacillin, and methicillin	**Same as penicillin *plus*** Penicillinase producing *Staphylococcus aureus*
	Aminopenicillins (extended-spectrum)	Ampicillin, amoxicillin	**Same as penicillin *plus*** *Enterococcus faecalis, Escherichia coli, Salmonella* and *Shigella*
	Ureidopenicillins	Ticarcillin, piperacillin	**Same as aminopenicillins *plus*** *Pseudomonas aeruginosa*
Cephalosporin	1st generation	Cefazolin, cephalexin	*Staphylococcus aureus, Escherichia coli,* and *Klebsiella*
	2nd generation	Cefuroxime, cefoxitin	Same as 1st generation *plus* gram-negative activity and anaerobic activity (cefoxitin)
	3rd generation	Ceftriaxone, cefotaxime Ceftazidime, cefoperazone	*Escherichia coli* and *Klebsiella* *Pseudomonas* (ceftazidime) Pneumococci, meningococci (ceftriaxone)
	4th generation	Cefepime	Good activity against gram-positive and negative bacteria including *Pseudomonas*
	5th generation	Ceftobiprole, ceftaroline	Same as 4th generation and MRSA
β-lactam + β-lactamase inhibitors		Amoxicillin-clavulanate* Cefoperazone-sulbactam Piperacillin-tazobactam* Ceftazidime-avibactam	Same as the spectrum of the respective β-lactam drug plus active against β-lactamase producing bacteria *Have excellent anaerobic coverage
Carbapenems		Imipenem, meropenem, doripenem	Broadest range of activity against most bacteria, which include gram-positive cocci, Enterobacteriaceae, *Pseudomonas, Listeria,* and anaerobes
Monobactam		Aztreonam	Gram-negative rods
Other cell wall inhibitors			
Glycopeptides		Vancomycin, teicoplanin	Active against most gram-positive bacteria including MRSA (drug of choice), and for *Clostridioides difficile*
Fosfomycin		Fosfomycin	Active against *Escherichia coli, Klebsiella, Enterococcus,* etc.
B. Protein Synthesis Inhibition			
Binds and inhibits 30S ribosomal subunit			
Aminoglycosides		Gentamicin, amikacin, tobramycin	Enterobacterales, *Pseudomonas, Acinetobacter* *Enterococcus*: Gentamicin *plus* cell wall active agent given
Tetracyclines		Tetracycline, doxycycline, minocycline	Rickettsiae, Chlamydiae, *Mycoplasma, Vibrio cholerae* Minocycline: *Acinetobacter, Burkholderia*
Glycylglycines		Tigecycline	*Acinetobacter, Enterococcus, Staphylococcus*

Contd...

Contd...

Class/mechanism	Drugs	Spectrum of activity
Binds and inhibits 50S ribosomal subunit		
Chloramphenicol	Chloramphenicol	*Haemophilus influenzae*, anaerobic infection
Macrolides	Erythromycin, azithromycin	*Streptococcus, Haemophilus influenzae, Mycoplasma*
Lincosamides	Clindamycin	*S. aureus*, streptococci, anaerobic infection
Oxazolidinones	Linezolid	Resistant gram-positives like MRSA and VRE infections
Streptogramins	Quinupristin-dalfopristin	MRSA and VRE infections
Mupirocin	Mupirocin	Topical ointment—skin infections, nasal carriers of MRSA
C. Nucleic Acid Synthesis Inhibitors		
DNA synthesis inhibitors		
Fluoroquinolones	Inhibit DNA gyrase and topoisomerase IV, thus inhibiting DNA synthesis	
1st generation	Norfloxacin, ciprofloxacin, ofloxacin	Enterobacterales
2nd generation	Levofloxacin, moxifloxacin, sparfloxacin	Others: *Haemophilus, Pseudomonas*
Nitroimidazoles (damage DNA)	Metronidazole, tinidazole	Anaerobic organisms, also active against protozoa: *Entamoeba, Giardia* and *Trichomonas*
RNA synthesis inhibitors		
Rifamycins	Rifampicin	Mycobacteria (*M. tuberculosis, M. leprae*, etc.)
D. Mycolic Acid Synthesis Inhibitors		
Isonicotinic acid hydrazide	Isoniazid (INH)	*M. tuberculosis*
E. Folic Acid Synthesis Inhibitors		
Bacteriostatic: Competitively inhibit enzymes involved in two steps of folic acid synthesis		
Antifolates (Sulfonamides and trimethoprim)	• Sulfadiazine • Cotrimoxazole (Trimethoprim + sulfamethoxazole)	**Sulfadiazine:** Used topically in burn wound surface **Cotrimoxazole** is indicated for: UTI pathogens (*E. coli, Klebsiella*, etc.) *Toxoplasma gondii, Pneumocystis jirovecii*
F. Antimicrobial Agents that Act on the Cell Membrane		
Lipopeptides	Daptomycin	Gram-positive bacteria including VRE and MRSA
Polymyxins	Polymyxin B and colistin	Multidrug-resistant gram-negative bacterial infections

Abbreviations: MRSA, methicillin-resistant *Staphylococcus aureus*; VRE, vancomycin-resistant *Enterococcus*

The emergence of resistance is a major problem worldwide in antimicrobial therapy. Infections caused by resistant microorganisms often fail to respond to the standard treatment, resulting in prolonged illness, higher healthcare expenditures, and a greater risk of death.

❖ Overuse and misuse of antimicrobial agents is the single most important cause of the development of acquired resistance

❖ The evolution of resistant strains is a natural phenomenon, which can occur among bacteria especially when an antibiotic is an overuse

❖ The use of a particular antibiotic poses selective pressure in a population of bacteria which in turn promotes resistant bacteria to thrive and the susceptible bacteria to die off **(Fig. 2.4.1)**

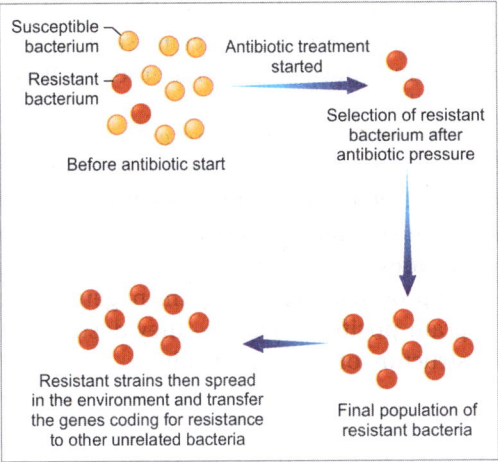

Fig. 2.4.1: Mechanism of development of acquired resistance.

❖ Thus the resistant bacterial populations flourish in areas of high antimicrobial use, where they enjoy a selective advantage over susceptible populations
❖ The resistant strains then spread in the environment and transfer the genes coding for resistance to other unrelated bacteria.

Other factors favoring the spread of antimicrobial resistance include—
❖ Poor infection control practices in hospitals, e.g. poor hand hygiene practices can facilitate the transmission of resistant strains
❖ Inadequate sanitary conditions
❖ Irrational use of antibiotics by doctors, not following antimicrobial susceptibility report
❖ Uncontrolled sale of antibiotics over the counters without prescription.

Mutational and Transferable Drug Resistance

In presence of selective antibiotic pressure, bacteria acquire new genes (i.e. acquired resistance) mainly by two broad methods.

Mutational Resistance

Resistance can develop due to mutation of the resident genes.
❖ It is typically seen in *Mycobacterium tuberculosis*, developing resistance to antitubercular drugs

Table 2.4.2: Mutational vs transferable drug resistance.

Mutational drug resistance	Transferable drug resistance
Resistance to one drug at a time	Multiple drugs resistance at the same time
Low-degree resistance	High-degree resistance
Resistance can be overcome by a combination of drugs	Cannot be overcome by drug combinations
Virulence of resistance mutants may be lowered	Virulence not decreased
Resistance is not transferable to other organisms	Resistance is transferable to other organisms
Spread to off-springs by vertical spread only	Spread by: Horizontal spread (conjugation, or rarely by transduction/transformation)

❖ Mutational drug resistance differs from transferable drug resistance in many ways (Table 2.4.2)
❖ Usually, it is a low-level resistance, developed to one drug at a time; which can be overcome by using a combination of different classes of drugs
❖ That is why multidrug therapy is used in tuberculosis using 4–5 different classes of drugs, such as isoniazid, rifampicin, pyrazinamide, ethambutol, and streptomycin.

Transferrable Drug Resistance

In contrast, transferrable drug resistance is plasmid coded and usually transferred by conjugation or rarely by transduction, or transformation (explained in Chapter 2.3)
❖ The resistance coded plasmid (called R plasmid) can carry multiple genes, each coding for resistance to one class of antibiotic
❖ Thus, it results in a high degree of resistance to multiple drugs, which cannot be overcome by using combination of drugs.

Mechanism of Antimicrobial Resistance

Bacteria develop antimicrobial resistance through several mechanisms.

Decreased Permeability across the Cell Wall

Certain bacteria modify their cell membrane porin channels; either in their frequency, size, or selectivity; thereby preventing the antimicrobial agents from entering the cell. This resistance mechanism has been observed in many gram-negative bacteria, such as *Pseudomonas, Enterobacter,* and *Klebsiella* species against drugs, such as imipenem, aminoglycosides, and quinolones.

Efflux Pumps

Certain bacteria possess efflux pumps that mediate expulsion of the drug(s) from the cell, soon after their entry; thereby preventing the intracellular accumulation of drugs. This strategy has been observed in:
- *Escherichia coli* and other Enterobacteriaceae against tetracyclines, chloramphenicol
- *Staphylococcus aureus* and *Streptococcus pneumoniae* against fluoroquinolones.

By Enzymatic Inactivation

Certain bacteria can inactivate the antimicrobial agents by producing various enzymes, such as:
- **β-lactamase** enzyme production: It breaks down the β-lactam rings, thereby inactivating the β-lactam antibiotics. There are various types of β-lactamase enzymes
  - Gram-positive bacteria produce: Penicillinase
  - Gram-negative bacteria produce enzymes such as extended-spectrum β-lactamase (ESBL), AmpC β-lactamase, and carbapenemases.
- **Aminoglycoside modifying enzymes** can be produced by both gram-negative and gram-positive bacteria—they destroy the structure of aminoglycosides.

By Modifying the Target Sites

Modification in the target sites of antimicrobial agents (which are within the bacteria) is a very important mechanism. It is observed in:
- **MRSA (Methicillin-resistant *Staphylococcus aureus*):** In these strains, the target site of penicillin, i.e. penicillin-binding protein (PBP) gets altered to PBP-2a. The altered PBP, coded by a chromosomally coded gene *mec A*, does not sufficiently bind to β-lactam antibiotics and therefore prevents them from inhibiting the cell wall synthesis
- **Vancomycin resistance in enterococci (VRE):** These strains have a change in the target site of vancomycin (i.e. D-alanine D-alanine side chain of peptidoglycan).

EXPECTED QUESTIONS

I. **Write short notes on:**
   1. Mechanism of antibiotic resistance.
   2. Mutational and transferable drug resistance.

II. **Multiple Choice Questions (MCQs):**
   1. **MRSA is mediated by:**
      a. Plasmid
      b. *mecA* gene
      c. Transposons
      d. None
   2. **All of the following antimicrobial agents act on the cell membrane, *except*:**
      a. Gramicidin
      b. Daptomycin
      c. Polymyxins
      d. Vancomycin
   3. **All of the following are true regarding transferrable drug resistance, *except*:**
      a. Multiple drugs resistance at the same time
      b. Virulence not decreased
      c. Low-degree resistance
      d. Cannot be overcome by drug combinations

Answers
1. b   2. d   3. c

CHAPTER 2.5

General Bacteriology: Normal Flora and Bacterial Pathogenesis

CHAPTER PREVIEW

- Microbiology of Normal Flora
- Mechanism of Bacterial Pathogenesis

MICROBIOLOGY OF NORMAL FLORA

Normal microbial flora refers to the diverse group of microbial populations that every human being harbors on skin and mucous membranes. They do not cause harm; rather they have a beneficiary effect on the host.

- Humans acquire the normal flora soon after the birth and then continue to harbor it until death
- In humans, the normal flora is located in various sites such as the gastrointestinal tract (GIT), respiratory tract, genitourinary tract, and skin
- Most of the normal flora predominantly contain bacteria and to a less extent some fungi and parasites
- GIT is the predominant site of normal flora, where the most common flora is *Bacteroides fragilis* (anaerobic flora). Among aerobes, *Escherichia coli* is the most common.

The microbiological profile of the normal flora in various sites of the human body is given in **Table 2.5.1**.

Role of Normal Flora

Various microorganisms present as the normal flora have a different relationship with the host. They may have a beneficiary effect on the host, or may be harmful to the host.

Table 2.5.1: Common normal flora of human host.

Anatomical site	Organisms as normal flora
Oral cavity	Nonsporing anaerobes Viridans streptococci, Yeast
Nasopharynx	Nonsporing anaerobes Streptococci, *Neisseria* (non-pathogenic) *Staphylococcus epidermidis*
Gastrointestinal tract	Nonsporing anaerobes (e.g. *Bacteroides fragilis*) Enterobacteriaceae and other gram-negative rods Enterococci *Candida* species Commensal *Entamoeba* species*
Vagina	Nonsporing anaerobes Diphtheroids *Lactobacillus* *Streptococcus agalactiae* *Candida*
Skin	Nonsporing anaerobes *Staphylococcus epidermidis* Diphtheroids, *Micrococcus*

*Parasites as a part of normal flora

Beneficial Effects

The normal microbial flora has several beneficial effects on the host:

- **Prevent colonization of pathogen:** By competing for attachment sites or essential nutrients
- **Synthesize vitamin:** Human enteric bacteria secrete several vitamins such as

vitamin K and B complex (e.g. vitamin B12) in excess
- ❖ **Waste produced antagonizes other bacteria:** Normal flora may inhibit or kill other nonindigenous organisms by producing a variety of waste substances such as—fatty acids, peroxides, lactic acid, etc.
- ❖ **Immune stimulation:** Normal microbiota being foreign to the host stimulates the host's immune system.

Disturbed Normal Flora Promote Infection

When the composition of normal flora is disturbed, it facilitates pathogenic organisms to enter and cause disease. Several mechanisms by which the normal flora is disturbed are as follows:
- ❖ **Injudicious use of broad-spectrum antimicrobial agent:** It may completely suppress the normal flora thus permitting the pathogen to take the upper hand and cause infection
- ❖ **Host factors** such as immune suppression, reduced peristalsis may promote the pathogen to grow
- ❖ **Physical destruction** of the normal flora by irradiations, chemicals, burns, etc.

Harmful Effects

Members of the normal flora may cause various endogenous disease.
- ❖ When the host immunity is lowered, *or*
- ❖ If they enter the wrong site or tissue—then even the resident flora can produce disease **(Table 2.5.2)**.

Probiotics

The term "Probiotics" is defined as the live microorganisms (part of normal flora) that, when administered in adequate amounts, confer a health benefit to the host.
- ❖ They are extremely useful in the conditions where the normal intestinal flora is suppressed
- ❖ Probiotics are commercially available in the form of capsules or sachets, consisting of a mixture of some important beneficiary bacteria and yeast of human intestinal flora such as *Bifidobacterium, Lactobacillus,* etc.
- ❖ Probiotics are found to have a beneficiary role in treating the following conditions:
    - Gastroenteritis due to any cause
    - Antibiotic-associated diarrhea
    - Lactose intolerance
    - Irritable bowel syndrome and colitis
    - Necrotizing enterocolitis
    - *Helicobacter pylori* infection.

Table 2.5.2: Diseases produced by normal flora.

Diseases	Anatomical site from which the flora is transferred
Urinary tract infection	Intestinal flora such as *Escherichia coli, Klebsiella*
Endocarditis	Oral flora (Viridans streptococci)
Dental caries	Oral flora
Peritonitis	Intestinal flora

MECHANISM OF BACTERIAL PATHOGENESIS

The ability of bacteria to produce disease or tissue injury is referred to as 'pathogenesis'. It involves several steps such as—transmission of the organism, infective dose, adhesion, invasion, intracellular survival, and expression of several virulence factors (like toxins and enzymes, etc.).

Route of Transmission

The route of transmission of infection plays a crucial role in the pathogenesis of certain bacteria. This difference is probably related to the modes by which different bacteria can initiate tissue damage and establish themselves **(Table 2.5.3)**.

Infective Dose

The infective dose of the bacteria is referred to as the minimum inoculum size that is capable of initiating an infection.
- ❖ **Low infective dose:** Certain organisms require a relatively small inoculum to initiate infection
    - *Shigella*: Very low (as low as 10 bacilli)
    - *Campylobacter jejuni* (500 bacilli).

CHAPTER 2.5 ♦ General Bacteriology: Normal Flora and Bacterial Pathogenesis

Table 2.5.3: Mode of transmission of bacterial infections.

Transmission	Bacterial agents/diseases
Contact	Multi-drug resistant organisms in hospitals such as *S. aureus, E. coli, Klebsiella*, etc.
Droplet	Meningococcus, *C. diphtheriae* Pneumococcus
Aerosol	*M. tuberculosis*
Ingestion	*Salmonella* and *Shigella* *Vibrio* and diarrheagenic *E. coli*
Vector-borne	Rickettsiae and *Borrelia*
Sexual	Gonococcus, *Chlamydia trachomatis* *Treponema pallidum*
Vertical	*Treponema pallidum*
Birth canal	*Listeria, Streptococcus agalactiae*

- **Large infective dose:** In contrast, bacteria with a high infective dose can initiate the infection only when the inoculum size exceeds a particular critical size
  - *Salmonella* (10^2–10^5 bacilli)
  - *Vibrio cholerae* (10^6–10^8 bacilli).

The infective dose varies depending upon the factors, such as:
- **Virulence of the organism:** Higher the virulence, the lower is the infective dose
- Host's age and overall immune status
- The ability of the organism to resist gastric acidity: *Shigella* can survive gastric acidity, even a low infective dose can initiate the infection. In contrast, *Vibrio* is extremely acid labile, hence requiring a heavy inoculum to bypass the gastric barrier.

Adhesion

Adhesion of the bacteria to body surfaces is the initial event in the pathogenesis of the disease. It is mediated by specialized molecules called adhesins that bind to specific host cell receptors.
- **Fimbriae or pili:** They are the most important adhesins present in some bacteria. They directly bind to the sugar residues on host cells
- **Other adhesins:** Apart from pili, there are other adhesins found in certain bacteria, such as M protein (*Streptococcus pyogenes*), lipoteichoic acid (gram-positive cocci), etc.

- **Biofilm formation:** It is another mechanism by which certain bacteria mediate strong adherence to certain structures, such as catheters, prosthetic implants, and heart valves. Biofilm is a group of bacterial cells which stick to each other on a surface and are embedded within a layer of a self-produced matrix of the glycocalyx.

Invasion

Invasion refers to the entry of bacteria into host cells, leading to its spread within the host tissues.
- Highly invasive pathogens produce spreading or generalized lesions (e.g. streptococcal infections)
- While less invasive pathogens cause localized lesions (e.g. staphylococcal abscess).

Important virulence factors that help in invasion include:
- Virulence marker antigen or invasion plasmid antigens in *Shigella*
- **Enzymes:** The invasion of bacteria is enhanced by many enzymes such as hyaluronidase, collagenase, streptokinase, IgA proteases.

Intracellular Survival

Some organisms survive in the intracellular environment. They are grouped into obligate and facultative intracellular organisms (**Table 2.5.4**). Various bacterial strategies that inhibit phagocytosis are:
- The bacterial capsule prevents the phagocyte from adhering to the bacterium. Examples of capsulated bacteria—*Neisseria meningitidis* and *Streptococcus pneumoniae*
- Inhibition of phagolysosome fusion by *Mycobacterium tuberculosis*

Table 2.5.4: Intracellular bacteria.

Facultative intracellular bacteria	Obligate intracellular
Salmonella typhi, *Brucella*	*Mycobacterium leprae*
Legionella, Listeria	*Rickettsia*
Neisseria meningitidis	*Chlamydia*
Mycobacterium tuberculosis	*Coxiella burnetii*

- Resistance to lysosomal enzymes by *Coxiella* species and *Mycobacterium leprae*.

Toxins

Endotoxins

Endotoxins are the lipid A portion of lipopolysaccharide (LPS).
- They are present as an integral part of the cell wall of gram-negative bacteria
- They are released from the bacterial surface by lysis of the bacteria
- They are responsible for various biological effects in the host such as—macrophage activation, platelet activation, activation of complement and coagulation pathway leading to disseminated intravascular coagulation (DIC) and septic shock and possibly death.

Exotoxins

They are heat-labile proteins; secreted by certain species of both gram-positive and gram-negative bacteria (examples are given in **Table 2.5.5**).
- **High potency:** Exotoxins are highly potent even in minute amounts
- **Used for vaccine:** Exotoxins can be converted into toxoids by treatment with formaldehyde
- **Specific action:** They are highly specific for a particular tissue, e.g. tetanus toxin for CNS.

Exotoxins differ from endotoxins in several ways **(Table 2.5.6)**.

Table 2.5.5: Bacterial exotoxins.

Organisms	Toxins (Exotoxins)
Staphylococcus aureus	Exfoliative toxin Enterotoxin Toxic shock syndrome toxin
Streptococcus pyogenes	Pyrogenic exotoxin
Corynebacterium diphtheriae	Diphtheria toxin
Bacillus anthracis	Anthrax toxin
Clostridium tetani	Tetanus toxin
Clostridium botulinum	Botulinum toxin
Diarrheagenic E. coli	Heat labile toxin Heat stable toxin Verocytotoxin
Shigella	Shiga toxin
Vibrio cholerae	Cholera toxin
Pseudomonas	Exotoxin-A

Table 2.5.6: Differences between bacterial endotoxins and exotoxins.

Endotoxins	Exotoxins
Lipopolysaccharides in nature	Proteins in nature
Part of the cell wall of gram-negative bacteria	Secreted both by gram-positive and gram-negative bacteria
Produce nonspecific action (fever, shock, etc.)	Specific action on particular tissues
Less potent	More potent
Poorly antigenic	Highly antigenic
No effective vaccine is available using endotoxin	Toxoid forms are used as a vaccine, e.g. tetanus toxoid

EXPECTED QUESTIONS

I. **Write short notes on:**
   1. Mechanisms of bacterial pathogenesis.
   2. Differences between endotoxins and exotoxins.

II. **Multiple Choice Questions (MCQs):**
   1. The chemical nature of endotoxin is:
      a. Protein
      b. Lipopolysaccharide
      c. Carbohydrate d. None
   2. The following are exotoxins, *except*:
      a. Botulinum toxin
      b. Anthrax toxin
      c. Diphtheria toxin
      d. Lipid A portion of LPS
   3. Obligate intracellular bacteria are all, *except*:
      a. *M. leprae* b. *Rickettsia*
      c. *Chlamydia* d. *M. tuberculosis*

Answers
1. b   2. d   3. d

CHAPTER 3

General Virology

CHAPTER PREVIEW

- Morphology of Virus
- Classification
- Viral Replication
- Pathogenesis of Viral Infections
- Laboratory Diagnosis of Viral Diseases
- Treatment
- Immunoprophylaxis

Viruses are the smallest unicellular organisms that are obligate intracellular. They differ from bacteria and other prokaryotes in many ways.

- They possess either DNA (deoxyribonucleic acid) or RNA (ribonucleic acid), but never both
- They cannot be grown on artificial cell-free media
- They do not have a cell wall or cell membrane or cellular organelles
- They lack the enzymes necessary for protein and nucleic acid synthesis
- They are not susceptible to antibacterial antibiotics.

MORPHOLOGY OF VIRUS

The virus particle comprises a **nucleic acid** surrounded by a protein coat called as **capsid**, together known as the nucleocapsid. Some viruses also have an outer **envelope (Figs. 3.1A and B)**.

- **Nucleic acid:** Viruses have only one type of nucleic acid, either DNA or RNA but never both. Accordingly, they are classified as DNA viruses and RNA viruses. The nucleic acid may be single or double-stranded, segmented, or unsegmented
- **Capsid:** It is composed of several protein subunits called capsomeres. It protects the nucleic acid core from the external environment
- **Symmetry:** It is the arrangement of capsomeres with respect to the surrounding nucleic acid, which can be of three types
  1. *Icosahedral symmetry:* The capsomeres are arranged surrounding the nucleic acid in a cubical shape; e.g. all DNA viruses (except poxviruses) and most of the RNA viruses **(Fig. 3.1A)**
  2. *Helical symmetry:* The capsomeres are coiled surrounding the nucleic acid in the form of a helix or spiral. Examples include—myxoviruses, rhabdoviruses, etc. **(Fig. 3.1B)**
  3. *Complex symmetry:* Poxviruses possess complex symmetry.
- **Envelope:** Certain viruses possess an envelope surrounding the nucleocapsid. The envelope is lipoprotein in nature
  - The envelope is lipoprotein in nature. The protein spikes (called peplomers) are embedded into the lipid layer
  - Peplomers bind to specific receptors on the host cells, thus facilitating the entry of the virus
  - Peplomers are antigenic; therefore, antibodies against them are protective
  - **Examples** of enveloped viruses include—influenza virus, hepatitis B, and coronavirus.

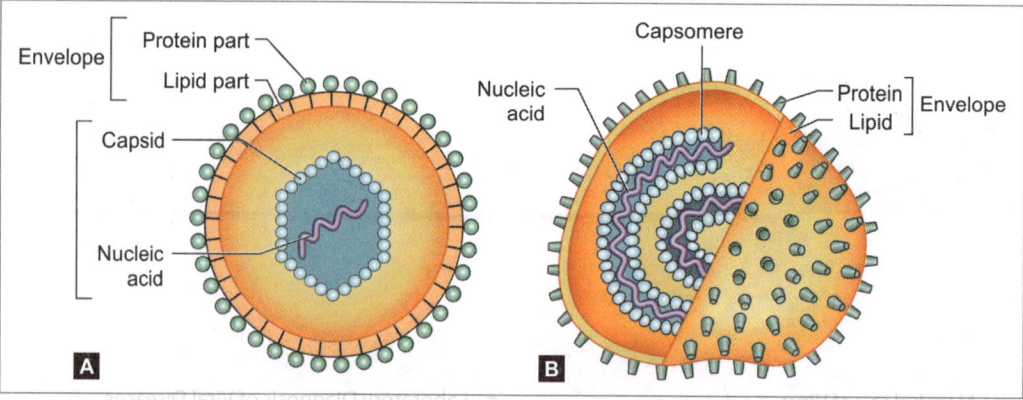

Figs. 3.1A and B: Structure and symmetry of virus: **A.** Enveloped virus with icosahedral nucleocapsid; **B.** Enveloped virus with helical nucleocapsid.

- **Size of the viruses:** Viruses are extremely small, and vary from 20–400 nm in size. The smallest virus is parvovirus (20 nm) and the largest is poxvirus (400 nm)
- **Shape of the viruses:** Mostly animal viruses are spherical shaped, with some exceptions:
  - Rabies virus: Bullet-shaped
  - Poxvirus: Brick-shaped
  - Adenovirus: Space vehicle-shaped
  - Rotavirus: Wheel-shaped.

CLASSIFICATION

There are various DNA and RNA virus groups, which further comprise several important viruses infecting humans as enlisted in **Table 3.1**.

VIRAL REPLICATION

Viruses undergo a complex way of cell division. Replication of viruses passes through seven sequential steps:

> Attachment → Penetration → Uncoating → Biosynthesis → Assembly → Maturation → Release.

1. **Adsorption/attachment:** It is the most specific step of viral replication. It involves receptor interactions between virus and host surface receptors
2. **Penetration:** After attachment, the virus particles penetrate into the host cells
3. **Uncoating:** Lysis of capsid due to host lysozymes and release of the nucleic acid
4. **Biosynthesis** of various viral components: i) nucleic acid, ii) capsid protein, iii) enzymes iv) other regulatory proteins
5. **Assembly:** Viral nucleic acid and proteins are packaged together to form progeny viruses (nucleocapsids)
6. **Maturation:** Following assembly, maturation of daughter virions takes place either in the nucleus or cytoplasm, or membranes
7. **Release** of daughter virions occurs either by:
   - Lysis of the host cells
   - Budding through the host cell membrane.

PATHOGENESIS OF VIRAL INFECTIONS

Most of the viral infections progress through the following steps inside the human body:
- Transmission (entry into the body)
- Primary site of replication
- Spread to a secondary site
- Manifestations of the disease.

Transmission

Viruses enter the human body through various routes **(Table 3.2)**.

Primary Site of Replication

- Some viruses are restricted to the portal of entry where they multiply and produce local diseases

Table 3.1: Important DNA and RNA viruses infecting humans.

DNA Virus Groups	DNA Viruses
Herpesviruses	Herpes simplex virus 1 and 2, Varicella-zoster virus, Cytomegalovirus (CMV), Epstein-Barr virus (EBV), Human herpesvirus-6, 7 and 8
Poxviruses (largest virus in size)	Variola virus (smallpox), Molluscum contageosum virus
Papovaviruses	Human papillomavirus
Parvoviruses (smallest virus in size)	Parvovirus B19
Hepadnavirus	Hepatitis B virus
Adenoviruses	Human adenovirus

RNA Virus Groups	RNA Viruses
Myxoviruses	Influenza viruses—A, B, and C Parainfluenza viruses, mumps virus, measles virus, respiratory syncytial virus, Nipah virus
Coronaviruses	Coronaviruses (SARS-CoV, MERS-CoV and SARS-CoV-2)
Arboviruses	Dengue virus, yellow fever virus, chikungunya virus, Kyasanur forest disease virus, Japanese B encephalitis virus, Zika virus
Retroviruses	HIV (human immunodeficiency virus)
Rabies virus	Rabies virus
Picornaviruses	Poliovirus, Coxsackievirus, enterovirus, rhinovirus
RNA hepatitis viruses	Hepatitis A, C, D, E viruses
RNA viruses causing gastroenteritis	Rotavirus, calicivirus, Norwalk virus, astrovirus
Miscellaneous RNA viruses	Filoviruses—Marburg virus and Ebola virus, Rubella virus

Table 3.2: Mode of transmission of viruses.

Transmission	Viruses
Respiratory route (probably the most common route)	• Myxoviruses such as influenza virus • Coronaviruses such as SARS-CoV-2 • Rhinovirus • Varicella-zoster virus • Cytomegalovirus • Rubella virus • Parvovirus • Smallpox virus
Oral route	• Rotavirus and other viral agents causing gastroenteritis • Poliovirus and other enteroviruses • Hepatitis viruses—A and E
Cutaneous route	• Herpes simplex virus-1 • Human papillomavirus • Molluscum contagiosum virus
Vector bite	Arboviruses such as: • Dengue virus (*Aedes*) • Chikungunya virus (*Aedes*) • Japanese encephalitis virus (*Culex*) • Yellow fever virus and Zika virus (*Aedes*) • Kyasanur Forest disease virus (Tick)
Animal bite	Rabies virus
Sexual route	• Herpes simplex virus-2 • Human papillomavirus • Hepatitis B, C and rarely D viruses • Human immunodeficiency virus (HIV)
Blood transfusion	• Hepatitis B, C and rarely D viruses • HIV
Needle-stick injury	• Hepatitis B, C and rarely D viruses • HIV
Mother-to-child transmission (including transplacental route)	• Rubella virus • Cytomegalovirus • Herpes simplex virus • Varicella-zoster virus • Parvovirus B19 • Hepatitis B and C viruses • HIV

❖ On the other hand, most of the viruses first multiply locally to initiate a silent local infection, which is followed by the spread via lymphatics to regional lymph nodes (most viruses) or via blood (e.g. poliovirus) or via neuronal spread to reach the central nervous system or CNS (e.g. rabies virus).

Spread of Virus

❖ **Primary viremia:** Viruses spread to the bloodstream either from the primary sites or from the lymph nodes

- **Secondary site of replication:** Viruses are then transported to the reticuloendothelial system (bone marrow, endothelial cells, spleen and liver) where further multiplication takes place
- **Secondary viremia:** From the spleen and liver, viruses spill over into the bloodstream leading to secondary viremia which results in the onset of non-specific symptoms
- **Target organs:** Via the bloodstream, they reach the target organs (lung, brain, skin, etc.). Certain viruses (e.g. rabies) affect the brain, there is no viremia. Instead, the virus reaches the target organ via neuronal spread
- **Tropism** of the viruses for specific organs determines the pattern of systemic illness; e.g. hepatitis viruses have tropism for hepatocytes and thus produce hepatitis
- **Shedding:** Following infection viruses escape the host by shedding either at the portal of entry (e.g. influenza virus) or in the blood (e.g. dengue virus) or near the target organ (e.g. salivary gland for mumps).

Manifestations of Viral Infections

- **Incubation period:** It is the time interval between the entry of the virus into the body and the appearance of the first clinical manifestation
    - The incubation period is shorter if the virus produces lesions near the site of entry, e.g. influenza virus
    - It is longer if the target organ is much far from the site of entry, e.g. poliovirus and rabies virus.
- **Clinical manifestations:** Persons infected with viruses develop either an inapparent (subclinical) infection or apparent (clinical) infection. The symptoms developed depend on the target body sites where the virus multiplies
    - Respiratory viruses such as influenza and coronaviruses produce respiratory infections
    - Gastroenteritis: Produced by rotavirus
    - Neurotropic viruses can produce meningitis (enteroviruses) or encephalitis (rabies)
    - Hepatitis viruses produce hepatitis

LABORATORY DIAGNOSIS OF VIRAL DISEASES

Laboratory diagnosis of viral infections is useful for the following purposes:
- **To start antiviral drugs** for infections caused by herpes, CMV, HIV, influenza viruses, etc.
- **Screening of blood donors** for HIV, hepatitis B, and hepatitis C helps in the prevention of transfusion-transmitted infections
- **Surveillance purpose:** To assess the disease burden in the community
- **For outbreak or epidemic investigation:** To initiate appropriate control measures
- **To start post-exposure prophylaxis** of antiretroviral drugs to the health care workers following needle stick injury (Chapter 43)
- **To initiate certain measures:** For example, if the newborn is diagnosed to have hepatitis B infection, then immunoglobulins (HBIG) should be started within 12 hours of birth.

Direct Demonstration of Virus

- **Electron microscopy:** Detection of viruses by electron microscopy (EM) is increasingly used nowadays. Viruses can be identified based on their distinct appearances; for example:
    - Rabies virus—bullet-shaped
    - Rotavirus—wheel-shaped
    - Coronavirus—petal-shaped peplomers
    - Adenovirus—space vehicle-shaped
    - Astrovirus—star-shaped peplomers.
- **Fluorescent microscopy:** Direct immuno-fluorescence (Direct-IF) technique is useful to detect viral particles in clinical samples. Its clinical applications are:
    - Diagnosis of rabies virus antigen in skin biopsies, corneal smear of infected patients
    - Rapid diagnosis of respiratory infections caused by influenza virus, rhinoviruses, and respiratory syncytial virus
- **Light microscopy:** It is useful for demonstration of inclusion bodies by histopathological staining of tissue sections,

which helps in the diagnosis of certain viral infections (see highlight box below).

> **Inclusion Body**
> They are the aggregates of viral proteins and other products of viral replication that confer altered staining property to the host cell.
>
> **Role in Laboratory Diagnosis**
> Inclusion bodies are characteristic of specific viral infections. They have distinct size, shape, location and staining properties by which they can be demonstrated in virus infected cells under the light microscope.
>
> **Location**
> They may be present either in the host cell cytoplasm or nucleus or both
> - **Intracytoplasmic inclusion bodies:** They are seen as pink structures (acidophilic)
>   - Paschen bodies—variola virus
>   - Molluscum bodies—molluscum contagiosum virus
>   - Negri bodies— rabies
> - **Intranuclear inclusion bodies:** They are basophilic.
>   - Cowdry type A inclusions—e.g. Torres body in yellow fever
>   - Cowdry type B inclusions—in poliovirus and adenovirus
> - **Both intracytoplasmic and intranuclear inclusions**— in cytomegalovirus (owl's eye appearance) and measles.

Detection of Viral Antigens

Detection of viral antigens in serum and other samples can be done by techniques such as enzyme-linked immunosorbent assay (ELISA), immunochromatographic test (ICT), enzyme-linked fluorescence assay (ELFA), etc. Some important antigen detection tests include:
- HBsAg antigen detection for hepatitis B virus infection from serum
- SARS-CoV-2 antigen (nucleocapsid protein) detection in nasopharyngeal swabs.

Detection of Viral Antibodies

Antibody detection from serum is one of the most commonly used methods in diagnostic virology. Techniques such as ELISA, ELFA, ICT are widely used; for example:
- Anti-hepatitis C antibodies in serum
- Antibodies against HIV antigens from serum
- Anti-dengue IgM/IgG antibodies from serum.

Molecular Methods

Molecular techniques have eased the diagnosis of viral infections. They are more sensitive, specific and yield quicker results.
- **Polymerase chain reaction (PCR)** is useful to detect viral DNA in clinical specimens
- **Reverse transcriptase-PCR (RT-PCR)** is used for the detection of RNA viruses in clinical specimens
- **Multiplex PCR** can simultaneously detect genes of common organisms responsible for a clinical syndrome; for example, multiplex PCR for respiratory infection simultaneously detects genes of many respiratory viruses in clinical specimens
- **Real time-PCR (rt-PCR):** It is considered as the gold standard method for the diagnosis of several viral infections such as influenza, COVID-19, etc. It has several advantages such as—
  - Quantifying viral nucleic acid in the samples, hence used to monitor the treatment response
  - Takes lesser time
  - More sensitive and specific than PCR.

Isolation of Virus

Viruses cannot be grown on artificial culture media. They are cultivated by animal inoculation, embryonated egg inoculation, or tissue cultures.

Animal Inoculation

Animal inoculation is largely restricted only for research purposes and for limited diagnostic purposes such as—primary isolation of arboviruses and coxsackieviruses.

Egg Inoculation

The use of egg inoculation in viral diagnostics is greatly limited now. An embryonated hen's egg has four sites that are specific for the growth of certain viruses **(Fig. 3.2)**.

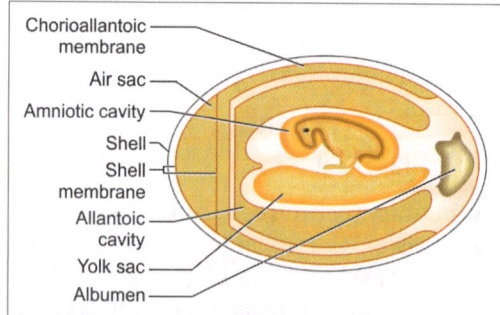

Fig. 3.2: Schematic diagram of an embryonated egg.

- **Yolk sac inoculation:** Used for arboviruses (e.g. JE virus) and some bacteria such as *Rickettsia* and *Chlamydia*
- **Amniotic sac:** Used for the isolation of influenza virus
- **Allantoic sac:** It is used for the production of viral vaccines such as—influenza vaccine, yellow fever (17D) vaccine
- **Chorioallantoic membrane:** Used for the isolation of poxviruses. They produce visible lesions over the chorioallantoic membrane called pocks.

Tissue Culture

The tissue culture technique was widely used in the past in diagnostic virology. It is of three types—(i) organ culture, (ii) explant culture, and (iii) cell line culture.

Cell line culture is the only isolation method that is in use now.

Types of Cell Lines

There are three types of cell lines —(i) primary cell lines, (ii) secondary cell lines, and (iii) continuous cell lines.

1. **Primary cell lines:** They are capable of very limited growth in culture, maximum up to 5–10 divisions. Examples include—human amnion cell line and chick embryo cell line
2. **Secondary cell lines:** They can divide a maximum of up to 10–50 divisions. Examples include—human fibroblast cell line and human embryonic lung cell starin
3. **Continuous cell lines:** They are derived from cancerous cell lines, and hence are capable of indefinite growth. Examples include—
   - HeLa cell line (human carcinoma of cervix cell line)
   - Vero cell line (vervet monkey kidney cell line).

Detection of Viral Growth in Cell Cultures

The following methods are used to detect the growth of the virus in cell cultures.

- **Cytopathic effect (CPE):** It is defined as the morphological change produced by the virus in the cell line detected by a light microscope. Examples of CPE effect produced by viruses include—
  - Syncytium formation by the measles virus
  - Granular clumps (like bunches of grapes) by adenovirus
  - Rapid crenation and degeneration of entire cell sheet by enteroviruses.
- **Other methods** to detect viral growth include—
  - Detection of viral antigens by direct immunofluorescence assay
  - Viral genes detection by using PCR.

TREATMENT OF VIRAL DISEASES

Only for limited viral diseases, effective antiviral drugs are available. Commonly used antiviral drugs for viral diseases are as follows:
- Acyclovir for herpes simplex virus and VZV infections
- Ganciclovir for CMV infections
- Oseltamivir for H1N1 flu
- Telbivudine, tenofovir, lamivudine for hepatitis B.

Interferons (IFNs)

IFNs-α, β have antiviral action; produced by many cell types such as macrophages (IFN-α) and fibroblasts (IFN-β). INF-γ does not have antiviral action.

- **Mechanism of action:** IFNs are part of innate immunity; the body's first line of antiviral defense. They are nonspecific in action; produced quickly following viral infection

- **Inducers:** Certain RNA viruses can induce IFN synthesis
- **Application:** IFN-α is used in the following clinical conditions:
  - Topically—used in rhinovirus infection, genital warts, and herpetic keratitis
  - Systemically—used in chronic hepatitis B, C, and D infections.

IMMUNOPROPHYLAXIS FOR VIRAL DISEASES

Viral Vaccines (Active Immunization)

Viral vaccines confer prolonged and effective immunity. Vaccines for viral infections may be available either in live, killed, or subunit forms.

Killed Viral Vaccines

Killed vaccines are available for various viral agents.
- **Preparation:** They are prepared by inactivating viruses with heat, phenol, formalin, or beta-propiolactone
- **Advantages:** They are more stable and are considered safe when given in immunodeficiency or pregnancy
- **Disadvantages:** Killed vaccines are associated with more adverse side effects due to reactogenicity
- **Examples:** Common killed viral vaccines for human use are:
  - Rabies non-neural vaccine—e.g. HDC (human diploid cell) vaccine
  - Killed injectable polio vaccine (IPV).

Subunit Vaccines

In subunit vaccines, only a particular antigen of the virus is used; prepared by DNA recombinant technology, e.g. hepatitis B vaccine.

Live Vaccines

Live vaccines are available for various viral agents.
- **Preparation:** They are prepared by attenuation by serial passages
- **Advantages:** Live vaccines provide a stronger and long-lasting immunity and are administered as a single dose (except OPV)
- **Disadvantages:** Live vaccines are risky in immunodeficiency or pregnancy. They are less stable than killed vaccines
- **Examples:** Common killed viral vaccines for human use are:
  - Live oral polio vaccine (OPV)
  - MMR vaccine for measles, mumps, and rubella.

Passive Immunization (Immunoglobulin)

Passive immunization is indicated when an individual is immunodeficient or when early protection is needed (i.e. for post-exposure prophylaxis). Currently, human immunoglobulins are available for many viral infections such as mumps, measles, hepatitis B, rabies, and varicella-zoster.

Combined Immunization

Simultaneous administration of vaccine and immunoglobulin in post-exposure prophylaxis is extremely useful. It is recommended for:
- Hepatitis B (neonates born to HBsAg positive mothers or for unvaccinated people following exposure)
- Rabies (for exposures to severe class III bites).

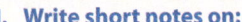

EXPECTED QUESTIONS

I. Write short notes on:
1. Laboratory diagnosis of viral infections.
2. Interferons.
3. Inclusion bodies.
4. Viral vaccines.

II. Multiple Choice Questions (MCQs):
1. **All of the following are RNA viruses, except:**
   a. Enterovirus
   b. Human adenoviruses

c. Coxsackievirus
d. Hepatitis A virus
2. **All of the following viruses are transmitted by the respiratory route, *except*:**
   a. Influenza virus
   b. Rotavirus
   c. Respiratory syncytial virus
   d. Rhinovirus
3. **All of the following are intracytoplasmic inclusion bodies, *except*:**
   a. Negri bodies
   b. Molluscum bodies
   c. Cowdry type A inclusions
   d. Guarnieri bodies
4. **Which of the following vaccine is a killed vaccine?**
   a. Mumps vaccine   b. Measles vaccine
   c. Rubella vaccine   d. IPV
5. **The largest virus in size is:**
   a. Herpes simplex virus
   b. Hepatitis B virus
   c. Poxvirus
   d. Adenovirus
6. **The smallest virus in size is:**
   a. Picornaviruses
   b. Parvovirus
   c. Hepatitis D virus
   d. Adenovirus
7. **Which of the following is continuous cell line?**
   a. HeLa cell line
   b. Amnion cell line
   c. Chick embryo cell line.
   d. Human fibroblast cell line
8. **Amniotic sac of embryonated hen's egg is used for isolation of:**
   a. HIV
   b. Influenza virus
   c. Hepatitis B virus
   d. Poliovirus

Answers
1. b   **2.** b   **3.** c   **4.** d   **5.** c   **6.** b   **7.** a   **8.** b

CHAPTER 4: General Parasitology

CHAPTER PREVIEW

- General Parasitology
- Life Cycle of Parasites
- Laboratory Diagnosis of Parasitic Diseases
- Treatment of Parasitic Diseases

Parasite is a living organism, which lives in or upon another organism (host) and derives nutrients directly from it, without giving any benefit to the host.

Medical Parasitology deals with the study of animal parasites, which infect and produce diseases in human beings. Parasites may be classified as—protozoans and helminths.

- ❖ **Protozoa:** They are unicellular eukaryotic cells that perform all the physiological functions
- ❖ **Helminths:** They are elongated flat or round worm-like parasites measuring few millimeters to as long as few meters. They are eukaryotic multicellular and bilaterally symmetrical.

Medically important protozoans and helminths are listed in **Table 4.1**.

LIFE CYCLE OF PARASITES

The life cycle of parasites depends upon three factors: host, mode of transmission, and infective form.

- ❖ **Host:** It is an organism, which harbors the parasite and provides the nourishment and shelter
    - Hosts can be classified into a *definitive host* (where the parasite undergoes a sexual cycle) or an *intermediate host* (where the parasite undergoes an asexual cycle)
    - Depending upon the number of hosts involved, the life cycle of the parasite may be direct or indirect

Table 4.1: Medically important protozoans and helminths.

Medically important protozoans

Amoebae
- *Entamoeba histolytica*
- Free-living amoebae: *Naegleria, Acanthamoeba, Balamuthia*

Flagellates
- Intestinal flagellate: *Giardia*
- Genital flagellate: *Trichomonas*
- Hemoflagellates: *Leishmania* and *Trypanosoma*

Apicomplexa
- Malaria parasites and *Babesia*
- Opportunistic coccidian parasites: *Toxoplasma, Cryptosporidium, Cyclospora,* and *Cystoisospora*

Miscellaneous protozoa: *Balantidium coli*

Medically important helminths

Cestodes
Diphyllobothrium, Taenia, Echinococcus, and *Hymenolepis*

Trematodes or flukes
Schistosoma, Fasciola, Clonorchis, Opisthorchis, Fasciolopsis, and *Paragonimus*

Intestinal nematodes
Trichuris, Enterobius, Hookworm, *Strongyloides,* and *Ascaris*

Somatic nematodes
Filarial nematodes, *Dracunculus* and *Trichinella*

- In the *direct life cycle,* the parasite requires only one host to complete its development
- In the *indirect life cycle,* the parasite requires two/or three hosts (one definitive host and another one or two intermediate host/s) to complete its development.

❖ **Infective form:** It is the morphological form of the parasite which is transmitted to man

❖ **Mode of transmission:** Parasites may be transmitted by various modes such as ingestion, skin penetration, vector-borne, sexual, vertical, blood transfusion, and autoinfection.

Details of the life cycle of some of the important human parasites have been described in Chapter nos. 27-34.

LABORATORY DIAGNOSIS OF PARASITIC DISEASES

Laboratory diagnosis plays an important role in establishing the specific diagnosis of various parasitic infections. Following are the techniques used in the diagnosis of parasitic infections.

Examination of Feces

Stool examination is the most common diagnostic technique used for the diagnosis of intestinal parasitic infections.

Specimen Collection

Stool specimens should be collected in wide-mouthed, clean, leak-proof, screw-capped containers (**Fig. 4.1**).

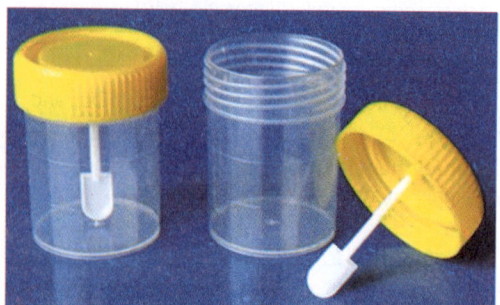

Fig. 4.1: Sample container for stool.

❖ **Timing:** Specimen should be collected before starting anti-parasitic drugs and closer to the onset of symptoms

❖ **Frequency:** At least three stool specimens collected on alternate days (within 10 days)

❖ **When to examine:** Liquid stool specimens should be examined within 30 minutes, semisolid stools within 1hr, and formed stools up to 24 hours after collection

❖ **For monitoring response to therapy:** Repeat stool examination can be done 3 to 4 weeks after the therapy for intestinal protozoan infection, and 5-6 weeks for *Taenia* infection

❖ **Specimens other than stool:**
  - *Perianal swabs* (cellophane tape or NIH swab): Useful for detecting eggs of *Enterobius vermicularis* deposited on the surface of the perianal skin
  - *Duodenal contents:* It is very useful for the detection of small intestine parasites like *Giardia intestinalis* and larva of *Strongyloides stercoralis*.

Macroscopic Examination

Macroscopic examination of stool may provide a clue about various parasitic infections.

❖ **Mucoid bloody stool:** Found in acute amoebic dysentery
❖ **Color:** Red-colored stool indicates gastrointestinal tract (GIT) bleeding
❖ **Frothy pale offensive stool** (containing fat) is usually found in giardiasis
❖ **Stool consistency:** In liquid stool, trophozoites are usually found; whereas in semi-formed stool both trophozoites and cysts are found and the cysts are mainly found in formed specimens.

Microscopic Examination

The microscopic examination includes direct wet mount examination and permanent staining methods.

Direct Wet Mount (saline and iodine mount)

Drops of saline and Lugol's iodine are placed on the left and right halves of the slide respectively (**Fig. 4.2**).

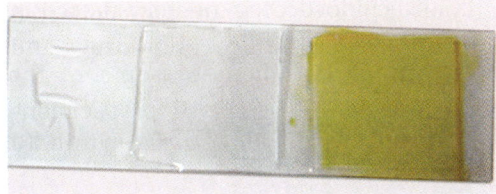

Fig. 4.2: Saline and iodine wet mount.
Source: Department of Microbiology, JIPMER, Puducherry (*with permission*).

- A small amount of feces is mixed with a stick to form a uniform smooth suspension
- A cover slip is placed on the mount and examined under a low power objective (10x) and then followed by a high power objective (40x) for the detection of protozoan cysts/trophozoites and ova of helminths
- **Normal constituents of stool specimen:** These include plant fiber, starch cells, muscle fibers, animal hair, pollen grains, yeast cells, bacteria, fat globules, air bubbles, etc.

Saline Mount

The saline mount is useful in the detection of trophozoites and cysts of protozoan parasites, and eggs and larvae of helminths. It has the following advantages over than iodine mount.
- The motility of trophozoites and larvae can be demonstrated
- Bile staining property can be appreciated—bile stained eggs appear golden brown and non-bile stained eggs appear colorless.

Note: Examples of non-bile stained eggs—*Enterobius*, hookworm, and *Hymenolepis nana* eggs.

Iodine Mount
- *Advantages:* Nuclear details of protozoan cysts, helminthic eggs, and larvae are better visualized, compared to saline mount
- *Disadvantages:* Iodine immobilizes and kills the parasites, hence motility of the trophozoites and helminthic larvae cannot be appreciated.

Concentration Techniques

If the parasite output is low in feces and direct examination may not be able to detect the parasites, then the stool specimens need to be concentrated.

Commonly used concentration techniques are:
- **Sedimentation techniques:** Example includes formalin-ether concentration technique
- **Flotation techniques:** Example includes saturated salt solution flotation technique.

Examination of Blood

Blood smear examination after staining with various Romanowsky stains such as Leishman's stain or Giemsa stain is useful in the diagnosis of infection caused by blood parasites like *Plasmodium*, *Trypanosoma*, *Leishmania*, *Wuchereria bancrofti*, *Brugia malayi*, etc.

Immunodiagnostic Methods

Immunodiagnostic methods involve the detection of parasite-specific antibodies in serum or the detection of circulating parasitic antigens in the serum.
- **Antibody detection tests:** Antibodies are detected in various parasitic infections; mainly from serum or from other specimens (like CSF in case of neurocysticercosis)
  - Antibodies can be detected by ELISA or immunochromatographic test (ICT)
  - Indications for antibody detection: Amoebic liver abscess, visceral leishmaniasis, toxoplasmosis, cysticercosis, hydatid disease, and lymphatic filariasis.
- **Antigen detection tests:** Indications for antigen detection in the diagnosis of parasitic diseases include—amoebiasis, malaria, and lymphatic filariasis.

Molecular Methods

Molecular methods most frequently used in diagnostic parasitology include—polymerase chain reaction (PCR) and real-time PCR.

TREATMENT OF PARASITIC DISEASES

Treatment of parasitic diseases primarily is based on chemotherapy and in some cases surgery.

- **Anti-parasitic drugs:** Various chemotherapeutic agents are used for the treatment and prophylaxis of parasitic infections
- **Surgical management:** It is useful for the management of parasitic diseases like cystic echinococcosis, neurocysticercosis, etc.

Details of treatment of some of the important human parasites have been described in Chapter nos. 27-34.

EXPECTED QUESTIONS

I. **Write short notes on:**
   1. Medically important parasites.
   2. Role of stool microscopy in the diagnosis of parasitic diseases.

II. **Multiple Choice Questions (MCQs):**
   1. **Advantages of the saline mount are all, except:**
      a. Useful in the detection of trophozoites and cysts of protozoan parasites and eggs and larvae of helminths
      b. Nuclear details of cysts are better visualized
      c. The motility of trophozoites and larvae can be seen
      d. Bile staining property can be appreciated
   2. **A stained peripheral blood smear is useful for the diagnosis of all of the following parasitic infections, except:**
      a. Malaria
      b. Filaria
      c. Hookworm disease
      d. Leishmania
   3. **All are non-bile stained eggs, except:**
      a. *Enterobius*
      b. Hookworm
      c. *Ascaris*
      d. *Hymenolepis*

Answers
1. b   2. c   3. c

CHAPTER 5: General Mycology

CHAPTER PREVIEW
- General Mycology
- Classification of Fungi
- Laboratory Diagnosis of Fungal Infections
- Treatment of Fungal Infections

GENERAL MYCOLOGY

Medical mycology is the branch of medical science that deals with the study of medically important fungi. The name 'fungus' is derived from Greek '*mykes*' meaning mushroom (a type of edible fungus). Some of the important properties of fungi are:

- Fungi are eukaryotic and they possess all the eukaryotic cell organelles
- They possess a rigid cell wall, composed of chitin, β-glucans, and other polysaccharides
- The fungal cell membrane contains ergosterol instead of the cholesterol
- They divide by asexual and/or sexual means by producing spores.

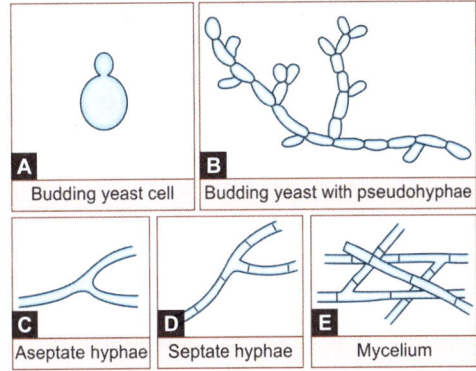

Figs. 5.1A to E: Morphological forms of fungi.

CLASSIFICATION OF FUNGI

Morphological Classification

Based on the morphological appearance, there are four main groups of fungi as follows (Figs. 5.1A to E):

1. **Yeast:** They grow as round to oval cells that reproduce by an asexual process called **budding** in which cells form protuberances that enlarge and eventually separate from the parent cells. An example includes — *Cryptococcus neoformans*
2. **Yeast-like:** In some yeasts (e.g. *Candida*), the bud remains attached to the mother cell, elongates, and undergoes repeated budding to form chains of elongated cells known as **pseudohyphae**.
3. **Molds:** They grow as long branching filaments of 2–10 μm width called **hyphae.**
   - Hyphae are either septate (i.e. form transverse walls) or nonseptate (there are no transverse walls)
   - Hyphae grow continuously and form a branching tangled mass of growth called **mycelium**
   - Molds reproduce by formation of different types of sexual and asexual spores
   - Examples of true molds include— Dermatophytes, *Aspergillus, Penicillium, Rhizopus, Mucor,* etc.

4. **Dimorphic fungi:** They exist as molds (hyphal form) at 25°C and as yeasts in human tissues at body temperature (37°C). Several medically important fungi are thermally dimorphic such as:
   - *Histoplasma capsulatum*
   - *Blastomyces dermatitidis*
   - *Coccidioides immitis*
   - *Paracoccidioides brasiliensis*
   - *Penicillium marneffei*
   - *Sporothrix schenckii*.

Clinical Classification of Fungal Diseases

Fungal infections (or mycoses) can be categorized into the following clinical types **(Table 5.1)**.

LABORATORY DIAGNOSIS OF FUNGAL INFECTIONS

The laboratory diagnosis of fungal diseases comprises the following:

Specimen Collection

It depends on the site of infection such as skin scraping, hair, nail, sputum, etc. For systemic mycoses, blood sample may also be collected. Cerebrospinal fluid (CSF) is collected for cryptococcal meningitis.

Microscopy

Microscopy is useful to demonstrate fungal elements in clinical specimens. Following microscopy techniques are used:

- **Potassium hydroxide (KOH) preparation**: Keratinized tissue specimens such as skin scrapings and plucked hair samples are treated with 10% KOH which digests the keratin material so that the fungal hyphae will be seen under the microscope **(Fig. 5.2A)**
- **Gram stain:** It is useful in identifying the yeasts (e.g. *Cryptococcus*) and yeast-like fungi (e.g. *Candida*). They appear as gram-positive budding yeast cells
- **India ink and nigrosin stains:** They are used as negative stains for demonstration of capsule of *Cryptococcus neoformans* **(Fig. 35.8A**, of Chapter 35)

Table 5.1: Classification of fungal diseases.

Fungal disease	Agents
Superficial mycoses	
Tinea versicolor	*Malassezia furfur*
Tinea nigra	*Hortaea werneckii*
Piedra	*Trichosporon beigelii, Piedraia hortae*
Dermatophytosis	*Trichophyton, Microsporum, Epidermophyton*
Subcutaneous mycoses	
Mycetoma	*Madurella mycetomatis*, and others
Sporotrichosis	*Sporothrix schenckii*
Chromoblastomycosis	*Phialophora* and others
Phaeohyphomycosis	*Exophiala* and others
Rhinosporidiosis	*Rhinosporidium seeberi*
Systemic mycoses	
Histoplasmosis	*Histoplasma capsulatum*
Blastomycosis	*Blastomyces dermatitidis*
Coccidioidomycosis	*Coccidioides immitis*
Paracoccidioidomycosis	*Paracoccidioides brasiliensis*
Opportunistic mycoses	
Candidiasis	*Candida albicans* and other species
Cryptococcosis	*Cryptococcus neoformans*
Zygomycosis	*Rhizopus, Mucor*
Aspergillosis	*Aspergillus flavus, Aspergillus fumigatus, Aspergillus niger*
Penicilliosis	*Penicillium marneffei*
Pneumocystosis	*Pneumocystis jirovecii*
Fusariosis	*Fusarium species*

- **Calcofluor white stain:** It is more sensitive than other stains; fungal elements fluoresce under UV light **(Fig. 5.2B)**
- **Histopathological stains:** They are useful for demonstrating fungal elements from biopsy tissues. This is useful for detecting invasive fungal infection
  - Periodic acid Schiff (PAS) stain
  - Gomori methenamine silver (GMS) stain
  - Hematoxylin and Eosin (H and E) stain.
- **Lactophenol cotton blue (LPCB):** It is used to study the microscopic appearance

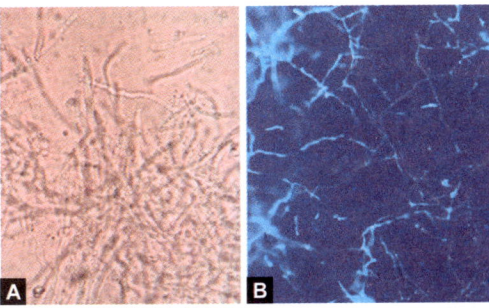

Figs. 5.2A and B: Fungal hyphae in: **A.** KOH mount; **B.** Calcofluor white stain mount.

Source: **A.** Dr Sherly Antony, Pushpagiri Medical College, Thiruvalla, Kerala; **B.** Department of Microbiology, JIPMER, Puducherry (*with permission*).

of the fungal isolates grown in culture. Fungal elements are stained blue colored.

Culture

A fungal culture is frequently performed for isolation and correct identification of the fungi.

Culture Media

- **Sabouraud's dextrose agar (SDA):** It is the most commonly used medium in diagnostic mycology
- **Brain heart infusion (BHI) agar and blood agar:** They are the enriched media, used for growing fastidious fungi like *Cryptococcus* and *Histoplasma*
- **Niger seed agar** and **bird seed agar:** They are used for the selective growth of *Cryptococcus*
- **CHROMagar *Candida* medium:** It is used for isolation as well as a differential medium for speciation of *Candida*.

Culture Condition

- **Temperature:** Most of the fungi grow well at 25–30°C except the dimorphic fungi that grow at both 25°C and 37°C
- **Incubation:** A special incubator called as **BOD incubators** (biological oxygen demand) are used for fungal culture and culture plates should be incubated for 2–3 weeks
- **Antibiotics** such as cycloheximide, and chloramphenicol can be added to the culture media to inhibit bacterial growth.

Culture Identification

The correct identification of the fungus is based on the macroscopic appearance of the colonies grown on culture and microscopic appearance (LPCB mount of colonies).

- **Macroscopic appearance of the colony:** Following growth characters are noted, such as—rate of growth (rapid/slow), pigmentation, texture and colony surface appearance.
- **Microscopic appearance of fungi:** Microscopic examination of the fungi can be done by:
  - **LPCB teased mount:** A bit of fungal colony is teased out from the culture tube and the LPCB mount is prepared.
  - **Slide culture:** It is done to demonstrate the most accurate in situ microscopic appearance of the fungal colony.

Immunological Methods

These tests are available to detect the antibody or antigen from serum and/or other body fluids.

- **Antibody detection** can be done by ELISA and agglutination test
- **Antigen detection:** Various fungal antigens can be detected in clinical specimens such as blood, CSF, urine, etc.
  - **Cryptococcal capsular antigen** from CSF by latex agglutination test
  - Detection of *Aspergillus* specific **galactomannan antigen** in patient's sera or urine (by ELISA)
  - **β-d-Glucan assay** by ELISA: It is a marker of all invasive fungal infections.

Automation

Automated identification systems such as MALDI-TOF and VITEK are revolutionary in the accurate identification of yeasts and to some extent molds.

Molecular Methods

Molecular methods useful in the diagnosis of fungal infections include—polymerase chain reaction (PCR), real-time PCR, and DNA sequencing methods.

TREATMENT OF FUNGAL INFECTIONS

Some of the commonly used antifungal agents include—amphotericin B, caspofungin, griseofulvin, fluconazole and voriconazole.

Treatment of the important human fungal infections has been described in Chapter no 35.

EXPECTED QUESTIONS

I. **Write short notes on:**
   1. Laboratory diagnosis of fungal infections.
   2. Dimorphic fungi.

II. **Multiple Choice Questions (MCQs):**
   1. All are yeast or yeast-like fungi, *except*:
      a. Candida
      b. Trichosporon
      c. Cryptococcus
      d. Trichophyton
   2. All of the following are microscopic techniques for the diagnosis of fungal diseases, *except*:
      a. KOH mount
      b. LPCB mount
      c. India ink staining
      d. CHROMagar identification
   3. All are systemic mycoses, *except*:
      a. Histoplasmosis
      b. Blastomycosis
      c. Dermatophytosis
      d. Coccidioidomycosis
   4. All are examples of molds, *except*:
      a. Aspergillus
      b. Penicillium
      c. Candida
      d. Rhizopus

Answers
1. d   2. d   3. c   4. c

CHAPTER 6

Epidemiology of Infectious Disease

CHAPTER PREVIEW

- Infection and Related-terminologies
- Epidemiological Patterns
- Eradication and Elimination
- Epidemiological Determinants of Disease Causation

The epidemiology branch of infectious disease deals with the distribution and determinants of infection-related health states in specified populations, and their application to the control of the disease.

INFECTION AND RELATED-TERMINOLOGIES

Following the entry of the microorganism into the body, it may lead to either infection or colonization; both the terms need to be distinguished.

- **Infection:** It is a process in which a pathogenic organism enters, establishes itself, multiplies, and invades the normal anatomical barrier of the host resulting in disease
- **Colonization:** Here, the pathogenic organism enters, multiplies but does not invade, and neither causes disease nor elicits a specific immune response
  - Colonizers are different from normal flora
  - They have pathogenic potential and may invade and cause disease in another host or the same host later.
- **Healthcare-associated infection (HAIs):** Defined as the new infections acquired in a healthcare facility (HCF) by a patient after 48 hours of admission, which was neither present nor incubating at the time of admission. (Chapter 36)
- **Community-associated infections:** Refers to the infections which developed in the community or within 48 hours of admission to a healthcare facility.

EPIDEMIOLOGICAL PATTERNS

Infectious diseases that are capable of directly transmitting to a man from another man, animal or environment are called communicable disease. The spread of communicable diseases in the community may occur in several epidemiological patterns—outbreak, epidemic, pandemic, hyperendemic and sporadic.

- **Outbreak** is a sudden rise in the number of cases in a limited geographic area
  - Cholera outbreak in Bengaluru in 2020, affecting 17 people
  - Nipah virus encephalitis outbreak in Kerala in 2018, resulting in 18 cases with 16 deaths.
- **Epidemic:** If the infection occurs at a much higher rate than usual in a particular geographical area, it is known as an epidemic. It usually affects a large number of people within a community, population, or region. The classical examples include:
  - SARS epidemic in China in 2003
  - Ebola epidemic in Africa in 2014.

- **Pandemic:** An infection that spreads rapidly to large areas of the world is known as a pandemic. Examples include:
  - COVID-19 pandemic in 2020 affecting >200 countries
  - Influenza pandemics: Several flu pandemics occurred so far including the H1N1 pandemic in 2009
  - Cholera: Seven pandemics of cholera have occurred so far in the past.
- **Endemic:** When a disease occurs at a persistent, usually low level in a certain geographical area, it is called an endemic. India is endemic to several diseases such as typhoid fever, cholera, filariasis, malaria, etc.
- **Sporadic:** Infections occur at irregular intervals or only in a few places; scattered or isolated. For example, several sporadic cases of cholera occur in India every year.

ERADICATION AND ELIMINATION

Eradication, elimination, and control of an infectious disease are related terminologies with distinct differences.

Eradication

It refers to the complete and permanent worldwide reduction to 'zero new cases' of the disease through deliberate efforts. If a disease has been eradicated, no further control measures are required.
- Smallpox was the only disease to be eradicated from the whole world (in 1980)
- Polio is on the verge of eradication. Most countries including India have already declared polio-free except Pakistan and Afghanistan.

Elimination

It refers to the 'reduction to zero' (or a very low defined target rate) of new cases in a defined geographical area. Elimination requires continued measures to prevent the re-establishment of disease transmission. The diseases which attained elimination in India include neonatal tetanus and leprosy.

Control

It refers to the reduction of disease incidence, prevalence, morbidity, or mortality to a locally acceptable level as a result of deliberate efforts. However, continued intervention measures are still required to maintain the reduction, e.g. diarrheal diseases.

EPIDEMIOLOGICAL DETERMINANTS OF DISEASE CAUSATION

The **Epidemiological Triad** depicts the causation of infectious disease. The triad consists of an external **agent**, a susceptible **host**, and an **environment** that brings the host and agent together.

Agent Factors

It refers to the infectious microorganism such as a virus, bacterium, parasite, or fungus that is responsible for the causation of the disease.
- Generally, the agent must be present for the disease to occur; however, the presence of that agent alone is not always sufficient to cause the disease
- A variety of agent-related factors influence whether the exposure to an organism will result in disease **(Table 6.1)**.

Table 6.1: Epidemiological determinants of disease causation.

Agent
• Organism's pathogenicity
• Infective dose
• Source and reservoir: Human or animal
• Mode of transmission: Contact, inhalation, ingestion, vector-borne, vertical transmission
• Infectivity or communicability

Host
• Age, gender, and race
• Underlying disease, pregnancy, etc.
• Underlying immune status and nutritional status
• Occupational status
• Personal practices: Hygiene and sexual practices
• Genetic make-up

Environment
• Seasonality
• Resistance to disinfectants
• Soil, moisture, rainfall

Organism's Pathogenicity

Pathogenicity refers to the ability of the organism to cause disease. Pathogenic microbes express various virulence factors that allow the organism to become established in a host and maintain the disease state.

Infective Dose

The infective dose is the minimum inoculum size that is capable of initiating an infection.
- **Low infective dose**: For example, *Shigella*, *Cryptosporidium parvum*. They require small inoculum to initiate infection
- **Large infective dose:** For example, *Salmonella* and *Vibrio cholerae*. They require a large inoculum size to initiate infection.

Source and Reservoir

The starting point for the occurrence of an infectious disease is known as a source or/and reservoir of infection.
- **Source:** It refers to a person, animal, or object from which the microorganism is transmitted to the host
- **Reservoir:** It is the natural habitat in which the organism lives, and multiplies. It may be a person, animal, arthropod, plant, soil, or substance on which the organism is dependent for its survival
- In tetanus infection, the reservoir and source of the agent (*Clostridium tetani*) are the same, i.e. the soil
- In hookworm infection, the reservoir is man, but the source of infection is the soil contaminated with the larva of hookworm.

The reservoir (and/or source) may be of three types.

Human Reservoir

By far the most important reservoir and/or source of infection for humans is man himself. The diseases that can be spread from one person to another are called **communicable diseases**. Human sources may be either cases or carriers.
- **Cases or patients:** They are the persons in a given population identified as having a particular disease
- **Carrier:** It refers to the persons who harbor the infectious agent in the absence of any clinical symptoms and shed the organism from the body via contact, air, or secretions. It results due to inadequate treatment or immune response. Different types of carriers are as follows:
  - **Incubatory carriers** are those who shed the organism during the incubation period of the disease, e.g. measles, mumps, polio, diphtheria, pertussis, influenza, etc.
  - **Healthy carriers** refer to the subclinical cases who develop into carriers without suffering from overt disease, e.g. polio, cholera, salmonellosis, diphtheria, etc.
  - **Convalescent carrier** is the one who has recovered from the disease and continues to harbor and shed the pathogen from his body
  - Carriers can be **temporary** (shed the organism for less than six months) or **chronic carriers** (shed the organisms for an indefinite period).

Animal Reservoir

The source of infection may sometime be animals and birds. The disease and the infections which are transmitted to man from vertebrates are called zoonoses. Common examples include:
- **From animals:** Rabies (from a dog), leptospirosis (from rodents), influenza (from pigs), etc.
- **Birds** may be the source of infection for various diseases like influenza, *Chlamydia psittaci* infection (psittacosis), histoplasmosis, etc.

Mode of Transmission

Microorganisms may be transmitted from the reservoir or source to a susceptible host in different ways.

Contact

This is the most common mode of transmission. Infection may be transmitted by direct or indirect contact.

- **Direct contact** is via the skin and mucosa of an infected person, e.g. through an unclean hand, kissing, or sexual contact. Organisms transmitted by direct contact include agents of common cold, skin infections, and sexually transmitted infections (STIs)
- **Indirect contact** is through the agency of fomites, which are inanimate objects, such as clothing, toys, etc. These may be contaminated by a pathogen and act as a vehicle for its transmission, e.g. face towels shared by various persons may lead to the spread of trachoma.

Inhalation

The inhalational route is the second most common mode of transmission. Transmission through respiratory route occurs either through droplets or aerosols.
- **Droplet transmission:** Transmission via large droplets requires close contact (<3 feet). Droplets may fall on surfaces and fomites present within 1 meter. People can subsequently acquire the infection when they touch the infected surfaces or fomites and then touch their nose, eyes, or mouth. Agents transmitted through droplets include:
  - Bacterial agents/diseases: Diphtheria, *H. influenzae*, meningococcus, pertussis, streptococcal pharyngitis
  - Viral agents/diseases: COVID-19, influenza, viral hemorrhagic fever (e.g. Ebola), mumps, parvovirus B19, rhinovirus, rubella, adenovirus.
- **Aerosol transmission:** Aerosols are small particles (<5 µm) generated by an infectious person during coughing, sneezing, or while performing certain aerosol-generating procedures (e.g. intubation). Infectious agents that are transmitted through aerosols include:
  - *Mycobacterium tuberculosis*
  - Measles virus
  - Varicella (chickenpox and zoster)
  - Smallpox (variola) virus.

Ingestion

Infectious agents can be transmitted by ingestion mode, either through contaminated water or food. Examples include:

- Intestinal infections like cholera, dysentery, diarrheagenic *E. coli* and intestinal parasitic infections, and viral agents of gastroenteritis, such as rotavirus
- Extraintestinal infections: In this type of infection, pathogens are transmitted by enteric route but produce disease manifestations elsewhere—*Salmonella* Typhi (typhoid fever), hepatitis A and E viruses, poliovirus, etc.

Inoculation

Pathogens, in some instances, may be inoculated directly into the skin or tissues of the host:
- **Animal bite**—for example, rabies virus is inoculated directly by the bite of a rabid animal
- **Inoculated directly into tissue**—spores of *Clostridium tetani* present in the soil, get deposited directly into the host tissues following severe wounds leading to tetanus.

Transmission of Blood-borne Infections

Blood-borne infections, such as hepatitis B, hepatitis C, and HIV may be transmitted by:
- Needle prick and other sharp injuries
- Blood transfusion
- Intravenous drug abuse (contaminated needles).

Vector Borne

Arthropod vectors, such as mosquitoes, flies, fleas, ticks, mites and lice are the vectors that transmit many diseases. Examples for vector-borne diseases include— *Anopheles* mosquito in malaria; *Culex* mosquito in filariasis, and arboviral infections.

Vertical Transmission

It refers to the transmission of infection from the mother to the fetus. It may be categorized into:
- **Transplacental transmission:** Infection transmitted via the placental barrier can lead to abortion, miscarriage, or stillbirth. If babies are born, they suffer from congenital malformations. The pathogens causing congenital infections are abbreviated as 'TORCH':
  - **T**oxoplasma gondii
  - **O**thers (*Treponema pallidum,* varicella-zoster virus, parvovirus, Zika virus)

- **R**ubella virus
- **C**ytomegalovirus
- **H**erpes simplex virus.

❖ **Transmission via the birth canal** without causing congenital malformation in the baby, e.g. include Group B *Streptococcus*, *Neisseria gonorrhoeae* and *Chlamydia trachomatis, Listeria,* and viruses (e.g. Hepatitis B, C, and HIV).

Infectivity or Communicability

It refers to the ability of an infectious agent to transmit from one person to another. A **period of communicability** is the time during which an infectious agent may be transferred directly or indirectly from an infected person to another person.

❖ **Measles:** From -4 to +4 days of onset of rash
❖ **Rubella:** From -1 to +1 week of onset of rash
❖ **COVID-19:** From -2 to +10 days of onset of symptoms.

Host Factors

Host refers to the human who can get the disease. A variety of factors intrinsic to the host, sometimes called risk factors, can influence an individual's exposure, susceptibility, or response to a causative agent.

❖ **Age:** Most viral infections are common at extremes of age, i.e. childhood and old age
❖ **Gender:** Most infections are either equally distributed or common in males
  - Males have a greater exposure risk to infections transmitted in work environments than females
  - Women are at greater risk of acquiring HIV and gonorrhea from sexual intercourse with an infected partner, as compared to men.
❖ **Pregnancy:** Certain diseases are common in pregnancy such as transplacental infections (e.g. CMV, rubella)
❖ **Host immune status:** Low immunity predisposes to many infections, such as CMV
❖ **Prior immunity:** Prior immunity to the agent due to vaccination or past infection can protect the individual from further infection. Some viral infections such as smallpox, chickenpox, measles, mumps, and rubella provide lifelong immunity
❖ **Nutritional status:** Malnutrition lowers the host immunity and thus predisposes to many viral infections, e.g. measles
❖ **Underlying comorbid disease**: People with diabetes, immunodeficiency disorders, or receiving steroid therapy are more prone to acquire various infections
❖ **Occupational status:** Sometimes, infectious diseases are more common in certain occupations; for example, zoonotic diseases such as anthrax are common among butchers, abattoirs, and farmers
❖ **Sexual practices:** People with multiple sex partners, men who have sex with men are more prone to develop various sexually-transmitted infections such as HIV
❖ **Hygiene:** Poor hygiene, poor sanitation, over-crowding, etc. predispose to several diseases such as acute diarrheal illness and typhoid fever
❖ **Genetic makeup:** Certain individuals are more prone to develop some microbial infections. This depends on the genetic makeup of the individual.

Environmental Factors

Environmental factors play an important role in disease causation.

❖ **Seasonality:** Many diseases are common in winters such as influenza and meningococcal meningitis; whereas vector-borne diseases such as malaria, dengue are more common in the rainy season
❖ **Disinfectants:** The organisms which are more resistant to the action of disinfectant can survive in the environment for longer. This is particularly important in the hospital environment where the multidrug-resistant organisms such as *Pseudomonas, Acinetobacter* and *Klebsiella,* etc. are widely prevalent
❖ **Soil:** Damp, sandy, or friable soil with vegetation is suitable for certain soil-transmitted helminths such as hookworm, *Ascaris,* and *Trichuris* than clay soil
❖ **Moisture:** Moisture is necessary for the survival of most microbes as dryness is rapidly fatal.

EXPECTED QUESTIONS

I. Write short notes on:
1. Epidemiological patterns.
2. Droplet versus aerosol transmission.

II. Multiple Choice Questions (MCQs):
1. If the infection occurs at a much higher rate than usual in a particular geographical area, it is known as:
   a. Epidemic   b. Pandemic
   c. Outbreak   d. Sporadic
2. Organisms with low infective dose include all, *except*:
   a. *Shigella*
   b. *Cryptosporidium parvum*
   c. *Giardia*
   d. *Vibrio cholerae*
3. Aerosol transmission occurs in all, *except*:
   a. *Mycobacterium tuberculosis*
   b. *Corynebacterium diphtheriae*
   c. Measles virus
   d. Varicella
4. Healthcare associated infection is defined as new infection acquired in a healthcare facility which was neither present nor incubating at the time of admission, within
   a. 24 hours   b. 48 hours
   c. 36 hours   d. 72 hours
5. The complete and permanent worldwide reduction to zero new cases of the disease through deliberate efforts is known as
   a. Reduction   b. Elimination
   c. Eradication d. Control
6. The person who harbors the infectious agent in the absence of any clinical symptoms and shed the organism to others is called
   a. Patient   b. Carrier
   c. Reservoir   d. Infectious

Answers
1. a   2. d   3. b   4. b   5. c   6. b

SECTION 2: Immunology

SECTION OUTLINE

7. Immunity, Components of Immune System, Immune Response
8. Antigen, Antibody and Complement
9. Antigen-Antibody Reaction
10. Hypersensitivity Reactions
11. Immunoprophylaxis and Immunization Schedule

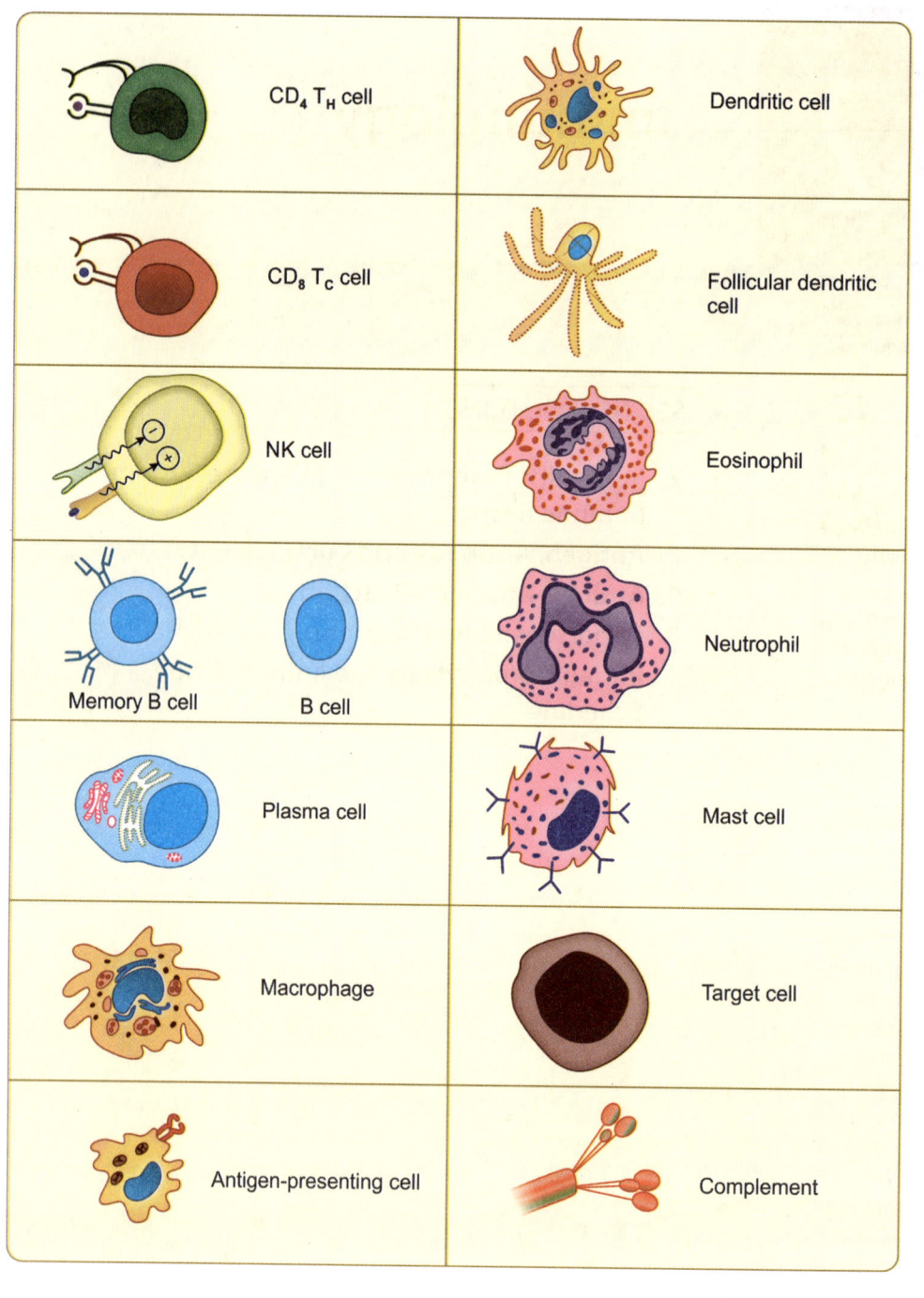

CHAPTER 7

Immunity, Components of Immune System, Immune Response

CHAPTER PREVIEW

- Innate Immunity
- Acquired Immunity
- Components of Immune System
- Immune Response

The term "immunity" is defined as the resistance offered by the host against microorganism(s) or any foreign substance(s). Immunity can be broadly classified into two types:
1. Innate immunity—present right from birth
2. Acquired/adaptive immunity—acquired during the course of life.

INNATE IMMUNITY

Innate immunity is the inborn resistance against infections that an individual possesses right from birth, due to his genetic or constitutional makeup.

Innate immunity has certain unique properties by which it can be differentiated from acquired immunity **(Table 7.1)**.

- **Acts in minutes:** Innate immunity is the **first line of host defense** against infections; occurs immediately after the microbial entry
- **Prior microbial exposure is not required:** Innate immunity is independent of prior exposure to the microbes; presents even before the first entry of the microorganism
- **Non-specific:** Cells of innate immunity are non-specific in their action; can be directed against any microbial antigen(s)
- **No memory:** Innate immunity does not have a memory component. Response to a repeat infection is identical to the primary response.

Mechanism of Innate Immunity

Following the exposure to microorganisms, several mediators of innate immunity are recruited to the site of infection. The first step that takes place is **attachment,** which involves binding the surface molecules of organisms to the receptors on the cells of innate immunity (e.g. Toll-like receptors).

Components of Innate Immunity

There are several mediators of innate immunity.

- **Anatomical barriers:** Such as skin and mucosal surfaces have a spectrum of antimicrobial activities
  - Mechanically prevents entry of microbes
  - Mucosa produces mucus which entraps microbes
  - Cilia present in the lower respiratory tract propel the microbes outside.
- **Physiological barriers** are also capable of inhibiting certain microbes; examples include:
  - Normal body temperature
  - Gastric acidity
  - Secretory products of mucosa such as saliva, tears, trypsin and bile salts, etc.

Table 7.1: Differences between innate and acquired immunity.

Properties	Innate immunity	Acquired/Adaptive immunity
Resistance to infection that an individual	Possesses right from birth	Acquires during his lifetime
Duration	The immune response occurs in minutes	The immune response occurs in days
Prior exposure to the antigen	Not required	Required
Immunological memory	Absent	Present
Host cell receptors	Non-specific, e.g. toll-like receptor	Specific, e.g. T cell receptors and B cell immunoglobulin receptors
Important components of innate immunity	<ul><li>Anatomical and physiological barriers</li><li>Host immune cells: Phagocytes, NK cells, mast cells, dendritic cells, etc.</li><li>Complement pathways—alternative and mannose-binding pathways</li><li>Normal resident flora</li></ul>	T cell B cell Classical complement pathway

- ❖ **Host immune cells:** Several immune cells such as phagocytes, NK cells, mast cells, and dendritic cells play a crucial role in innate immunity
   - *Phagocytes* such as neutrophils, and macrophages are the main components of innate immunity. They are rapidly recruited to the site of infection and mediate phagocytosis (i.e. engulfment of microbes and subsequent microbial killing
   - *Natural killer (NK) cells:* They are a class of lymphocytes that kill intracellular pathogens, virus-infected cells, and tumor cells
   - *Mast cells:* They are present in the epithelial lining of respiratory and other mucosa and are capable of killing the microbes by releasing several inflammatory meditators
   - *Dendritic cells:* They respond to microbes by producing numerous cytokines that initiate inflammation.
- ❖ **Complement pathways:** Alternative and mannose-binding pathways are the chief mediators of innate immunity
- ❖ **Normal resident flora** lining the intestinal, respiratory, and genital tract can compete with the pathogens for nutrition. They also produce antibacterial substances

- ❖ **Acute phase reactant proteins (APRs):** They are the proteins synthesized by liver at a steady concentration, but their synthesis increases exponentially during acute inflammatory conditions. Examples of APR include: C-reactive protein, serum amyloid A, complement proteins, coagulation protein, and mannose-binding protein.

> **C-Reactive Protein (CRP)**
> It is one of the most common markers of acute inflammation, used in most diagnostic laboratories.
> - The level of CRP rises in acute inflammatory conditions including bacterial infection
> - CRP is so named because it precipitates with the C-carbohydrate antigen of pneumococcus. However, it is not an antibody against the C-antigen of pneumococcus; it is non-specific, can be raised in any inflammatory conditions
> - It can be detected by latex agglutination test using latex particles coated with anti-CRP antibodies.

The differences between innate and acquired immunity are depicted in **Table 7.1**.

ACQUIRED IMMUNITY

Acquired immunity is defined as the resistance against the infecting foreign substance that

an individual acquires or adapts during the course of his life.
- ❖ **Mediators: T cells and B cells** are the chief mediators of acquired immunity. Other mediators include:
  - Classical complement pathway
  - Antigen-presenting cells
  - Cytokines (IL-2, IL-4, IL-5).
- ❖ **The response occurs in days:** Acquired immunity involves activation of T and B cells against the microbial antigens; which takes several days to weeks to develop, following the microbial entry
- ❖ **Requires prior microbial exposure:** Acquired immunity develops only after exposure to the microbes
- ❖ **Specific:** Acquired immunity is highly specific; directed against specific antigens of the microbes
- ❖ **Memory present:** Acquired immunity does have a memory component. A proportion of T and B cells become memory cells following primary contact with the microbe, which play an important role when the microbe is encountered subsequently
- ❖ **Host cell receptors** of acquired immunity are specific for a particular microbial antigen. Examples include T cell receptors and B cell immunoglobulin receptors.

Types of acquired immunity: Acquired immunity can be classified in two ways:
1. Active and passive immunity
2. Artificial and natural immunity.

Active Immunity

Active immunity is the resistance developed by an individual towards an antigenic stimulus.
- ❖ Here, the host's immune system is actively involved against the antigenic stimulus; leading to the activation of T and B cells, and the production of specific antibodies
- ❖ Active immunity may be induced naturally or artificially
  - **Natural active immunity** occurs following exposure to microbial infection (e.g. measles virus infection)
  - **Artificial active immunity** develops following exposure to an immunogen by vaccination (e.g. measles vaccine). Vaccines are discussed in Chapter 11.
- ❖ As the host's immune apparatus is actively involved, active immunity often fails to develop when the host is immunocompromised
- ❖ Active immunity **develops slower**; as there is an initial **lag phase**, required for activation of the T and B cells
- ❖ **Long-lasting:** Active immunity usually lasts for longer periods, but the duration varies depending on the type of pathogen.

Types of immune response in active immunity vary depending on the microbial exposure that occurs for the first time (called primary immune response) and subsequent time (called secondary immune response).

Passive Immunity

Passive immunity is defined as the resistance that is transferred passively to a host in a "readymade" form without the active participation of the host's immune system.
- ❖ Passive immunity can also be induced naturally or artificially
  - **Natural passive immunity** involves the IgG antibody transfer from mother to fetus across the placenta
  - **Artificial passive immunity** develops following the readymade transfer of commercially prepared immuno-globulin (e.g. Rabies immunoglobulin).
- ❖ Passive immunity plays a very important role in:
  - Immunodeficient individuals (as the host's immune apparatus is not effective), and
  - Post-exposure prophylaxis; when an immediate effect is warranted.
- ❖ Passive immunity **develops faster**; there is no lag phase
- ❖ There is no **immunological memory** as the memory cells are not involved
- ❖ **Booster doses are not effective:** As the memory component is absent, the effect produced following subsequent immunoglobulin administration is the

Table 7.2: Differences between active and passive immunity.

Properties	Active immunity	Passive immunity
Mechanism	Produced actively by host immune system	Immunoglobulins received passively
Induced by	• Infection (natural) • Vaccination (artificial)	• Mother to fetus IgG transfer (natural) • Readymade antibody transfer (artificial)
Duration	Long-lasting	Short-lasting
Lag period	Present	No lag period
Memory	Present	No memory
Booster doses	Useful	Less effective
In Immuno-deficient individuals	Not useful	Useful
Post-exposure prophylaxis	Less useful	Useful

same as the effect produced after the primary dose.

The differences between active and passive immunity are listed in **Table 7.2**.

OTHER TYPES OF IMMUNITY

Local (or Mucosal) Immunity

Local or mucosal immunity is the immune response that is active at the mucosal surfaces such as intestinal or respiratory or genitourinary mucosa.
❖ It is mediated by a type of IgA antibody called secretory IgA, which prevents the entry of microbes at the local site itself
❖ Local immunity can only be induced by natural infection or by live vaccination, e.g. live oral polio vaccine (but not by killed vaccines).

Herd Immunity

Herd immunity is defined as the overall immunity of a community (or herd) toward a pathogen.

❖ It plays a vital role in preventing epidemic diseases
❖ If herd immunity is good, that means a large population of the community is immune to a pathogen. Hence, epidemics are less likely to occur and eradication of the disease may be possible
❖ Herd immunity develops following effective vaccination against some diseases like:
   ▪ Diphtheria and pertussis vaccine
   ▪ Measles, mumps, and rubella (MMR) vaccine
   ▪ Polio (oral polio vaccine)
   ▪ Smallpox vaccine.

COMPONENTS OF THE IMMUNE SYSTEM

The immune system comprises lymphoid organs, cells of the immune system (lymphoid cells and other cells) and their soluble products called cytokines.

Lymphoid Organs

Lymphoid organs consist of central and peripheral lymphoid organs.

Central or Primary Lymphoid Organs

The central lymphoid organs are the site for the development of immune cells. Examples include:
❖ **Thymus:** It is the site of proliferation and maturation of T cells
   ▪ It has an outer cortex and an inner medulla
   ▪ Any defect in the thymus leads to a defect in the maturation of T-lymphocytes that in turn results in severe life-threatening immunodeficiency disorders.
❖ **Bone marrow:** It is the site of the development of B cells
   ▪ Almost all the cells in the blood have originated from pluripotent hematopoietic stem cells of bone marrow and the process is called hematopoiesis
   ▪ The progenitor T and B cells originate in the bone marrow. Further development

of B cells occurs in the bone marrow itself, whereas the progenitor T cells migrate to the thymus for further proliferation.

Peripheral or Secondary Lymphoid Organs

They host the T cells and B cells. Examples include:

- **Lymph node:** They are small bean-shaped organs; distributed along the lymphatic vessels
  - They host the mature B cells and T cells
  - Divided into the outer cortex, inner medulla, and in-between there is a paracortical area
  - Cortex is rich in lymphoid follicles containing B cells, whereas the paracortical area is rich in T cells
  - They act as physiological barriers; filter the microbial antigens carried to the lymph node by activating the T and B cells.
- **Spleen:** Spleen is the largest secondary lymphoid organ. It acts as a physiological barrier similar to the lymph node in clearing the microbial antigens through the stimulation of T and B cells
- **Mucosa-associated lymphoid tissue (MALT):** The group of lymphoid tissues lining the mucosal sites (e.g. respiratory or intestinal) is collectively known as MALT
  - They are present either as loose clusters of lymphoid cells or as organized structures such as tonsils, appendix, and Peyer's patches
  - They provide immunity at the local sites by encountering the pathogen entry.

Lymphoid Cells

Lymphoid cells consist of lymphocytes such as T cells, B cells, and NK cells.

T Lymphocytes

They constitute 70–80% of blood lymphocytes. They bear specialized surface receptors called T cell receptors (TCR). T cell development takes place in the thymus. There are two types of effector T cells—(1) $CD4^+$ helper T cells and (2) $CD8^+$ cytotoxic T cells.

- **Helper T cells:** Helper T cells (T_H) possess CD4 molecules as surface receptors
  - They recognize the antigenic peptides that are processed by antigen-presenting cells and presented along with MHC-II molecules (major histocompatibility complex)
  - Following antigenic stimulus, the helper T cells differentiate into either of the two types of cells—(1) $T_H 1$, and (2) $T_H 2$ subset
  - $T_H 1$ cells secrete specific cytokines such as IL-2, interferon-gamma which modulate the cellular humoral immune response
  - $T_H 2$ cells secrete specific cytokines such as IL-4, IL-5, and IL-6 which modulate the humoral immune response.
- **Cytotoxic T cells:** In contrast to T_H cells, cytotoxic T cells (T_C) possess CD8 molecules and recognize the intracellular antigens (e.g. viral antigens or tumor antigens) that are processed by any nucleated cells and presented along with MHC-I. In general, T_C cells are involved in the destruction of virus-infected cells and tumor cells.

B Lymphocytes

B lymphocytes are the mediators of humoral immunity; constitute 10–15% of blood lymphocytes. B cells proliferate through various stages, first in bone marrow, then in peripheral lymphoid organs. B cells produce five classes of antibodies, which in turn have various biological functions (discussed in Chapter 8).

NK Cells

Natural killer (NK) cells are large granular lymphocytes that constitute 10–15% of peripheral blood lymphocytes. They are derived from a separate lymphoid lineage. Similar to cytotoxic T cells, NK cells also are involved in the destruction of virus-infected cells and tumor cells.

Other Cells of the Immune System

Other cells of the immune system include phagocytes, such as

- ❖ **Macrophages:** They play a vital role in host defense by performing two important functions—
  1. *Phagocytosis:* The process by which the microbes are ingested and subsequently killed through producing various lysosomal enzymes and free radicals
  2. *Antigen presentation:* Macrophages capture the antigen, process it into smaller antigenic peptides, and present the antigenic peptides along with the MHC class II molecules to the helper T cells; thus facilitating helper T cell activation.

  Examples of macrophages present in various body sites include—(i) Kupffer cells in liver, (ii) microglial cells in brain, (iii) alveolar macrophages in lungs, etc.
- ❖ **Microphages:** Examples include granulocytes such as neutrophils, eosinophils, and basophils. They are the principal phagocytes; the mechanism of microbial killing is similar to that of macrophages
- ❖ **Dendritic cells:** They are non-phagocytic in nature. They help in antigen presentation; their main function is to capture, process, and present the antigenic peptides on their cell surface to the helper T cells
- ❖ **Mast cells:** They are present in various body sites, such as skin and respiratory mucosa. They contain cytoplasmic granules rich in histamine and other active substances and play an important role in the development of certain allergic (type I hypersensitivity) reactions.

Cytokines

They are the soluble products secreted from various cells of the immune system. They include interleukins (IL), interferons (IFN- α, β, γ), tumor necrosis factors (TNF), colony-stimulating factors (CSF), etc.

Major Histocompatibility Complex (MHC)

They are a group of host cell surface molecules that bind to peptide fragments derived from pathogens and display them on the host cell surface for recognition by the appropriate T cells.

- ❖ **MHC-I:** MHC-I proteins are located on the surface of all nucleated cells. They present the peptide antigen to CD8 T cells
- ❖ **MHC-II:** MHC-II proteins are located on the surface of antigen-presenting cells. They present the peptide antigen to CD4 T cells.

IMMUNE RESPONSE

Immune response refers to the highly coordinated reaction of the cells of the immune system and their products. It has two arms.

Cell-mediated Immune Response (CMI)

It plays a crucial role in protecting against intracellular microbes as well as tumor cells. Although CMI is mainly T cell-mediated (especially cytotoxic T cells); however, various other effector cells such as natural killer (NK) cells, macrophages, and granulocytes are also components of CMI.

Humoral or Antibody-mediated Immune Response (AMI)

It protects the host by secreting *antibodies*; that can bind and neutralize microbial antigens circulating free or present on the surface of the host cells and in the extracellular spaces, but have no role against intracellular antigens.

CHAPTER 7 ♦ Immunity, Components of Immune System, Immune Response

EXPECTED QUESTIONS

I. Write an essay on:
1. Define immunity. Describe in detail about the properties and mediators of innate immunity.

II. Write short notes on:
1. Herd immunity.
2. Differences between innate and acquired immunity.
3. Differences between active and passive immunity.

III. Multiple Choice Questions (MCQs):
1. Which is not a mediator of innate immunity?
    a. T cells
    b. NK cell
    c. Phagocytes
    d. Neutrophil
2. Which of the following about innate immunity is wrong?
    a. The immune response occurs in minutes
    b. Non-specific
    c. It is first line of defense
    d. Need prior contact with the antigen
3. Which of the following about active immunity is correct?
    a. No lag phase
    b. Booster doses are useful
    c. Useful in immunodeficient people
    d. No memory cells
4. The type of immunity that develops after infection is:
    a. Artificial immunity
    b. Acquired immunity
    c. Passive immunity
    d. Combined immunity
5. The immunity develops after the vaccination is an example for:
    a. Natural active immunity
    b. Artificial active immunity
    c. Natural passive immunity
    d. Artificial passive immunity

Answers
1. a 2. d 3. b 4. b 5. b

CHAPTER 8: Antigen, Antibody and Complement

CHAPTER PREVIEW
- Antigen
- Antibody
- Complement

ANTIGEN

Antigen (Ag) is defined as any substance that satisfies two distinct immunologic properties—immunogenicity and antigenicity.
1. **Immunogenicity:** It is the ability of an antigen to induce an immune response in the body
2. **Antigenicity (immunological reactivity):** It is the ability of an antigen to combine specifically with antibodies.

The substance that satisfies the first property, i.e. immunogenicity (inducing a specific immune response) is more appropriately called **"immunogen"** rather than using the word "antigen".

Hapten

Haptens are low molecular weight molecules that **lack immunogenicity** (cannot induce an immune response) but **retain antigenicity or immunological reactivity** (i.e. can bind to their specific antibody or T cell receptor). Haptens can become immunogenic when combined with a larger protein molecule called a **carrier**.

Epitope

Epitope or antigenic determinant is the smallest unit of an antigen that is capable of reacting with the specific site of an antibody. The specific site of an antibody that reacts with the corresponding epitope of an antigen is called **paratope**.

Factors Influencing Immunogenicity of Ag

There are various factors that influence the immunogenicity of an antigen.
- **Size of the antigen:** Larger is the size more potent is the molecule as an immunogen
- **Chemical nature of the antigen:** Proteins are stronger immunogens than carbohydrates or lipids
- **Susceptibility of antigen to tissue enzymes:** Only substances that are susceptible to the action of tissue enzymes are immunogenic
- **Structural complexity:** Polymers made up of at least two or more amino acids are immunogenic
- **Foreignness to the host:** Higher is the phylogenetic distance between the antigen and the host; more is the immunogenicity
- **Genetic factor:** Different individuals of a given species show different types of immune responses towards the same antigen due to genetic differences
- **Optimal dose of antigen:** An antigen is immunologically active only in the optimal dose range. A too little dose or too large dose fails to elicit an immune response

CHAPTER 8 ◆ Antigen, Antibody and Complement

- ❖ **Route of antigen administration:** In general, the immune response is better induced following the parenteral administration of an antigen
- ❖ **Sometimes, repeated doses of antigens** may be required to generate an adequate immune response.

> **Adjuvant**
> The term "adjuvant" refers to any substance that enhances the immunogenicity of an antigen. They are usually added to vaccines to increase the immunogenicity of the vaccine antigen.
>
> **Examples of Adjuvants**
> - **Alum** (aluminum hydroxide or phosphate)
> - **Lipopolysaccharide** (LPS) fraction of *Bordetella pertussis* is an excellent adjuvant for diphtheria and tetanus toxoids. This explains the reason for using combined immunization for diphtheria, pertussis and tetanus in the form of DPT vaccine.
>
> **Mechanism of Adjuvant Action:** Adjuvants act through the following steps:
> - Delaying the release of antigen
> - By activating phagocytosis
> - By activating T_H cells.

ANTIBODY

Antibody or immunoglobulin is a specialized glycoprotein, produced from activated B cells (plasma cells) in response to an antigen, and is capable of combining with the antigen that triggered its production.
- ❖ Immunoglobulin (Ig) constitutes 20–25% of total serum proteins
- ❖ There are five classes of Ig recognized—IgG, IgA, IgM, IgD, and IgE.

Structure of Antibody

An antibody molecule is a 'Y-shaped' heterodimer, composed of four polypeptide chains **(Fig. 8.1)**—two light (L) chains and two heavy (H) chains.
- ❖ **Bonds:** All four H and L chains are bound to each other by disulfide bonds, and by noncovalent interactions
- ❖ **Ends:** The chains have two ends—an amino-terminal end (NH_3) and a carboxyl-terminal end (COOH)

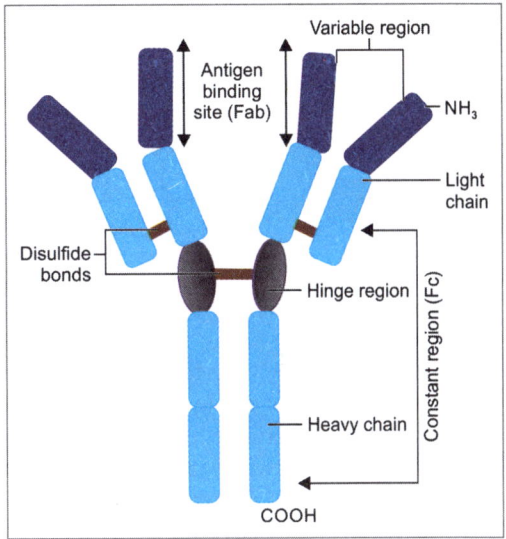

Fig. 8.1: General structure of an antibody.

Table 8.1: Type of heavy chain in each immunoglobulin class.	
Immunoglobulin class	**Heavy chain type**
IgG	γ (gamma)
IgA	α (alpha)
IgM	μ (mu)
IgD	δ (delta)
IgE	ε (epsilon)

- ❖ **H chain classes:** There are five classes of H chains. Each Ig has one type of H class. The five classes of Igs (IgG, IgA, IgM, IgD, and IgE) are classified based on the type of H chains they possess **(Table 8.1)**.

Variable and Constant Regions

Each H and L chain comprises two regions—variable and constant region.
1. **Variable region:** Contains a variable sequence of amino acids. It is the antigen-binding region of an antibody
   - It comprises a hypervariable region called paratope, which makes actual contact with the epitope of the antigen
   - Antibodies produced against various antigens differ from each other in the amino acid sequences of the variable region.

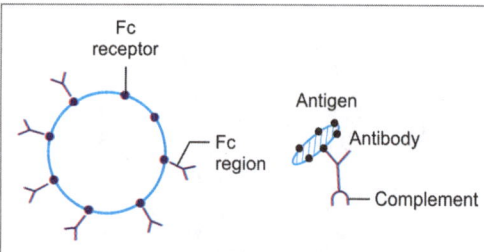

Fig. 8.2: Function of the constant region (Fc) of antibody.

2. **Constant region (Fc):** It constitutes the remaining part of an Ig molecule other than that of the variable region
   - The amino acid sequence of the Fc region shows a uniform pattern
   - The Fc region of the antibody mediates various effector functions such as binding to the complements, and various other cell types such as phagocytes, lymphocytes, mast cells, NK cells, eosinophils, etc. **(Fig. 8.2)**
   - These cells bear Fc receptors (FcR) that bind to the Fc region of immunoglobulins.

Immunoglobulin Classes

There are five classes of immunoglobulins.

Immunoglobulin G (IgG)

It constitutes about 70–80% of total Ig in the body. It mediates various functions.
- IgG can **cross the placenta**; hence providing immunity to the fetus and newborn
- **Complement fixing:** Fc region of IgG can bind to complement factors; thus activating the classical pathway of the complement system
- **Phagocytosis:** IgG bind to Fc receptors present on phagocytes (macrophages, neutrophils) and enhances the phagocytosis (opsonization) of antigen bound to them
- It mediates precipitation and neutralization reactions
- IgG is raised after a long time following infection and represents chronic or past infection (recovery).

Immunoglobulin M (IgM)

Among all Ig, IgM has the highest molecular weight. It is present only in the intravascular compartment, not in body fluids or secretions. It exists either in monomeric form with 2 valencies or pentameric form (5 Ig joined together with a valency of 10 **(Fig. 8.3A)**. IgM mediates various functions.
- **Acute infection:** IgM is the first antibody to be produced following an infection; represents acute or recent infection. It is also called a primary immune response antibody
- **Complement fixing:** It is the most potent activator of the classical complement pathway
- It is also present on B cell surface in monomeric form and serves as **B cell receptor** for antigen binding
- It acts as an **opsonin**; binds to an antigen which is then easily recognized and removed (opsonization)
- **Fetal immunity:** It is the first antibody to be synthesized in fetal life; thus provides immunity to the fetus
- Protection against **intravascular organisms**: IgM being intravascular, is responsible for protection against blood invasion by microorganisms
- IgM mediates **agglutination** reaction.

Immunoglobulin A (IgA)

IgA is the second most abundant class of Ig next to IgG, constituting about 10–15% of total serum Ig. It exists in both monomeric and dimeric forms.
- **Serum IgA:** IgA in serum is predominantly in monomeric form
- **Secretory IgA:** It is dimeric in nature, with a valency of four **(Fig. 8.3B)**
  - *Location:* Secretory IgA is the predominant antibody found in body secretions like milk, saliva, tears, intestinal and respiratory tract mucosal secretions
  - *Function:* The secretory IgA mediates **local or mucosal immunity**; protects against pathogens by cross-linking the

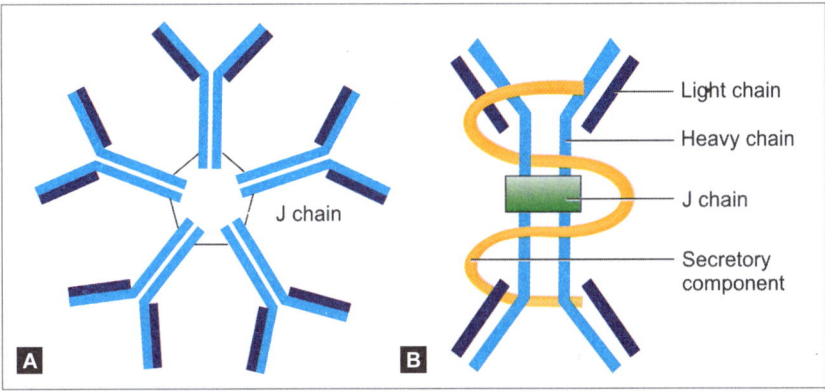

Figs. 8.3A and B: A. Pentameric IgM; **B.** Dimeric IgA.

antigens and preventing their entry through the mucosal surfaces.

Immunoglobulin E (IgE)

Among all Ig, IgE is having the lowest serum concentration. It is also the only heat-labile antibody.
- IgE is highly potent and mediates **type I hypersensitivity** reactions by binding to the mast cells (Chapter 10)
- IgE is elevated in **helminthic infections**.

Immunoglobulin D (IgD)

IgD is found as membrane Ig on the surface of B cells and acts as a B cell receptor along with IgM.

Monoclonal Antibody

Monoclonal antibodies (mAb) are defined as the antibodies derived from a single clone of plasma cell; all having the same antigen specificity, i.e. produced against a single epitope of an antigen.
- **Production:** Monoclonal antibodies are produced by a method called as hybridoma technique
  - In the hybridoma technique, antibody-forming mouse splenic B cells are fused with myeloma cells (cancerous plasma cells) to produce hybridoma cells
  - These hybridoma cells can grow and survive long producing the desired antibody.
- **Uses:** mAb has various uses such as:
  - *Diagnostic reagents:* The widest application of mAb is the detection of antigens. The antigen detection kits employ various mAb tagged with detection molecules, such as an enzyme, which detects the specific antigens in the clinical specimens by using various formats like ELISA, rapid tests, etc.
  - *Passive immunity:* For post-exposure prophylaxis against various infections, mAb targeting specific antigens of infecting organisms can be administered. Examples include—immunoglobulins against hepatitis B, rabies, and tetanus
  - *Therapeutic use:* Monoclonal antibodies are used in the treatment of various inflammatory conditions, allergic diseases, and cancers.

COMPLEMENT

The term 'complement' (C) represents a group of proteins normally found in the serum in an inactive form, but when activated by a microbial antigen, they augment the immune response and cause microbial cell lysis.
- The complement system is grouped into complement components (nine proteins, C1 to C9), and the properdin system
- The majority of the complement proteins are synthesized in the liver

❖ Complements are species nonspecific and heat-labile.

Complement Activation

There are three pathways of complement activation:
1. **Classical pathway:** This is an antibody-dependent pathway. The pathway is triggered by the formation of antigen-antibody complex, i.e. when the host antibody binds to antigens present on the microbial cell surface. The complements bind to the F_c region of the antibody. The nine complements (C1 to C9) bind to the antibody, one after the other in a sequential manner
2. **Alternative pathway:** This is an antibody-independent pathway. This pathway is triggered directly by the antigen (e.g. bacterial endotoxin) to which the complements and properdin proteins bind in a sequential manner
3. **Lectin pathway:** This is a recently described pathway. It resembles the classical pathway, but it is antibody independent. It is mediated through lectin proteins of the host that interact with mannose residues present on microbial surfaces. Subsequently, complement proteins bind sequentially.

Stages of Complement Activation

There are four main stages in the activation of any of the complement pathways.
1. Initiation of the pathway
2. Formation of C3 convertase
3. Formation of C5 convertase
4. Formation of membrane attack complex (MAC):

The three pathways differ from each other only in the first two stages (i.e. till the formation of C3 convertase). The steps involved in the remaining stages are exactly same in all three pathways.

The final stage is formation of **membrane attack complex** (MAC) by binding of C5 to C9. MAC forms pores in the target cell (i.e. microbial surface), which leads to cell lysis and death **(Fig. 8.4)**.

Effector Functions of Complement

The effector functions of complement products are as follows:
❖ **Target cell lysis by MAC:** As already explained, bacteria, enveloped viruses, damaged cells, tumor cells, etc. are killed by complement-mediated cell lysis
❖ **Inflammatory response:** The complement by-products such as C3a, C4a, and C5a induce mast cell degranulation leading to

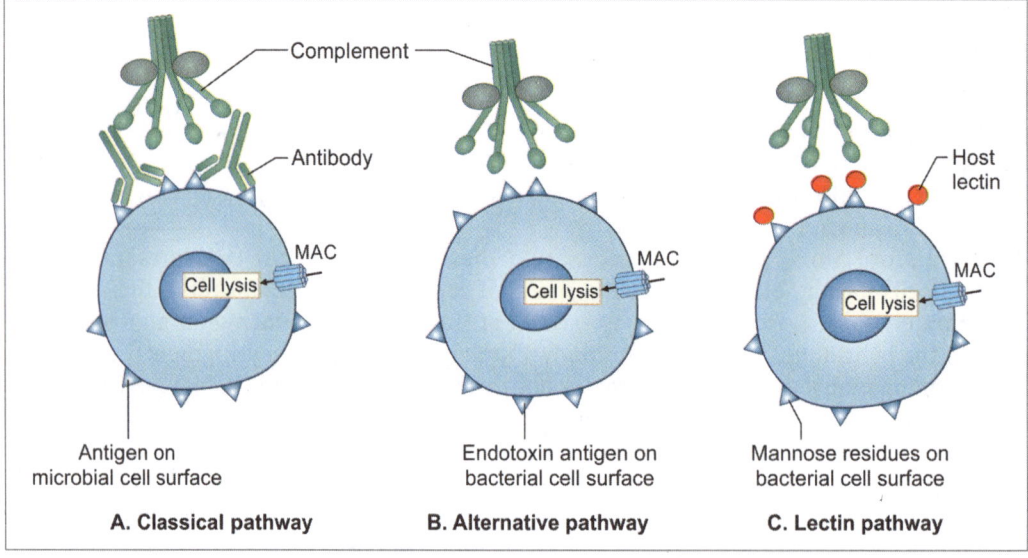

Fig. 8.4: The complement pathways.

vasoconstriction, and increased vascular permeability
* **Opsonization:** Some complement by-products (C3b and C4b) act as major opsonins and facilitate phagocytosis
* Complement helps in removing the immune complexes from blood
* **Viral neutralization:** Complements play a crucial role in the neutralization of viruses.

EXPECTED QUESTIONS

I. **Write an essay on:**
1. Define antibody. Describe in detail the structure and functions of various types of antibodies.

II. **Write a short note on:**
1. Monoclonal antibodies and their applications.
2. The structure and function of IgG antibody.
3. The structure and function of IgA.
4. The structure and function of IgM.

III. **Multiple Choice Questions (MCQs):**
1. Which antibody crosses the placenta?
   a. IgA   b. IgG
   c. IgE   d. IgM
2. What is the total vacancies of IgM?
   a. 10   b. 5
   c. 2   d. 1
3. Which antibody is elevated in acute infection?
   a. IgA   b. IgG
   c. IgE   d. IgM
4. Which antibody mediates mucosal immunity?
   a. IgA   b. IgG
   c. IgE   d. IgM
5. The smallest determinant of antigenicity is called as:
   a. Antigen   b. Immunogen
   c. Epitope   d. Paratope
6. 70-80% total antibody is constituted by:
   a. IgA   b. IgE
   c. IgG   d. IgM
7. The most potent activator of classical complement pathway is:
   a. IgA   b. IgM
   c. IgG   d. IgE
8. Complement mediated cell lysis is done by:
   a. Anaphylatoxins
   b. Activation of apoptosis
   c. Membrane attack complex
   d. Inhibition of protein synthesis

Answers
1. b   2. a   3. d   4. a   5. c   6. c   7. b   8. c

CHAPTER 9

Antigen–Antibody Reaction

CHAPTER PREVIEW

- General Properties
- Conventional Immunoassays
  - Precipitation Reaction
  - Agglutination Reaction
- Newer Techniques
  - ELISA and ELFA
- Immunofluorescence Assay
- Chemiluminescence Immunoassay
- Rapid Tests

GENERAL PROPERTIES

The antigen (Ag)–antibody (Ab) reaction refers to the binding of antigen and antibody with each other specifically and in an observable manner.

- **Specific:** Ag-Ab reaction involves specific interaction between the epitope of an antigen with the corresponding paratope of its homologous antibody
- **Noncovalent interactions:** The union of antigen and antibody requires the formation of a large number of non-covalent interactions between them
- **Immunoassays:** Because Ag-Ab reactions are specific and observable, they are extensively used in laboratories for the diagnosis of infectious diseases. Such assays are called immunoassays
  - *Antigen detection assays:* Detect antigens in the patient's sample by employing a specific antibody
  - *Antibody detection assays:* Detect antibodies in a patient's sample by employing a specific antigen.
- **Serological tests:** Immunoassays can be developed for the detection of antigens or antibodies in various clinical specimens, the most common being serum specimen. The immunoassays that are designed specifically for testing on serum specimens are called **serological tests**
- **Titer:** The exact amount of antibody in serum can be estimated by serial dilution of the patient's serum and mixing each dilution of the serum with a known quantity of antigen. The measurement of antibodies is expressed in terms of titer
  - The antibody titer of serum is the highest dilution that shows an observable reaction with the antigen
  - Antigen titer can also be similarly measured in the sera by testing the series of diluted sera against a known quantity of antibodies.

Lattice Hypothesis

When the sera-containing antibody is serially diluted (in normal saline), the antibody level gradually decreases.

- When a fixed quantity of antigen is added to such a set of test tubes containing serially diluted sera, then it is observed that the Ag-Ab reaction occurs at its best only in the middle test tubes where the amount

CHAPTER 9 ♦ Antigen–Antibody Reaction

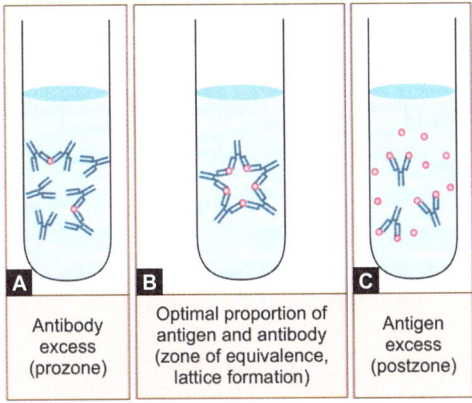

Figs. 9.1A to C: A. Prozone; **B.** Zone of equivalence; **C.** Postzone.

CONVENTIONAL IMMUNOASSAYS

PRECIPITATION REACTION

When a **soluble antigen** reacts with its antibody in the presence of optimal temperature, pH, and electrolytes (NaCl), it leads to the formation of the Ag–Ab complex in the form of:

- **Insoluble precipitation band** when gel or agar containing medium is used (called immunodiffusion), or
- **Insoluble floccules** when the liquid medium is used (called flocculation test).

Earlier, precipitation reactions were one of the widely used serological tests. However, with the advent of simple and rapid newer techniques, their application is greatly reduced. There are only limited situations where precipitation reactions are still in use, such as:

- **Slide flocculation test** (for syphilis): For example, VDRL (Venereal Disease Research Laboratory) and RPR (Rapid Plasma Reagin) tests
- **Elek's gel precipitation test:** Used for detecting diphtheria toxin.

of antigen and antibody are equivalent to each other (*zone of equivalence*)
- The Ag–Ab reaction is weak or fails to occur when the number of antigens and antibodies are not proportionate to each other **(Figs. 9.1A to C)**
  - In the earlier test tubes, *antibodies are excess*, hence the Ag–Ab reaction does not occur: This is called as **prozone phenomenon**
  - In the later test tubes, *antigen is excess*, hence the Ag–Ab reaction fails to occur: This is called as **postzone phenomenon**.

TYPES OF ANTIGEN-ANTIBODY REACTIONS

The Ag–Ab reactions used in diagnostic laboratories are based on various techniques which are broadly classified as conventional techniques and newer techniques.
- **Conventional techniques:** Examples include precipitation and agglutination reactions
- **Newer techniques:** Examples include—
  - Enzyme-linked immunosorbent assay
  - Enzyme-linked fluorescent assay
  - Immunofluorescence assay
  - Chemiluminescence immunoassay
  - Rapid tests
  - Western blot.

AGGLUTINATION REACTION

When a **particulate** or **insoluble** antigen is mixed with its antibody in the presence of electrolytes at a suitable temperature and pH, the particles are clumped or agglutinated.
- **Advantages:** Agglutination is more sensitive than the precipitation test and the clumps are better visualized and interpreted as compared to bands or floccules
- **Types:** Agglutination reactions are classified as direct, indirect (passive) tests. All these agglutination tests are performed either on a slide or in a tube or on a card or sometimes in microtiter plates.

Direct Agglutination Test

Here, the antigen directly agglutinates with the antibody.

Slide Agglutination

It is usually performed to confirm the identification and serotyping of bacterial colonies grown in culture. It is also the method used for blood grouping and cross-matching.

> A bacterial colony is mixed with a drop of saline on a slide to form a uniform smooth milky white suspension
> ↓
> To this, a drop of the antiserum (serum-containing appropriate antibody) is added and the slide is shaken thoroughly (manually or by rotator) for a few seconds
> ↓
> A positive result is indicated by visible clumping with the clearing of the suspension (**Fig. 9.2**)
> or
> If the milky white suspension remains unchanged, indicates a negative result (**Fig. 9.2**)

Tube Agglutination

This is a quantitative test done for estimating antibody in serum. The **antibody titer** can be estimated as the highest dilution of the serum which produces a visible agglutination.

> A fixed volume of a particulate antigen suspension is added to an equal volume of serial dilutions of a serum sample (containing appropriate antibody) in test tubes
> ↓
> A positive test indicates agglutination (clump formation at the bottom of the tube with the clearing of the supernatant)
> or
> A negative test indicates agglutination has not occurred (Ag suspension forms button at the bottom of the tube)

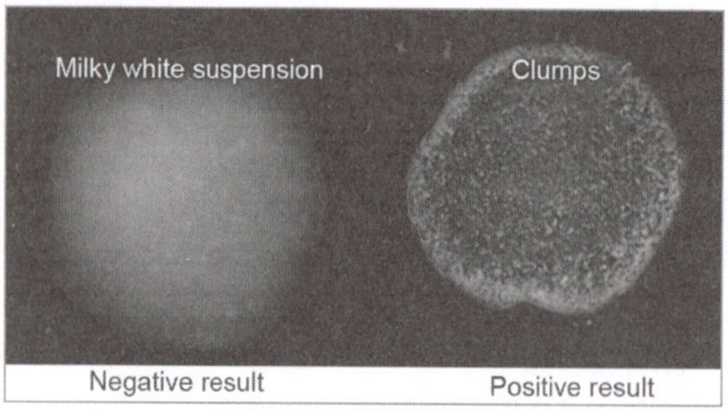

Fig. 9.2: Slide agglutination test.
Source: Department of Microbiology, JIPMER, Puducherry (*with permission*).

Tube agglutination is routinely used for the serological diagnosis of various diseases, such as:

- **Typhoid fever (Widal test):** It detects antibodies against both H (flagellar) and O (somatic) antigens of *Salmonella* Typhi
- Acute brucellosis (standard agglutination test)
- Coombs antiglobulin test
- Heterophile agglutination tests:
  - Typhus fever (Weil Felix reaction)
  - Infectious mononucleosis (Paul Bunnell test)
  - *Mycoplasma* pneumonia (Cold agglutination test).

Microscopic Agglutination

Here, the agglutination test is performed on a microtiter plate and the result is read under a microscope. The classical example is microscopic agglutination test (MAT) done for leptospirosis.

Indirect or Passive Agglutination Test (for Antibody Detection)

As the agglutination test is more sensitive and better interpreted than the precipitation test, an attempt has been made to convert a precipitation reaction into an agglutination reaction. This is possible by coating the soluble antigen on the surface of a carrier molecule (e.g. RBC or latex) so that the antibody binds to the coated antigen and agglutination takes place on the surface of the carrier molecule.

Latex Agglutination Test (LAT) for Antibody Detection

Here, latex particles are used as carrier molecules that are capable of adsorbing several types of antigens. For a better interpretation of the result, the test is performed on a black color card.

- A drop of patient's serum (containing antibody) is added to a drop of latex solution coated with the antigen and the card is rotated for uniform mixing
- A positive result is indicated by the formation of visible clumps (**Fig. 9.3**)

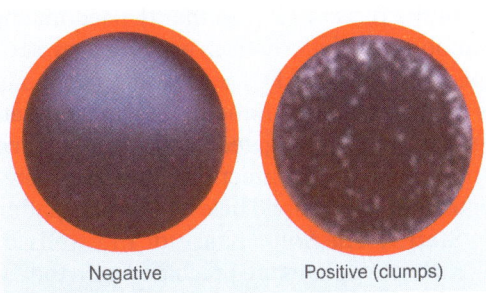

Fig. 9.3: Passive (latex) agglutination test.
Source: Department of Microbiology, JIPMER, Puducherry (*with permission*).

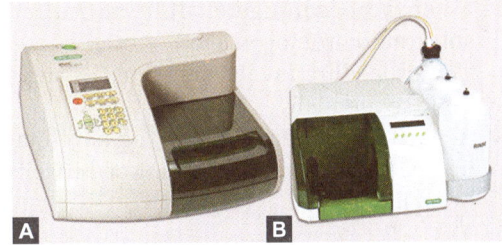

Figs. 9.4A and B: A. ELISA reader (Biorad); **B.** ELISA washer.
Source: Biorad Pvt. ltd (*with permission*).

- LAT is one of the most widely used tests at present as it is very simple and rapid
- It is used for the detection of ASO (antistreptolysin O antibody).

Reverse Passive Agglutination Test (for Antigen Detection)

In this test, the antibody is coated on a carrier molecule that detects antigen in the patient's serum. The classical example is **the latex agglutination test for antigen detection**: It is used widely for the detection of CRP (C reactive protein), RA (rheumatoid arthritis factor), capsular antigen detection in CSF (for pneumococcus, meningococcus, and *Cryptococcus*) and streptococcal grouping.

NEWER IMMUNOASSAYS

ENZYME-LINKED IMMUNOSORBENT ASSAY (ELISA)

ELISA is an immunoassay that detects either antigen or antibodies in the specimen, by using an enzyme-substrate–chromogen system for detection.

Principle of ELISA

ELISA is so named because of its two components:
- **Immunosorbent:** Here, a microtiter plate of absorbing material is used (e.g. polystyrene, polyvinyl) that specifically absorbs the antigen or antibody present in the serum
- **Enzyme** is used to label one of the components of immunoassay (i.e. antigen or antibody).

Substrate-chromogen system: It is added at the final step of ELISA. The enzyme reacts with the substrate, which in turn activates the chromogen to produce a color. The color change is detected by spectrophotometry in an ELISA reader **(Fig. 9.4A)**.

> (Ag-Ab complex)-enzyme + substrate → activates the chromogen → color change → detected by spectrophotometry (ELISA reader, **Fig. 9.4A**)

Procedure of ELISA

ELISA is performed on a microtiter plate containing 96 wells **(Fig. 9.5)**, made up of polystyrene, or polyvinyl material.
- ELISA kits are commercially available; contain all necessary reagents (such

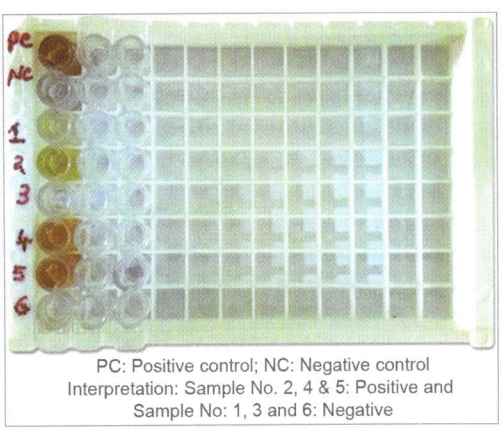

PC: Positive control; NC: Negative control
Interpretation: Sample No. 2, 4 & 5: Positive and Sample No: 1, 3 and 6: Negative

Fig. 9.5: ELISA for HBsAg.
Source: Department of Microbiology, Pondicherry Institute of Medical Sciences, Puducherry (*with permission*).

as enzyme conjugate, dilution buffer, substrate/chromogen, etc.)
- The procedure involves a series of steps done sequentially
- At each step, a reagent is added and then incubated, followed by washing of the wells by an ELISA washer **(Fig. 9.4B)**.

Types of ELISA

There are several types of ELISA, which differ from each other in their principles.

Direct ELISA

It is used for the detection of antigen in test serum. Here, the primary antibody (targeted against the serum antigen) is labeled with the enzyme **(Fig. 9.6A)**.
- **Step 1:** Wells of the microtiter plate are empty, not precoated with Ag or Ab
- **Step 2:** Test serum (containing antigen) is added into the wells. Antigen becomes attached to the solid phase by passive adsorption
- **Step 3:** After washing, the enzyme-labeled primary antibodies (raised in rabbits) are added
- **Step 4:** After washing, a substrate-chromogen system is added and the color is measured.

> Well + Ag (test serum) + primary Ab-enzyme + substrate-chromogen → color change **(Fig. 9.6A)**.

Indirect ELISA

It is used for the detection of antibody or less commonly antigen in serum. It differs from the direct ELISA in that the secondary antibody is labeled with an enzyme instead of the primary antibody. The secondary antibody is an anti- species antibody, e.g. anti-human Ig (an antibody targeted to the Fc region of any human Ig). Indirect ELISA for antibody detection is described below **(Fig. 9.6B)**.
- **Step 1:** The solid phase of the wells of microtiter plates are precoated with the Ag
- **Step 2:** Test serum (containing primary Ab specific to the Ag) is added to the wells. Ab gets attached to the Ag coated on the well
- **Step 3:** After washing, enzyme-labeled secondary Ab (anti-human immunoglobulin) is added
- **Step 4:** After washing, a substrate-chromogen system is added and the color is developed.

> Wells are coated with Ag + primary Ab (test serum) + secondary Ab-enzyme + substrate-chromogen → development of color **(Fig. 9.6B)**.

Other types of ELISA include:
- **Sandwich ELISA:** It detects the antigen in test serum. It is so named because the antigen gets sandwiched between a capture antibody (coated on the well) and a detector antibody
- **IgM antibody capture (MAC) ELISA:** This is an enzymatically amplified sandwich-type immunoassay. This format of ELISA is widely used for dengue, Japanese B encephalitis and West Nile virus, scrub typhus, leptospirosis, toxoplasmosis, etc.
- **Competitive ELISA:** It is so named because the antigen in the test serum competes with another antigen of the same type coated on the well to bind to the primary antibody.

Advantages of ELISA

ELISA is the method of choice for detection of antigens/antibodies in serum in modern days, especially in big laboratories as a large number of samples can be tested together using the 96 well microtiter plate.
- It is economical, takes 2–3 hours for performing the assay

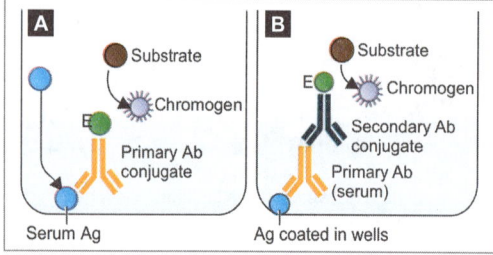

Figs. 9.6A and B: A. Direct ELISA (for antigen detection); **B.** Indirect ELISA (for antibody detection).

- ELISA has a high sensitivity; that is why it is commonly used for performing screening tests at blood banks and tertiary care sites
- Its specificity used to be low. But now, with the use of more purified recombinant and synthetic antigens, and monoclonal antibodies, ELISA has become more specific.

Disadvantages of ELISA

- In small laboratories having less sample load, ELISA is less preferred than rapid tests as the latter can be performed on individual samples
- It takes more time (2–3 hours) compared to rapid tests which take 10–20 minutes
- It needs expensive equipment such as an ELISA washer and reader.

Applications of ELISA

ELISA can be used both for antigen and antibody detection.
- ELISA used for antigen detection: Hepatitis B [hepatitis B surface antigen (HBsAg) and precore antigen (HBeAg)], NS1 antigen for dengue, etc.
- ELISA can also be used for antibody detection against hepatitis B, hepatitis C, HIV, dengue, herpes simplex virus, Epstein Barr virus, toxoplasmosis, leishmaniasis, etc.

ENZYME-LINKED FLUORESCENT ASSAY (ELFA)

It is a modification of ELISA, which differs from ELISA in two ways: (i) automated system, all steps are performed by the instrument itself, and (ii) Ag-Ab-enzyme complex is detected by the fluorometric method. VIDAS and miniVIDAS (bioMérieux) are commercially available systems based on ELFA technology.

IMMUNOFLUORESCENCE ASSAY (IFA)

It is a technique similar to ELISA, but differs by the use of fluorescent dye instead of enzyme

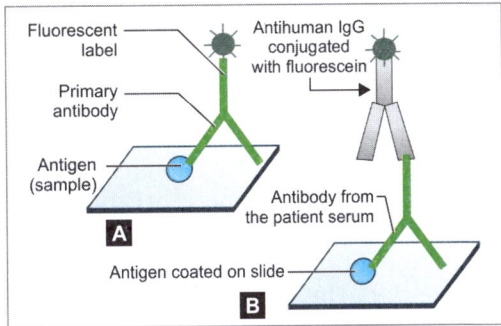

Figs. 9.7A and B: Immunofluorescence assay: **A.** Direct; **B.** Indirect.

for labeling the antibody. It is of two types: direct and indirect.

Direct Immunofluorescence Assay

- **Step 1:** Sample containing cells carrying surface antigens is smeared on a slide
- **Step 2:** Primary antibody specific to the antigen, tagged with a fluorescent dye is added
- **Step 3:** The slide is washed to remove the unbound antibodies and then viewed under a fluorescence microscope **(Fig. 9.7A)**.

Indirect Immunofluorescence Assay

This detects antibodies in the sample. Slides smeared with cells carrying known antigens are commercially available.
- **Step 1:** Test serum-containing primary antibody is added to the slide
- **Step 2:** The slide is washed to remove the unbound antibodies. A secondary antibody (antihuman antibody conjugated with fluorescent dye) is added
- **Step 3:** The slide is washed and then viewed under a fluorescence microscope **(Fig. 9.7B)**.

Applications: Immunofluorescence assay has various applications, such as:
- Detection of autoantibodies (e.g. antinuclear antibodies) in autoimmune diseases
- Detecting microbial antigens, e.g. rabies antigen in corneal smear
- Detection of viral antigens in cell lines inoculated with the specimens.

CHEMILUMINESCENCE IMMUNOASSAY

The principle of chemiluminescence immunoassay (CLIA) is similar to that of ELISA; however, the chromogenic substance is replaced by chemiluminescent compounds (e.g. luminol and acridinium ester) that generate light during a chemical reaction (luxogenic). The light (photons) can be detected by a photomultiplier, also called as luminometer (**Fig. 9.8**).

> (Ag-Ab complex)-enzyme + chemiluminescent substrate → product + light (photons) → detected by luminometer or photomultiplier.

Advantages of CLIA

❖ CLIA claims to be 10 times more sensitive than ELISA
❖ Individual specimens can be tested in CLIA in contrast to ELISA which is preferred for testing multiple samples at a time.

Applications

CLIA has limited applications in diagnostic microbiology compared to ELISA. Currently, it is available for the detection of antigens or antibodies against various infections such as hepatitis viruses, HIV, and biomarkers such as procalcitonin.

WESTERN BLOT

Western blot detects specific proteins (antibodies) in a sample containing mixture of antibodies each targeted against different antigens of same microbe.

❖ **Procedure:** It has three steps: (i) separation of antigen mixture into individual fragments by *gel electrophoresis*, (ii) transfer of antigen fragments onto a *nitrocellulose membrane*, (iii) detection of individual antibodies in serum against each antigenic fragments by *enzyme immunoassay*
❖ **Advantages:** It has an excellent specificity. Hence, it is often used as a supplementary test to confirm the result of ELISA or other immunoassays having higher sensitivity
❖ **Applications:** Western blot formats are available to detect antibody in various diseases such as HIV, cysticercosis, hydatid disease, etc.

RAPID TESTS

Rapid tests are revolutionary in the diagnosis of infectious diseases. They are very simple to perform (one-step method), rapid (takes 10–20 minutes), require minimal training, and do not need any sophisticated instruments.

❖ These tests are also called **Point-of-care** (POC) tests because unlike ELISA and other immunoassays, the POC tests can

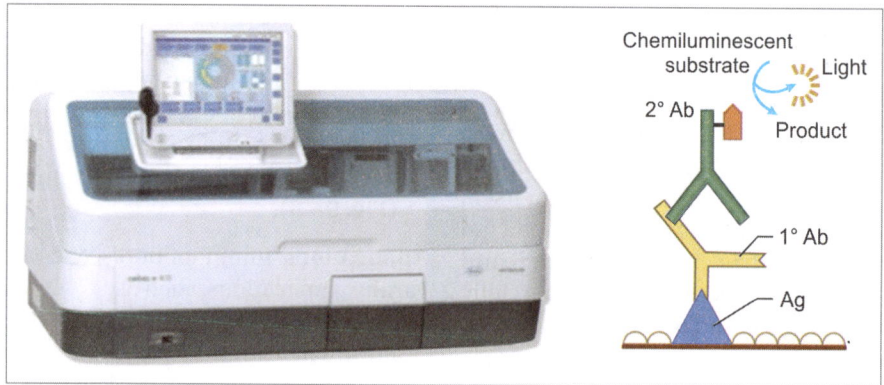

Fig. 9.8: Chemiluminescence system (CLIA) and its principle.
Source: Department of Microbiology, JIPMER, Puducherry (*with permission*).

be performed independent of laboratory equipment and deliver instant results
- Two principles of rapid tests are available—lateral flow assay and flow-through assay
- Both formats are available for the diagnosis of various diseases such as malaria, hepatitis B, hepatitis C, HIV, leptospirosis, etc.

Immunochromatographic Test (Lateral Flow Assay)

The immunochromatographic test (ICT) is based on the lateral flow technique. It is widely used in diagnostic laboratories because of its simplicity, low cost, and rapidity. It can be used for both antigen and antibody detection in the sample. The principle of the antigen detection method is described below.

Principle of ICT (Antigen Detection)

The test system consists of a nitrocellulose membrane (NCM) and an absorbent pad. Two formats are available: cassette or strip **(Figs. 9.9A and B)**. The NCM is coated at two places in the form of lines—a test line, coated with monoclonal antibody targeted against the test antigen, and a control line, coated with anti-species immunoglobulin. Specific Ab against the target Ag labeled with a chromogenic marker (specific Ab tagged with *colloidal gold* or *silver*, a visually detectable marker) is infiltrated in the absorbent pad lining the sample window.

- The sample (serum) containing the test antigen is added to the sample well; it reacts with antibody labeled with a chromogenic marker (*colloidal gold* or *silver*, a visually detectable marker)
- Both 'Ag-specific Ab-colloidal gold complex' as well as the 'free colloidal gold-labeled Ab' move laterally along the nitrocellulose membrane
- **Test band:** At the test line, the Ag-labeled Ab complex is immobilized by binding to the monoclonal Ab in the test line to form a colored band **(Figs. 9.9A and B)**
- **Control band:** The free colloidal gold-labeled Ab can move further and binds to the anti-human Ig to form a color control band. If the control band is not formed, then the test is considered invalid irrespective of whether the test band is formed or not **(Figs. 9.9A and B)**.

Flow-through Assay

Flow-through tests are another type of rapid diagnostic assays that differ from ICT in two aspects: (1) protein A is used for labeling antibody instead of gold conjugate, and (2) the sample flows vertically through the nitrocellulose membrane (NCM) as compared to lateral flow in ICT.

Flow-through tests can be used for both antigen and antibody detection. HIV TRI-DOT test is a classical example (described below, **Fig. 9.10A**). It detects antibodies to HIV-1 and 2 separately in patient's serum.

- The test system is in a cassette format, consisting of a NCM and an absorbent pad. The NCM is coated at three regions—two test regions coated with HIV-1 and 2 antigens and a third control region coated with antihuman Ig
- Sample and buffer reagents are added sequentially from the top following which they pass through the membrane and excess fluid is absorbed into the underlying absorbent pad
- As the patient's sample passes through the membrane, HIV antibodies, if present bind to the immobilized antigens **(Fig. 9.10B)**

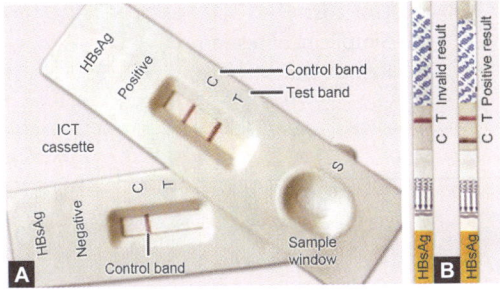

Figs. 9.9A and B: ICT for HBsAg detection: **A.** Cassette format; **B.** Strip format.

Source: Department of Microbiology, Pondicherry Institute of Medical Sciences, Puducherry (*with permission*).

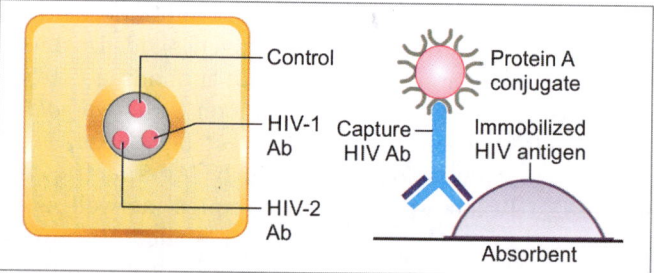

Figs. 9.10A and B: Flow-through assays: **A.** HIV TRI-DOT assay for HIV-1 and 2 antibodies detection; **B.** Principle of HIV TRI-DOT.

- **Test dots:** Protein-A conjugate (present in buffer) binds to the Fc portion of the HIV antibodies to give distinct pinkish-purple DOT(s), separately for HIV-1 and 2 antibodies

- **Control dot:** Irrespective of whether the HIV antibodies are present or not, protein-A can bind to any IgG present in serum and the IgG-protein A complex can further bind to the antihuman Ig at the control line to give a pinkish purple DOT.

EXPECTED QUESTIONS

I. Write an essay on:
1. Enumerate the properties and types of antigen-antibody reactions. Describe in detail the principle, types, and applications of ELISA?

II. Write short notes on:
1. Precipitation reaction.
2. Agglutination reactions.
3. Indirect immunofluorescence assay.
4. Immunochromatographic test.
5. Chemiluminescence immunoassay (CLIA).

III. Multiple Choice Questions (MCQs):
1. **The Prozone phenomenon is due to:**
   a. Excess antigen
   b. Excess antibody
   c. Hyperimmune reaction
   d. Both antigen and antibody excess

2. **All are agglutination reactions,** *except*:
   a. VDRL test
   b. Standard agglutination test
   c. Widal test
   d. Paul Bunnell test

3. **The following methods of diagnosis utilize labeled antibodies,** *except*:
   a. ELISA
   b. CLIA
   c. Precipitation test
   d. Immunofluorescence

4. **All of the following are true about immunochromatographic tests,** *except*:
   a. Require experienced personnel
   b. Low cost
   c. Simplicity of testing
   d. Rapid results

Answers
1. b   2. a   3. c   4. a

CHAPTER 10

Hypersensitivity Reactions

CHAPTER PREVIEW

- Definition and Classification
- Type I Hypersensitivity Reaction
- Type II Hypersensitivity Reaction
- Type III Hypersensitivity Reaction
- Type IV Hypersensitivity Reaction

The purpose of immune response is to eliminate the foreign antigens that have entered into the host. In most instances, immune response leads to only a subclinical or localized inflammatory response which just eliminates the antigen without causing significant damage to the host. However, at times, this response becomes abnormal; leading to an exaggerated inflammatory response that causes extensive tissue damage or sometimes even death.

DEFINITION AND CLASSIFICATION

The term hypersensitivity (HSN) or allergy refers to the injurious consequences in the sensitized host, following contact with specific antigens. Gell and R Coombs classified HSN reactions into four types **(Table 10.1)**.

- ❖ **Immediate HSN reactions:** These reactions occur immediately, within minutes to few hours of antigen contact, as a result of an abnormal exaggerated humoral response (antibody-mediated). This can be further classified into three types (HSN type I, II, and III), based on the type of effector mechanisms
- ❖ **Delayed HSN reaction:** It occurs after few days of antigen contact, as a result of an abnormal cell-mediated immune response. This is also called type IV HSN reaction. It is mediated by a specific subset

Table 10.1: Features of various types of hypersensitivity reactions.				
	Type I	**Type II**	**Type III**	**Type IV**
Immune response altered	Humoral	Humoral	Humoral	Cell-mediated
Immediate or delayed	Immediate	Immediate	Immediate	Delayed
The duration between the appearance of symptoms and antigen contact	2–30 minutes	5–8 hours	2–8 hours	24–72 hours
Antigen	Soluble	Cell surface bound	Soluble	Soluble or bound
Mediator	IgE	IgG	Ag-Ab complex	T_{DTH} cell
Effector mechanism	Mast cell degranulation	ADCC Complement-mediated cytolysis	Complement activation and inflammatory response	Macrophage activation leads to phagocytosis or cell cytotoxicity

Abbreviation: ADCC, antibody-dependent cellular cytotoxicity.

of T_H cells called delayed hypersensitivity T cells or T_{DTH} cells.

TYPE I HYPERSENSITIVITY REACTION

Type I HSN reaction involves the production of IgE by sensitized B cells following contact with an allergen which in turn induces mast cell degranulation. Type I reaction occurs in various clinical conditions such as anaphylaxis and asthma.

Mechanism of Type I Hypersensitivity

Type I HSN reaction occurs through two phases; the sensitization and effector phases, both occurring with an interval of 2–3 weeks **(Fig. 10.1)**.

Sensitization Phase

This occurs when an individual is exposed for the first time to the sensitizing or priming dose of an allergen.
- In susceptible individuals, very minute doses can be sufficient to sensitize the host cells
- The antigenic peptides are presented by antigen-presenting cells to the CD4 helper T cells
- Activated T_H cells are differentiated into T_H2 cells which in turn secrete interleukin 4 (IL-4)
- IL-4 induces the B cells to differentiate into IgE producing plasma cells and memory cells
- Secreted IgE migrates to the target sites, and coat on the surface of mast cells. Such sensitized mast cells (coated with IgE) will be waiting for interaction with the subsequent antigenic challenge.

Effector Phase

When the same allergen is introduced subsequently (shocking dose), it directly encounters with the IgE antibodies coated on mast cells.
- IgE cross-linkage initiates the mast cell activation and degranulation. Granules in turn release several pharmacologically

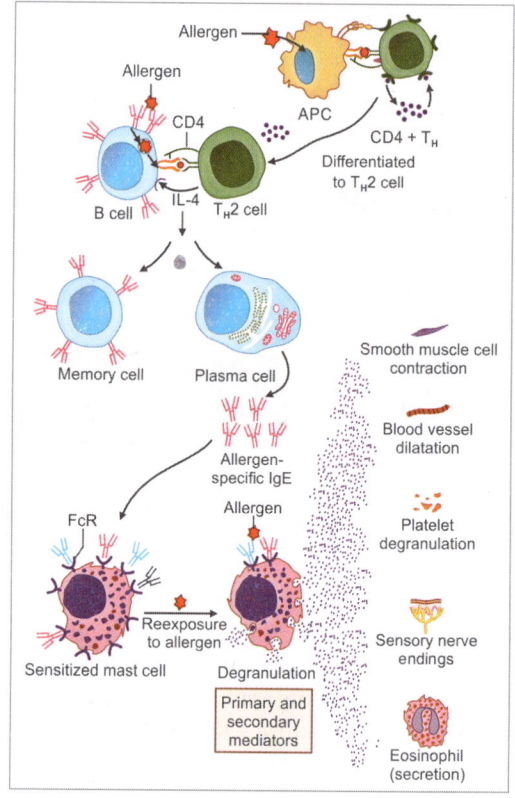

Fig. 10.1: Mechanism of type I hypersensitivity reaction.

active chemical mediators that lead to various manifestations of type-1 reaction
- **Degranulation occurs in two phases**: Mast cells undergo degranulation in two phases
  1. Primary mediators: The preformed chemical mediators which are already synthesized by mast cells are immediately released, e.g. histamine and serotonin
  2. Secondary mediators: The mast cells synthesize them following stimulation by allergen and release, e.g. prostaglandins and leukotrienes.
- **Pharmacological actions:** The chemical mediators perform several pharmacological actions, such as bronchial and other smooth muscle contraction, increased vascular permeability, and vasodilation
- **Symptoms:** These actions in combinations, produce symptoms such as breathlessness, hypotension, and shock leading to death at times.

Manifestations of Type I Reaction

There are various manifestations of type I HSN reaction.

- **Systemic anaphylaxis:** It is an acute medical emergency condition, characterized by severe dyspnea, hypotension, and vascular collapse leading to death at times
  - A wide range of allergens such as penicillin have been shown to trigger anaphylaxis in susceptible humans
  - Epinephrine (adrenalin) is the drug of choice for systemic anaphylactic reactions.
- **Localized anaphylaxis (Atopy):** Here, the reaction is limited to a specific target tissue or organ, mostly the epithelial surfaces at the entry sites of allergen. They almost always run in families (i.e. inherited). Examples include:
  - *Allergic rhinitis (or hay fever):* Exposure to airborne allergens with the conjunctiva and nasal mucosa leads to conjunctival watering, sneezing, and coughing
  - *Asthma:* Exposure to allergens to lower respiratory mucosa results in contraction of bronchial smooth muscles, bronchoconstriction, and dyspnea
  - *Food allergy:* The food allergens (e.g. nuts, eggs, seafood, etc.) can stimulate the mast cells lining the gut mucosa to cause GI symptoms such as diarrhea and vomiting
  - *Atopic dermatitis* (allergic eczema): Characterized by erythematous skin eruptions
  - *Drug allergy* by various drugs such as penicillin, sulfonamides, etc.

Detection of Type I Hypersensitivity

Type I HSN reaction can be demonstrated by various tests such as:
- Skin prick test
- Detection of total serum IgE antibody by various enzyme immunoassay
- Detection of allergen-specific IgE by various immunoassay formats.

Treatment

Treatment of type I HSN reaction includes:
- Avoidance of contact with known allergens
- **Hyposensitization:** Repeated exposure to increased subcutaneous doses of allergens can reduce or eliminate the allergic response to the same allergen
- Monoclonal anti-IgE antibody
- Drugs such as antihistamines, epinephrine (adrenaline), and cortisone.

TYPE II HYPERSENSITIVITY REACTION

In type II reactions, the host injury is mediated by **antibodies** (IgG or rarely IgM), which interact with various types of antigens, such as:
- Host cell surface antigens (e.g. RBC membrane antigens like blood group and Rh antigens)
- Extracellular matrix antigens, or
- Exogenous antigens absorbed on host cells (e.g. a drug coating on the RBC membrane).

Various clinical conditions where type II HSN reactions occur are as follows:
- Complement-dependent reaction, e.g. ABO or Rh incompatibility, hemolytic anemia (autoimmune or drug-induced)
- Antibody-dependent cellular cytotoxicity (ADCC)
- Antibody-dependent cellular dysfunction, e.g. Graves' disease and myasthenia gravis.

TYPE III HYPERSENSITIVITY REACTION

Type III HSN reactions develop as a result of the excess formation of immune complexes (Ag-Ab complexes) which initiate an inflammatory response through activation of the complement system leading to tissue injury. Type III reactions occur either in localized or generalized forms.
- **Localized or arthus reaction:** It is defined as a localized area of tissue necrosis due to vasculitis resulting from acute immune complex deposition at the site of inoculation of antigen
  - In skin: Following insect bites

- In lungs: Farmer's lungs, following inhalation of actinomycetes.
- ❖ **Systemic reaction:** Here, the small-sized soluble Ag-Ab complexes are carried in circulation and deposited in various distant sites. Examples include:
  - Connective tissue disorders such as systemic lupus erythematosus and rheumatoid arthritis
  - **Serum sickness:** This condition is not seen nowadays, it was seen in the past, following serum therapy, i.e. administration of foreign serum, e.g. horse anti-tetanus serum, to treat tetanus cases.

TYPE IV HYPERSENSITIVITY REACTION

Type IV HSN reactions differ from other types in various ways:
- ❖ **Delayed type:** It is delayed-type (occurs after 48–72 hours of antigen exposure)
- ❖ **T_{DTH} cells:** It is cell-mediated; characteristic cells called T_{DTH} cells (delayed type of hypersensitivity T cells) are the principal mediators of type IV reactions
- ❖ **Activated macrophages:** Tissue injury occurs predominantly due to activated macrophages
- ❖ **Mechanism:** The type IV HSN reaction occurs in two phases:
  1. *Sensitization phase:* This is the initial phase of 1–2 weeks, that occurs following antigenic exposure. The antigen-presenting cells process and present the antigenic peptides to the helper T cells. T_H cells are differentiated to form T_{DTH} cells
  2. *Effector phase:* The T_{DTH} cells, on subsequent contact with the antigen, secrete a variety of cytokines (e.g interferon-γ) which attract and recruit various inflammatory cells (e.g. macrophages) at the site of DTH reaction.
- ❖ **Granuloma formation:** Pathology of type IV reaction involves granuloma formation: Granuloma consists of an inner zone of epithelioid cells, typically surrounded by a collar of lymphocytes and a peripheral rim of fibroblasts and connective tissue
- ❖ **Common examples** of type IV reaction include:
  - Skin tests such as tuberculin test and lepromin test
  - Contact dermatitis, following exposure to nickel, etc.

► EXPECTED QUESTIONS ◄

I. **Write short notes on:**
1. Type I hypersensitivity reaction.
2. Type II hypersensitivity reaction.
3. Immune complex-mediated hypersensitivity reaction.
4. Type IV hypersensitivity reaction.

II. **Multiple Choice Questions (MCQs):**
1. **Type I hypersensitivity is mediated by which of the following immunoglobulins?**
   a. IgA   b. IgG
   c. IgM   d. IgE

2. **All are early hypersensitivity reactions, except:**
   a. Type I hypersensitivity
   b. Type II hypersensitivity
   c. Type III hypersensitivity
   d. Type IV hypersensitivity

3. **A positive tuberculin test is an example of:**
   a. Type I hypersensitivity
   b. Type II hypersensitivity
   c. Type III hypersensitivity
   d. Type IV hypersensitivity

Answers
1. d   2. d   3. d

CHAPTER 11: Immunoprophylaxis and Immunization Schedule

CHAPTER PREVIEW
- Active Immunoprophylaxis
- Passive Immunoprophylaxis
- National Immunization Schedule

Immunoprophylaxis against microbial pathogens can be classified into active immunoprophylaxis (or vaccination) and passive immunoprophylaxis (or immunoglobulin administration).

VACCINATION (ACTIVE IMMUNOPROPHYLAXIS)

Vaccine is an immunobiological preparation that provides specific protection against a given disease. Following vaccine administration, the immunogen (active ingredient of the vaccine) stimulates the immune system of the body to produce active immunity in the form of protective antibody and/or immunocompetent T cell response.

Vaccines may be of various types based on their method of preparation by using live modified organisms, inactivated or killed organisms, extracted or cellular fractions, toxoids, subunit or combinations of all these. Vaccines of future prospects include DNA vaccine and viral vector vaccine.

Live Attenuated Vaccine

Live vaccines, such as BCG **(Table 11.1)** are prepared from live (usually attenuated) organisms.
- ❖ The live attenuated organisms lose their ability to induce full blown disease, but retain their immunogenicity
- ❖ Attenuation is achieved by passing the live organisms serially through a foreign host, such as chick embryo/tissue culture or live animals
- ❖ Live vaccines in general, are more potent immunizing agents compared to killed vaccines
- ❖ They are capable of inducing mucosal immunity by stimulating secretory IgA antibody production at the local mucosal sites.

Precautions while Using Live Attenuated Vaccines

- ❖ **Contraindications:** Live vaccines should not be administered in individuals with immunodeficiency diseases or any conditions that suppresses the immunity, such as leukemia, lymphoma, malignancies, on corticosteroid or any other immunosuppressive drug therapy
- ❖ **Pregnancy** is another contraindication, unless the risk of infection exceeds the risk of harm to the fetus by giving the live vaccine
- ❖ When **two live vaccines** are required to be given; they should be administered with an interval of at least 4 weeks
- ❖ **Dosage:** Most live vaccines are given in single dose format as effective immunity is achieved with a single dose. Exception is oral polio vaccine (OPV) which is given

SECTION 2 ♦ Immunology

Table 11.1: Example of commonly used vaccines.

Bacterial	Viral
Live attenuated vaccines	
BCG vaccine	Measles vaccine
Typhoral vaccine	Mumps vaccine
	Rubella vaccine
	Live attenuated influenza vaccine
	Chickenpox vaccine
	Oral polio vaccine (OPV)
	Rotavirus vaccine
	Yellow fever 17D vaccine
	Hepatitis A vaccine
	Japanese B encephalitis vaccine (14-14-2 strain)
Killed/inactivated vaccine	
Typhoid vaccine	Injectable polio vaccine (IPV)
Cholera vaccine	Killed influenza vaccine
Pertussis vaccine	Rabies vaccine
Plague vaccine	Covaxin for COVID-19
Toxoid vaccine	**Subunit vaccine**
DT (Diphtheria toxoid)	Hepatitis B vaccine
TT (Tetanus toxoid)	HPV (Human papillomavirus) vaccine
Cellular fraction	**DNA/RNA vaccine**
Meningococcal vaccine	COVID-19 vaccines such as Moderna or Pfizer vaccines
Pneumococcal vaccine	**Viral vector vaccine**
Haemophilus influenzae type b (Hib) vaccine	Covishield vaccine (COVID-19)
Combined vaccine	
DPT vaccine (Diphtheria, pertussis and tetanus)	Mumps, measles, rubella (MMR) vaccine
Pentavalent vaccine (DPT + Hib + Hepatitis B)	

Note: Details about individual vaccine is discussed in the respective chapters.

as multiple doses at spaced intervals to achieve effective immunity
* **Risk of gaining the virulence:** The attenuation of the live vaccine has to be done in an effective way otherwise there is always a risk of gaining the virulence back
* **Storage:** Live vaccines must be stored cautiously to retain effectiveness, especially the OPV and measles vaccine.

Inactivated or Killed Vaccine

It consists of organisms, which are grown in culture under controlled conditions and then killed using methods, such as heat or formaldehyde.
* They are generally safer but less efficacious than live vaccines
* Compared to the live vaccines, killed vaccines require large doses, adjuvants, and multiple doses to confer immunity. In most cases, a booster dose is also needed
* Adjuvants increase the immunogenicity of the vaccine antigen (e.g. alum is used as adjuvant in DPT vaccine)
* Killed vaccines are usually administered in subcutaneous or intramuscular routes. The only absolute contraindication is a severe local or general reaction to the previous dose. Various characteristics of killed and live vaccines are given in **Table 11.2**.

Toxoid Vaccine

The exotoxins produced by certain bacteria can be detoxicated to form toxoid by treating with acidic pH, formalin or by prolonged storage.
* Toxoid is a form of toxin that loses its virulence property but retains immunogenicity
* When a toxoid preparation is given as vaccine, it induces formation of neutralizing antibodies that are capable of neutralizing the toxin moiety produced during an infection; rather than acting upon the organism
* Examples include diphtheria toxoid (from *Corynebac-terium diphtheriae*) and tetanus toxoid (from *Clostridium tetani*).

Extracted or Cellular Fractions Vaccine

Vaccines, in certain instances, are prepared from extracted cellular fractions;

Table 11.2: Characteristics of killed and live vaccines.

Characteristics	Killed vaccine	Live vaccine
Number of doses	Multiple	Single*
Need for adjuvant	Yes	No
Duration of immunity	Shorter	Longer
Effectiveness of protection	Lower	Greater
Mimics natural infection	Less closely	More closely
Immunoglobulins produced	IgG	IgA and IgG
Mucosal immunity	Absent	Induced
Cell-mediated immunity	Poor	Induced
Reverts back to virulent form	No	Possible
Stability at room temperature	High	Low
Immunodeficiency and pregnancy	Safe	Unsafe

*Exception is oral polio vaccine (OPV), which is given as multiple doses at spaced intervals to achieve effective immunity.

examples include meningococcal vaccine, pneumococcal vaccine and *Haemophilus influenzae* type b vaccine—all are prepared from the capsular polysaccharide antigens of the respective organism.

Subunit Vaccines

For certain viruses, only a particular subunit of the virus is necessary to initiate the immunity, e.g. hepatitis B surface antigen (HBsAg) is the immunogenic component of hepatitis B virus. So, this viral component alone can be used as vaccine rather than the whole virus.
- Examples of subunit vaccines include hepatitis B vaccine and human papillomavirus (HPV) vaccine.
- DNA recombinant technology is used for the preparation of such sub-viral components.

Combinations

If more than one immunizing agents are included in a vaccine preparation, it is called combined vaccine. The aim of the combined vaccine is to—
- Simplify administration and
- Augment the immunogenicity of the immunogen. For example, in DPT vaccine, the pertussis component acts as an adjuvant, which increases the immunogenicity of both diphtheria toxoid and tetanus toxoid.

Newer Vaccine Approaches

DNA or RNA Vaccine

DNA or RNA vaccines have recently been marketed. They have many advantages such as cost effectiveness and mounting a stronger and wider range of immune response.

The small pieces of DNA or RNA containing genes from the pathogenic microorganism are injected into the host. The gene of interest gets integrated with the host cell genome and starts transcribing the proteins against which the host mounts an immune response. The classical examples are COVID-19 vaccines such as Moderna or Pfizer vaccines.

Viral Vector Vaccines

The classical example is Covishield vaccine for COVID-19. These vaccines use a safe virus (e.g., Adenovirus) to encode the desired gene (e.g. S gene). Such vaccine when injected cannot cause disease but serves as a platform to produce proteins (e.g. spike proteins) that will stimulate the host immune system.

Cold Chain

"Cold chain" refers to a system of transport, storage, and handling of vaccines, starting at the manufacturer level and ending with the site of administration of the vaccine to the client. The optimum temperature for refrigerated vaccines is between +2°C and +8°C. For frozen vaccines the optimum temperature is –15°C or lower. In addition, protection from light is a necessary condition for some vaccines. Improper cold chain maintenance is one of the most common causes of vaccine failure;

especially oral polio vaccine which is the most sensitive vaccine to heat; must be stored at −20°C.
- ❖ Vaccines which must be stored in the freezer compartment are polio and measles vaccines
- ❖ Vaccines which must be stored in the COLD part but never allowed to freeze are—DPT, TT, Td, BCG, hepatitis B, *H. influenzae* type b and diluents.

Vaccine Vial Monitor

Vaccine vial monitor is a tool to monitor the stability/potency of a vaccine and to check the efficiency of cold chain.

It is heat sensitive label lining the vaccine vial. It contains an outer blue circle and an inner white square. With time and exposure to higher temperature, the inner square changes its color gradually from white towards blue, whereas the outer circle is not heat sensitive; it remains blue throughout **(Table 11.3 and Fig. 11.1)**.

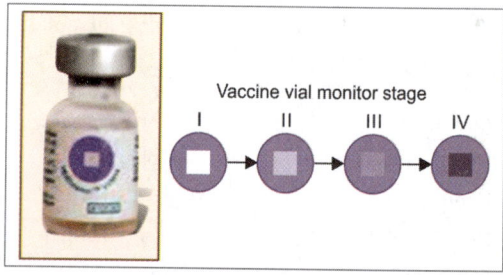

Fig. 11.1: Various stages of vaccine vial monitor (Vaccine is usable up to stages I and II and should be discarded for stages III and IV)

Source: Pondicherry Institute of Medical Sciences, Puducherry (*with permission*).

NATIONAL IMMUNIZATION SCHEDULE (NIS)

Immunization is one of the most logical and cost effective strategies of any country for the prevention of childhood sicknesses and disabilities and is thus a basic need for all children. The following is the national immunization schedule recommended by the Ministry of Health, Government of India and it includes those vaccines that are given free of cost to all children of our country **(Table 11.4)**.

PASSIVE IMMUNOPROPHYLAXIS (IMMUNOGLOBULINS)

Passive immunoprophylaxis is given in the form of commercially available ready made **immunoglobulins** prepared against the pathogenic microorganism. Unlike vaccines, immunoglobulins act faster, without involvement of host immune apparatus.

Passive immunization is useful in the following circumstances:
- ❖ For immunocompromised individuals who cannot synthesize antibodies
- ❖ For post-exposure prophylaxis to achieve an immediate effect.

For the treatment of toxin mediated diseases to ameliorate the effect of toxin. Antibiotics cannot neutralize the toxin; hence, they cannot be used for the treatment of toxin mediated diseases.

Passive immunoprophylaxis available against various microbial diseases is given in **Table 11.5**.

Table 11.3: Staging of vaccine vial monitor.

	Inner square	Outer circle	Vaccine
Stage 1	White	Blue	Can be used
Stage 2	Light blue	Blue	Can be used
Stage 3	Blue	Blue	Discard
Stage 4	Dark blue	Blue	Discard

Table 11.4: National Immunization Schedule (NIS) for infants, children and pregnant women.

Vaccine	When to give	Maximum age	Dose	Dilution	Route	Site
For pregnant women						
TT/Td-1	Early in pregnancy		0.5 mL	No	IM	Upper arm
TT/Td-2	4 weeks after TT/Td-1*	<36 weeks of pregnancy (if missed, can be given later)	0.5 mL	No	IM	Upper arm
TT/Td- Booster	If received 2 TT/Td doses in a pregnancy within the last 3 years*		0.5 mL	No	IM	Upper arm
For infants						
BCG	At birth or as early as possible	Till 1 year	0.05 mL (0.1 mL for >1 month)	Saline	ID	Left upper arm
Hepatitis B - Birth dose	At birth or as early as possible	Within 24 hour	0.5 mL	No	IM	Anterolateral side of mid-thigh
OPV-0	At birth or as early as possible	Within first 15 days	2 drops	No	Oral	Oral
OPV 1, 2 and 3	At 6 weeks, 10 weeks and 14 weeks	5 years of age	2 drops	No	Oral	Oral
Pentavalent# 1, 2 and 3	At 6 weeks, 10 weeks and 14 weeks	1 year of age	0.5 mL	No	IM	Anterolateral side of mid-thigh
PCV^ (3 doses)	At 6 weeks and 14 weeks, booster at 9-12 months	–	0.5 mL	–	IM	Anterolateral side of mid-thigh
Rotavirus##	At 6 weeks, 10 weeks and 14 weeks	1 year of age	5 drops	No	Oral	Oral
IPV	Two fractional doses at 6 and 14 weeks of age	1 year of age	0.1 mL	No	ID	Right upper arm
Measles /MR 1st Dose	9 completed months–12 months	5 years of age (only measles vaccine)	0.5 mL	Sterile water	SC	Right upper arm
JE - 1**	9 completed months–12 months	15 years of age	0.5 mL	Phosphate buffer	SC	Left upper arm
Vitamin A (1st dose)	At 9 completed months, given along MR vaccine	5 years of age	1 mL (1 lakh IU)	No	Oral	Oral

Contd...

Contd...

Vaccine	When to give	Maximum age	Dose	Dilution	Route	Site
For Children						
DPT booster-1	16–24 months	7 years of age	0.5 mL	No	IM	Anterolateral side of mid-thigh
MR 2nd dose$	16–24 months	5 years of age	0.5 mL	Sterile water	SC	Right upper arm
OPV Booster	16–24 months	5 years of age	2 drops	No	Oral	Oral
JE-2	16–24 months	–	0.5 mL	Phosphate buffer	SC	Left upper arm
Vitamin A*** (2nd to 9th dose)	16–18 months. Then one dose every 6 months up to the age of 5 years	5 years of age	2 mL (2 lakh IU)	No	Oral	Oral
DPT Booster-2	5–6 years	7 years of age	0.5 mL	No	IM	Upper arm
TT/Td	10 years and 16 years		0.5 mL	No	IM	Upper arm

***TT/Td:** Tetanus toxoid (TT) is given alone, or in combination with adult diphtheria toxoid (Td). The second or booster dose is ideally given before 36 weeks of pregnancy, but should be given even if presented late in pregnancy or during labor.
***JE Vaccine** is introduced in selected endemic districts after the campaign: UP, Bihar, Assam, West Bengal and Karnataka.
*** The 2nd to 9th doses of Vitamin A can be administered to children 1–5 years old during biannual rounds, in collaboration with ICDS (Integrated Child Development Services).
#**Pentavalent** vaccine- contains combination of DPT, hepatitis B and *H.influenzae* type b vaccines. Interval between two doses of pentavalent vaccine or OPV should never be less than 1 month.
##**Rotavirus vaccine:** Given in selected states such as Andhra Pradesh, Assam, Haryana, Himachal Pradesh, Jharkhand, Madhya Pradesh, Odisha, Rajasthan, Tamil Nadu, Tripura and Uttar Pradesh.
^**Pneumococcal conjugate vaccine (PCV):** Given in selected states such as Bihar, Himachal Pradesh, Madhya Pradesh, Uttar Pradesh (12 districts) & Rajasthan (9 districts).
$**Children who have not been received a single vaccine coming after 1 year:** Will be given 3 doses of DPT at an interval of 4 weeks; Measles-1st dose, JE-1st dose (wherever applicable) up to 2 years of age.
Abbreviations: IM, intramuscular; SC, subcutaneous; ID, intradermal; TT/Td, Tetanus and adult diphtheria toxoid; BCG, Bacillus Calmette-Guerin; PCV, Pneumococcal conjugate vaccine.

Table 11.5: Passive immunoprophylaxis.

Immunoglobulin preparations	Source	Indications
Diphtheria antitoxin	Equine	Treatment of respiratory diphtheria
Tetanus immune globulin (TIG)	Equine, Human	Treatment of tetanus as PEP, for people not adequately immunized with tetanus toxoid
Botulinum antitoxin	Equine, Human	Treatment of botulism
Varicella-zoster immune globulin (VZIG)	Human	PEP for immunosuppressed contacts of acute cases or newborn contacts
Rabies immunoglobulin (RIG)	Equine, Human	Treatment of rabies and PEP in people not previously immunized with rabies vaccine
Hepatitis B immunoglobulin (HBIG)	Human	PEP for percutaneous or mucosal or sexual exposure Newborn of mother with HBsAg +ve
Rubella	Human	Women exposed during early pregnancy
Measles	Human	Infants or immunosuppressed contacts of acute cases exposed <6 days previously

Abbreviation: PEP, post-exposure prophylaxis.

EXPECTED QUESTIONS

I. Write short notes on:
1. Live vaccines vs. killed vaccines.
2. National Immunization Schedule.
3. Passive immunoprophylaxis.

II. Multiple Choice Questions (MCQs):
1. All of the following are live attenuated vaccines, *except:*
   a. MMR
   b. Yellow fever 17D
   c. Salk polio
   d. Sabin polio
2. All the following vaccines are given at birth, *except:*
   a. BCG
   b. Hepatitis B
   c. DPT
   d. OPV
3. Example for subunit vaccine is:
   a. *H. influenza* b vaccine
   b. Hepatitis B vaccine
   c. Meningococcal vaccine
   d. Pertussis vaccine
4. Vaccine administered intradermally is:
   a. MMR
   b. DPT
   c. BCG
   d. Salk polio vaccine

Answers
1. c 2. c 3. b 4. c

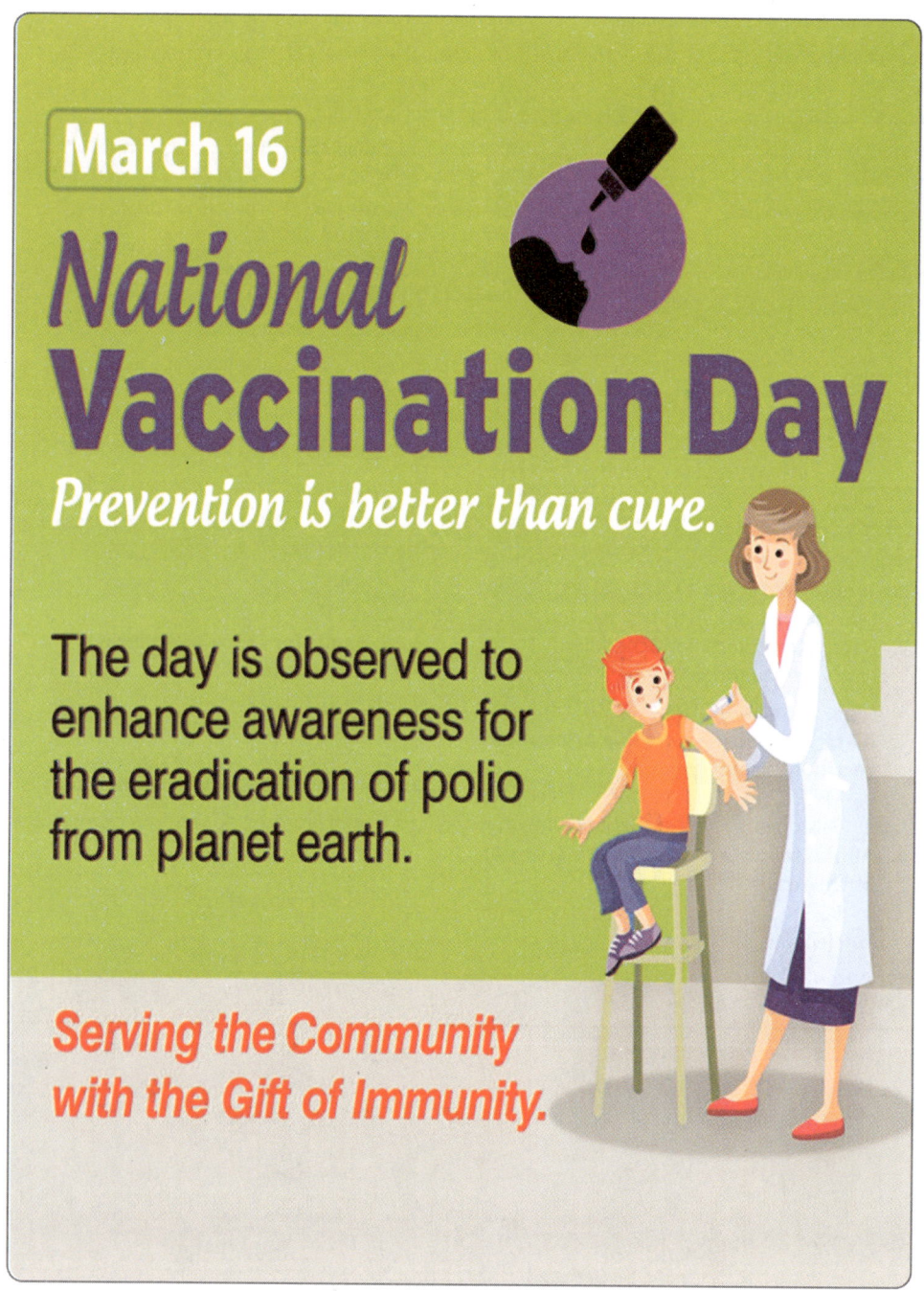

SECTION 3: Bacterial Infections

SECTION OUTLINE

12. Gram-positive and Gram-negative Cocci Infections: *Staphylococcus, Streptococcus, Pneumococcus, Enterococcus* and *Neisseria*
13. Gram-positive Bacilli Infections: *Corynebacterium* and *Bacillus*
14. Anaerobic Infections
15. Mycobacteria Infections
16. Gram-negative Bacilli Infections-I: Enterobacterales and *Vibrio*
17. Gram-negative Bacilli Infections-II: Nonfermenters, Fastidious and Others
18. Miscellaneous Bacterial Infections

ANTIBIOTIC RESISTANCE

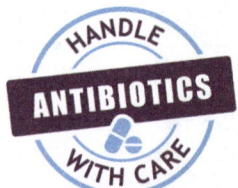

Antibiotic resistance happens when bacteria change and become resistant to the antibiotics used to treat the infections they cause. This is compromising our ability to treat infectious diseases and undermining many advances in medicine.

We must handle antibiotics with care so they remain effective for as long as possible.

WHAT HEALTH WORKERS CAN DO

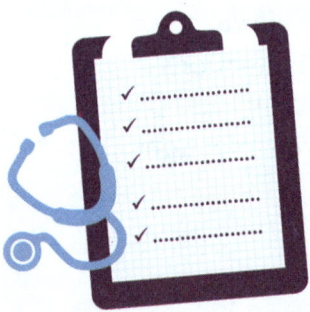

1. **Prevent infections** by ensuring your hands, instruments and environment are clean
2. Keep your patients' **vaccinations** up to date
3. If you think a patient might need antibiotics, where possible, **test to confirm** and find out which one
4. Only prescribe and dispense antibiotics when they are **truly needed**
5. Prescribe and dispense the **right antibiotic** at the right dose for the right duration

www.who.int/drugresistance

#AntibioticResistance

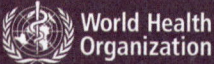

CHAPTER 12

Gram-positive and Gram-negative Cocci Infections

CHAPTER PREVIEW

Gram-positive cocci
- *Staphylococcus*
- *Streptococcus*
- *Enterococcus*

Gram-negative cocci
- Meningococcus
- Gonococcus

GRAM-POSITIVE COCCI INFECTIONS

Gram-positive cocci that are of human importance include:
- *Staphylococcus*: *S. aureus* and coagulase-negative staphylococci (CoNS)
- *Streptococcus*: β-hemolytic streptococci, Viridans streptococci, *S. pneumoniae* (pneumococcus)
- *Enterococcus*: *E. faecalis* and *E. faecium*.

The gram-positive cocci infecting man can be differentiated from each other by various laboratory findings **(Table 12.1)**.

STAPHYLOCOCCUS

Staphylococci can be classified into *S. aureus*, the most pathogenic species to man and other species called coagulase-negative staphylococci (CoNS) that are less pathogenic to man.

Staphylococcus aureus

Staphylococcus aureus is the most common gram-positive cocci infecting humans. It can cause both community and nosocomial acquired infections that may range from relatively milder skin and soft tissue infections to life-threatening systemic infections.

Virulence Factors

The pathogenic potential of *S. aureus* is due to the expression of several virulence factors which include:
- **Toxins** such as hemolysins, exfoliative toxin, enterotoxin, and toxic shock syndrome toxin
- **Extracellular enzymes** such as coagulase, heat-stable thermonuclease, staphylokinase, hyaluronidase, etc.
- **Cell wall-associated factors** such as peptidoglycan layer, teichoic acid, clumping factor, and protein A.

Clinical Manifestations

The clinical spectrum of *S. aureus* includes **(Figs. 12.1A and B)**:
- Skin and soft tissue infections such as folliculitis, furuncle, cellulitis, abscess, impetigo, etc.
- Musculoskeletal infections such as osteomyelitis, septic arthritis, and pyomyositis
- Respiratory tract infections such as pneumonia
- Bacteremia, sepsis, and infective endocarditis
- Urinary tract infections (UTI).

Toxin-mediated infections: *S. aureus* can also cause several toxin-mediated diseases such as:

Organism	Catalase	Gram-positive cocci	Culture finding on blood agar	Other tests
S. aureus	Positive	Arranged in clusters	Pinhead-shaped colonies with a narrow zone of complete (β) hemolysis and golden yellow pigmentation	Coagulase test: positive
CoNS	Positive	Arranged in clusters	Pinhead-shaped colonies without hemolysis and no pigmentation	Coagulase test: negative
β-hemolytic streptococci	Negative	Arranged in short chains	Pinpoint colonies with a wide zone of complete (β) hemolysis	**S. pyogenes:** Bacitracin (S), CAMP test negative **S. agalactiae:** Bacitracin (R), CAMP test positive
Viridans streptococci	Negative	Arranged in long chains	Minute α-hemolytic (green-colored) colonies	Bile solubility test: negative Inulin: not fermented Optochin: resistant
S. pneumoniae	Negative	Arranged in pairs, lanceolate-shaped	Draughtsman-shaped or carom coin-shaped colonies with partial (α) hemolysis	Bile solubility test: positive Inulin: fermented Optochin: sensitive
Enterococcus	Negative	Arranged in pairs, spectacle eye-shaped	Small, translucent, non-hemolytic colonies	Bile esculin test: positive E. faecalis: Arabinose not fermented E. faecium: Arabinose fermented

Abbreviation: CoNS, coagulase-negative staphylococci; S, sensitive; R, resistant; CAMP test, Christie–Atkins–Munch-Peterson test.

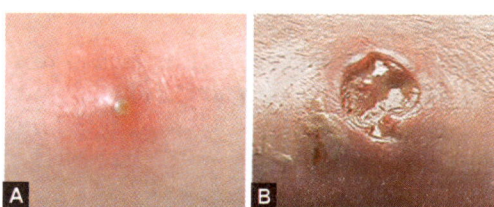

Figs. 12.1A and B: A. Staphylococcal folliculitis; **B.** Staphylococcal abscess (ruptured).

Source: Centers for Disease Control and Prevention (CDC), Atlanta (*with permission*).

- **Scalded skin syndrome:** Mediated by exfoliative toxin (or epidermolytic toxin), characterized by localized tender blisters and bullae formation and exfoliation of the skin
- **Food poisoning:** Mediated by enterotoxin. It is a *preformed toxin* (i.e. secreted in food before consumption) so that it can act rapidly. As a result, the *incubation period is short* (1-6 hours)
- **Toxic shock syndrome:** Mediated by toxic shock syndrome toxin (TSS)
  - It is common among women using vaginal tampons during menstruation
  - The toxin is absorbed into circulation to cause a potentially fatal multisystem disease with erythematous rashes.

HAI: Overall, *S. aureus* is a leading cause of healthcare-associated infections (HAI). The hospital staff are the potential carriers of *S. aureus*. Hospital strains are often multidrug-resistant, spread to patients either from hospital staff/other patients/environment or also from patients' skin flora.

Laboratory Diagnosis

The various specimens collected depend on the nature of the lesion such as pus, wound swab, sputum, midstream urine, and blood.

CHAPTER 12 ♦ Gram-positive and Gram-negative Cocci Infections

- **Direct smear microscopy:** Reveals gram-positive cocci in clusters and pus cells **(Fig. 12.2A)**
- **Culture:** Incubation at 37°C for 24h reveals the following growth:
  - Nutrient agar—produces golden yellow-pigmented colonies
  - Blood agar—shows pin-head colonies with a narrow zone of complete (β) hemolysis **(Fig. 12.3)**
  - Selective media such as mannitol salt agar—produces yellow colonies.
- **Culture smear microscopy** from the colonies reveals gram-positive cocci in clusters **(Fig. 12.2B)**
- **Biochemical identification:** Various tests which help in the identification of *S. aureus* are:
  - Catalase test—positive (differentiates staphylococci from streptococci)
  - Coagulase test—positive (differentiates *S. aureus* from CoNS). Two test formats are available: slide coagulase and tube coagulase tests **(Figs. 12.4A to C)**
  - Protein A detection (differentiates *S. aureus* from CoNS).
- **Automated identification systems** such as VITEK and MALDI-TOF can be performed for rapid and accurate identification of *S. aureus*
- **Antimicrobial susceptibility testing** can be performed by disk diffusion method (on Mueller–Hinton agar) or MIC-based method (VITEK).

TREATMENT — S. aureus

S. aureus is primarily treated by anti-staphylococcal penicillins such as cloxacillin.

However, for MRSA infections (see below), vancomycin is the drug of choice. Others include clindamycin, doxycycline, co-trimoxazole, or linezolid, etc.

MRSA

Methicillin-resistant *S. aureus* (MRSA) is a resistant phenotype, that has been increasingly reported over the last few decades. It shows resistance to all β-lactam antimicrobials and thus possesses a great therapeutic challenge. It is widespread in hospital settings, causing several outbreaks.

Contd...

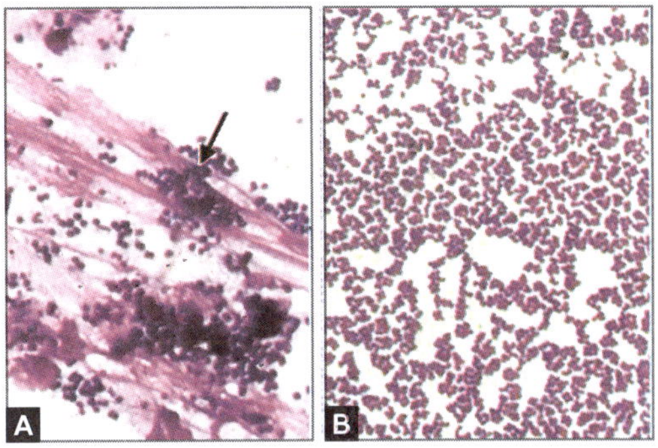

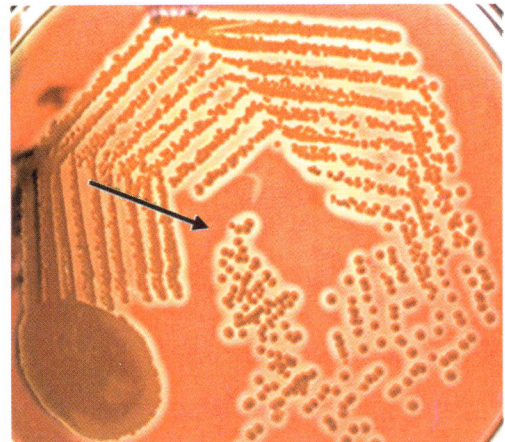

Figs. 12.2A and B: A. Direct smear: arrow showing gram-positive cocci in clusters with pus cells; **B.** Culture smear showing gram-positive cocci in clusters.

Source: Department of Microbiology, JIPMER, Puducherry (*with permission*).

Fig. 12.3: Colonies of *S. aureus*: Blood agar—arrow shows a narrow zone of beta-hemolysis surrounding the colonies.

Source: Department of Microbiology, Pondicherry Institute of Medical Sciences, Puducherry (*with permission*).

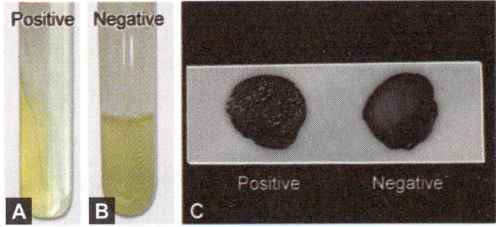

Figs. 12.4A to C: Coagulase test: **A.** Tube coagulase test (positive); **B.** Tube coagulase test (negative); **C.** Slide showing coagulase test.

Source: Department of Microbiology, Pondicherry Institute of Medical Sciences, Puducherry (*with permission*).

Contd...

- **Mechanism:** Mediated by a gene called ***mecA gene***, which alters penicillin-binding protein (PBP) present on *S. aureus* cell wall to PBP2a.
  - PBP is an essential protein needed for the cell wall synthesis of bacteria. β-lactam drugs bind and inhibit this protein, thereby inhibiting the cell wall synthesis
  - The altered PBP2a of MRSA strains have less affinity for β-lactam antibiotics; hence, MRSA strains are resistant to all β-lactam antibiotics
- **Epidemiology:** MRSA rate is very high, accounting for 30-40% of *S. aureus* infections in India
- **Detection:** By performing a susceptibility test for oxacillin or cefoxitin
- **Treatment:** Vancomycin or linezolid are recommended for serious infections, whereas doxycycline or cotrimoxazole can be given for nonlife-threatening infections.

Control Measures

Prevention of spread of *S. aureus* infections in hospitals involves:

- Ensure proper **infection control measures** such as hand hygiene (most efficient way to prevent hospital spread), isolation of the patients and all other measures of **contact precautions** (described in detail in Chapter 38)
  - **Screening of MRSA carriers** among hospital staff should be done when there is an outbreak
  - **Treatment of carriers** is done by use of topical 2% mupirocin (for nasal carriers) and chlorhexidine body bath (for skin carriers)
  - **Stoppage of antibiotic misuse** in hospitals.

Coagulase-negative Staphylococci (CoNS)

Other species of *Staphylococcus* do not produce coagulase enzyme and are called as coagulase-negative staphylococci (CoNS).

- They are usually harmless skin commensals and rarely pathogenic to man
- They are less virulent than *S. aureus* and may cause infections in immunocompromised patients, infections in prosthetic devices associated, and surgical site infections
- *S. epidermidis* is the most common CoNS infecting man
- Others include—*S. saprophyticus, S. lugdunensis, S. schleiferi,* and *S. haemolyticus.*

STREPTOCOCCUS

Streptococci can be classified based on the pattern of hemolysis they produce on blood agar.

- **α or partial hemolysis**: Greenish discoloration surrounding the colonies; e.g. Viridans streptococci and *S. pneumoniae*
- **β or complete hemolysis:** Yellowish discoloration surrounding the colonies; e.g. β-hemolytic streptococci such as *S. pyogenes* and *S. agalactiae*
- **γ hemolysis:** No hemolysis surrounding the colonies; e.g. *Enterococcus* (now it is separated from the genus *Streptococcus*).

Lancefield grouping: The β-hemolytic streptococci are further classified based on the C-carbohydrate antigen in the cell wall into 20 serological groups. The majority of streptococci causing human infection include—group A streptococci (*S. pyogenes*) and group B streptococci (*S. agalactiae*).

Streptococcus pyogenes

Streptococcus pyogenes (group A *Streptococcus*) is one of the leading cause of pyogenic infections in humans.

Virulence Factors

The virulence factors of *S. pyogenes* include:
- Cell wall antigens such as C-carbohydrate antigens, M protein, capsule, etc.
- Toxins such as streptococcal pyrogenic exotoxin and hemolysins
- Various enzymes such as streptokinase, streptodornase, hyaluronidase, etc.

Clinical Manifestations

Streptococcus pyogenes is associated with a variety of suppurative and non-suppurative manifestations.

- **Suppurative manifestations** include:
  - Sore throat (pharyngitis): *S. pyogenes* is the most common bacterial cause of pharyngitis in children
  - Superficial skin and soft-tissue infections: Such as impetigo, cellulitis, and erysipelas
  - Necrotizing fasciitis: Involves extensive necrosis of subcutaneous tissue, fascia, and muscles
  - Bacteremia
  - Toxic shock syndrome (mediated by streptococcal pyrogenic exotoxin)
  - Puerperal sepsis, following vaginal delivery.
- **Non-suppurative manifestations** are acute rheumatic fever (affecting the heart) and post-streptococcal glomerulonephritis (affecting the kidney). The underlying pathogenesis is due to *molecular mimicry*; where, the antibodies produced against previous streptococcal infections cross-react with human tissues (heart or kidneys) to produce lesions.

Laboratory Diagnosis

The specimen to be collected depends on the site of the infection. Common specimens are pus, throat swab, blood, etc.
- **Direct smear microscopy:** Reveals pus cells with gram-positive cocci in short chains **(Fig. 12.5A)**

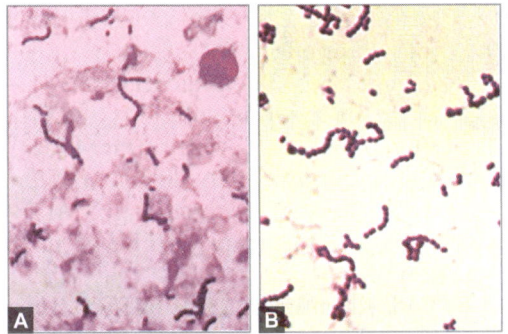

Figs. 12.5A and B: Streptococci: **A.** In Gram-stained smear of pus; **B.** In culture smear showing gram-positive cocci in short chains.

Source: Department of Microbiology, Pondicherry Institute of Medical Sciences, Puducherry (*with permission*).

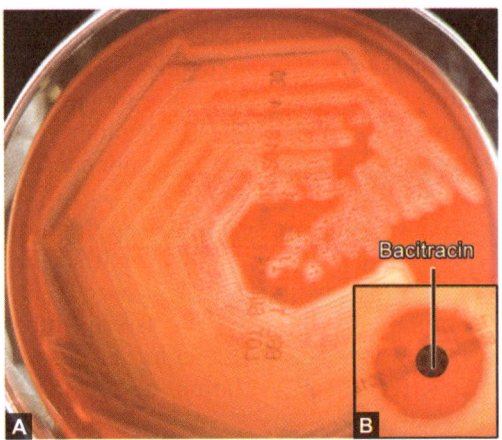

Figs. 12.6A and B: *Streptococcus pyogenes:* **A.** Growth on blood agar with a wide zone of beta-hemolysis around the pinpoint colonies; **B.** Bacitracin sensitive.

Source: Department of Microbiology, JIPMER, Puducherry (*with permission*).

- **Culture** on blood agar reveals pinpoint colonies with a wide zone of β-hemolysis **(Fig. 12.6A)**
- **Culture smear** microscopy from the colonies reveals gram-positive cocci in short chains **(Fig. 12.5B)**
- **Biochemical identification:** Various tests which help in the identification of *S. pyogenes* are:
  - Catalase negative
  - Susceptible to bacitracin **(Fig. 12.6B)**
  - CAMP (Christie, Atkins, and Munch-Peterson) test: Negative.
- **Lancefield grouping** shows group A *Streptococcus*
- **Automated ID systems** such as VITEK and MALDI-TOF can be performed for rapid and accurate identification of *S. pyogenes*
- **Serology:** ASO (anti-streptolysin O) antibodies and anti-DNase B antibodies are elevated
- **Antimicrobial susceptibility testing** can be performed by disk diffusion method (on Mueller–Hinton blood agar) or MIC-based method (VITEK).

TREATMENT — S. pyogenes

The infections caused by *S. pyogenes* are primarily treated by penicillin. Erythromycin can be given in case of penicillin allergy.

Streptococcus agalactiae

Streptococcus agalactiae colonizes the female genital tract and therefore the infection is common in neonates and in pregnancy.
- It has been recognized as a major cause of neonatal sepsis and meningitis
- Infections in pregnancy can lead to peripartum fever, endometritis, and puerperal sepsis
- Similar to *S. pyogenes*, it also produces β-hemolytic pinpoint colonies, gram-positive cocci in chains, and catalase negative
- But it differs from *S. pyogenes*, being bacitracin resistant, CAMP test positive and Lancefield grouping showing group B *Streptococcus*
- Penicillin/ampicillin plus gentamicin are the drug of choice for all *S. agalactiae* infections.

Viridans streptococci

Viridans streptococci are commensals of the mouth and upper respiratory tract.
- However, occasionally they can cause infections such as dental caries, subacute bacterial endocarditis and suppurative infections
- They appear as long chains of gram-positive cocci and produce minute α-hemolytic colonies on blood agar
- They are usually susceptible to penicillin and vancomycin.

Streptococcus pneumoniae (Pneumococcus)

Streptococcus pneumoniae, commonly referred to as pneumococcus is the leading cause of lobar pneumonia, otitis media in children, and meningitis in all ages.
- **Clinical manifestations:** *S. pneumoniae* can cause both invasive infections such as lobar pneumonia, bloodstream infection, pyogenic meningitis, septic arthritis and non-invasive infections such as otitis media and sinusitis
- **Risk factors** for pneumococcal infection include—children less than two years, splenectomy, underlying comorbid conditions (e.g. chronic lung, kidney, and liver disease), etc.
- **Laboratory diagnosis:** Clinical specimens include CSF, blood, sputum, etc. depending on the system involved
  - *Gram stain:* Pneumococci appear as capsulated gram-positive cocci in pair, lanceolate-shaped **(Fig. 12.7)**
  - *Antigen detection:* Detection of capsular antigens in CSF by latex agglutination test
  - *Culture:* On blood agar, pneumococci produce characteristic draughtsman or carom coin-shaped α-hemolytic colonies **(Fig. 12.8A)** and on chocolate agar, it produces greenish discoloration (bleaching effect)
  - *Identification:* Pneumococcus shows—(i) a positive bile solubility test, (ii) susceptibility to optochin **(Fig. 12.8B)**, and (iii) positive for inulin fermentation. Automated ID systems (e.g. MALDI-TOF or VITEK) can also be used for identification
  - **Antimicrobial susceptibility testing:** It can be performed by disk diffusion method (on Mueller–Hinton blood agar) or MIC-based method (VITEK).
- **Treatment:** Meningitis and bacteremia cases respond well to penicillin-G.

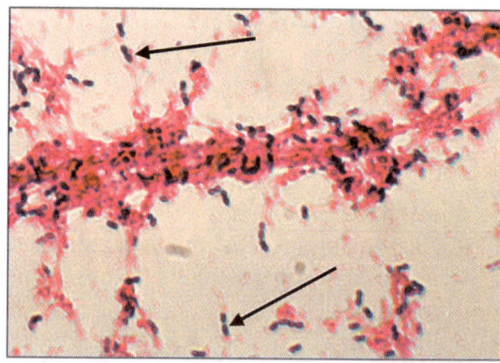

Fig. 12.7: Pneumococci in Gram stained smear of sputum [lanceolate shaped gram-positive cocci in pair surrounded by clear halo (capsule)].

Source: Public Health Image Library, ID#/2896/Dr Mike Miller/Centers for Disease Control and Prevention (CDC), Atlanta (*with permission*).

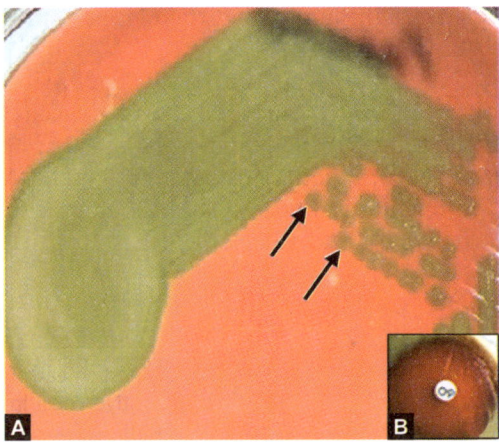

Figs. 12.8A and B: Properties of pneumococci: **A.** α-hemolytic draughtsman-shaped colonies on blood agar; **B.** Sensitive to optochin.

Source: Department of Microbiology, Pondicherry Institute of Medical Sciences, Puducherry (*with permission*).

Ceftriaxone or vancomycin can be given in case of penicillin resistance
- Meningitis cases require early treatment as are associated with high fatality
- Pneumonia cases can be treated with oral amoxicillin or levofloxacin or IV ceftriaxone.

❖ **Infection control measures** such as droplet precautions should be followed in hospitals (refer Chapter 38)

❖ **Vaccine**: There are two vaccines available for pneumococcus:
- 23-valent pneumococcal polysaccharide vaccine (PPSV23)—given to high-risk adults such to old age, immunodeficiency, splenic dysfunction, etc., but not to children. It is less immunogenic and provides short-term immunity
- Pneumococcal conjugate vaccine (PCV13)—given both to children and high-risk adults. It is more immunogenic and provides longer immunity.

ENTEROCOCCUS

Enterococci are part of the normal flora of the human intestine. *E. faecalis* and *E. faecium* are the common species infecting man.

❖ **Clinical manifestations:** Enterococci can cause various infections ranging from UTI, chronic prostatitis, bacteremia, endocarditis, and intra-abdominal infections

❖ **Laboratory diagnosis**: Enterococci have the following laboratory features.
- *Gram stain:* They appear oval-shaped gram-positive cocci in pairs; at an angle to each other
- *Culture:* Produce non-hemolytic translucent colonies on blood agar
- *Identification:* Enterococci show a positive bile esculin hydrolysis test. *E. faecalis* and *E. faecium* are differentiated by the arabinose test. Automated ID systems can also be used for identification
- **Antimicrobial susceptibility testing:** It can be performed by disk diffusion method (on Mueller–Hinton agar) or MIC-based method (VITEK).

❖ **Treatment**: Enterococci can be treated with ampicillin ± gentamicin, vancomycin, and fosfomycin.

GRAM-NEGATIVE COCCI INFECTIONS

Gram-negative cocci that are pathogenic to man are *Neisseria meningitidis* and *Neisseria gonorrhoeae*.

NEISSERIA MENINGITIDIS

N. meningitidis (or meningococci) are capsulated gram-negative diplococci— one of the important causes of pyogenic meningitis.

❖ **Virulence factors:** Pathogenesis of meningococcal infection is due to the expression of several virulence factors
- Important virulence factors are—polysaccharide capsule, endotoxin, and outer membrane proteins
- Based on the capsule, meningococci can be typed into several serotypes
- Serotypes A, B, C, X, Y and W135 cause invasive disease.

❖ **Clinical manifestations:** Meningococcus is transmitted by droplet inhalation
- The majority of infections result in a nasopharyngeal carriage

- In susceptible children, it spreads through the hematogenous route to CNS to cause pyogenic meningitis
- Systemic spread can cause fatal septicemia and complication such as Waterhouse–Friderichsen syndrome—characterized by adrenal hemorrhage, disseminated intravascular coagulation, purpuric rashes, and shock.
- **Epidemiology**: Meningococcus causes several patterns of invasive disease ranging from sporadic infection, to endemic, and explosive epidemics
  - The serogroups distribution varies among various regions of the world
  - The sub-Saharan belt of Africa is the most prevalent area.
- **Laboratory diagnosis**: Useful specimens are CSF and blood for cases and nasopharyngeal swab for carriers
  - *Gram stain* reveals gram-negative diplococci, capsulated, lens-shaped **(Fig. 12.9)**
  - *Useful culture media* are—blood agar and chocolate agar (for CSF specimen), blood culture bottles (for blood), and Thayer Martin media (for nasopharyngeal swab)
  - *Identification:* It is catalase and oxidase-positive, ferments glucose and maltose.
- **Treatment:** Third-generation cephalosporins such as ceftriaxone are the drug of choice. Meningitis cases are associated with high fatality and therefore warrant early treatment
- **Vaccines:** Capsular polysaccharide vaccine and conjugated capsular vaccine are available for meningococcus
- **Infection control measures** such as droplet precautions should be followed in hospitals (refer Chapter 38).

NEISSERIA GONORRHOEAE

Neisseria gonorrhoeae causes a sexually transmitted infection (STI), known as 'gonorrhea'.
- **Virulence factors** of *N. gonorrhoeae* that mediate pathogenesis include—pili (helps in adhesion) and outer membrane protein
- **Clinical manifestations:** Gonorrhea commonly manifests as:
  - In males: Acute urethritis, characterized by purulent urethral discharge
  - In females: Mucopurulent cervicitis is the most common presentation
  - In both sexes: Anorectal and pharyngeal gonorrhea
  - Among neonates: Transmission during delivery from the maternal genital tract to the baby can cause conjunctivitis *(ophthalmia neonatorum)* in the newborn
  - Disseminated gonococcal infection: Presents as polyarthritis, and endocarditis.
- **Laboratory diagnosis**: Urethral swabs (for males) and endocervical swabs (for females) are the ideal specimens. Specimens should be collected in charcoal-coated swabs (Stuart's transport medium)
  - They appear gram-negative intracellular kidney-shaped diplococci **(Fig. 12.10)**
  - For culture, selective media such as Thayer-Martin medium and modified New York City medium are used
  - It is oxidase-positive, and ferments only glucose, but not maltose.
- **Treatment:** Third-generation cephalosporin such as ceftriaxone is the drug of choice. Both sexual partners should be treated.

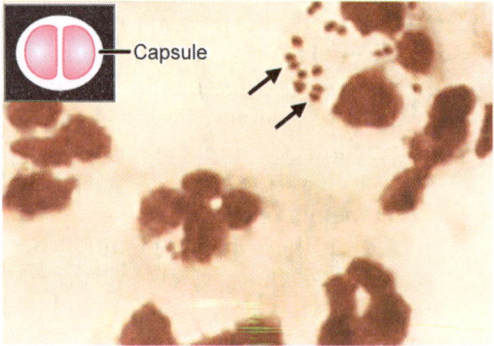

Fig. 12.9: Meningococci in CSF smear (gram-negative diplococci, lens-shaped) (arrows showing).
Source: Centers for Disease Control and Prevention (CDC), Atlanta *(with permission)*.

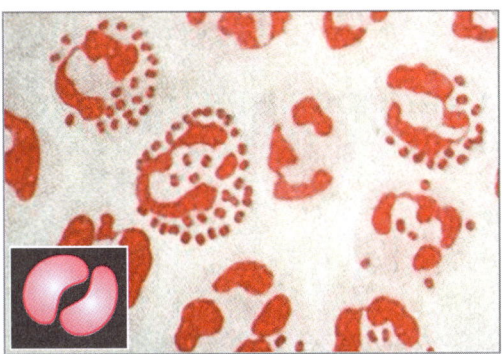

Fig. 12.10: Gonococcus (gram-negative diplococci, kidney-shaped).
Source: Public Health Image Library, ID# /2108, Centers for Disease Control and Prevention (CDC), Atlanta *(with permission)*.

EXPECTED QUESTIONS

I. Write an essay on:
1. Discuss the manifestations, laboratory diagnosis, and treatment of staphylococcal infections.

II. Write short notes on:
1. Infections are caused by *S. pyogenes*.
2. Laboratory diagnosis and treatment of pneumococcal infections.
3. Methicillin-resistant *Staphylococcus aureus* (MRSA).
4. Meningococcal meningitis.
5. Clinical manifestations and laboratory diagnosis of gonorrhea.
6. Write briefly on clinical spectrum and laboratory diagnosis of enterococci infections.

III. Multiple Choice Questions (MCQs):
1. Scalded skin syndrome is mediated by:
    a. Hemolysin
    b. Coagulase
    c. Enterotoxin
    d. Exfoliative toxin
2. All of the above can be given for the treatment of MRSA, *except*:
    a. Meropenem b. Vancomycin
    c. Cotrimoxazole d. Linezolid
3. *Streptococcus pyogenes* can be differentiated from *S. agalactiae* by testing susceptibility to:
    a. Optochin b. Bacitracin
    c. Polymyxin d. Novobiocin
4. Pneumococcus can be identified by testing susceptibility to:
    a. Polymyxin b. Novobiocin
    c. Optochin d. Bacitracin
5. Carrom coin appearance of colonies is seen for:
    a. *S. pyogenes*
    b. Viridans streptococci
    c. *S. agalactiae*
    d. *S. pneumoniae*
6. Serotyping of meningococci are based on:
    a. Outer membrane proteins
    b. Endotoxin
    c. Capsular polysaccharide
    d. Transferrin binding proteins
7. Which of the following is the property of enterococci?
    a. Bacitracin sensitive
    b. CAMP positive
    c. Bile esculin hydrolysis
    d. Optochin sensitive

Answers
1. d   2. a   3. b   4. c   5. d   6. c   7. c

CHAPTER 13

Gram-positive Bacilli Infections

CHAPTER PREVIEW

- *Corynebacterium* species
- *Bacillus* species
- Other Gram-positive Bacilli Infections

Gram-positive bacilli of human importance include:
- *Corynebacterium* species
- *Bacillus* species
- *Clostridium* species: Discussed in Chapter 14, along with other anaerobic infections
- Mycobacteria (discussed in Chapter 15)
- Others: *Listeria* and Actinomycetes (discussed later in this chapter).

CORYNEBACTERIUM SPECIES

Corynebacteria are club-shaped gram-positive bacilli. *C. diphtheriae* is the most important species pathogenic to man; other species called *diphtheroids* are mainly skin commensals, and occasionally can be pathogenic to man.

Corynebacterium diphtheriae

Corynebacterium diphtheriae is the causative agent of **diphtheria**—a contagious disease, characterized by pseudomembrane formation over the tonsil. It commonly affects unvaccinated children.

Virulence Factors

The pathogenesis of diphtheria is mediated by diphtheria toxin; which acts by inhibiting protein synthesis.
- **Diphtheria toxin** is a bacteriophage coded toxin, comprises of two fragments—A and B
  - *Fragment B* binds to the host cell receptors and helps in the entry of fragment A
  - *Fragment A* is the active fragment, that gets internalized into the host cell and causes inhibition of protein synthesis by inhibiting elongation factor 2 (EF-2).
- **Transmission** occurs through inhalation of respiratory droplets (by coughing or sneezing)
- **Spread:** Organism does not invade, multiplies only at the local site, and secrets toxin. It is the toxin that enters the circulation and goes to various sites to produce various clinical manifestations.

Clinical Manifestations

Respiratory diphtheria is the most common form; characterized by—the presence of a tough leathery greyish white pseudomembrane, formed over the tonsils.

The **other manifestations** are cutaneous diphtheria and less commonly, toxic systemic complications such as myocarditis and neurologic manifestations.

Epidemiology

The incidence of diphtheria is greatly reduced after the introduction of widespread immunization. However, there are reports of a resurgence of cases in older children with incomplete booster doses. India still accounts for the maximum number of cases globally. The main source of infection is the carriers (nasal and throat), which is common in children.

Laboratory Diagnosis

The role of laboratory diagnosis is to: (i) confirmation of clinical diagnosis, (ii) initiate the control measures, and (iii) for epidemiological purposes. However, treatment should promptly be started, not be delayed for obtaining laboratory results.

- **Specimens:** Throat swabs containing fibrinous exudates and a portion of pseudomembrane are the ideal specimens
- **Direct microscopy** of the specimen reveals:
  - *Gram stain:* Shows club-shaped gram-positive bacilli in Chinese letter or cuneiform arrangement, i.e. V- or L-shaped, due to dividing bacilli attached at an angle to each other at their ends **(Fig. 13.1A)**
  - *Albert's stain:* Shows characteristic green bacilli with bluish-black metachromatic granules at the poles **(Fig. 13.1B)**.
- **Culture:** Important culture media are:
  - Enriched media such as blood agar and Loeffler's serum slope **(Fig. 13.2A)**
  - *Potassium tellurite agar:* It is a selective media. *C. diphtheriae* produces black colored colonies after 48h of incubation **(Fig. 13.2B)**.
- **Identification** of the *C. diphtheriae* grown in culture is confirmed by various biochemical tests (e.g. serum sugar fermentation test) or by automated ID systems such as MALDI-TOF or VITEK
- **Toxin demonstration:** As *C. diphtheriae* can also be found as a colonizer in throat, demonstration of toxin (DT) production following isolation is important to establish the pathogenesis. Toxin demonstration can be done by:
  - Elek's gel precipitation test
  - Detection of DT by immunoassays
  - Detection of gene coding DT by PCR.

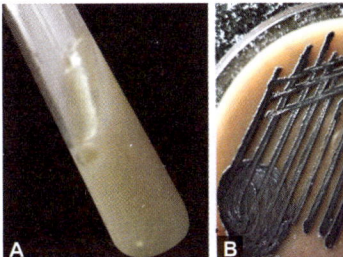
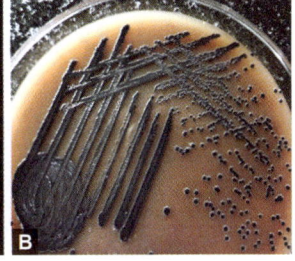

Figs. 13.2A and B: A. Loeffler's serum slope; **B.** Potassium tellurite agar shows black colonies.
Source: Department of Microbiology, **A.** JIPMER, Puducherry; **B.** PIMS, Puducherry (*with permission*).

| TREATMENT | Diphtheria |

Diphtheria is a medical emergency, and should be treated at the earliest. The treatment regimen comprises:
- **Anti-diphtheritic serum:** Passive immunization with anti-diphtheritic horse serum is the treatment of choice as it neutralizes the toxin.
- **Antibiotics** such as penicillin or erythromycin: It has a role if given early in treatment before toxin release. Antibiotics are also useful for the treatment of carriers.

Infection Control Measures

Patient should be placed in isolation room and all the steps of droplet precaution should be followed for the prevention of transmission of *C. diphtheriae* in hospitals (refer Chapter 38).

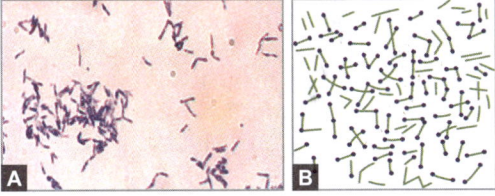

Figs. 13.1A and B: *Corynebacterium diphtheriae*: **A.** Gram-stained smear shows V- or L-shaped bacilli with cuneiform arrangement; **B.** Albert's stain shows dark blue metachromatic granules at the ends of the green bacilli (schematic).
Source: **A.** Public Health Image Library, ID# /1943; Centers for Disease Control and Prevention (CDC), Atlanta (*with permission*).

Vaccine

The diphtheria vaccine (toxoid) is given under the national immunization schedule as a combined vaccine along with pertussis and tetanus (DPT vaccine).

- **Children:** A total of seven doses are given
  - Three doses of pentavalent vaccine (DPT + hepatitis B+ *Haemophilus influenzae* b) at 6, 10, and 14 weeks of birth, followed by
  - Two booster doses of DPT at 16–24 months and 5 years, and
  - Another two booster doses of Td (tetanus toxoid, adult dose of diphtheria toxoid) at 10 years and 16 years.
- **A pregnant woman** also should receive two doses of Td at one month interval
- **Site:** DPT is given deep intramuscularly (IM) at the anterolateral aspect of the thigh
- **Thiomersal** (0.01%) is used as a preservative
- **Storage:** DPT should be kept at 2–8°C; if accidentally frozen then it has to be discarded
- **Protective titer:** Following vaccination, an antitoxin titer of ≥ 0.01 IU/mL is said to be protective.

BACILLUS SPECIES

Bacillus species are gram-positive spore-bearing bacilli.
- The important pathogens are *B. anthracis* (causes anthrax) and *B. cereus* (causes food poisoning)
- Other *Bacillus* species (called as anthracoid bacilli) are common laboratory contaminants.

Bacillus anthracis

Bacillus anthracis is the causative agent of anthrax, an important zoonotic disease transmitted by occupational exposure to infected animals such as cattle and sheep.

Pathogenesis

The pathogenesis of anthrax is mediated by two important virulence factors—
1. **Capsule:** It is polypeptide in nature, and acts by inhibiting phagocytosis
2. **Anthrax toxin:** It has three fragments; edema factor, protective factor and lethal factor.

Clinical Manifestations

B. anthracis is transmitted in three modes—contact, inhalation and ingestion. Accordingly anthrax in humans manifests in three forms.
1. **Cutaneous anthrax** (Hide porter's disease): It is the most common form (95%), characterized by black eschar surrounded by non-pitting called **malignant pustule** (Fig. 13.3)
2. **Pulmonary anthrax:** Wool sorter's disease (as commonly seen in workers of wool factory), characterized by hemorrhagic mediastinitis
3. **Intestinal anthrax** is very rare.

Laboratory Diagnosis

The useful specimens include—pus, sputum, blood, and CSF.
- **Gram stain:** *B. anthracis* appears as long chains of gram-positive bacilli with non-bulging spores, described as bamboo stick appearance
- **McFadyean's reaction:** Shows amorphous purple capsule surrounding blue bacilli (polychrome methylene blue stain)
- **Culture media:** Culture properties useful for identification are:
  - Medusa head appearance colonies on nutrient agar (seen under 10x microscope)
  - Dry wrinkled, nonhemolytic colonies on blood agar

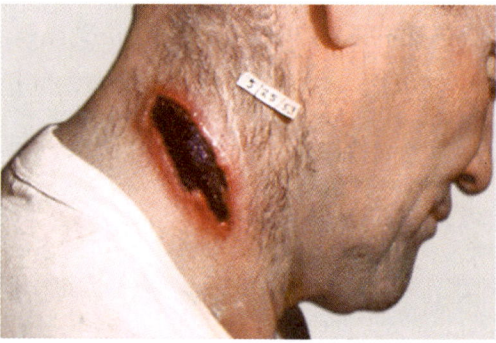

Fig. 13.3: Malignant pustule.
Source: Public Health Image Library, ID# 1934/Centers for Disease Control and Prevention (CDC), Atlanta (*with permission*).

- Inverted fir tree appearance growth on gelatin stab agar.

> **TREATMENT** — Anthrax
>
> Ciprofloxacin or doxycycline are the drugs of choice, given for:
> - 7-10 days for treatment of anthrax
> - 60 days for post-exposure prophylaxis (along with anthrax vaccine)

Vaccine

Two important vaccines are available for anthrax.
- Live attenuated, non-capsulated spore vaccine
- Adsorbed (alum precipitated) toxoid vaccine containing the protective factor.

Bacillus cereus Food Poisoning

Bacillus cereus is a normal habitant of soil, also widely isolated from food items. It is an important agent of food poisoning in man; mediated by producing two types of toxins—
1. **Emetic toxin:** causes emetic type of food poisoning
   - It is a preformed toxin (like *S. aureus* enterotoxin), that acts immediately after food intake, and therefore the incubation period is short (1–6 hours)
   - Associated with the consumption of contaminated fried rice with emetic toxin.
2. **Diarrheal toxin:** causes a diarrheal type of food poisoning. Organism secretes this toxin only after entering the intestine, hence the incubation period is longer (8–16 hours).

OTHER GRAM-POSITIVE BACILLI INFECTIONS

Listeria

Listeria monocytogenes is a food-borne pathogen that can cause serious infections, particularly in neonates (neonatal meningitis and sepsis), pregnant women, and elderly people.
- Laboratory diagnosis involves CSF and blood culture
- Ampicillin is the drug of choice, given for 2–3 weeks in combination with gentamicin.

Actinomycetes

Actinomycetes are a diverse group of gram-positive bacilli arranged in chains or branching filaments. Important genera include:
- *Actinomyces:* They are anaerobe and non-acid fast; produce a clinical condition called actinomycosis, characterized by a painless, slow-growing mass with a cutaneous fistula in the cervicofacial region
- *Nocardia:* They are aerobe and acid-fast; cause pulmonary infection and a subcutaneous infection called actinomycetoma.

EXPECTED QUESTIONS

I. **Write short notes on:**
   1. Laboratory diagnosis of diphtheria.
   2. Diphtheria vaccine.
   3. Clinical forms of anthrax.

II. **Multiple Choice Questions (MCQs):**
   1. Chinese letter pattern is observed in microscopy for_____?
      a. *C. diphtheriae*
      b. *Bacillus anthracis*
      c. *Clostridium* species
      d. Mycobacteria
   2. Bamboo stick appearance is observed in microscopy for_____?
      a. Mycobacteria
      b. *Bacillus anthracis*
      c. *C. diphtheriae*
      d. *Clostridium* species
   3. Selective medium used for *C. diphtheriae* is _____?
      a. Blood agar
      b. Chocolate agar
      c. LJ medium
      d. Potassium tellurite agar

Answers
1. a   2. b   3. d

CHAPTER 14

Anaerobic Infections

> **CHAPTER PREVIEW**
> - *Clostridium* Species
> - Non-sporing Anaerobes

The obligate anaerobic bacteria infecting man can be grouped into spore-bearing (e.g. *Clostridium*) and non-sporing anaerobes.

CLOSTRIDIUM SPECIES

Clostridia are gram-positive bacilli with bulging spores, commonly found as saprophytes in soil and commensals in the intestine of man and animals. However, few members can cause a variety of infections in humans.
- *Clostridium perfringens*: causes gas gangrene
- *Clostridium tetani*: causes tetanus
- *Clostridium botulinum*: causes botulism
- *Clostridioides difficile*: causes pseudomembranous colitis.

Clostridium perfringens

It is an intestinal commensal and also a soil saprophyte. It is the causative agent of **gas gangrene**, a rapidly spreading edematous myonecrosis.

Pathogenesis

The pathogenesis is due to its invasiveness and liberation of a variety of toxins including α-toxin (lecithinase), which is the principal virulence factor.

Clinical Manifestations

Clostridium perfringens infections are mostly polymicrobial involving other clostridia species. Various manifestations include:
- **Clostridial wound infections:** It occurs in three stages—(i) simple wound contamination, (ii) anaerobic cellulitis, (iii) anaerobic myositis or gas gangrene

> **Gas gangrene**
> It is rapidly spreading, edematous myonecrosis, occurring in association with severely crushed wounds contaminated with pathogenic clostridia:
> - **Agents:** *C. perfringens* is the most common causative agent (60%), followed by *C. novyi* and *C. septicum* (20–40%)
> - **Predisposing factors:** Crushing injuries of muscles (e.g. road traffic accidents or bullet injuries) lead to interruption in the blood supply and anoxic muscle necrosis.
> - **Clinical Manifestations include**—the incubation period is about 10–48 hours. Characterized by sudden onset of excruciating pain at the affected site, rapid development of a foul-smelling thin serosanguineous discharge and gas bubbles **(crepitus)** in the muscle planes.

- **Clostridial enteric infections** such as food poisoning, necrotizing enterocolitis, and gangrenous appendicitis

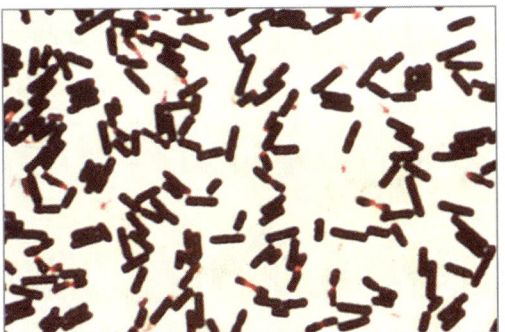

Fig. 14.1: Gram-stained smear of *Clostridium perfringens*.

Source: Public Health Image Library/ID# 11196, Don Stalons/Centers for Disease Control and Prevention (CDC), Atlanta (*with permission*).

- Skin and soft-tissue infections
- Bacteremia.

Laboratory Diagnosis

- **Specimen:** Necrotic tissues, muscle fragments, and exudates from deeper parts of the wound
- **Direct microscopy:** Thick, stubby, boxcar-shaped gram-positive bacilli without spore are suggestive of *C. perfringens* **(Fig. 14.1)**
- **Culture:** Culture media such Robertson cooked meat (RCM) broth, egg yolk agar, etc. are used, which are incubated anaerobically by GasPak or Anoxomat, etc.
- **Identification**: *C. perfringens* is identified by:
  - Target hemolysis (double zone of hemolysis)
  - Nagler's reaction: Opalescence surrounding the streak line on egg yolk agar
  - Reverse CAMP test: Positive
  - Automated ID method such as MALDI-TOF is the current method of choice for rapid and accurate identification.

> **TREATMENT** — Gas gangrene
>
> Surgical debridement is the mainstay of treatment. All devitalized tissues should be widely resected to remove conditions that produce an anaerobic environment. Other treatment modalities include:
>
> *Contd...*

Contd...

> **TREATMENT** — Gas gangrene
>
> - Hyperbaric oxygen
> - Antibiotics such as penicillin plus clindamycin
> - Passive immunization with anti-α-toxin antiserum.

Clostridium tetani

It is the causative agent of 'tetanus'—an acute disease, manifested by skeletal muscle spasm and autonomic nervous system disturbance.

- **Transmission:** Tetanus bacilli enter through wounds (accidents or surgical incision) or neonates through umbilical stumps
- **Pathogenesis:** It produces a powerful neurotoxin *tetanospasmin*, which blocks the release of neurotransmitters glycine and GABA (gamma-aminobutyric acid) from the inhibitory neuron terminals, thereby causing spastic contraction of muscles **(Fig. 14.2A)**
- **Clinical manifestation:** The incubation period is about 6–10 days. Muscles of the face and jaw are often affected first (called trismus or lockjaw) followed by painful muscle spasms → leading to descending spastic paralysis
  - *Abnormal posture:* The patient may develop an opisthotonos position due to generalized spastic contraction of the extensor muscles **(Fig. 14.2B)**
  - *Autonomic disturbance* may occur leading to alerted blood pressure, tachycardia, intestinal stasis, sweating, etc.
- **Laboratory diagnosis:** Excised tissue bits from the necrotic depths of wounds are more reliable than wound swabs
  - *Gram staining* reveals gram-positive bacilli with terminal and round spores (drum stick appearance) **(Fig. 14.2C)**
  - *Culture* using Robertson cooked meat broth, followed by toxigenicity test.
- **Treatment:** The treatment modalities of tetanus include:

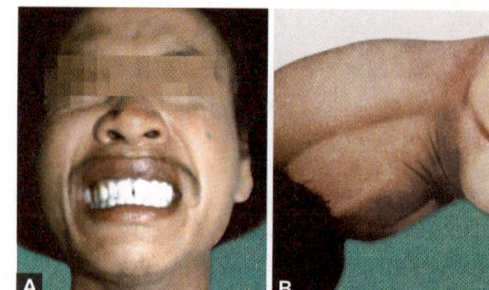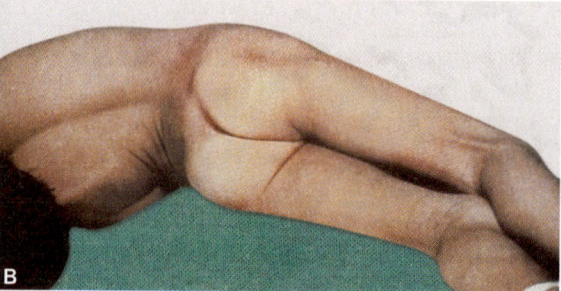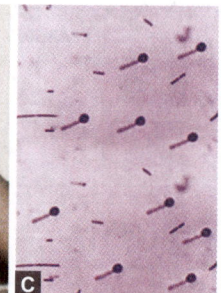

Figs. 14.2A to C: A. Lockjaw and facial spasms; **B.** Patient with opisthotonos seen in tetanus; **C.** Gram-stained smear of *Clostridium tetani* showing round terminal spore-bearing gram-positive bacilli.
Source: **A.** Wikia/Hoidkempuhtust; **B.** Public Health Image Library, ID# 6373; **C.** ID# 12056/Dr Holdeman/Centers for Disease Control and Prevention (CDC), Atlanta (*with permission*).

- Passive immunization by tetanus immunoglobulin
- The first dose of TT (if unvaccinated)
- Antibiotics: Metronidazole or penicillin.
❖ **Vaccine:** The tetanus toxoid (TT) vaccine is the most effective way of prevention of tetanus. TT is given along with DPT vaccine under the childhood immunization program (refer Chapter 13 for details).

Clostridium botulinum

It produces a powerful neurotoxin *botulinum toxin*, which acts by blocking the release of acetylcholine from nerve terminals and thereby causing flaccid paralysis of voluntary muscles. Botulism occurs in three clinical types.
1. **Food-borne botulism**: It results from the consumption of foods (e.g. canned food) contaminated with preformed botulinum toxin
2. **Wound botulism:** It results from contamination of wounds with *C. botulinum* spores
3. **Infant botulism:** It is the most common type; (75%); usually affects infants following ingestion of contaminated food (usually **honey**). Manifestations include floppy neck, and extreme weakness (hence called **floppy child syndrome**). It is usually self-limiting.

Clostridioides difficile Infection (CDI)

Clostridioides difficile (old name *Clostridium difficile*) is an important cause of healthcare-associated infection. It is responsible for a unique colonic disease—**pseudomembranous colitis**, which occurs almost exclusively in association with prolonged antimicrobial use in hospitals; therefore, called as antibiotic-associated diarrhea.
❖ **Risk factors:** *Clostridioides difficile* is associated with the following risk factors
  - **Prolonged antibiotics use:** Cephalosporins, clindamycin, ampicillin and fluoroquinolones are frequently responsible for this condition
  - Advanced age (>65 years)
  - Immunosuppression and cancer chemotherapy
  - Malignancies and gastrointestinal surgeries.
❖ **Laboratory diagnosis:** Various methods to detect CDI include:
  - Culture on special media such as CCFA (cycloserine cefoxitin fructose agar)
  - Cell culture cytotoxin neutralization assay
  - Detection of antigen (GDH, toxin A/B) in stool (by rapid test)
  - PCR detecting toxin gene (toxin A/B).
❖ **Treatment:** Oral vancomycin or metronidazole are given for treatment
❖ **Prevention (infection control measures)** followed are:
  - Broad spectrum antimicrobials should be stopped at the earliest
  - Infection control measures of contact precaution (see Chapter 38) should be

followed such as: strict hand hygiene and patient isolation
- Ensure proper disinfection of floor, surfaces, toilets and other soiled areas using 1% freshly prepared hypochlorite solution.

NON-SPORING ANAEROBES

Non-sporing anaerobes are often a part of the normal flora of the mouth, GIT, and genital tract of man and animals. Medially important non-sporing anaerobes include:
- Gram-positive cocci: *Peptostreptococcus*
- Gram-negative cocci: *Veillonella*
- Gram-positive bacilli: *Bifidobacterium, Propionibacterium,* and *Mobiluncus*
- Gram-negative bacilli: *Bacteroides, Prevotella, Porphyromonas, Fusobacterium.*

Bacteroides fragilis

Bacteroides fragilis is recognized as the most common commensal in the human intestine; it is also the most frequent anaerobe isolated from clinical specimens. It causes peritonitis and intra-abdominal abscess following bowel injury (most common manifestation), pelvic inflammatory disease (PID), brain abscesses, bacteremia, and empyema.

EXPECTED QUESTIONS

I. **Write short notes on:**
   1. Gas gangrene.
   2. Tetanus.
   3. Botulism.
   4. Antibiotic-associated diarrhea.

II. **Multiple Choice Questions (MCQs):**
   1. Naegler's reaction is positive for?
      a. *Clostridium perfringens*
      b. *Clostridium tetani*
      c. *Clostridium botulinum*
      d. *Clostridioides difficile*
   2. Pseudomembranous colitis is caused by__?
      a. *Clostridium perfringens*
      b. *Clostridium tetani*
      c. *Clostridium botulinum*
      d. *Clostridioides difficile*
   3. The most common type of botulism?
      a. Food botulism
      b. Infant botulism
      c. Wound botulism
      d. Iatrogenic botulism
   4. Which of the following produces a toxin that inhibits release of GABA and glycine neurotransmitters?
      a. *Clostridium perfringens*
      b. *Clostridium tetani*
      c. *Clostridium botulinum*
      d. *Clostridioides difficile*
   5. The most effective way of preventing tetanus:
      a. Hyperbaric oxygen
      b. Antibiotics
      c. Tetanus toxoid
      d. Surgical debridement and toilet

Answers
1. a   2. d   3. b   4. b   5. c

CHAPTER 15

Mycobacteria Infections

CHAPTER PREVIEW

- Mycobacterium tuberculosis
- Mycobacterium leprae
- Nontuberculous Mycobacteria

Mycobacteria are acid-fast obligate aerobes. They can be classified into:
- *Mycobacterium tuberculosis* complex: It is responsible for tuberculosis in man
- *Mycobacterium leprae* (Hansen's bacillus): causes leprosy
- Nontuberculous mycobacteria (NTM): causes cutaneous, and pulmonary infections.

MYCOBACTERIUM TUBERCULOSIS

Mycobacterium tuberculosis complex causes tuberculosis, which is one of the oldest disease of mankind and is a major cause of death worldwide. It usually affects the lungs, although other organs are also involved. India accounts for the highest burden of tuberculosis (20% of total TB cases) worldwide.

Pathogenesis

- **Transmission:** *M. tuberculosis* is mainly transmitted by inhalation of aerosols (<5μm), generated while coughing or sneezing by infected patients
- **Bacillary load:** At least 10^4 bacilli/mL in sputum is required for an effective transmission
- A fraction of small droplet nuclei containing bacilli reaches the lungs, where the bacilli are phagocytosed by the alveolar macrophages
- *M. tuberculosis* is an obligate intracellular pathogen, that survives inside the macrophage by inhibition of phagolysosome fusion
- **CMI:** Host's cell-mediated immune response to *M. tuberculosis* is critical to contain the infection
- **Macrophage-activating response:** If the host mounts a good immune response, the activated macrophages kill the tubercle bacilli and form characteristic granuloma called tubercles
- **Tissue-damaging response:** In case bacilli are more virulent and the host mounts a delayed hypersensitivity reaction (DTH) to contain the infection, which leads to lung tissue destruction.

Clinical Forms

Tuberculosis occurs both in pulmonary and extrapulmonary forms.

Pulmonary Tuberculosis (PTB)

It is the most common type, presents either as primary PTB in children or as post-primary PTB in adults.
- **Primary PTB:** It is characterized by fibrotic nodular lesions (Ghon focus) in the lungs and associated hilar lymphadenopathy—

together referred to as primary complex. The middle and lower lobes of the lungs are commonly affected
- **Post-primary PTB:** It usually occurs in adults, where the apical lobe of the lungs gets involved. Common features observed are hematogenous spread, cavitation, and caseating granuloma formation
- **Clinical features:** Patients usually present with fever, productive cough (±hemoptysis) and occasionally pleuritic chest pain, night sweating, weight loss, etc.

Extrapulmonary Tuberculosis (EPTB)

EPTB results from hematogenous dissemination of tubercle bacilli to various organs. In HIV patients, the occurrence of EPTB is much higher. The common types of EPTB include—tuberculous lymphadenitis (35%), pleural tuberculosis (20%), genitourinary tuberculosis, skeletal tuberculosis, tuberculous meningitis, gastrointestinal tuberculosis, and tuberculous skin lesions.

Epidemiology

About a quarter of the current world population is infected asymptomatically with *M. tuberculosis*, of which 5–10% develop the clinical disease during their lifetime.
- **World:** The WHO has estimated 10 million new cases of TB occurred in 2018 with a global incidence of 130 new cases per one lakh population per year
- Countries with high TB burden are **India, China, Indonesia, Philippines, Pakistan, Nigeria, Bangladesh and South Africa**
- **India:** In 2018, about 27 lakh cases occurred India; with highest burden from Uttar Pradesh (20% of total TB cases) followed by Maharashtra
- TB is one of the top 10 causes of death worldwide and the leading cause among infectious diseases.

Laboratory Diagnosis

The specimens collected for the diagnosis of tuberculosis depend upon the clinical forms.
- In PTB, a minimum of *two sputum specimens* are examined—early morning and spot
- Whereas in EPTB, the specimens vary depending on the site involved such as pleural fluid, CSF, urine, etc.

Microscopy

Acid-fast staining is the microscopic method performed for the detection of *M. tuberculosis*.
- **Digestion and decontamination:** The sputum specimens are prior subjected to digestion (to liquefy the thick pus) and decontamination by treatment with sodium hydroxide (Petroff's method) or N-acetyl L-cysteine (NALC)
- **Methods:** The various acid-fast staining methods available are:
  - Ziehl–Neelsen (ZN) staining (hot method) using 25% sulfuric acid as the decolorizer—*M. tuberculosis* appears as long slender, beaded, red colored acid-fast bacilli **(Fig. 15.1A)**
  - Kinyoun's cold acid-fast staining
  - Fluorescent (auramine phenol) staining—is more sensitive and smears can be screened more rapidly than ZN staining. Tubercle bacilli appear bright brilliant green against the dark background **(Fig. 15.1B)**.
- **Grading** of the sputum smear is done (0 to 3+) which helps to determine the severity of disease, and infectiousness and also to monitor the response to treatment
- **Detection limit:** At least 10^4 bacilli/mL in sputum is required for the bacilli to be detected in acid-fast stained smear.

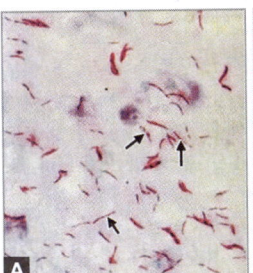 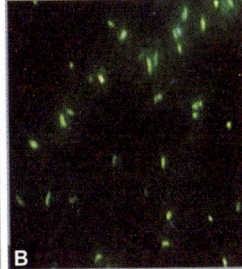

Figs. 15.1A and B: A. ZN staining of sputum smear showing long, slender and beaded red colored acid–fast bacilli; **B.** Auramine phenol staining of sputum smear—Tubercle bacilli appear bright brilliant green against the dark background.

Source: **A and B.** Department of Microbiology, JIPMER, Puducherry (*with permission*).

Culture

Culture is more sensitive than microscopy, with a detection limit of 10-100 bacilli/mL. Various culture methods/media available are:

- **Conventional media** such as Lowenstein-Jensen (LJ) medium: *M. tuberculosis* produces rough, tough, and buff-colored colonies after an incubation of 6-8 weeks **(Fig. 15.2A)**
- **Automated culture systems,** e.g. MGIT (Mycobacteria growth indicator tube): Takes less time than LJ culture (3 weeks). It can also be used for drug susceptibility testing **(Fig. 15.2B)**
- **Identification** of *M. tuberculosis* in culture is made by:
  - Automated identification—by MALDI-TOF
  - Antigen detection by ICT—detecting MPT 64 antigen.

Molecular Methods

As culture is time-consuming, and microcopy is less sensitive, the diagnosis of TB greatly relies on molecular methods. Various molecular methods available are:

- **Cartridge-based nucleic acid amplification test (e.g. GeneXpert):** It is an automated real-time PCR system that has completely revolutionized the diagnosis of TB
  - *Uses:* It serves two purposes—(i) detection of *M. tuberculosis* complex in the specimen, and (ii) detection of rifampicin resistance
  - *Advantages:* It is rapid, takes <2h of time, and is highly sensitive (detection limit 131 bacilli/mL of the specimen).
- **Chip-based NAAT: Truenat** is a chip-based real-time PCR system, developed in India, that works in a similar principle as GeneXpert
- **Line probe assay (LPA):** It involves probe-based detection of amplified DNA in the specimen
  - *Uses:* (i) Identification of MTB complex, (ii) detection of resistance to first-line and second-line antitubercular drugs
  - *Disadvantages:* It takes 2-3 days. It is less sensitive, and can be performed only on smear-positive specimens.

Drug Susceptibility Test (DST)

Universal-DST refers to performing DST for all TB patients—first performing CBNAAT to determine rifampicin susceptibility; followed by line probe assay (LPA) or MGIT to detect susceptibility to other anti-tubercular drugs.

Diagnosis of Latent Tuberculosis

Latent tuberculosis is diagnosed by demonstration of delayed or type IV hypersensitivity reaction against the tubercle bacilli antigens.

- **Two methods** are available: (1) tuberculin skin test (or Monteux test), (2) IFN-γ release assay
- **A positive test** indicates prior exposure to *M. tuberculosis*, but cannot differentiate between past exposure and active infection. However, in infants, it can suggest an active infection.

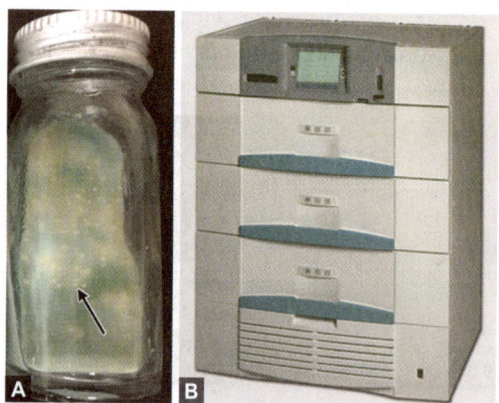

Figs. 15.2: Culture media/culture systems for *M. tuberculosis*: **A.** Lowenstein-Jensen medium (arrow showing rough, tough and buff-colored colonies); **B.** BACTEC MGIT.

Source: Department of Microbiology, JIPMER, Puducherry (with permission).

TREATMENT — Tuberculosis

Treatment of tuberculosis involves a multidrug regimen of first-line agents, given for a longer duration (6 months) and under the direct supervision:

Contd...

Contd...

> **TREATMENT** — **Tuberculosis**
>
> - Intensive phase (2 months) with four drugs (HRZE): Isoniazid, rifampicin, pyrazinamide, and ethambutol
> - Continuation phase (4 months) with three drugs (HRE): Isoniazid, rifampicin, and ethambutol
> - FDC: All drugs must be given in fixed-dose combination (FDC) tablets as per body weight
> - Daily-oral regimen: The FDC tablets should be taken orally, once a day.

Drug Resistance

Failure to adhere to the multidrug regimen is a common practice in patients, which often leads to the emergence of drug resistance in *M. tuberculosis*. The common pattern of drug resistance are:

- ❖ **MDR-TB:** Defined as resistance to both isoniazid and rifampicin with or without resistance to other first-line drugs
- ❖ **XDR-TB:** Defined as MDR-TB plus resistance to second-line agents such as at least one injectable aminoglycoside and one fluoroquinolone.

National TB Elimination Programme

The National Tuberculosis Elimination Programme (NTEP) is the national program implemented in India for the control of tuberculosis. It was earlier called as Revised National Tuberculosis Control Programme (RNTCP).

Nikshay: It is a web portal for surveillance of TB, where all health care facilities need to notify all new TB cases through this web.

Infection Control Measures

Airborne precautions (e.g. negative pressure isolation room, N95 respirator, etc.) must be followed (Chapter 38).

Vaccine

Bacillus Calmette-Guérin (BCG) is a live attenuated vaccine for tuberculosis.
- ❖ **Strain:** In India, WHO recommended Danish 1331 strain of BCG is used. It is prepared in Central BCG laboratory, Guindy, Chennai
- ❖ **Indication:** It is given to newborn, at birth
- ❖ **Administered** by intradermal route above the insertion of left deltoid. If properly given, a permanent tiny round scar is developed in 6-12 weeks of time
- ❖ **Protection:** BCG has a variable efficacy of 0–80% and only up to 15–20 years. However, it surely gives protection against the development of complications such as tuberculous meningitis and disseminated tuberculosis
- ❖ **Contraindications to BCG include:** Child born to a TB-positive mother or child with low immunity or HIV-positive.

MYCOBACTERIUM LEPRAE

Mycobacterium leprae (Hansen's bacillus) causes leprosy; characterized by anesthetic skin lesions, bony deformities, and disfigurement.

- ❖ Due to fear, ignorance, superstitious beliefs, and characteristic disfigurement produced in the patients, leprosy remained as a social stigma over many years and patients have been socially outcasted
- ❖ However today, with early diagnosis and effective treatment, patients can lead a productive life in the community and the deformities can largely be prevented.

Clinical Manifestations

Based on the number of skin lesions, presence of nerve involvement and identification of bacilli in the slit-skin smear, leprosy can be classified into two categories. This classification is used by the leprosy control program for the treatment of patients (described later).

- ❖ **Paucibacillary (PB) leprosy:** A case of leprosy that fulfills all the criteria—(i) 1 to 5 skin lesions, (ii) no nerve involvement, and (iii) slit-skin smear-negative for lepra bacilli
- ❖ **Multibacillary (MB) leprosy:** A case of leprosy that fulfills any one of the criteria—(i) >5 skin lesions; or (ii) nerve involvement (neuritis); or (iii) slit-skin smear-positive for lepra bacilli.

Table 15.1: Differences between lepromatous leprosy and tuberculoid leprosy.

Characters	Lepromatous leprosy (LL)	Tuberculoid leprosy (TT)
Bacillary load	Multibacillary	Paucibacillary
Skin lesions	• Many, symmetrical • Margin is irregular	• One or few, asymmetrical • Margin is sharp
Nerve lesion	Appear late	• Early anesthetic skin lesion • Enlarged thickened nerves
CMI	Low	Normal
Lepromin test	Negative	Positive
Humoral immunity	Exaggerated	Normal

Abbreviation: CMI, cell-mediated immunity.

Leprosy is a bipolar disease. Depending upon the host cell-mediated immune response (CMI), the patient can develop various clinical forms ranging from lepromatous, borderline, or tuberculoid forms
❖ There are various **classification schemes** described in the literature such as Ridley-Jopling, Madrid, and Indian classification
❖ The **differences** between lepromatous leprosy (LL) and tuberculoid leprosy (TT) are depicted in **Table 15.1**.

Epidemiology

Unlike its superstitious beliefs, leprosy is not a highly communicable disease. Intimate and prolonged contact is necessary for transmission. Only about 5% of spouses living with leprosy patients develop the disease.
❖ **Transmission:** *M. leprae* is transmitted mainly through:
  ▪ Nasal droplet inhalation (common mode)
  ▪ Contact transmission (skin).
❖ **Leprosy elimination:** As per WHO, leprosy is said to be eliminated if the caseload is <1 case per 10,000 population. Many countries have achieved this target including India
❖ **The situation in World**: Once leprosy was worldwide in distribution, but now, it is almost exclusively confined to the developing nations of Asia, and Africa
❖ **The situation in India**: Although India has achieved leprosy elimination in 2005, cases still occur in various pockets of India such as Bihar, Chhattisgarh, etc. India still accounts for the highest-burden of leprosy in the world.

Laboratory Diagnosis

Smear Microscopy

Smear microscopy is done to demonstrate the acid-fast bacilli in the lesions.
❖ **Specimens:** A total of six samples are collected; four from the skin (forehead, cheek, chin, and buttock), one from the ear lobe and nasal mucosa by nasal blow/scraping. Skin specimens are collected by a technique called slit-skin smear
❖ **Acid-fast stain** using 5% sulfuric acid: *M. leprae* appears red acid-fast bacilli arranged in cigar-like bundles to form globi, found inside the foamy macrophages **(Fig. 15.3)**.

Other Methods

The other methods for diagnosis of leprosy include:
❖ **Mouse footpad cultivation:** *M. leprae* is not cultivable in culture media or in tissue culture, but can grow in mouse foot pads

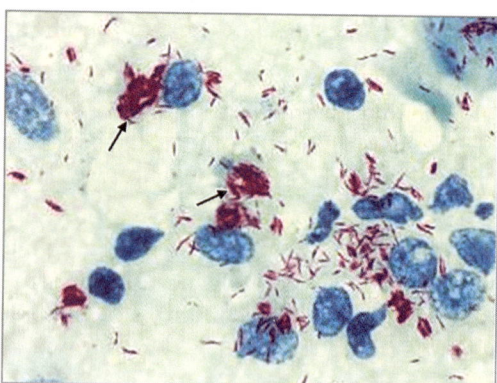

Fig. 15.3: Acid-fast stained slit skin smear showing numerous *Mycobacterium leprae* singly or in globi (arrows).

Source: Dr Isabella Princess, Apollo Hospital, Chennai (*with permission*).

- **Antibody detection** by FLA-ABS (fluorescent leprosy antibody absorption test)
- **Lepromin test:** It is a skin test, similar to the tuberculin test. A positive test indicates CMI is intact and good prognosis, while a negative test indicates low CMI and poor prognosis.

TREATMENT — Leprosy

Multidrug therapy (MDT) is recommended for the treatment of leprosy, because of the risk of development of drug resistance to a single drug.
- **3-drug regimen:** WHO recommends a 3-drug regimen of rifampicin, dapsone and clofazimine for all leprosy patients
- **Duration of treatment**—6 months for paucibacillary leprosy and 12 months for multibacillary leprosy
- **Follow-up** is conducted annually for 2 years for paucibacillary leprosy and 5 years for multibacillary leprosy cases.

NONTUBERCULOUS MYCOBACTERIA (NTM)

They are a diverse group of mycobacteria, exist either as saprophytes or commensals, but can occasionally cause opportunistic infection in man. The various NTMs can be classified, as follows:

- **Photochromogens:** Produce pigments only in light, e.g.
  - *M. marinum:* It causes skin ulcers known as **swimming pool granuloma** or fish tank granuloma
  - *M. kansasii:* It causes chronic pulmonary disease resembling tuberculosis.
- **Scotochromogens:** Produce pigments both in light and dark, e.g.
  - *M. scrofulaceum:* It causes scrofula (cervical lymphadenitis) in children
  - *M. gordonae:* It is often found as commensal in tap water.
- **Non-chromogens:** Do not produce pigments, e.g. *M. avium-intracellulare* complex (MAC). It causes opportunistic infection, especially in HIV-infected people such as lymphadenitis, respiratory infection, and disseminated disease
- **Rapid growers:** Grow within one week, e.g. *M. chelonae, M. fortuitum,* they cause post-trauma injection abscess and catheter-related infections.

EXPECTED QUESTIONS

I. **Write an essay on:**
   1. Discuss the pathogenesis, clinical manifestations and laboratory diagnosis of pulmonary tuberculosis.

II. **Write short notes on:**
   1. Clinical manifestations of leprosy.
   2. Nontuberculous mycobacteria (NTM) infections.
   3. BCG vaccine.
   4. Drug resistance in TB.

III. **Multiple Choice Questions (MCQs):**
   1. How much bacillary load in sputum is required for effective transmission of *M. tuberculosis*?
      a. 10 bacilli/mL
      b. 100 bacilli/mL
      c. 1,000 bacilli/mL
      d. 10,000 bacilli/mL
   2. Survival of *M. tuberculosis* inside the macrophages is due to:
      a. Inhibition of entry into the host cell
      b. Inhibition of entry into the phagosome
      c. Inhibition of phagosome-lysosome fusion
      d. Inhibits degradation by lysosomal enzymes
   3. GeneXpert can detect resistance to:
      a. Isoniazid   b. Rifampicin
      c. Pyrazinamide   d. Ethambutol
   4. Which of the following is a rapid grower mycobacteria?
      a. *M. marinum*
      b. *M. kansasii*
      c. *M. scrofulaceum*
      d. *M. chelonae*

Answers
1. d   2. c   3. b   4. d

CHAPTER 16

Gram-negative Bacilli Infections-I

CHAPTER PREVIEW

- Enterobacterales
  - E. coli
  - Klebsiella
- Shigella
- Salmonella
- Vibrio

ENTEROBACTERALES

Enterobacterales include the commensal bacteria in the human intestine called coliform bacilli. They have the following general properties:
- They are gram-negative bacilli
- Aerobes and facultative anaerobes
- Nonfastidious, can grow in basal media like nutrient agar
- Ferment glucose and reduce nitrate
- All are catalase-positive, but oxidase test negative.

Based on the fermentation of lactose, Enterobacterales can be classified into:
- **Lactose fermenters (LF)**: Ferment lactose, and produce pink colonies on MacConkey agar; e.g. *Escherichia*, *Klebsiella*, *Enterobacter*, and *Citrobacter*
- **Non-lactose fermenters (NLF)**: Do not ferment lactose, produce pale colonies on MacConkey agar; e.g. *Salmonella*, *Shigella*, Proteeae (*Proteus*, *Morganella*, *Providencia*), and *Yersinia*.

Escherichia coli

Escherichia coli is the most common pathogen encountered clinically. It is also the most common aerobe to be harbored in the gut of humans.

Clinical Manifestations

Various strains of *E. coli* have been associated with various manifestations.

UTI by UPEC

Urinary tract infection (UTI) is caused by a strain of *E. coli* known as uropathogenic *E. coli* (UPEC), which is the most common cause (70–75%) of UTI. Infection to the bladder is usually spread by ascending route through the urethra, from the perineal flora.

Diarrhea (Diarrheagenic *E. coli*)

Diarrhea is caused by a strain of *E. coli* known as diarrheagenic *E. coli*, which further comprises six pathotypes.

1. **Enteropathogenic *E. coli* (EPEC)**: It causes infantile diarrhea. It is nontoxigenic and noninvasive
2. **Enterotoxigenic *E. coli* (ETEC)**: It causes traveler's diarrhea. Pathogenesis is mediated by producing toxins such as:
   - Heat labile toxin (LT): Acts by increasing cyclic AMP (similar to cholera toxin)
   - Heat stable toxin (ST): Acts by increasing cyclic GMP.
3. **Enteroinvasive *E. coli* (EIEC)**: It is not toxigenic, but invasive and causes bloody diarrhea (i.e. dysentery)

4. **Enterohemorrhagic *E. coli* (EHEC):** The most common serotype associated with EHEC is O157:H7
   - Its pathogenesis is mediated by a toxin called verocytotoxin (or Shiga-like toxin)
   - It also causes dysentery, similar to EIEC
   - Verocytotoxin damages the endothelial cells causing capillary microangiopathy which may lead to complications such as hemolytic uremic syndrome (HUS) and hemorrhagic colitis.
5. **Enteroaggregative *E. coli* (EAEC):** It causes persistent and acute diarrhea
6. **Diffusely adherent *E. coli* (DAEC):** It causes diarrhea in children aged 2–6 years.

Other Infections

Apart from UTI and diarrhea, *E. coli* can cause several pyogenic infections such as:
- **Abdominal infections:** Bacterial peritonitis (primary or secondary), visceral abscesses, such as hepatic abscess
- Pneumonia (especially in hospitalized patients—ventilator-associated pneumonia)
- Bloodstream infection (especially in hospitalized patients)
- Meningitis (especially neonatal meningitis)
- Wound and soft tissue infections such as cellulitis, infection of ulcers and wounds, especially in patient with diabetic foot.

Laboratory Diagnosis

Sample collection depends on the site of infection—urine, stool, pus, wound swab, blood, CSF, etc.
- **Direct smear microscopy:** Shows gram-negative bacilli, and pus cells
- **Culture:** Incubation at 37°C for 24h reveals the following growth:
  - Blood agar: Gray, moist colonies
  - MacConkey agar: Flat, pink LF colonies **(Fig. 16.1A)**
  - **Culture smear and motility:** Motile gram-negative bacilli **(Fig. 16.1B)**.
- **Biochemical identification:** Various biochemical tests which help in the identification of *E. coli* are:
  - Catalase positive and oxidase negative

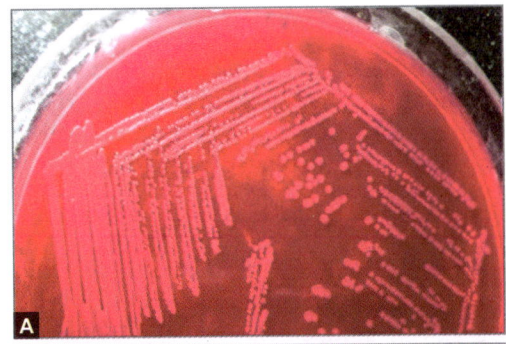
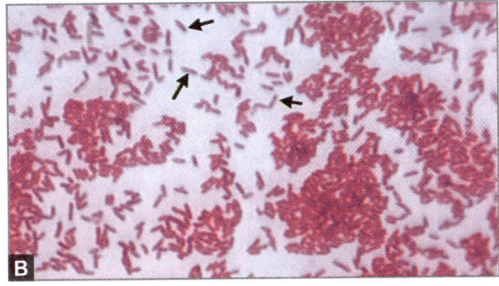

Figs. 16.1A and B: A. Flat pink lactose fermenting colonies of *E. coli* on MacConkey agar; **B.** Slender gram-negative bacilli (arrows showing).

Source: Department of Microbiology, Pondicherry Institute of Medical Sciences, Puducherry (*with permission*).

  - ICUT tests: Indole, Citrate, Urease, Triple sugar iron (TSI) test are useful for identification.
- **Automated ID systems** such as VITEK and MALDI-TOF can be performed for rapid and accurate identification of *E. coli*
- **Antimicrobial susceptibility testing** can be performed by disk diffusion method (on Mueller-Hinton agar) or MIC-based method (VITEK).

TREATMENT	*E. coli* and *Klebsiella*

Treatment is essentially based upon an antimicrobial susceptibility test report. The majority of isolates in hospitals are multi-drug resistant (MDR) and require treatment with any of the following higher antimicrobials if found susceptible:
- Carbapenems such as meropenem
- β-lactam/β-lactamase inhibitor combinations (BL/BLIs) such as piperacillin-tazobactam or cefoperazone-sulbactam
- Aminoglycosides such as amikacin
- Polymyxins such as colistin
- Others: Fosfomycin or tigecycline, etc.

Preventive Measures

Infection control measures (contact precaution) such as hand hygiene are crucial to limit the spread of infection by multi-drug resistant Enterobacterales (refer Chapter 38).

Klebsiella pneumoniae

Similar to *E. coli*, *Klebsiella pneumoniae* can cause UTI, lobar pneumonia, meningitis (in neonates), septicemia, pyogenic infections such as abscesses, and wound infections.

- ❖ **Laboratory diagnosis:** Similar to *E. coli*, *K. pneumoniae* is also a lactose fermenter
  - It differs from *E.coli* in being non-motile, capsulated, and produces mucoid colonies **(Fig. 16.2)**
  - Identification can be done by various conventional biochemical tests such as catalase, oxidase, indole, citrate, urease, TSI or by automated ID systems such as VITEK and MALDI-TOF.
- ❖ **Treatment** for *K. pneumoniae* is the same as discussed for *E. coli*.

Other *Klebsiella* species include:
- ❖ *Klebsiella granulomatis:* It causes granuloma inguinale, a type of genito-ulcerative disease
- ❖ *K. rhinoscleromatis* and *K. ozaenae:* Produce infections of the nasal cavity, called rhinoscleroma and atrophic rhinitis respectively.

Enterobacter species

Enterobacter species are similar to *Klebsiella* in clinical manifestations and also in most of the biochemical reactions except for being motile. *E. aerogenes* and *E. cloacae* are the most commonly isolated species from the clinical specimens. Treatment of *Enterobacter* infections is same as discussed for *E. coli*.

Citrobacter species

Citrobacter species are environmental contaminants, but species such as. *C. freundii* and *C. koseri* can cause human infections.
- ❖ **Manifestations:** They occasionally cause urinary tract, gallbladder and middle ear infections and neonatal meningitis

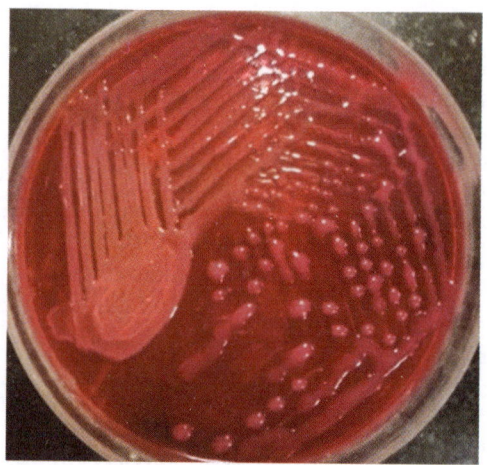

Fig. 16.2: *Klebsiella pneumoniae*; on MacConkey agar showing mucoid pink-colored lactose-fermenting colonies.

Source: Department of Microbiology, Pondicherry Institute of Medical Sciences, Puducherry (*with permission*).

- ❖ **Identification** is made either by automated identification systems such as MALDI-TOF or VITEK; or by conventional biochemical tests
- ❖ **Treatment:** Most *Citrobacter* isolates are MDR, and the guideline for treatment is the same as that used for *E. coli*.

Salmonella

Salmonellae are broadly classified into two groups, based on the clinical disease produced:
1. **Typhoidal *Salmonella*:** It includes serotypes *S.* Typhi and *S.* Paratyphi. They are restricted to human hosts, in whom they cause enteric fever.
2. **Non-typhoidal salmonellae or NTS:** The remaining serotypes can colonize the intestine of a broad range of animals, including mammals, reptiles, birds, and insects. They also infect humans causing food-borne gastroenteritis and septicemia.

Enteric Fever

Enteric fever is a potentially fatal multisystem illness caused by *Salmonella* Typhi (typhoid fever) and, *S.* Paratyphi A, B and C (paratyphoid fever).

Pathogenesis

Salmonellae are transmitted by oral route, through ingestion of contaminated food or water.

- The infective dose of *Salmonella* is higher than that of *Shigella*. Minimum 10^3–10^6 bacilli are needed to initiate the infection
- **Risk factors** that promote transmission include the conditions that decrease gastric acidity and intestinal integrity
- **Primary bacteremia:** The bacilli enter through a specialized epithelial cell lining the intestinal mucosa—called M cells. Following this, they are internalized by macrophages and are carried to the bloodstream
- **Spread:** Then, the bacilli disseminate throughout the body such liver, spleen, lymph nodes and bone marrow, etc. where further multiplication takes place and then seeded back into the bloodstream (**secondary bacteremia**), which leads to the onset of clinical disease.

Clinical Manifestations of Enteric Fever

The incubation period is about 10–14 days. Enteric fever is named after the mode of transmission (enteric route) of its causative agent. However, the manifestations seen are largely extraintestinal.

- **Fever (step ladder pattern of remittent fever):** Fever rises gradually to a higher level with every spike; then falls, but does not touch normal
- **Other symptoms:** Headache, chills, cough, sweating, myalgia, and arthralgia
- **Rashes (called rose spots):** Faint, salmon-colored, blanching, maculopapular rash on the trunk and chest seen in 30% of patients at the end of the first week
- **Early intestinal manifestations** such as abdominal pain, nausea, vomiting, constipation or diarrhea, and anorexia
- **Important signs** include hepatosplenomegaly, epistaxis, and relative bradycardia
- **Complications:** Gastrointestinal bleeding and intestinal perforation can occur mostly in the third and fourth weeks of illness
- **Neurologic manifestations** occur rarely which include meningitis, and neuropsychiatric symptoms such as delirium, etc.

Laboratory Diagnosis

(A) Blood Culture (First week of illness)

In the first week of illness, a blood culture is recommended.

- **Conventional blood culture** on media such as brain heart infusion (BHI) broth (monophasic media) or BHI broth/agar (biphasic media)
- **Automated blood culture systems**—such as BACTEC or BacT/ ALERT
- **Blood culture positivity** is >90% in the first week and thereafter it gradually declines
- If blood culture is found negative, bone marrow culture or culture from duodenal aspirate may be performed in the first week of illness.

(B) Stool/urine Culture (in 3–4 weeks of illness)

Stool or urine culture is indicated in 3-4 weeks of illness, and also for detection of carriers:

- For **stool culture** the following media are used:
  - Enrichment broth such as Selenite F broth, tetrathionate broth, and gram-negative broth
  - Low selective medium such as MacConkey agar: Produces translucent NLF colonies
  - Highly selective media: DCA (deoxycholate citrate agar), XLD agar (xylose lysine deoxycholate), and Wilson Blair's Bismuth sulphite medium are used.
- A **urine culture** can be performed on media such as MacConkey agar.

(C) Identification

Salmonellae are motile, gram-negative bacilli.

- Identification from the colonies grown in culture is made either by automated ID system such as VITEK or by conventional biochemical tests such as—catalase, oxidase, indole, citrate, urease and TSI
- **A slide agglutination test** is performed to confirm the serotype.

(D) Widal test (Serum antibody detection)
Widal test is indicated in 2–3 weeks of illness. It is a tube agglutination test, that detects antibodies in the patient's serum against antigens of *Salmonella* Typhi and *S.* Paratyphi.

- **Antigens:** In the Widal test, four different antigens are used such as:
    - O antigen of *S.* Typhi (TO): It is cross-reactive to O antigens of *S.* Paratyphi A and B. Therefore, TO antigen can detect O antibody of *S.* Typhi, as well as *S.* Paratyphi A and B
    - H antigen of *S.* Typhi (TH)
    - H antigen of *S.* Paratyphi A (AH)
    - H antigen of *S.* Paratyphi B (BH)
- **Procedure:** Serial dilutions of patient serum are mixed with four different *Salmonella* antigens (TO, TH, AH, and BH) and the tubes are incubated in the water bath at 37°C for 24 hours
- **Result:** The result is read using a concave mirror. If corresponding antibodies are present, then an agglutination reaction will occur leading to matt formation. The absence of antibodies would lead to button formation **(Fig. 16.3)**
    - *O antibodies:* Produce granular chalky clumps when reacts with O Ag
    - *H antibodies:* Produce cottony woolly clumps when react with H Ag.
- **Significant titer:** H antibody titer of >1:200 is considered significant, whereas significant titer for O antibody is taken as >1:100. Low titers may be produced in cross-reacting infections and therefore should be ignored **(Fig. 16.4)**
- **Interpretation:** The results are interpreted as below:
    - In *S.* Typhi infection: Antibodies to TO and TH antigens are raised
    - In *S.* Paratyphi A infection: Antibodies to TO and AH antibodies are raised
    - In *S.* Paratyphi B infection: Antibodies to TO and BH antibodies are raised.
- **False-negative:** The Widal test may produce a false-negative result in a very early stage (1st week) or due to prior antimicrobial therapy or due to prozone phenomena (antibody excess)
- **False-positive:** Widal test may produce a false-positive result in presence of cross-reacting infections (called anamnestic reactions).

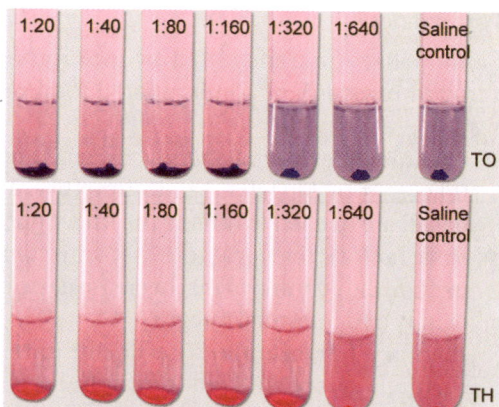

Fig. 16.4: Widal test showing titre of TO 1:160 and TH 1:320.

Abbreviation: TO and TH, antibody titre to *S.*Typhi O and H antigens in patient's serum.

Source: Department of Microbiology, Pondicherry Institute of Medical Sciences, Puducherry *(with permission).*

(E) Other Tests
- **Antigen detection (serum and urine):** By ELISA
- **Molecular methods:** PCR detecting *flagellin* gene, *iro B* and *fli C* gene
- **Nonspecific findings:** For example, neutropenia
- **Antimicrobial susceptibility testing** can be performed by disk diffusion test or by MIC-based automated system (e.g. VITEK).

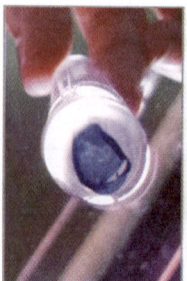 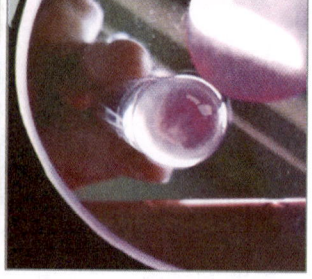

Fig. 16.3: O and H agglutination in Widal test (reading taken in a mirror).

Source: Department of Microbiology, Pondicherry Institute of Medical Sciences, Puducherry *(with permission).*

TREATMENT — Enteric fever

Third-generation cephalosporins such as ceftriaxone is the drug of choice for empirical treatment.
   Alternative drugs are azithromycin, ciprofloxacin, chloramphenicol, ampicillin, and cotrimoxazole.

Vaccines for Typhoid Fever

There are two types of typhoid vaccines available currently.
1. **Vi antigen vaccine:** It is composed of purified Vi capsular polysaccharide antigen derived from *S.* Typhi strain Ty2
   - It is given as a single dose, by IM or subcutaneous route
   - The vaccine confers protection for 2 years; a booster is given every 2 years.
2. **Typhoral:** It contains live attenuated *S.* Typhi Ty21a strain
   - It is given orally as enteric-coated capsules
   - Four doses, given on alternate days
   - Revaccination is recommended every 5 years.

Shigella

Shigella is the causative agent of bacillary dysentery. It comprises four species—*S. dysenteriae, S. flexneri, S. boydii* and *S. sonnei*.
- **Transmission** of infection occurs by ingestion through contaminated fingers (most common), food, water, or rarely flies. Risk factors include overcrowding, poor hygiene, and children, etc.
- **Minimum infective dose:** As low as 10–100 bacilli are capable of initiating the disease, probably because of their ability to survive in gastric acidity
- **Pathogenesis** is due to the expression of various toxins such as—*Shigella* enterotoxin (by *S. flexneri*), Shiga toxin (by *S. dysenteriae*) endotoxin (by all species)
- **Clinical features:** Bacillary dysentery is characterized by the passage of loose stool mixed with blood and mucus
   - Shiga toxin (*S. dysenteriae*) is similar to verocytotoxin (of EHEC) and is associated with complications such as hemolytic uremic syndrome and hemorrhagic colitis
   - Rarely, may be associated with intestinal complications such as toxic megacolon, perforations, and rectal prolapse.
- ❖ **Laboratory diagnosis** includes isolation of organism from diarrheic stool specimen using enrichment medium such as selenite F medium and selective media such as DCA (deoxycholate citrate agar) or XLD (xylose lysine deoxycholate) agar; followed by identification by using appropriate biochemical reactions or automated ID method (like VITEK)
- ❖ **Antimicrobial susceptibility testing** can be performed by disk diffusion test or VITEK.
- ❖ **Treatment** of shigellosis includes fluid replacement and antimicrobials such as ciprofloxacin.

Tribe Proteeae

Tribe Proteeae comprises three genera: *Proteus, Morganella,* and *Providencia*.
- ❖ Although they are saprophytes and commensals; they can also cause opportunistic infections such as urinary tract infections,

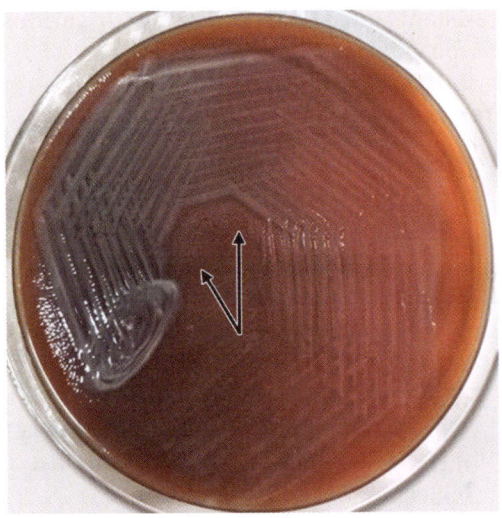

Fig. 16.5: *Proteus* on blood agar, showing swarming growth (arrows showing).
Source: Department of Microbiology, JIPMER, Puducherry (*with permission*).

wound and soft tissue infections, septicemia and nosocomial outbreaks. *Proteus* is also involved in the pathogenesis of renal stones (struvite/phosphate stones)
- **Laboratory diagnosis:** *Proteus* produces characteristic swarming growth on blood agar **(Fig. 16.5)**. Identification of various members are made based on conventional biochemical tests or automated ID methods such as MALDI-TOF and VITEK. Antimicrobial susceptibility testing can be performed by disk diffusion test or VITEK
- **Treatment** is the same as discussed for *E. coli*, except that Tribe Proteeae are intrinsically resistant to certain antimicrobial agents (e.g. colistin, tigecycline, etc.) which should be avoided in the treatment
- The somatic antigen of certain non-motile *Proteus* strains (called X strains) can be used to detect cross-reacting heterophile antibodies in sera of patients suffering from rickettsial infections (Weil-Felix reaction).

Serratia

Serratia marcescens is usually a saprophyte in the environment, and typically produces a red non-diffusible pigment called prodigiosin. However, the hospital strains of *S. marcescens* are often non-pigmented and multiple drug-resistant and are associated with various nosocomial infections.

Yersinia species

Yersinia pestis (Plague)

It is the causative agent of plague, a fulminant systemic zoonosis; transmitted from rodents by the arthropod vector, the rat flea.
- **Epidemiology:** Plague was one of the greatest killer known to mankind; caused several pandemics in the ancient days producing millions of deaths. In India, the Surat epidemic (in 1994) has witnessed more than 6,000 suspected plague cases with 60 deaths
- **Clinical forms:** Human plague occurs in three clinical forms—(1) bubonic plague (most common form, characterized by enlarged and tender regional lymph nodes), (2) pneumonic plague, and (3) septicemic plague
- **Laboratory diagnosis:** Depending upon the type of plague, the specimens collected are: pus or fluid aspirated from buboes, sputum and blood
- **Direct microscopy:** Reveals gram-negative oval coccobacilli and pus cells
  - **Wayson staining** demonstrates *bipolar* or *safety pin* appearance of the bacilli
  - **Culture media** used are: Blood agar (non-hemolytic colonies) and MacConkey agar (NLF colonies)
  - **Identification** from colonies is either by automated identification systems (e.g. MALDI-TOF) or by conventional biochemical tests.
- **Treatment:** Streptomycin or gentamicin is recommended for treatment.

Yersiniosis

Infections due to other *Yersinia* species such as *Y. enterocolitica* or *Y. pseudotuberculosis* are called yersiniosis. They are enteropathogenic and cause gastroenteritis, terminal ileitis, and mesenteric lymphadenitis.

VIBRIO CHOLERAE

Vibrio cholerae is the causative agent of an acute diarrheal disease called cholera. It differs from Enterobacterales being oxidase-positive.

Typing

Typing of *Vibrio cholerae* can be done as follows:
- **Serogroups:** Based on the somatic O antigen, *V. cholerae* can be typed into several serogroups (>200). Out of which, serogroups O1 is the most common group to cause cholera, followed by serogroups O139
- **Biotypes:** Serogroup O1 can be typed based on biochemical reactions into two biotypes—classical and El Tor
  - Classical biotype is more virulent whereas El Tor biotype is more resistant to environmental stresses
  - Therefore classical biotype produces more severe illness, whereas El Tor

biotype produces milder cases but more number of carriers.
- **Serotypes:** Serogroup O1 can be typed based on minor differences in O antigen into three serotypes—Ogawa, Inaba, Hikojima.

Epidemiology

The world has witnessed several cholera pandemics in the past; resulting in several thousands of deaths.
- **Seven pandemics** have been reported till date—first six were due to classical biotype and the seven one was due to El Tor biotype
- **Currently**, cholera occurs as sporadic and limited outbreaks. Majority of cases are due to El Tor, but cases due to classical biotype still occur in small proportion.

Pathogenesis

Pathogenesis of *V. cholerae* is due to a potent enterotoxin, called cholera toxin and a pilus (TCP).
- **Toxin-coregulated pilus (TCP):** It helps in the adhesion of the bacilli to the intestinal epithelium
- **Cholera toxin:** It is similar to the heat-labile toxin of *E. coli*, and has two fragments A and B
  - Fragment B binds to GM1 ganglioside receptors on the intestinal epithelium
  - Fragment A is the active unit, acts by increasing cyclic AMP
  - Cyclic AMP inhibits the absorption sodium and activates the secretion chloride, which lead to the accumulation of sodium chloride and water in the intestinal lumen and finally results in watery diarrhea.

Clinical Manifestations

Cholera manifests as painless watery diarrhea, described as a **rice-water stool**.
- **Mild fluid loss** may lead to features such as weakness, postural hypotension, tachycardia, and decreased skin turgor
- **Severe dehydration** can result in renal failure and fluid loss leading to—oliguria, weak or absent pulses, sunken eyes, wrinkled ("washerwoman") skin and even coma.

Laboratory Diagnosis

Useful specimens are watery stool (for cases) or rectal swabs (for carriers).
- **Transport media:** Specimens should be sent in appropriate transport media such as VR medium (Venkatraman-Ramakrishnan), and Cary-Blair medium
- **Direct microscopy** of the stool specimen reveals:
  - Gram stain: Gram-negative rods, short curved comma-shaped (fish in stream appearance)
  - Hanging drop method: Demonstrates **darting motility**—extremely active motility with rapid changing direction.
- **Culture:** Various culture media used for *V. cholerae* are:
  - **Enrichment broth:** Alkaline peptone water, Monsur's taurocholate tellurite peptone water
  - **Selective media**: (i) Bile salt agar, (ii) Monsur's gelatin taurocholate tellurite (GTT) agar, and (iii) thiosulfate citrate bile salts sucrose (TCBS) agar
  - **TCBS agar:** It is the most common selective media used for *V. cholerae*, which produces typical yellow colonies **(Fig. 16.6)**
  - **MacConkey agar:** *V. cholerae* produces translucent NLF colonies.
- **Culture smear and motility testing**—reveal short curved gram-negative bacilli and darting motility
- **Identification:** *V. cholerae* produces hemodigestion on blood agar and gives positive string test. Identification of *V. cholerae* from the colonies can be performed by following tests:
  - Conventional biochemical tests such as oxidase, catalase, indole, citrate, urease and TSI test
  - Automated methods such as MALDI-TOF and VITEK.
- **Typing:** After being identified as *V. cholerae*, it is further subjected to various typing methods

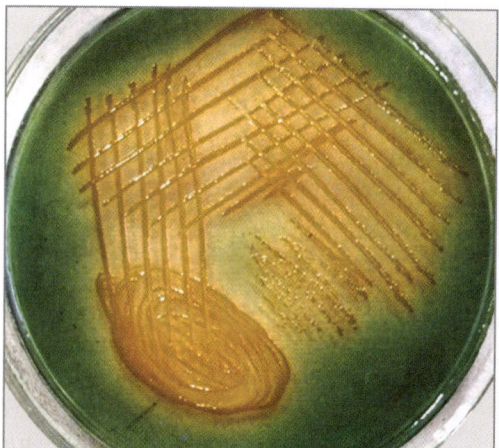

Fig. 16.6: Thiosulfate citrate bile salts sucrose (TCBS) agar with yellow-colored colonies of *Vibrio cholerae*.
Source: Department of Microbiology, Pondicherry Institute of Medical Sciences, Puducherry (*with permission*).

- *Biotyping:* To differentiate classical and El Tor
- *Serogrouping:* To differentiate O1 and O139
- *Serotyping:* To differentiate Ogawa, Inaba, and Hikojima serotypes of serogroup O1.
❖ **Antigen detection** can be done by tests such as cholera dipstick assay
❖ **Molecular method:** Multiplex PCR can be used to detect common diarrheal pathogens

❖ **Antimicrobial susceptibility testing** can be performed by disk diffusion test or by automated methods (e.g. VITEK).

> **TREATMENT** Cholera
>
> Fluid replacement is the mainstay of treatment of cholera. Antibiotics such as macrolides (azithromycin) or doxycycline can be given to severely dehydrated patients.

Cholera Vaccine

Oral cholera vaccines (OCV) are currently in use for the prevention of cholera. They usually give short-term protection (6 months or so). Two types of OCVs are available.
1. **Killed whole-cell vaccine,** e.g. include whole-cell (WC) vaccine (e.g. Shanchol) and whole-cell recombinant B subunit vaccine (e.g. Dukoral)
2. **Oral live attenuated vaccines,** e.g. CVD 103-HgR vaccine.

   Injectable killed vaccines which were used before are no longer used.

Halophilic Vibrio

The *Vibrio* species other than *V. cholerae* that grow in higher salt concentrations are called **halophilic *Vibrios*;** examples include *V. parahaemolyticus, V. alginolyticus* and *V. vulnificus.* They cause intestinal and extraintestinal manifestations.

EXPECTED QUESTIONS

I. **Write essay on:**
   1. Discuss the pathogenesis, clinical manifestations, laboratory diagnosis, and treatment of enteric fever.
   2. Discuss the epidemiology, clinical manifestations, laboratory diagnosis and treatment of cholera.

II. **Write short notes on:**
   1. Diarrheagenic *E. coli*.
   2. *Klebsiella pneumoniae* infections.
   3. Shigellosis.
   4. Plague.

III. **Multiple Choice Questions (MCQs):**
   1. TCBS agar is used for_____?
      a. *Vibrio cholerae*   b. *Salmonella*
      c. *Shigella*   d. *Mycobacteria*
   2. Which of the following exhibits darting motility?
      a. *Salmonella*   b. *Shigella*
      c. *Vibrio cholerae*   d. *E. coli*
   3. In first week of illness, enteric fever is diagnosed by_____?
      a. Widal test   b. Blood culture
      c. Stool culture   d. Urine culture

Answers
1. a   2. c   3. b

CHAPTER 17

Gram-negative Bacilli Infections-II

CHAPTER PREVIEW
- Nonfermenter GNBs
- Fastidious GNBs
- Miscellaneous GNBs

This chapter deals with gram-negative bacilli (GNB) infections caused by the following organisms:
- **Nonfermenter GNBs:** Such as *Pseudomonas*, *Acinetobacter*, and *Burkholderia*
- **Fastidious GNBs:** Such as *Haemophilus*, *Brucella*, and *Bordetella*
- **Miscellaneous GNBs:** Such as *Campylobacter*, *Helicobacter pylori*, *Legionella*, *Gardnerella vaginalis*, and *Streptobacillus moniliformis*.

NONFERMENTING GRAM-NEGATIVE BACILLI

Nonfermenters do not ferment any carbohydrates but utilize them oxidatively. Important human pathogens are discussed below.

Pseudomonas aeruginosa

P. aeruginosa is a major pathogenic species, causing infections among hospitalized patients and in patients with cystic fibrosis.

Pathogenesis

The pathogenesis is greatly attributed to its ability to develop widespread resistance to multiple antibiotics and disinfectants and produce several virulence factors.
- **Toxins**, e.g. exotoxin A. It acts by inhibiting protein synthesis
- **Enzymes**, e.g. phospholipases, elastases, etc.
- **Pigments:** *Pseudomonas* produces various pigments such as:
  - Pyocyanin: It is a blue-green pigment, produced only by *P. aeruginosa*
  - Pyoverdin: It is greenish-yellow pigment, produced by most species
  - Pyorubin: This pigment imparts red color.

Clinical Manifestations

Most of the infections are encountered in hospitalized patients who get colonized with the organisms either from the heavily contaminated hospital environment or from the hospital staff (through contaminated hands). Colonized patients develop the disease in the presence of underlying risk factors such as burn wounds, patients with immunosuppression, and post surgeries. The manifestations are as follows:
- **Healthcare-associated infections** such as—(i) ventilator-associated pneumonia (VAP), (ii) central-line associated bloodstream infection (CLABSI), (iii) catheter-associated urinary tract infection (CAUTI), (iv) surgical site infection (SSI)
- **Chronic respiratory tract infections:** It occurs in patients with underlying conditions that cause airway damage such as cystic fibrosis, or bronchiectasis

- **Bacteremia** leading to sepsis and septic shock
- **Infective endocarditis (native valves):** It occurs among IV drug abusers
- **Ear infections:** The infections are either mild, such as **swimmer's ear** (among children), or serious necrotizing form designated as **malignant otitis externa** (in elderly diabetic patients)
- **Eye infections** such as corneal ulcers (in contact lens wearers) and endophthalmitis secondary to bacteremia
- **Shanghai fever:** It is a mild febrile illness resembling typhoid fever
- **Skin and soft tissue infections** such as burns wound infection, ecthyma gangrenosum, green nail syndrome, and cellulitis with blue-green pus
- **Other infections:** Bone and joint infections such as osteomyelitis and septic arthritis and meningitis (in postoperative or post-traumatic patients).

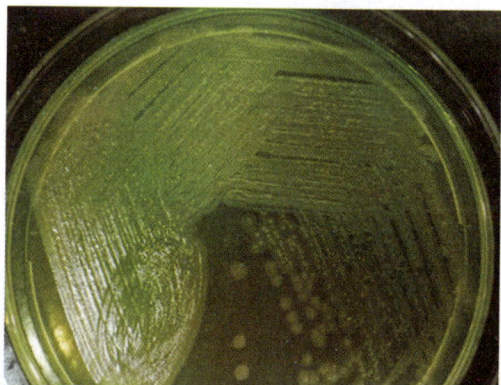

Fig. 17.1: *Pseudomonas aeruginosa* on nutrient agar showing: large irregular colonies with metallic sheen and green color pigmentation.

Source: Department of Microbiology, Pondicherry Institute of Medical Sciences, Puducherry (*with permission*).

Laboratory Diagnosis

Specimen collection depends upon the site of infection, such as—pus, blood, tracheal aspirate, sputum, wound swab, urine, etc.
- **Direct smear:** Reveals gram-negative bacilli, and pus cells
- **Culture:** Incubation at 37°C aerobically for 24 h yields the following growth
  - Nutrient agar: Opaque, irregular colonies with metallic sheen (iridescence) and blue green diffusible pigments **(Fig. 17.1)**
  - Blood agar: β-hemolytic gray moist colonies
  - MacConkey agar: Non-lactose fermenting (NLF) colonies
  - Selective media such as cetrimide agar may be used.
- **Culture smear and motility:** Motile, gram-negative bacilli
- **Identification** from the colonies is made by automated ID systems such as MALDI-TOF or VITEK or by conventional biochemical tests such as—catalase (positive), oxidase (positive), indole, citrate, urease, TSI, etc.
- **AST:** Antimicrobial susceptibility testing is performed by disk diffusion test or by automated MIC detection method (e.g. VITEK).

> **TREATMENT** *P. aeruginosa*
>
> - *Pseudomonas aeruginosa* is intrinsically resistant to ceftriaxone, amoxicillin-clavulanate, ertapenem, tetracyclines, tigecycline, etc. Therefore, these drugs should not be used in the therapy
> - Only limited agents have good anti-pseudomonal action such as ceftazidime, piperacillin-tazobactam, carbapenems, amikacin, quinolones (ciprofloxacin or levofloxacin), etc.

Preventive Measures

Infection control measures (contact precaution) such as hand hygiene are crucial to limit the spread of *Pseudomonas* infection in the hospitals (see Chapter 38).

Acinetobacter species

They are saprophytic bacilli, can cause widespread healthcare-associated infections, especially in patients with underlying diseases and immunosuppression.
- **Clinical manifestations:** *Acinetobacter baumannii* causes widespread healthcare associated infections such as:

- Ventilator associated pneumonia
- Central line associated bloodstream infection
- Catheter-associated UTI
- Wound and soft tissue infections
- Infections in burn patients.

❖ **Laboratory diagnosis:** It is a nonfermenter, but differs from *P. aeruginosa*, by being nonmotile, oxidase negative, does not produce any pigment. Antimicrobial susceptibility testing is performed by disk diffusion test or by VITEK

❖ **Treatment** for *Acinetobacter* is similar to that of *Pseudomonas*, except that it responds to certain additional agents such as minocycline or tigecycline

❖ **Prevention:** Infection control measures such as improved hand hygiene are essential to prevent nosocomial infections due to *Acinetobacter* (refer contact precaution, Chapter 38).

Burkholderia species

Important species that are pathogenic to man include *B. cepacia* complex and *B. pseudomallei*.

❖ ***B. cepacia* complex:** It inhabits a moist hospital environment and intravenous fluids; can cause fatal respiratory infections and septicemia in hospitalized patients with underlying diseases and immunosuppression

❖ ***B. pseudomallei*:** It is the causative agent of **melioidosis**; which presents in various clinical forms ranging from acute localized infection, subacute pulmonary infection, bloodstream infection, and chronic suppurative infection
- **Diagnosis:** It shows bipolar staining in Gram-stained smear, intrinsically resistant to polymyxin B, and grows on selective media such as Ashdown's medium
- **Treatment:** Compromises of— (i) intensive phase (2 weeks) with ceftazidime or meropenem, followed by (ii) maintenance phase (12 weeks) with oral cotrimoxazole.

FASTIDIOUS GRAM-NEGATIVE BACILLI

Fastidious gram-negative bacilli include *Haemophilus, Bordetella,* and *Brucella*.

Haemophilus species

Haemophilus species are pleomorphic gram-negative bacilli that require special growth factors (such as X factor or V factor or both).

Haemophilus influenzae

It is the most pathogenic species; causes pneumonia and meningitis in children. It requires both X and V factors for its growth.

❖ **Pathogenesis:** It is capsulated, which is the main virulent factor. Based on capsular polysaccharide antigen, it can be typed into 6 serotypes (a to f)—serotype b being the most pathogenic and invasive

❖ **Clinical manifestations:** The spectrum of illness can be divided into:
- Invasive infections such as pneumonia, bacteremia, meningitis, and epiglottitis
- Noninvasive infection such as otitis media, sinusitis, etc.

❖ **Laboratory diagnosis:** It is fastidious, grows in chocolate agar, not in blood agar
- But it can grow on blood agar, adjacent to the *Staphylococcus aureus* streak line—a unique property described as **satellitism**. Factor X (hemin) is present in blood agar and factor V is released from *S. aureus*. Therefore larger colonies are formed adjacent to *S. aureus* streak line and size of the colonies decreases gradually away from the *S. aureus* streak line **(Fig. 17.2)**
- Identification is confirmed by disk test for X and V requirements or automated ID systems such as MALDI-TOF.

❖ **Treatment:** Ceftriaxone is given for treatment

❖ **Vaccine:** Hib conjugate vaccine (*H. influenzae* type b) is available for children. Under the national immunization program, it is given as a part of the pentavalent vaccine at 6, 10, and 14 weeks.

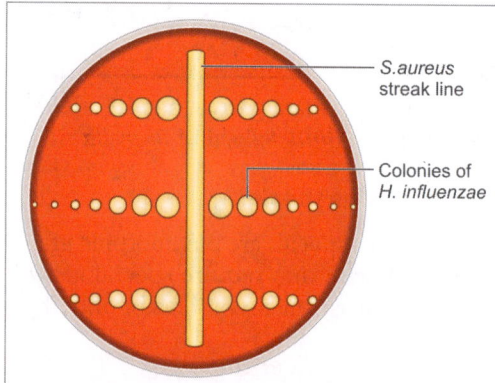

Fig. 17.2: Satellitism of *Haemophilus influenzae* (schematic diagram).

Haemophilus ducreyi

It is the causative agent of soft chancre (chancroid); a sexually transmitted infection characterized by painful genital ulcers and enlarged tender inguinal lymph nodes (bubo).

HACEK Group

They represent a group of highly fastidious gram-negative bacilli, which are found as the normal commensal of the oral cavity but can cause serious infections such as endocarditis. They include—*Haemophilus* species, *Aggregatibacter* species, *Cardiobacterium hominis*, *Eikenella corrodens* and *Kingella kingae*.

Bordetella pertussis

Bordetella pertussis is the causative agent of **whooping cough**; a highly contagious toxin-mediated disease, characterized by paroxysmal cough ending in a high pitched inspiratory sound described as "whoop".

- **Pathogenesis** is mediated by the expression of several virulence factors such as pertussis toxin, tracheal cytotoxin, adhesins, etc.
- **Laboratory diagnosis:** Nasopharyngeal aspirate collected by alginate swabs can be subjected to culture on special media such as Regan-Lowe or Bordet-Gengou media. It produces mercury drops or bisected pearls colony
- **Treatment:** Macrolide such as azithromycin is the drug of choice
- **Prevention:** Two vaccines are available—(1) whole-cell pertussis vaccine: which is given as a part of DPT under the national immunization schedule (see Chapter 13 for detail), and (2) acellular pertussis vaccine.

Brucella species

Brucellosis is a highly contagious zoonotic febrile illness called undulant fever or Malta fever.

- **Agents:** *Brucella melitensis* is the most common species, affects sheep and goat. Other species are *B. abortus* (cattle), *B. canis* (dog), etc.
- **Transmission:** Transmitted from infected animals to man by various modes such as direct contact or by eating or drinking unpasteurized/raw dairy products
- **Clinical manifestations:** Overall brucellosis resembles typhoid-like illness. It manifests as a triad of fever, arthralgia, and hepatosplenomegaly
  - Fever is undulating in nature, i.e. afebrile period between febrile periods
  - Musculoskeletal involvement is common such as vertebral osteomyelitis or septic arthritis.
- **Laboratory diagnosis:** Specimen collected are blood or bone marrow
  - *Culture:* Blood culture or bone marrow culture is performed either by using (i) conventional blood culture bottles, or (ii) Castaneda's biphasic media (BHI broth/agar), or (iii) automated blood culture systems like BacT/ALERT
  - Detection of antibodies by serological tests such as standard agglutination test (SAT) or ELISA.
- **Treatment:** Comprises of doxycycline, in combination with rifampicin or streptomycin, given for a longer duration (6 weeks).

MISCELLANEOUS GRAM-NEGATIVE BACILLI

Campylobacter

Campylobacter jejuni is an important agent of inflammatory diarrhea or dysentery.

- **Transmission** is mainly by ingestion of raw or undercooked food products

- **Clinical manifestations:** Characterized by inflammatory diarrhea, abdominal pain, and fever. Extraintestinal complications can also be occasionally seen (mainly due to other species such as *C. fetus*) such as bacteremia, sepsis, meningitis, etc.
- **Diagnosis:** Stool culture can be done using selective media such as Skirrow's, Butzler's media and incubating in microaerophilic (5%O_2) conditions. Gram stain reveals a curved gram-negative rod
- **Treatment:** Fluid and electrolyte replacement is the mainstay of treatment. Oral macrolides are the drug of choice (erythromycin or azithromycin).

Helicobacter pylori

Helicobacter pylori is a curved gram-negative rod that colonizes the stomach.
- **Clinical manifestations:** *H. pylori* is associated with the pathogenesis of the following conditions:
  - Acute gastritis involving the antrum region
  - Peptic ulcer disease (duodenal and gastric ulcers): It presents with epigastric pain with a burning sensation; develops either following a meal (as in duodenal ulcer) or in an empty stomach (as in gastric ulcer)
  - Adenocarcinoma of stomach
- **Diagnosis:** Urea breath test and biopsy urease test are the preferred methods. Other diagnostic modalities include:
  - Fecal antigen (coproantigen) assay
  - Culture using Skirrow's media and chocolate agar and incubating the plates at 37°C under microaerophilic condition
- **Treatment** includes a triple-drug regimen, comprising omeprazole, clarithromycin, and metronidazole; given for 7–14 days.

Legionella

L. pneumophila is a fastidious, pleomorphic gram-negative short rod, associated with two clinical syndromes—(i) Pontiac fever (an acute, milder flu-like self-limited illness), and (ii) Legionnaires' disease (a severe form of interstitial pneumonia)
- **Transmission:** Aspiration of the organism from oropharyngeal colonization or directly via the drinking of contaminated water is the most common mode. Aerosols from contaminated air conditioners, nebulizers, and humidifiers are another mode of transmission
- **Laboratory diagnosis** includes—(i) isolation of the organism in buffered charcoal, yeast extract (BCYE) agar, or (ii) urinary antigen detection
- **Treatment:** Macrolides (e.g. azithromycin) and respiratory quinolones are now the antibiotics of choice.

Gardnerella vaginalis

It causes profuse watery vaginal discharge—a condition called bacterial vaginosis. It is diagnosed if any 3 of the following 4 findings are present (Amsel's criteria):
1. **Discharge:** Thin white homogeneous vaginal discharge uniformly coated on the vaginal wall
2. **pH** of vaginal discharge more than 4.5
3. **Whiff test:** Accentuation of a distinct fishy odor of vaginal secretions, when mixed with 10% solution of KOH
4. **Clue cells:** They are vaginal epithelial cells coated with coccobacilli, which have a granular appearance and indistinct borders observed on a wet mount **(Fig. 17.3)**.

Treatment of bacterial vaginosis involves oral metronidazole, given twice daily for 7 days.

Streptobacillus moniliformis

It causes a zoonotic systemic illness transmitted by rodents; called **rat-bite fever**. This condition is also caused by another gram-negative bacillus called *Spirillum minus*.

SECTION 3 ♦ Bacterial Infections

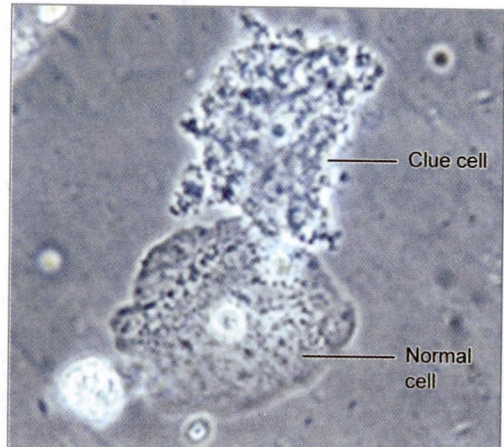

Fig. 17.3: Wet mount of vaginal secretion depicting clue cell.
Source: Public Health Image Library/ID#: 14574/ M. Rein/Centers for Disease Control and Prevention (CDC), Atlanta (*with permission*).

▶ EXPECTED QUESTIONS ◀

I. Write short notes on:
1. Infections caused by *Pseudomonas*.
2. Laboratory diagnosis of *H. influenzae*.
3. Melioidosis.
4. Pertussis.
5. Infections caused by *Acinetobacter*.

II. Multiple Choice Questions (MCQs):
1. **Satellitism is observed in culture for___?**
   a. Bordetella
   b. *H. influenzae*
   c. Brucella
   d. Pseudomonas
2. **Undulant fever is caused by _____?**
   a. Burkholderia
   b. Helicobacter
   c. *H. influenzae*
   d. Brucella
3. **Urea breath test is done _____?**
   a. Campylobacter
   b. Burkholderia
   c. Helicobacter
   d. *H. influenzae*
4. **Melioidosis is caused by_____?**
   a. Burkholderia pseudomallei
   b. Burkholderia cepacia
   c. Burkholderia mallei
   d. Pseudomonas aeruginosa
5. **Ecthyma gangrenosum is caused by:**
   a. Pseudomonas
   b. Bordetella
   c. Brucella
   d. *H. influenzae*

Answers
1. b   2. d   3. c   4. a   5. a

CHAPTER 18: Miscellaneous Bacterial Infections

CHAPTER PREVIEW

- Spirochetes: *Treponema*, *Borrelia* and *Leptospira*
- Rickettsiae and Related Genera
- Chlamydiae
- Mycoplasma

SPIROCHETES

Spirochetes are thin, flexible, elongated spirally coiled helical bacilli; e.g. *Treponema*, *Borrelia* and *Leptospira*.

Treponema pallidum (Syphilis)

Treponema pallidum is the causative agent of a sexually transmitted infection called as syphilis. It is a genitoulcerative disease, transmitted by sexual contact, but rarely by non-venereal modes such as direct contact, blood transfusion or transplacental transmission. The incubation period is about 9-90 days.

Clinical Stages

The clinical course of syphilis passes through four clinical stages.
1. **Primary syphilis**: It is characterized by:
   - *Genital ulcer*: Painless, firm, non-suppurative genital ulcers (called hard chancre), and
   - *Lymphadenopathy* (usually inguinal): Painless firm, non-suppurative, and often bilateral.
2. **Secondary syphilis**: It usually develops 6-12 weeks after the healing of the primary lesion. It presents as:
   - Skin rashes on palms and soles
   - Mucosal patches
   - *Condylomata lata*: Mucocutaneous papules are seen in the perianal region, vulva, and scrotum.
3. **Latent syphilis**: It is a clinically silent phase between secondary and late syphilis. It is characterized by the absence of clinical manifestations with positive serological tests for syphilis
4. **Late syphilis**: It occurs several decades after the initial infection, and is associated with skin, CVS, and CNS manifestations
   - *Skin lesions* are called gummata: They are destructive granulomatous lesions
   - *CVS manifestations*: It is characterized by aneurysm of ascending aorta and aortic regurgitation
   - *CNS manifestations*: Common manifestations include—chronic meningitis, general paresis of the insane, and tabes dorsalis.

Congenital syphilis: Mother-to-fetus transmission can lead to the development of various congenital manifestations such as—Hutchinson's teeth (notched central incisors), mulberry-shaped molar, saddle nose, etc.

Laboratory Diagnosis

Syphilis is mainly diagnosed by the following diagnostic modalities.

Direct Microscopy

Treponemes can be demonstrated from the superficial lesions of primary, secondary, and congenital syphilis. The surface of the genital ulcer is cleaned with saline, gentle pressure is applied at the base of the lesion, and a drop of exudate is collected on a slide and examined by any of the following methods:

- Dark ground microscopy (DGM) **(Fig. 18.1A)**
- Direct fluorescent antibody staining for *T. pallidum* (DFA-TP)
- Silver impregnation staining—such as Levaditi stain and Fontana stain: *Treponema* do not take up ordinary stains as they are extremely thin and delicate. Therefore, silver impregnation methods can be used to increase their thickness **(Fig. 18.1B)**.

Cultivation

Pathogenic treponemes including *T. pallidum* cannot be grown in artificial culture media but are maintained by subcultures in susceptible animals such as rabbit testes (e.g. Nichols strain).

Serology (Antibody Detection)

As microscopy is difficult and culture methods are not available, antibody detection methods are of paramount importance in the diagnosis of syphilis. Depending upon the type of antigen used, two types of tests are available to detect antibodies in a patient's sera.

Non-treponemal Tests

These tests detect non-specific reagin antibody by using cardiolipin antigen derived from the bovine heart. These tests work on the principle of slide flocculation (precipitation reaction).

- **Venereal disease research laboratory (VDRL) test:** The patient's serum is mixed with a drop of VDRL antigen on a concave slide, which is then mixed by rotating the slide. A positive test is indicated by the formation of medium to large clumps of Ag-Ab complexes; visualized by focusing the slide under the microscope **(Figs. 18.2A and B)**
- **Rapid plasma reagin (RPR):** It is similar to the VDRL test, except that it does not require a microscope to take the reading. RPR is preferred to test individual samples (less sample load); whereas VDRL is preferred when samples are tested in batches (large sample load).

Treponemal Tests

These tests detect species-specific antibody by using *T. pallidum*-specific antigen; which is polysaccharide in nature. Various tests are:

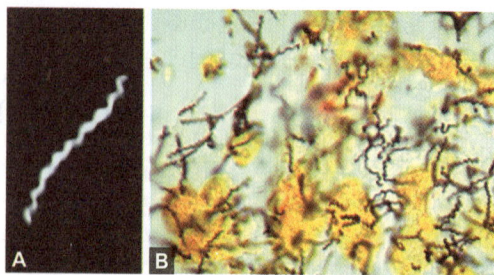

Figs. 18.1 A and B: Direct microscopy of *T. pallidum:* **A.** Dark ground microscope; **B.** Silver impregnation method.

Source: Public Health Image Library, **A.** ID# 2043; **B.** ID# 836, Centers for Disease Control and Prevention (CDC), Atlanta (*with permission*).

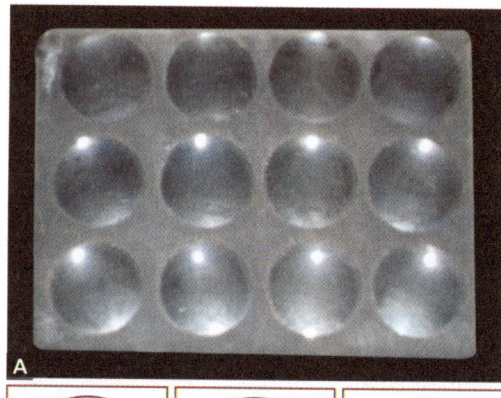
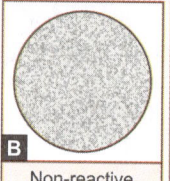
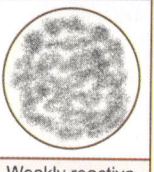
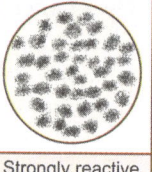

Figs. 18.2A and B: A. VDRL slide; **B.** VDRL test results.

Source: Department of Microbiology, JIPMER, Puducherry (*with permission*).

- TPI: *T. pallidum* immobilization test
- FTA-ABS: Fluorescent treponemal antibody absorption test
- TPHA: *T. pallidum* hemagglutination test
- TPPA: *T. pallidum* particle agglutination test
- Western blot and enzyme immunoassay.

> **TREATMENT** — Syphilis
>
> Penicillin is the drug of choice for treating all stages of syphilis. Doxycycline can be used alternatively in case of penicillin allergy.

Nonvenereal Treponema species

Endemic or nonvenereal treponematoses are caused by three close relatives of *T. pallidum*; producing primary mucocutaneous lesions in non-genital sites (e.g. extremities, oral mucosa).
- *T. pertenue*: Causes yaws
- *T. endemicum*: Causes endemic syphilis
- *T. carateum*: Causes pinta.

Borrelia species

Most of the species of *Borrelia* occur as commensals on the buccal and genital mucosa. Few are pathogenic to man, such as:
- *B. recurrentis* causes epidemic relapsing fever
- *B. duttonii* and *B. hermsii* cause endemic relapsing fever
- *B. burgdorferi* is the agent of Lyme disease
- *B. vincentii* causes Vincent's angina in association with fusiform bacilli.

Leptospira interrogans

Leptospira interrogans is the causative agent of leptospirosis; a zoonotic disease transmitted, by direct contact with the urine of infected animals such as rodents.

Leptospira interrogans is antigenically complex and comprises 26 serogroups; which are further typed into >300 serovars. The serogroups and serovars differ in their geographical distribution and severity of infection.

Clinical Manifestations

Leptospira interrogans produces two types of illnesses.

- The majority (90%) of leptospirosis cases present as mild anicteric febrile illness
- Few cases (10%) progress to severe form hepatorenal hemorrhagic syndrome or **Weil's disease**; characterized by icterus, high-grade fever, hemorrhagic manifestations, and impaired renal functions.

Laboratory Diagnosis

Laboratory diagnosis of leptospirosis involves the following modalities. Specimens include blood and CSF (in the early stage) and urine (in the late stage).
- **Dark ground microscopy** of clinical specimens such as blood or CSF reveals spirally coiled bacilli (tightly) with hooked ends **(Figs. 18.3A and B)**
- **Culture:** Can be performed on special media such as Ellinghausen-McCullough-Johnson-Harris (EMJH) medium and incubated at 30°C for 4–6 weeks
- **Serology for antibody detection:** Various tests are available such as :
  - *Genus specific tests:* Latex agglutination test, ELISA, ICT (immunochromatographic test)

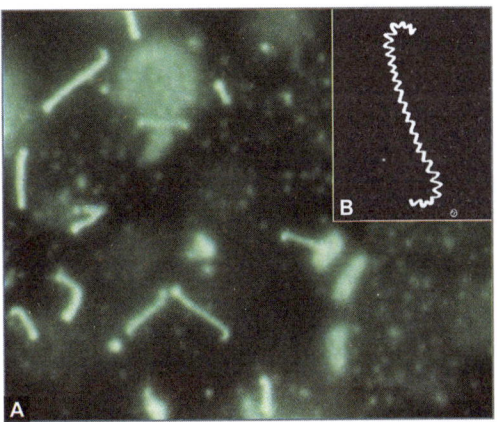

Figs. 18.3A and B: *Leptospira interrogans* (spirally coiled bacilli with hooked ends): **A.** Dark ground microscopy of the mount following microscopic agglutination test; **B.** Schematic diagram (viewed under a dark-ground microscope).

Source: **A.** Public Health Image Library/ID#: 2888/ Mrs M Gatton, Centers for Disease Control and Prevention (CDC), Atlanta (*with permission*).

- *Serovar specific test:* **Microscopic agglutination test**. It serves as the gold standard reference method for the diagnosis of leptospirosis.

> **TREATMENT** — Leptospirosis
>
> Oral doxycycline is given for mild leptospirosis; whereas severe cases are treated with penicillin.

RICKETTSIAE AND RELATED GENERA

Rickettsiaceae comprise of two genera—*Rickettsia* and *Orientia*; both possess the following properties:

- They are obligate intracellular organisms
- They are not cultivable in artificial media, although they can grow in cell lines, or by animal and egg inoculation
- They are transmitted by arthropod vectors, such as tick, mite, flea, or louse.

The various members of Rickettsiae are:

- *R. prowazekii:* It is the causative agent of epidemic typhus, transmitted by louse
- *R. typhi:* It causes endemic typhus, transmitted by flea
- *R. rickettsii:* It is the causative agent of Rocky Mountain spotted fever, transmitted by tick
- *R. conorii:* It causes Indian tick typhus, transmitted by tick
- *R. akari:* It is the causative agent of rickettsialpox, transmitted by mite
- *Orientia tsutsugamushi:* It is the causative agent of scrub typhus, transmitted by mite.

Clinical Manifestations

For all Rickettsiae, the final target site is the endothelial cells. Clinically the rickettsial infections may manifest as a combination of one or more of the following features—fever, rashes, headache, myalgia, eschar, lymphadenopathy, etc.

Other genera related to *Rickettsia* are:

- *Ehrlichia:* It produces an acute febrile illness called ehrlichiosis, transmitted by ticks. It infects leukocytes such as granulocytes, monocytes; producing intracellular inclusions, called **morula**
- *Coxiella burnetii:* It causes **Q fever**, transmitted by inhalational mode; characterized by atypical pneumonia, hepatitis and on chronic stage, produces endocarditis. Rashes are typically absent
- *Bartonella:* It has there important species, which are associated with distinct clinical conditions
  - *B. bacilliformis* is the causative agent of a systemic disease called Carrion's disease and a local cutaneous lesion called verruga peruana
  - *B. quintana* causes trench fever
  - *B. henselae* is the agent of cat-scratch disease.

Laboratory Diagnosis

Laboratory diagnosis of rickettsial infection includes:

- **Weil Felix test:** It is a heterophile agglutination test, where rickettsial antibodies are detected by using non-specific cross-reacting *Proteus* antigens such as OX2, OX19, and OXK antigens
  - In epidemic and endemic typhus—sera agglutinate mainly with OX19 and sometimes with OX2
  - In tick-borne spotted fever—antibodies to both OX19 and OX2 are elevated
  - In scrub typhus—antibodies to OXK are raised
  - The test is negative in rickettsialpox, Q fever, ehrlichiosis and bartonellosis.
- **Specific antibody detection test,** e.g. indirect immunofluorescence test and ELISA.

> **TREATMENT** — Rickettsial infections
>
> Doxycycline is the drug of choice in the majority of rickettsial infections.

CHLAMYDIAE

Chlamydiae are obligate intracellular bacteria that cause a spectrum of diseases in man infecting the eye, genital organs, and lungs.

Clinical Manifestations

Chlamydiae have three pathogenic species infecting man, which are associated with various clinical manifestations.

Chlamydia trachomatis

Chlamydia trachomatis comprise of 19 serovars, which cause various infections in man such as:
- **Trachoma:** It is a type of chronic kerato-conjunctivitis, caused by serotypes A, B, and C
- **Genital chlamydiasis:** Caused by serotypes D to K, presents as urethral discharge (urethritis) and mucopurulent cervicitis, etc.
- **Inclusion conjunctivitis:** Caused by serotypes D to K. It presents mucopurulent discharge from the eyes. It can affect adults (swimming pool conjunctivitis) or neonates (ophthalmia neonatorum)
- **Infant pneumonia:** Caused by serotypes D to K, presents as interstitial pneumonia in infants
- **LGV (lymphogranuloma venerum):** It is a sexually transmitted infection, caused by serotypes L1, L2, and L3. It is characterized by painless genital ulcers and painful inguinal lymphadenopathy.

Chlamydia psittaci

It is a pathogen of birds. Infection in man can range from mild influenza-like syndrome to fatal atypical pneumonia. It comprises of several serotypes.

Chlamydia pneumoniae

It is an exclusively human pathogen, that causes atypical interstitial pneumonia. It is also associated with the pathogenesis of atherosclerosis. It has only one serotype.

Laboratory Diagnosis

Specimens collected depend upon the types of infection associated— (1) Scrapings or swabs from infected sites: Urethral swab for urethritis, endocervical swab for cervicitis, or conjunctival swabs for ocular infections, (2) Nasopharyngeal aspirate and respiratory secretions for suspected pneumonia, or (3) Bubo aspirate for LGV.

- **Microscopy:** Useful for detection of chlamydial inclusion bodies. Common staining methods used are Gram staining, Lugol's iodine, and direct immuno-fluorescence test
- **Antigen detection:** Enzyme immunoassays are available for the detection of LPS antigens
- **Culture:** It was the gold standard method in the past. Various culture methods available are:
  - Egg inoculation (yolk sac)
  - Mice inoculation
  - Cell line culture by using McCoy, HeLa (for *C. trachomatis*), or HEp2 (for *C. pneumoniae*).
- **Nucleic acid amplification tests (NAAT)**, e.g. PCR
  - This is considered as the most sensitive and specific method
  - Currently the diagnostic assay of choice for chlamydial infections.
- **Serology (antibody detection):** Two formats are available
  - ELISA using group-specific LPS antigen
  - Micro-immunofluorescence test detects antibody against species and serovar-specific MOMP (major outer membrane protein) antigen of *C. trachomatis*.

> **TREATMENT — Chlamydial infections**
> - Azithromycin is the drug of choice
> - Alternatively, doxycycline, tetracycline, erythromycin or ofloxacin can be used.

Prevention

Control measures for the prevention of chlamydial genital infections include:
- Periodic screening of high-risk groups, such as young women having multiple sex partners
- Treatment of both the sex partners
- Use of barrier methods of contraception such as condoms
- Abstain from sex till 7 days after starting the treatment.

MYCOPLASMA

Mycoplasmas are the smallest microbes capable of free-living in the environment. They lack rigid cell wall and therefore, are resistant to cell wall-acting antibiotics such as beta-lactams.

- ❖ **M. pneumoniae** is the pathogenic species, which is the causative agent of **primary atypical pneumonia** (community acquired pneumonia)
  - ■ *Clinical manifestations:* M. pneumoniae produces upper respiratory tract infection (manifests as pharyngitis, tracheobronchitis), **atypical pneumonia** (community acquired interstitial pneumonia) and extrapulmonary manifestations (e.g. septic arthritis, Guillain–Barre syndrome or neurologic manifestations)
  - ■ *Laboratory diagnosis* involves detection of antibodies (e.g. ELISA) or isolation of the organism in specific culture media such as PPLO broth
  - ■ *Treatment:* Macrolides are the drug of choice.
- ❖ **Urogenital mycoplasmas** include *M. hominis, M. genitalium* and *Ureaplasma urealyticum.* They cause urethritis.

EXPECTED QUESTIONS

I. Write short notes on:
1. Clinical manifestations of syphilis.
2. Laboratory diagnosis of syphilis.
3. Leptospirosis.
4. Infections produced by Chlamydiae.
5. Rickettsial infections.

II. Multiple Choice Questions (MCQs):
1. **Weil's disease is caused by___?**
   a. Leptospira interrogans
   b. Borrelia recurrentis
   c. Orientia tsutsugamushi
   d. Mycoplasma pneumoniae
2. **VDRL test is done for___?**
   a. Leptospirosis
   b. Lyme disease
   c. Scrub typhus
   d. Syphilis
3. **Primary atypical pneumonia is caused by ____?**
   a. Leptospira interrogans
   b. Borrelia recurrentis
   c. Mycoplasma pneumoniae
   d. Orientia tsutsugamushi
4. **Lyme disease is caused by____?**
   a. Leptospira interrogans
   b. Borrelia recurrentis
   c. Borrelia vincenti
   d. Borrelia burgdorferi

Answers
1. a   2. d   3. c   4. d

SECTION 4: Viral Infections

SECTION OUTLINE

19. Herpes and Other DNA Virus Infections
20. Myxoviruses and Rubella Virus Infections
21. Coronavirus Infections including COVID-19
22. Arbovirus Infections
23. Rabies and Polio
24. HIV/AIDS
25. Viral Hepatitis
26. Miscellaneous RNA Virus Infections

Vaccinate and keep your life safe from

Hepatitis B

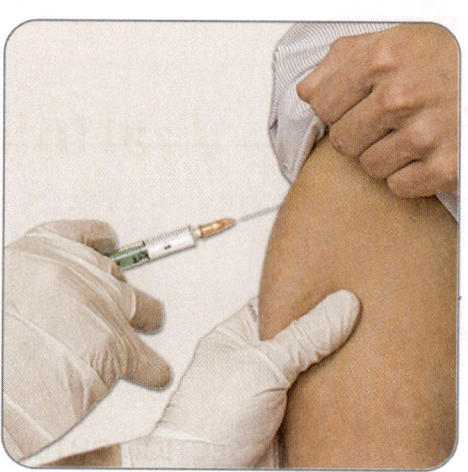

Healthcare workers are at highest risk of contracting Hepatitis B virus

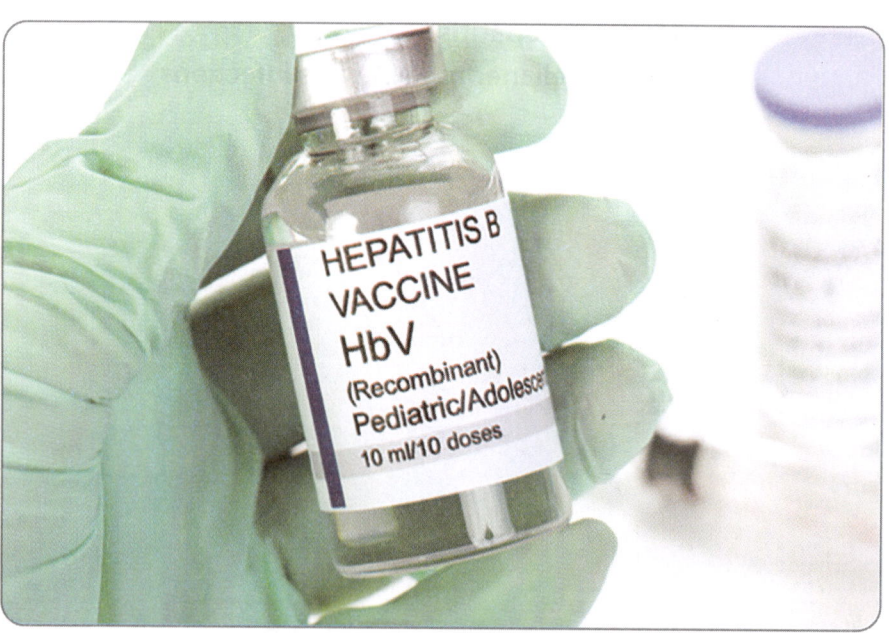

CHAPTER 19

Herpes and Other DNA Virus Infections

CHAPTER PREVIEW

- Herpesviruses
- Other DNA Virus Infections

DNA viruses include herpesviruses, parvoviruses, papilloma and polyomaviruses, poxviruses, adenoviruses, bacteriophages, and hepatitis B virus. The hepatitis B virus is discussed in Chapter 25, along with other hepatitis viruses. Other DNA viruses are discussed here.

HERPESVIRUSES

Herpesviruses are a group of DNA viruses that possess a unique property of establishing latent or persistent infections in their hosts and later on undergoing periodic reactivation. Based on the site of latency, they can be further grouped into three subfamilies.

1. **α-herpesviruses:** They undergo latency in neurons. Examples include—Herpes simplex viruses (HSV-1 and HSV-2), Varicella-zoster virus
2. **β-herpesviruses:** They undergo latency in glands and kidneys. An example includes cytomegalovirus
3. **γ-herpesviruses:** They undergo latency in lymphoid tissues. An example includes Epstein-Barr virus.

Herpes Simplex Virus

Herpes simplex viruses (HSV) are of two distinct types; HSV-1 and HSV-2.

Pathogenesis

The pathogenesis of HSV-1 and HSV-2 involves the following steps.

- ❖ **Transmission:** Infection is transmitted through abraded skin or mucosa—oropharyngeal contact is common for HSV-1, whereas sexual contact is common for HSV-2
- ❖ **Primary infection:** HSV replicates at the local site of infection and can produce lesions anywhere, but more commonly in:
  - HSV-1 lesions are confined to areas above the waist (most common site—around the mouth)
  - HSV-2 produces lesions below the waist (most common site—genital area).
- ❖ **Latency:** They invade the local nerve endings and migrate to dorsal root ganglia where they undergo latency (HSV-1 in trigeminal ganglia and HSV-2 in sacral ganglia)
- ❖ **Recurrent infections:** Reactivation of the latent virus can occur following various provocative stimuli, such as fever, stress, etc., which leads to the spread of the virus via the nerves back to the peripheral site (skin or mucosa or organs) producing secondary lesions. The recurrent lesions are typically less severe than the primary lesions.

Clinical Manifestations

HSV are extremely widespread and can cause a spectrum of diseases—involving skin, mucosa, and various organs.

- ❖ **Oral-facial mucosal lesions**: They are the most common manifestation of HSV

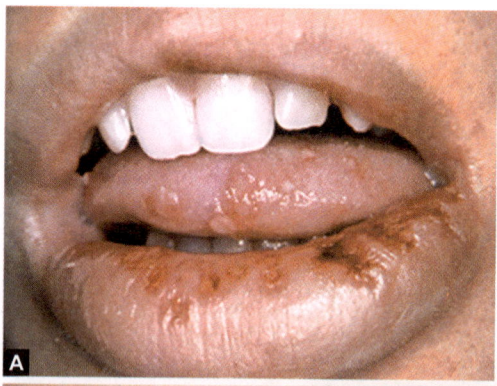

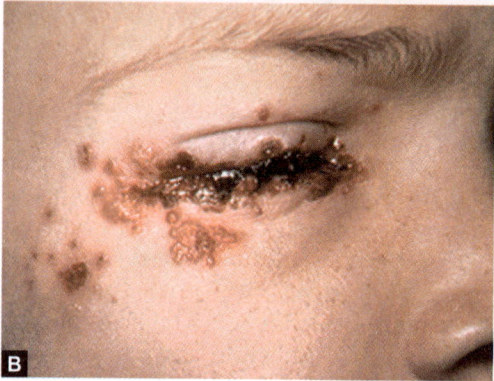

Figs. 19.1A and B: A. Vesicular lesions on lips and tongue due to HSV-1 infection; **B.** Periocular vesicular lesions due to HSV-1 infection.

Source: Public Health Image Library, **A.** ID# 12616 (Robert E Sumpter), **B.** ID# 6492 (Dr KL Hermann)/Centers for Disease Control and Prevention (CDC), Atlanta (*with permission*).

infections, characterized by painful vesicular lesions **(Figs. 19.1A and B)**
- The most commonly affected site is buccal mucosa
- The most frequent primary lesions are gingivostomatitis and pharyngitis
- The most frequent recurrent lesion is herpes labialis (painful vesicles near lips) **(Fig. 19.1A)**.

❖ **Cutaneous lesions:** HSV usually infects abraded skin and causes various cutaneous lesions
- Herpetic whitlow: Small blisters on fingers and lips
- Febrile blisters: Fever due to any other cause can provoke HSV to cause recurrent blisters
- Herpes gladiatorum: Mucocutaneous lesions present on the body of wrestlers
- Eczematous lesion called eczema herpeticum
- Erythema multiforme.

❖ **CNS infections:** Various CNS infections such as:
- Encephalitis: HSV is the most common cause of acute sporadic viral encephalitis
- Chronic meningitis (called Mollaret meningitis).

❖ **Genital lesions:** HSV-2 is more common than HSV-1 to produce genital lesions; described as bilateral, painful, multiple, tiny vesicular ulcers

❖ **Ocular lesions:** HSV produces various ocular manifestations such as kerato-conjunctivitis, corneal ulcer (called dendritic ulcers), and blindness

❖ **Neonatal herpes:** Transmission of infection during birth can lead to neonatal herpes. Transmission is more common during birth than in utero. Neonates can present with either local lesions or disseminated infection or CNS infections.

Laboratory Diagnosis

Laboratory diagnosis of HSV infections includes the following modalities.

❖ **Cytopathology:** Giemsa staining of scrapping obtained from the lesions (Tzanck smear preparation) detects inclusion bodies, called Lipschutz body) and formation of multinucleated giant cells

❖ **Viral isolation** in various cell lines (e.g. McCoy cell line) to demonstrate characteristic cytopathic effect such as diffuse rounding and ballooning of cell lines

❖ **Viral antigen detection** in the specimen by direct immunofluorescence (DIF)

❖ **HSV DNA detection** by PCR and real-time PCR (detecting glycoprotein B and UL 30 genes)

❖ **Antibody detection** by ELISA or other formats-detecting antibodies to glycoprotein G.

TREATMENT — HSV infections

Antiviral drugs such as acyclovir are effective for HSV infections. In case of acyclovir resistance, foscarnet is the drug of choice.

Prevention

General measures can be taken such as:
- Use of condom to prevent genital herpes
- Neonatal herpes can be prevented by prior administration of acyclovir to mothers during third trimester of pregnancy or delivery by elective cesarean section.

Infection control measures: Patients with mucocutaneous herpes in hospitals, should be kept on contact precautions until lesions are dry and crusted (refer Chapter 38).

Varicella-zoster Virus

Varicella-zoster virus (VZV) produces vesicular eruptions (rashes) on the skin and mucous membranes in the form of two clinical entities:

Chickenpox

It occurs following primary infection, usually affecting children, characterized by:
- **Rashes:** Generalized diffuse bilateral vesicular rashes, centripetal in distribution and appear in multiple crops **(Fig. 19.2A)**
- **Complications:** More common in adults and immunocompromised individuals
  - *The most common* complications are secondary bacterial infections of the skin and CNS involvement (encephalitis and meningitis, etc.)
  - *Most serious* complication: varicella pneumonia

- *Reye's syndrome* can occur secondary to VZV infection. It is characterized by fatty degeneration of the liver following salicylate (aspirin) intake.
- **Epidemiology:** Chickenpox is a highly contagious disease
  - Common in children between 1 to 14 years of age
  - **Period of infectivity:** Child is infectious from 2 days before the onset of rash to 5 days thereafter, until the vesicles are crusted
  - **Source of infection:** Patients are the only source, there are no carriers.
- **Pregnancy:** Infection during early pregnancy can cause congenital malformations in the fetus such as cicatricial skin lesions and limb hypoplasia (congenital varicella syndrome).

Zoster or Shingles

Zoster usually occurs following reactivation of latent VZV present in the trigeminal ganglia that occurs mainly in old age or immunocompromised individuals.
- **Rashes:** They are unilateral and segmental, confined to the area of skin supplied by the affected nerves **(Fig. 19.2B)**. Head, neck, and trunk are the most common affected sites
- **Complications:** Zoster may present with complications such as:
  - *Zoster ophthalmicus:* Unilateral painful crops of skin rashes surrounding the eye
  - *Ramsay Hunt syndrome:* It develops when the facial nerve is involved; presents as facial paralysis, and vesicles on the face and ears
  - *Post-herpetic neuralgia*: Pain at the local site lasting for months; most common complication in elderly patients.

Laboratory diagnosis and treatment of varicella-zoster virus are similar to as discussed for HSV.

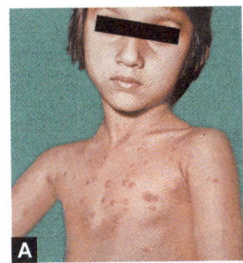 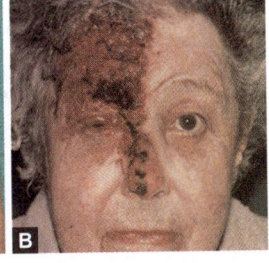

Figs. 19.2A and B: A. Rashes of chickenpox; **B.** Segmental distribution of rashes of Zoster.

Source: **A.** Public Health Image Library, ID#/2882/JD Millar/Centers for Disease Control and Prevention (CDC), Atlanta (*with permission*); **B.** Recommendations of the Advisory Committee on Immunization Practices [ACIP]. MMWR Morb Mortal Wkly Rep 2008;57[RR-5]:1 (*with permission*).

Infection Control Measures

Patients infected with VZV should be kept in isolation. Airborne precautions (e.g. negative air-flow rooms) plus contact precautions must be followed until lesions are dry and crusted (Chapter 38). For localized zoster in an immunocompetent host, contact precaution alone can be followed.

Cytomegalovirus

Cytomegalovirus (CMV) causes an array of clinical syndromes such as:
- Congenital infection called cytomegalic inclusion disease
- Perinatal infections
- Severe infection in immunocompromised (HIV) and transplant recipients
- It can also cause a mononucleosis-like syndrome in adults following blood transfusion.

Laboratory diagnosis of CMV infections include:
- **Inclusion bodies:** Detection of perinuclear inclusion bodies (with owl's eye appearance) in urine specimen
- **Virus isolation** in human fibroblasts cell line: cytopathic effect can be demonstrated after 2–3 weeks
- **Antibody detection** (by ELISA): Detects IgM and IgG antibodies against various viral antigens
- **Antigen detection** (e.g. pp65 antigen) by indirect immunofluorescence test using specific monoclonal antibody
- **Molecular methods** (by PCR): Detects various genes targets such as glycoprotein B (UL55).

> **TREATMENT** — **CMV infections**
>
> CMV does not respond to acyclovir. Drugs such as ganciclovir, valganciclovir, foscarnet and cidofovir are used for the treatment of CMV infections.

Epstein-Barr Virus

Epstein-Barr Virus (EBV) is transmitted by oropharyngeal contact through infected salivary secretions.
- **Pathogenesis:** They infect the B-lymphocytes. The infected B cells become immortalized and produce a large number of polyclonal immunoglobulins. In response to this, the bystander CD8 T lymphocytes are stimulated and appear atypical
- **Clinical manifestations:** EBV is associated with several manifestations
    - *Infectious mononucleosis:* It is characterized by pharyngitis, cervical lymphadenopathy, and atypical lymphocytosis
    - *Malignancies:* EBV is associated with the pathogenesis of several malignancies such as Burkitt's lymphoma and nasopharyngeal carcinoma, Hodgkin's, and non-Hodgkin's lymphoma.
    - *Other conditions associated with EBV:* Lymphoproliferative disorder and oral hairy leukoplakia (wart-like growth of epithelial cells of the tongue developed in some HIV-infected patients and transplant recipients).
- **Laboratory diagnosis of EBV infections include:**
    - Detection of nonspecific heterophile antibody to sheep RBC antigens (by Paul Bunnell test)
    - Detection of specific anti-EBV antibodies: ELISA and indirect IF assay detect antibodies specific to viral capsid antigen, EBNA (nuclear antigen), and early antigen.

> **TREATMENT** — **EBV infections**
>
> - **Supportive measures** such as analgesics are used in the treatment of infectious mononucleosis
> - **Acyclovir** is useful in the treatment of oral hairy leukoplakia, though relapse is common. It reduces EBV shedding from the oropharynx.
> - **Antibody to CD20** (rituximab) has been effective in some cases.

Less Common Herpesviruses

- **HHV 6 and 7:** Human herpesvirus (HHV) 6 and 7 infect T-lymphocytes. HHV-6 produces an exanthematous disease called as sixth disease, (exanthem subitum or roseola infantum)
- **Human herpesvirus 8:** It infects B-lymphocytes, and can cause a malignancy

called Kaposi's sarcoma in HIV-infected individuals.

OTHER DNA VIRUSES

Parvoviruses

Parvovirus is the smallest virus infecting man and produces the following infections.
- **Erythema infectiosum** (fifth disease): It is a common childhood exanthema, characterized by rashes on the face, described as slapped cheek appearance
- They infect RBC precursors to cause non-immune hydrops fetalis and aplastic anemia.

Papillomaviruses

Human papillomavirus (HPV) has several serotypes, each other is associated with specific infections.
- **Benign lesions (warts):** They are small, hard, rough growth on the skin—e.g. common warts, plantar warts, anogenital warts, etc.
- **Epidermodysplasia verruciformis:** It is a benign skin condition with malignant potential. It is seen with serotypes 5, 8, 9, etc.
- **Malignant neoplasia,** e.g. carcinoma of the cervix and other genital mucosa, larynx, or esophagus
  - Serotypes 16 and 18 have high malignant potential for carcinoma cervix
  - Serotypes 6 and 11 are associated with a pre-malignant condition of the cervix called cervical intraepithelial neoplasia (CIN).
- **Vaccine:** Nine-valent (e.g. Gardasil) and bivalent (e.g. Cervarix) vaccines are available for the prevention of HPV infections. It is recommended for all adolescent boys and girls aged 11–12 years.

Polyomaviruses

They usually infect animals; only a few are human pathogens such as JC virus and BK virus. Both are named after the initials of the patients in whom they were described first.

- **JC virus:** Causes progressive multifocal leukoencephalopathy (PML); a slow virus disease infecting the brain
- **BK virus:** Causes nephropathy in kidney transplant recipients.

Adenoviruses

Adenoviruses infect and replicate in the epithelial cells and produce various infections such as:
- **Respiratory infections:** Upper respiratory tract infection, pneumonia
- **Ocular infections:** Pharyngoconjunctival fever, and epidemic keratoconjunctivitis (or shipyard eye)
- **Infantile diarrhea:** Caused by serotypes 40 and 41
- **Hemorrhagic cystitis:** Caused by serotypes 11 and 21.

Poxviruses

Poxviruses are the largest among all the viruses infecting man. They possess single dsDNA and replicate in the cytoplasm.
- **Smallpox virus** (*Variola*): It is the agent of a highly contagious severe exanthematous disease 'smallpox'; which was the first infectious disease to be eradicated from the world
  - The rashes were typically deep-seated, appeared in one stage, and were centrifugally distributed (extremities were affected first)
  - The introduction of live-attenuated *Vaccinia* vaccine was one of the reasons for its successful eradication.
- **Molluscum contagiosum virus** is another poxvirus that infects humans
  - **Lesions:** It produces pink pearly wart-like lesions, umbilicated with a characteristic dimple at the center
  - **Inclusion bodies:** Histopathological stain of skin scrapings demonstrates typical intracytoplasmic inclusions called molluscum bodies.
- **Monkeypox virus:** Can produce vesicular rash similar to smallpox but milder. Infection can be prevented by smallpox vaccination.

Bacteriophages

Bacteriophages are viruses that infect bacteria. They are **tadpole-shaped**; measure about 28–100 nm in size. They possess a hexagonal head (capsid) enclosing a dsDNA with a tail ending with tail fibers **(Fig. 19.3)**.

Life Cycle

Bacteriophages exhibit two different types of life cycles.
- **Lytic cycle** (or virulent cycle): After the phage infects the bacterium, the phage DNA replicates in the cytoplasm. The daughter phages produced are subsequently released from the bacteria by causing lysis of the bacterial cell
- **Lysogenic cycle** (or temperate cycle): Here, the phage DNA gets integrated into the bacterial chromosome (called lysogenic conversion). But when they want to come out, they get excised from the bacterial chromosome, then transform into lytic phages, multiply in the cytoplasm, and are released by lysis.

Significance/Uses of Bacteriophages

Bacteriophages have been used for various purposes.
- **Phage typing:** Useful for classifying bacteria beyond species level (e.g. for *S. aureus*). It was in use before, now less commonly used
- **Used in treatment (phage therapy):** Lytic phages can kill the bacteria, therefore may be used for the treatment of bacterial infections such as post-burn and wound infections
- **Used as a cloning vector:** Bacteriophages have been used as cloning vectors in recombinant DNA technology
- **Transfer drug resistance:** Temperate phages can transfer bacterial genes from one bacterium to another by **transduction** (e.g. transfer of plasmids coding for β-lactamases)
- **Code for toxins:** The phage genomes code for the following bacterial toxins—diphtheria toxin, cholera toxin, Shiga toxin, etc.

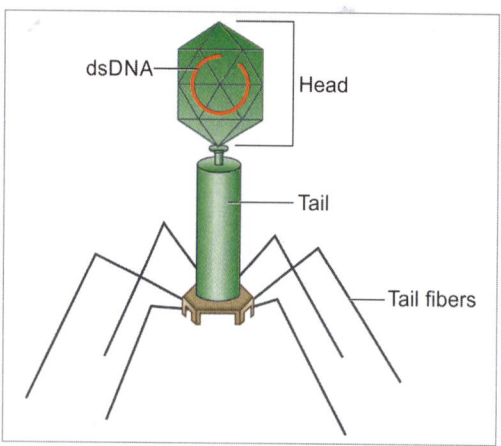

Fig. 19.3: Morphology of bacteriophage.

EXPECTED QUESTIONS

I. Write an essay on:
1. Discuss the pathogenesis, clinical manifestations, and laboratory diagnosis of herpes simplex virus infections.

II. Write short notes on:
1. Chickenpox.
2. Cytomegalovirus infections.
3. Epstein-Barr virus infections.
4. Bacteriophage.

III. Multiple Choice Questions (MCQs):
1. Erythema infectiosum is caused by___?
    a. Parvovirus
    b. Human herpesvirus-6
    c. *Orientia tsutsugamushi*
    d. *Mycoplasma pneumoniae*
2. Paul-Bunnell test is done for___?
    a. Toxic shock syndrome
    b. Infectious mononucleosis
    c. Chicken pox
    d. Hemorrhagic cystitis
3. Which of the following toxin is phage coded?
    a. Tetanus toxin   b. Botulinum toxin
    c. Cholera toxin   d. Pneumolysin

Answers
1. a   2. b   3. c

CHAPTER 20: Myxoviruses and Rubella Virus Infections

CHAPTER PREVIEW

- Orthomyxoviruses: Influenza Virus
- Paramyxoviruses: Parainfluenza, Measles, Mumps, RSV
- Rubella Virus

MYXOVIRUSES

Myxoviruses are a group of viruses that bind to mucin receptors on the surface of RBCs. They are divided into two groups:

1. **Orthomyxoviruses:** They possess segmented RNA; e.g. influenza virus (**Fig. 20.1**)
2. **Paramyxoviruses:** They possess non-segmented RNA; e.g. parainfluenza virus, mumps, measles, Nipah, Hendra, and respiratory syncytial virus.

Influenza Virus

Influenza viruses are one of the major cause of morbidity and mortality and have been responsible for several epidemics and pandemics of respiratory diseases in the last two centuries, caused by various serotypes; of which the latest pandemic was caused by A/H1N1 serotype in 2009.

❖ **Types:** Influenza virus has two unique antigens on their envelope—hemagglutinin (HA) and neuraminidase (NA) antigen (**Fig. 20.1**)
  - Based on these antigens, influenza virus can be divided into four serotypes (A to D)
  - Influenza A is further divided into various subtypes—e.g. A/H1N1, H5N1, H3N2, etc.

❖ **Antigen variation:** Influenza virus has a unique property of undergoing frequent antigen variations; which may be either a minor genetic variation—called antigenic drift or a major genetic change—called antigen shift (**Table 20.1**). Antigenic variation is responsible for pandemics and outbreaks of cases.

Pathogenesis

Pathogenesis of influenza involves the transmission of the virus, followed by spread to the respiratory epithelium.

❖ **Transmission:** It is transmitted by (i) **inhalation of respiratory droplets** generated by coughing and sneezing, (ii) **via contact with surfaces or fomites** infected with respiratory droplets, and then touching the nose, eyes, or mouth

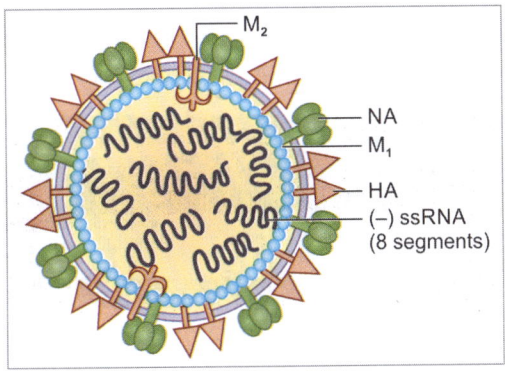

Fig. 20.1: Influenza virus (schematic diagram).

Table 20.1: Differences between antigenic drift and drift.

Antigenic drift	Antigenic shift
It is a major genetic change	It is a minor genetic change
Occurs due to point mutations	Occurs due to genetic assortment between the viruses
Results in outbreaks and minor periodic epidemics	Results in pandemics and major epidemics (e.g. A/H1N1 pandemics of 2009)
Occurs more frequently, every 2–3 years	Occurs less frequently every 10–20 years
Seen in both influenza virus type—A and B	Seen only in influenza A

- **Spread:** The virus infects the respiratory epithelial cells by binding of viral HA antigens to specific sialic acid receptors on the respiratory mucosa
- **Avian flu:** Bird flu strains are highly lethal to chickens causing an economic loss in poultry
  - A/H5N1 is the most common avian flu strain that has been endemic in the world
  - **Transmission** from birds to humans is rare. If transmitted, the disease in man is more severe than A/H1N1.
- **A/H1N1 flu:** In 2009, influenza A/H1N1 caused a global pandemic affecting several countries, including India
  - A/H1N1 2009 flu originated by genetic reassortment of four strains (1 human strain + 2 swine strains + 1 avian strain) and the mixing had occurred in pigs
  - It can be transmitted from human to human, which has accounted for its rapid spread
  - Currently, it is a seasonal flu strain in India.
- **Seasonal flu:** Influenza outbreaks are common during winters. The currently circulating strains causing seasonal flu are influenza A/H1N1, A/H3N2, and influenza B.

Clinical Manifestations

The majority of individuals develop mild flu-like symptoms such as chills, headache, and dry cough, followed by high-grade fever, myalgia, and anorexia.
- Minor cases can develop pneumonia—secondary bacterial pneumonia or rarely viral pneumonia
- Patients with risk factors such as elderly patients (≥65 years), chronic pulmonary, cardiac, renal, and hematologic diseases, and immunosuppression are more prone to develop complications.

Epidemiology

Influenza viruses cause seasonal flu epidemics worldwide almost every year, however they differ widely in severity and the extent of spread.
- **Global pandemics** of novel influenza A subtypes occur every 10–40 years, which can cause much higher mortality than seasonal flu
- **Seasonality:** Influenza outbreaks are common during winters
- **Epidemiological pattern:** It depends upon the nature of antigenic variation that occurs in the influenza types (as described earlier).

Laboratory Diagnosis

The nasopharyngeal swab is the ideal specimen, collected by dacron or polyester flocked swabs in viral transport media **(Fig. 20.2)**.
- **Molecular test:** Detection of viral RNA (HA or NA genes) in nasopharyngeal swabs by real-time reverse transcriptase PCR remains the gold standard method of diagnosis
  - It is highly sensitive and specific with a turnaround time of 2–3 hours

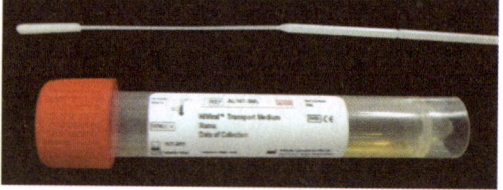

Fig. 20.2: Viral transport medium and swab.
Source: Department of Microbiology, JIPMER, Puducherry (with permission).

- It simultaneously detects the three common seasonal flu strains (A/H1N1, A/H3N2, and type B).
- **Direct immunofluorescence test:** Viral antigens coated onto epithelial cells can be directly detected in nasal aspirates
- **Isolation of virus** in embryonated eggs and primary monkey kidney cell lines was in use in the past
- **Antibody detection** in patient serum is mainly useful for epidemiology purposes, not for clinical diagnosis.

> **TREATMENT — Influenza**
>
> Specific antiviral agents given for the treatment of influenza are neuraminidase inhibitors (e.g. oseltamivir) or matrix protein M2 inhibitors (e.g. amantadine).

Prevention

General Preventive Measures

Measures of droplet precaution (Chapter 38) should be followed:
- **Strict hand hygiene**
- **Isolation room:** Patients should be kept in isolation room or cohorting to be followed
- **Containment of coughs and sneezes**
  - Respiratory hygiene and cough etiquette
  - Use of personal protective equipment (PPE) such as gloves, 3-ply masks, gown and googles for a HCW. Patient should wear a mask.
- **Work restriction:** CDC recommends that people with influenza-like illness remain at home until at least 24 hours after they are free of fever (<100°F) without the use of fever-reducing medications.

Influenza Vaccine

Both live attenuated and injectable vaccines are available for influenza.
- **Strains:** The seasonal flu strains are usually included in the vaccine such as A/H1N1, A/H3N2, and influenza B strain
- **Schedule:** It is taken as a single dose, every year before the winter season begins
- **Injectable vaccines:** There are three types of injectable vaccines
  - Inactivated influenza vaccine
  - Cell culture-based inactivated influenza vaccine
  - Recombinant influenza vaccine.
- **Live attenuated influenza vaccine:** It is administered by intranasal spray.

Parainfluenza Viruses

Human parainfluenza viruses are one of the major cause of respiratory tract disease in young children; producing various respiratory tract infections such as:
- Mild common cold syndrome
- Croup (laryngotracheobronchitis)
- Lower respiratory tract infections such as pneumonia or bronchiolitis.

It has four serotypes; all are transmitted by the respiratory route.

Measles Virus

Measles is an acute, highly contagious exanthematous childhood disease.

Pathogenesis

Measles is transmitted via the respiratory route either by—droplets inhalation or small-particle aerosols. It multiplies locally and subsequently spreads through the bloodstream to various target sites, including the skin, respiratory tract, and conjunctiva.

Clinical Manifestations

Symptoms appear after an incubation period of about 10 days. The disease can be divided into the following stages.

1. **Prodromal stage:** This stage lasts for 4 days and is characterized by manifestations such as:
   - **Fever** is the first manifestation (appears on the 10th day), followed by Koplik's spots (i.e. on the 12th day)
   - **Koplik's spots:** They are pathognomonic of measles, characterized by the bluish white spot on buccal mucosa **(Fig. 20.3A)**
   - **Non-specific symptoms** may be present such as cough, cold, nasal discharge, redness of eye, etc.
2. **Eruptive stage:** This stage starts on the 14th day, characterized by exanthematous

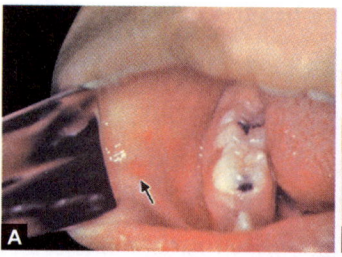 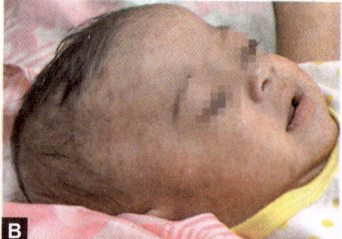 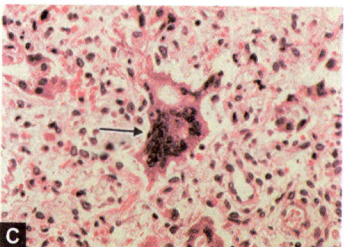

Figs. 20.3A to C: A. Koplik spot in the buccal mucosa (measles) (arrow showing); **B.** Measles rashes (on face); **C.** Multinucleated giant cell of measles infected cell lines (arrow showing).
Source: **A.** Public Health Image Library, ID# 6111; **B.** ID# 17980; **C.** ID# 859/Centers for Disease Control and Prevention (CDC), Atlanta (*with permission*).

rashes **(Fig. 20.3B)**, which begin from behind the ears → then spread to the face, arm, trunk and legs → then fade in the same order after 4 days of onset.

Fever (10th day) → Koplik's spot (12th day) → rashes (14th day)

Complications

Patients with risk factors such as age <5 or >20 yrs, pregnant women, and immunocompromised hosts, etc. are more prone to develop complications.
- **Secondary bacterial infections** such as otitis media and bronchopneumonia
- **Giant-cell pneumonitis** (Hecht's pneumonia) occurs due to the virus itself
- **Diarrhea** leads to malnutrition
- **CNS complications** such as subacute sclerosing panencephalitis (SSPE). This is a rare, but severe complication of measles.

Laboratory Diagnosis

Nasopharyngeal swab, conjunctival swab, respiratory secretions, etc. are the ideal specimens.
- **Antigen detection** in the infected cells by using anti-nucleoprotein antibodies (by direct IF test)
- **Virus isolation:** Using monkey or human kidney cells and demonstrating cytopathic effect such as multinucleated giant cells (Warthin-Finkeldey cells) containing both intranuclear and intracytoplasmic inclusion bodies **(Fig. 20.3C)**
- **Antibody detection:** Demonstration of raised titers of anti-measles antibody in the CSF is diagnostic of SSPE
- **RT-PCR** is available targeting measles-specific N gene (nucleoprotein) in the clinical specimens.

TREATMENT — Measles

- There is no specific antiviral therapy available for measles
- Treatment is symptomatic and consists of general supportive measures.

Prevention

General Preventive Measures

Airborne precautions such as isolation in negative pressure room, use of PPEs such as N95 respirator, etc. must be followed while handling measles cases (Chapter 38 for detail).

Measles Vaccine

Live attenuated vaccine is available for measles using Schwartz strain or Edmonston-Zagreb strain.
- It is available as a monovalent vaccine or along with mumps and rubella vaccine (MMR vaccine) or with rubella vaccine (MR vaccine)
- **Indication:** Under the national immunization schedule of India, the measles-rubella (MR) vaccine is given at 9 completed months to 12 months along with vitamin A supplements, and the second dose of MR vaccine at 16–24 months
- **Post-exposure prophylaxis:** Susceptible contacts may be protected against measles

if the vaccine is given within 3 days of exposure. Measles immunoglobulin (Ig) can also be given within 3 days. However, both vaccine and Ig should not be given together.

Mumps Virus

Mumps virus is the most common cause of parotid gland enlargement in children.
- **Transmission:** It is transmitted through the respiratory route via droplets, saliva, and fomites
- **Target sites:** Mumps virus has a special affinity for glandular epithelium. The classic sites include salivary glands, testes, pancreas, ovaries, CNS, etc.
- **Clinical manifestations:** Causes bilateral parotitis, although it can also infect other salivary glands. In severe cases, it can cause complications such as orchitis, pancreatitis, oophoritis, and aseptic meningitis
- **Epidemiology:** Mumps is endemic worldwide, epidemics occur every 3–5 years; typically associated with unvaccinated people living in overcrowded areas
    - **Period of communicability:** Patients are infectious from 1 week before to 1 week after the onset of symptoms
    - **Source:** Cases (both clinical and subclinical cases) are the source of infection
    - **Age:** Children of **5–9 years** of age are most commonly affected.
- **Laboratory diagnosis:** The buccal or oral swab specimens are most ideal
    - Direct viral antigen detection can be done by using mumps-specific fluorescent staining
    - Virus isolation using monkey kidney cell line
    - Serum antibodies detection: ELISA
    - Reverse-transcription PCR is available to detect mumps specific N gene (nucleoprotein).
- **Vaccine:** Live attenuated vaccine using Jeryl Lynn strain is available for the prevention of mumps. It is available either as monovalent or more commonly as a part of the trivalent MMR vaccine.

Respiratory Syncytial Virus

Respiratory syncytial virus (RSV) is a major respiratory pathogen of young children and is the most common cause of bronchiolitis in infants. It can also cause pneumonia and tracheobronchitis in infants.
- **Transmission:** It is transmitted by direct contact of eyes with contaminated fingers or by droplet inhalation
- **Clinical manifestations:** It is the most common cause of bronchiolitis, and tracheobronchitis in infants
- **Laboratory diagnosis:** (i) Antigen detection in respiratory secretions by direct-IF, (ii) isolation of virus using HeLa and HEp-2 cell line and demonstration of typical cytopathic effect—syncytium formation (multinucleated giant cell), (iii) RT-PCR amplifying viral RNA (such as nucleoprotein N gene)
- **Treatment:** Ribavirin is the drug of choice.

Nipah and Hendra Viruses

They cause an emerging viral infection, affecting CNS (producing encephalitis).
- **Transmission** to man is through direct contact with infected bats, pigs, or persons
- The **case-fatality rate** is very high (50–70%)
- The **latest outbreak** of Nipah encephalitis occurred in Kerala, India in 2018, which witnessed 18 cases with 16 deaths
- **Laboratory diagnosis:** Real-time PCR from the throat and nasal swabs, CSF, urine, and blood performed in the early stages of the disease confirms the diagnosis
- **Treatment:** No effective antiviral treatment is available.

RUBELLA

Rubella virus produces a childhood exanthema similar to that of measles. Therefore, rubella is also known as **German measles**. However, unlike measles, it is highly teratogenic; can cause congenital rubella syndrome.
- Rubella is not a Myxovirus but belongs to the Togavirus family. It is discussed here because of its clinical resemblance to measles

- Rubella may present in two clinical forms—postnatal infection and congenital infection.

Postnatal Rubella Infection

Postnatal rubella may occur during neonatal age, childhood, and adult life. The virus is acquired by respiratory droplets.
- The incubation period is about 14 days
- **Rashes** are often the first manifestations in children. Rashes start on the face, extend to the trunk and extremities, and disappear in 3 days
- **Lymphadenopathy** (occipital and post-auricular) is the most striking feature
- **Forchheimer spots** may be seen in some cases. They are petechiae spots developed on the soft palate and uvula.

Congenital Rubella Syndrome

The most serious consequence of rubella virus infection is congenital rubella syndrome.
- **Triad:** Rubella is highly teratogenic; affects three primary organs
  1. *Ear:* Sensory neural deafness (most common defect)
  2. *Eyes:* Salt and pepper retinopathy and cataract, and
  3. *Heart:* Patent ductus arteriosus.
- **Severity:** The severity is maximum if the mother acquires the infection in the first trimester.

Laboratory Diagnosis

Nasopharyngeal or throat swab taken 6 days before and after the onset of rash is the ideal specimen.
- **Isolation of virus:** Monkey or rabbit origin cell lines may be used
- **Serology (antibody detection):** ELISA is the preferred method for rubella diagnosis. It detects both IgM and IgG separately. Detection of IgM antibody is useful for the diagnosis of congenital rubella
- **Molecular test:** RT-PCR is available for detecting rubella-specific RNA (nucleoprotein N gene) in clinical specimens.

Rubella Vaccine

Live attenuated vaccine is available for rubella using **RA 27/3** strain. It is available singly or in combination with mumps and measles (MMR vaccine)
- **Indication:** In India, rubella vaccine is indicated to all women of reproductive age (first priority group) followed by all children (1–14 years). Under the national immunization schedule, rubella vaccine is given along with measles (MR vaccine) at 9–12 months of age and a second dose at 16–24 months in selected states
- **Precautions:** Vaccine is contraindicated in pregnancy. If received, women should avoid pregnancy for at least 4 weeks following vaccination.

EXPECTED QUESTIONS

I. **Write an essay on:**
   1. Discuss the clinical manifestations, laboratory diagnosis, and prevention of influenza.

II. **Write short notes on:**
   1. Mumps parotitis.
   2. Measles.
   3. Congenital rubella syndrome.

II. **Multiple Choice Questions (MCQs):**
   1. **The classical triad in congenital rubella syndrome is characterized by all, *except*:**
      a. Cataract   b. Deafness
      c. Cardiac defect d. Hepatitis
   2. **Avian flu strain is___?**
      a. A/H5N1   b. A/H3N2
      c. A/H1N1   d. Influenza B
   3. **Seasonal flu strain includes all, *except*?**
      a. A/H5N1   b. A/H3N2
      c. A/H1N1   d. Influenza B
   4. **SSPE is a complication seen with___?**
      a. Influenza   b. Measles
      c. Mumps   d. Rubella

Answers
1. d   2. a   3. a   4. b

CHAPTER 21

Coronavirus Infections including COVID-19

CHAPTER PREVIEW

- Epidemiology
- Pathogenesis
- Clinical Manifestations
- Laboratory Diagnosis
- Treatment
- Vaccine and Infection Control

Coronaviruses (CoV) cause respiratory tract infections in man; illness ranging from mild common cold to severe disease like pneumonia. The coronaviruses that caused explosive outbreaks of severe respiratory disease with higher mortality are as follows.

- **SARS-CoV** (Severe acute respiratory syndrome coronavirus): It has caused an explosive epidemic called 'SARS' in China in 2003
- **MERS-CoV** (Middle East respiratory syndrome coronavirus): It has caused an explosive epidemic called 'MERS' in Middle East (Saudi Arabia) in 2012
- **SARS-CoV-2** (Severe acute respiratory syndrome coronavirus-2): It is the causative agent of an ongoing explosive pandemics affecting the whole world in 2019-20; called COVID-19.

CORONAVIRUS DISEASE (COVID)-2019

Coronavirus disease-2019 (COVID-19) is an acute respiratory disease caused by severe acute respiratory syndrome coronavirus-2 (SARS-CoV-2). It has caused an explosive catastrophic pandemic that affected almost all parts of the world and produced significant loss of lives and financial crisis.

Epidemiology

SARS-CoV-2 originated from China (Wuhan city) in December 2019 and subsequently spread rapidly to affect the rest of the world over 3-4 months—pandemic was declared on 11th March 2020 by WHO.

- **Highest cases:** USA accounted for the maximum number of cases, followed by India, Brazil, UK, and France
- **Mortality rate:** It varies among the countries and also across different time spans of the pandemic—with an overall mortality rate of 1.6 to 1.8%
- **India:** Accounts for the second-highest number of cases. However, the pandemic had a slower growth curve to reach its peak in India. India witnessed three distinct waves of the explosive surge in cases
  - First wave was around September 2020
  - Second wave was around April 2021 (due to delta variant)
  - Third-wave was around January 2022 (due to the omicron variant).

Morphology

The SARS-CoV-2 is a RNA virus, that comprises of a nucleocapsid with a helical symmetry, surrounded by an envelope. It possesses 4 structural proteins **(Fig. 21.1)**.

1. Nucleocapsid (N) protein

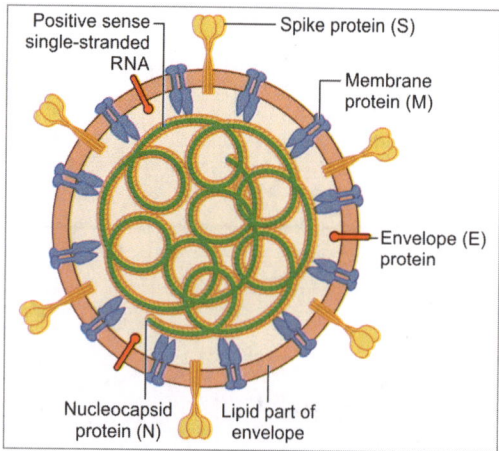

Fig. 21.1: Structure of SARS-CoV-2.

2. Spike protein (S): Helps in the attachment to the host cells
3. Membrane glycoprotein (M)
4. Envelope protein (E).

Pathogenesis

Pathogenesis of COVID-19 involves the following sequential steps.

- ❖ **Transmission:** COVID-19 virus is primarily transmitted via any of the following routes
  - *Respiratory droplets* can fall on the mouth, nose, or eyes (if present within 1 meter), and
  - *Contact routes:* (i) direct contact with infected people, or (ii) indirect contact with the surfaces or objects in the immediate environment. Following contact, the virus can only be transmitted by touching the contaminated hand to a person's mouth, nose, or eyes
  - *Aerosol transmission* can occur in specific settings in which aerosol-generating procedures are performed (e.g. endotracheal intubation).
- ❖ **Host cell entry:** The virus enters the host cell by binding of its spike (S) antigen with the host cell receptor of SARS-CoV-2 called, i.e. angiotensin-converting enzyme-2 (ACE-2)
  - ACE-2 is highly expressed on mucosal epithelial cells of the eye, nose, and oral cavity
  - Subsequently, the virus is carried to the pharynx and then to the lungs.
- ❖ **Development of influenza-like illness (ILI):** At the initial stage, SARS-CoV-2 infects the pharyngeal epithelium, and induces inflammation. This accounts for the influenza-like illness (ILI) which occurs at the beginning stage of most of the symptomatic cases
- ❖ **Development of ARDS:** Certain patients with COVID-19 with comorbidity progress into acute respiratory distress syndrome (ARDS). The underlying mechanisms are due to
  - Reduced pulmonary surfactants from type-II alveolar cells
  - The massive release of pro-inflammatory cytokines causes cytokine storm.

Clinical Manifestations

The incubation period for COVID-19 (time between infection and symptom onset) is about 5-6 days but can be as long as 14 days. The majority of the infections remain asymptomatic. Symptomatic patients may present with different stages of severity—mild, moderate, and severe disease **(Table 21.1)**.

Laboratory Diagnosis

Laboratory diagnosis is necessary only in specific indications as per the Government of India, such as symptomatic patients,

Table 21.1: Clinical severity of COVID-19 disease.

Clinical stage	Clinical presentations
Mild disease	
ILI ((influenza-like illness)	Mild URT symptoms such as fever, cough, sore throat, malaise, headache without dyspnea (SpO$_2$ ≥94%)
Moderate disease	
Pneumonia	ILI plus any one: (1) dyspnea, (2) SpO$_2$ ≤93%, (3) respiratory rate ≥24 per minute
Severe disease : Called as severe acute respiratory illness (SARI)	
Severe pneumonia	Clinical signs of pneumonia plus any one: (i) Respiratory rate >30/min, or (ii) SpO$_2$ <90%
Complications	Acute respiratory distress syndrome (ARDS), sepsis, septic shock and other nonrespiratory complications

asymptomatic contacts with high-risk exposure, or recent international travel.
- **Specimens:** Throat swabs and nasal swabs are the ideal specimens, collected by Dacron or polyester flocked swabs and then dipped into the viral transport media
- **Real-time RT-PCR:** Real-time reverse-transcriptase PCR testing is the gold standard method for diagnosis of COVID-19
  - *Formats:* (i) conventional real-time PCR—useful if sample load is high, takes more time (4-6h), (ii) automated real-time PCR formats (GeneXpert and Truenat)—useful in laboratories with lesser sample load, takes less time (1-2h)
  - *Gene targets:* Current guidelines recommend that the real-time PCT kits target **at least two genes** of SARS-CoV-2, among the following genes:
    - Spike protein (S)
    - Envelope protein (E)
    - Membrane protein (M)
    - Nucleocapsid protein (N)
    - RNA-dependent RNA polymerase (RdRp)
    - Open reading frames (ORF1a/b).
- **CRISPR-based assay** (clustered regularly interspaced short palindromic repeats): It is a low-cost, rapid, point-of-care test, which can identify the RNA of the SARS-CoV-2 virus
- **Antigen detection assay:** Point-of-care test; detects nucleocapsid protein antigen in nasopharyngeal swab by immunochromatographic test (ICT)
- **Antibody (IgG) detection assay:** Used for surveillance purposes in a high-risk and vulnerable group; not for clinical diagnosis
- **Sequencing:** Useful to determine mutations in the viral genome (e.g. omicron)
- **Omicron detection:** Specific real-time PCR kit are available, which can detect the precise mutations in S gene that occurs in omicron variants
- **Viral culture:** Used for research purpose
- **Nonspecific tests** include:
  - Radiology (chest CT scan): Ground-glass appearance
  - Biomarkers: IL-6, D-dimer.

TREATMENT — COVID-19

COVID-19 cases can be managed either by:
- **Home isolation:** Indicated for the asymptomatic or mild case without risk factors), or
- **Hospitalization:** Indicated for moderate to severe cases or with risk factors like diabetes, immunosuppression, etc.

Symptomatic management: such as
- **Respiratory support:** (i) Supplemental oxygen to maintain $SpO_2 > 94\%$, (ii) Mechanical ventilation
- **Others:** Steroid, anticoagulant (like heparin) to prevent coagulopathies and management of shock, etc.
- **Antiviral drugs:** Although not very promising, but following drugs are approved for use in COVID-19
- **Remdesivir:** Interferes with viral RNA polymerase, given in moderate to severe cases
- **Tocilizumab:** Monoclonal antibody against IL-6 receptor, given in severe disease to reduce the cytokine storm.

Vaccine

Several vaccines are available for COVID-19. Three vaccines are licensed in India so far—Covaxin, Covishield and Sputnik V.
- **Indication:** COVID-19 vaccination is indicated for all aged ≥15 years
- **Covaxin:** It is a whole-virion inactivated vaccine, which uses spike protein as a target. It is administered in two doses (4-6 weeks apart) by IM route
- **Covishield:** It is based on a non-replicating adenovirus vector expressing spike protein. It is administered in two doses (12–16 weeks apart) by IM route
- **Sputnik V vaccine:** It is a Russian vaccine, also based on adenovirus vector. It is given in two doses (by IM route), at a gap of 3 weeks
- **Precaution dose:** A third dose of the COVID-19 vaccine is recommended to use for the high-risk groups
- **Interchangeability** between the vaccines is not permitted
- **Storage:** Covaxin and Covishield can be stored at 2–8°C, whereas Sputnik V needs to be stored at –18°C

- **Other non-COVID-19 vaccines** can be administered only after a 14 days gap of COVID vaccination
- **Efficacy:** COVID-19 vaccines induce an adequate immune response (of 70–90% efficacy) in about 2–3 weeks after the second dose.

Infection Prevention and Control

Infection prevention and control (IPC) is the most effective method for the prevention of COVID-19.

In Community-settings

The recommended IPC practices are:
- Hand hygiene after contact with other individuals, in high-touch areas, in public places, etc.
- The physical distance of at least one meter
- Use of non-medical masks in public places
- Respiratory hygiene and cough etiquette
- Quarantine of asymptomatic individuals with high-risk exposure.

In Healthcare-settings

The recommended IPC practices are:
- **Use of appropriate PPE** when giving care to COVID-19 patients (Chapter 37). The recommended PPE are gown, 3-ply mask, goggles, and gloves. N95 respirator may be necessary when working in places where aerosol-generating procedures are carried out such as ICUs or operation theatres
- **Environmental cleaning** of floor and surfaces, equipment, high-touch areas, etc. with appropriate disinfectants such as hypochlorite or alcohol
- **Biomedical waste management** should be carried out as per the 2016 guideline (Chapter 42). However, additional precautions are taken such as the use of a double bag, label as 'COVID-19 waste', and disinfecting the outer bag with hypochlorite before handing over
- **Laundry management:** Washing linens at 60-90°C with laundry detergent followed by soaking in 0.1% sodium hypochlorite.

EXPECTED QUESTIONS

I. **Write an essay on:**
1. Discuss the pathogenesis, clinical manifestations, and laboratory diagnosis of COVID-19.

II. **Write short notes on:**
1. COVID-19 vaccines.
2. Infection prevention and control practices recommended for COVID-19.
3. Treatment strategies for COVID-19.

III. **Multiple Choice Questions (MCQs):**
1. While examining a stable patient with COVID-19, all the following PPE are required, *except*:
   a. N 95 mask
   b. Gown
   c. Goggles
   d. Gloves
2. Gene targets for COVID -19 detection include all, *except*:
   a. Spike protein (S)
   b. Envelope protein (E)
   c. Membrane protein (M)
   d. Reverse transcriptase gene
3. Which of the following is not used for clinical diagnosis of COVID-19 disease:
   a. Real-time RT-PCR
   b. Truenat
   c. Antigen detection
   d. Antibody detection

Answers
1. a   2. d   3. d

CHAPTER 22

Arbovirus Infections

CHAPTER PREVIEW

- Chikungunya Virus
- Dengue Virus
- Kyasanur Forest Disease Virus
- Japanese B Encephalitis
- Yellow Fever Virus
- Zika Virus

Arboviruses are a diverse group of RNA viruses that are transmitted by arthropod (insect) vectors from one vertebrate host to another. Viruses must multiply inside the insects and establish a lifelong harmless infection in them.

- ❖ **Geographical distribution:** Arboviruses vary greatly in their geographical distribution which in turn depends on various factors such as climatic conditions and the presence of vectors
- ❖ **Arbovirus found in India:** Although over 40 arboviruses have been detected in India, few of them are highly endemic and produce several outbreaks every year, which include:
  - Dengue virus: Produces hemorrhagic fever
  - Chikungunya virus: Produces fever and arthralgia, rarely hemorrhagic fever
  - Kyasanur forest disease virus: Produces hemorrhagic fever
  - Japanese B encephalitis and West Nile encephalitis viruses: Produce encephalitis.
- ❖ **Arbovirus not found in India:** There are over 100 arboviruses prevalent in various parts of the world other than India. Few of them are of global significance and hence have been discussed in this chapter (yellow fever virus and Zika virus).

DENGUE

Dengue virus is the most common arbovirus found in India. It has four serotypes (DEN-1 to DEN-4). *Aedes aegypti* is the principal vector followed by *Aedes albopictus.* They usually bite during the daytime.

Pathogenesis

The pathogenesis of dengue is different in the first infection from that of subsequent infections.

- ❖ **Primary dengue infection** occurs when a person is infected with the dengue virus for the first time with any one serotype
- ❖ **Secondary dengue infection:** Months to years later, a more severe form of dengue illness may appear, due to infection with another second serotype which is different from the first serotype causing primary infection
  - *Mechanism:* The severity of secondary infection is due to a mechanism called **antibody-dependent enhancement**. Antibodies against the first serotype combine with the second serotype and instead of neutralizing the virus, they protect the second serotype from the host immune response

- *Complications:* The risk of hemorrhagic fever and shock is more in secondary dengue infection
- *The sequence of infection:* Among all serotype combinations, serotype 1 followed by 2 produces the most severe disease.

Clinical Classifications

The incubation period is about 5 days. Dengue can occur in three clinical stages:

1. **Dengue fever (DF):** It is characterized by abrupt onset of high fever (also called biphasic fever, break-bone fever, or saddleback fever). Other features are rashes, headache, myalgia, joint pain, lymphadenopathy, retro-orbital pain, loss of appetite, nausea and vomiting
2. **Dengue hemorrhagic fever (DHF):** It is characterized by:
   - High-grade continuous fever
   - Hepatomegaly
   - Thrombocytopenia (platelet count <1 lakh/mm^3)
   - Raised hematocrit (packed cell volume) by 20%
   - Evidence of hemorrhages can be detected by:
     - Positive tourniquet test (>20 petechial spots per square inch area in the cubital fossa
     - Spontaneous bleeding from skin, nose, mouth, and gums.
3. **Dengue shock syndrome (DSS):** Here, all the above criteria of DHF are present, and in addition manifestations of shock are present, such as:
   - Rapid and weak pulse
   - Narrow pulse pressure (<20 mm Hg) or hypotension
   - Presence of cold and clammy skin
   - Restlessness.

WHO has described a classification which grades dengue into two stages based on the severity.
1. Dengue with or without warning signs
2. Severe dengue.

Epidemiology

Globally, dengue is endemic in more than 100 countries with 2.5 billion people at risk.
- ❖ Tropical countries of Southeast Asia and the Western Pacific are at the highest risk
- ❖ **The situation in India:** Disease is prevalent throughout India affecting almost 31 states/Union territories
  - In 2019: >1.37 lakh cases were reported with >130 deaths; the maximum was from Karnataka and Gujarat
  - All serotypes have been reported from India, but DEN-1 and DEN-2 serotypes are widespread.

Laboratory Diagnosis

The laboratory diagnosis of dengue comprises of the following modalities.
- ❖ **NS1 Antigen detection** by ELISA and ICT formats. NS1 antigen becomes detectable from day 1 of fever and remains positive up to 7 days
- ❖ **Antibody detection** by ELISA: It detects IgM and IgG separately. For IgM, a special type of ELISA is available called IgM antibody capture (MAC) ELISA
  - In primary infection: IgM antibody usually appears after 5 days of fever and is suggestive of active infection
  - In secondary infection: Rapid rise of IgG antibody titer is suggestive of active infection.
- ❖ **Detection of specific genes of viral RNA** by real-time RT-PCR: It is the most sensitive and specific assay, and can be used for the detection of serotypes and quantification of viral load in blood. Viral RNA can be detected in blood from −1 to +5 days of onset of symptoms.

TREATMENT
Dengue

There is no specific antiviral therapy. Treatment is symptomatic and supportive such as:
- Replacement of plasma losses
- Correction of electrolyte and metabolic disturbances
- Platelet transfusion if needed

Dengue Vaccine (CYD-TDV)

This vaccine has been licensed for human use since 2015.
- It is a live-attenuated, Chimeric Yellow Fever-Dengue-Tetravalent Dengue Vaccine (CYD-TDV); commercially available as dengvaxia
- It uses live attenuated yellow fever 17D virus as a vaccine vector in which the target genes of all four dengue serotypes are integrated by recombinant technique
- **Age:** It is indicated for 9–45 years of age
- **Schedule:** 3 doses given subcutaneously at 6-month intervals
- In India, it is not available yet because of its safety issues.

CHIKUNGUNYA

Chikungunya fever is a re-emerging disease characterized by acute fever with severe arthralgia.
- **Transmission:** It is transmitted by *Aedes aegypti*, which usually bites during day time
- **Clinical manifestations:** The incubation period is about 5 days (3–7 days). The most common symptoms are fever and severe joint pain (due to arthritis), worsened in the morning
  - **Arthritis** is polyarticular, migratory, and edematous (joint swelling), predominantly affecting the small joints of the wrists and ankles
  - Symptoms are often confusing with that of dengue. In general, Chikungunya is less severe, less acute, and hemorrhagic manifestations are rare compared to dengue.
- **Epidemiology:** Chikungunya is a classic example of re-emerging disease as it was clinically quiescent for a long time (1973–2005) in most parts of the world. Currently, it has been reported in India, and other Southeast Asian and African countries, where it is associated with several outbreaks
- **Laboratory diagnosis** of Chikungunya comprises of the following modalities
  - **Serum antibody detection by ELISA:** Detection of IgM or a fourfold rise in IgG titer is suggestive of infection. MAC ELISA is available for the detection of IgM antibodies
  - **Reverse-transcriptase PCR** has been developed to detect specific genes in blood.

> **TREATMENT** — Chikungunya
>
> Treatment of Chikungunya is only by supportive measures; no specific antiviral drugs or vaccination are available.

KYASANUR FOREST DISEASE (KFD) VIRUS

KFD virus is named after the place where the disease is prevalent—Kyasanur Forest in Shimoga district of Karnataka, India.
- **Transmission:** Hard ticks are the primary vector of KFD virus; whereas monkeys are the amplifier hosts, where the virus multiplies exponentially
- **Clinical manifestations:** The incubation period varies from 3 to 8 days. The disease occurs in two stages
  - The first stage (hemorrhagic fever)
  - The second stage in the form of meningoencephalitis.
- **Epidemiology:** KFD is currently endemic in five districts of Karnataka—Shimoga, North Kannada, South Kannada, Chikkamagaluru, and Udupi
- **Laboratory diagnosis:** Diagnosis is made by detection of IgM antibody by ELISA or real-time RT-PCR has been developed to detect viral RNA
- **Treatment** of KFD is only by supportive measures; no specific antiviral drugs are available
- **Vaccine:** A formalin-inactivated killed vaccine has been developed. It is recommended in endemic areas of Karnataka (villages within 5 km of endemic foci).

JAPANESE B ENCEPHALITIS

Japanese B encephalitis virus is the leading cause of vaccine-preventable viral encephalitis in Asia, including India.

- **Transmission:** JE virus is transmitted by the bite of the *Culex* mosquito. *C. tritaeniorhynchus* is the primary vector, followed by *C. vishnui*
- **Host:** JE virus has several animal and bird hosts—pigs are the amplifier host; others being cattle and buffalo
- **Clinical manifestations:** The clinical course of the disease can be divided into three stages:
  1. Prodromal stage of febrile illness
  2. Acute encephalitis stage
  3. Sequelae: Some cases (up to 50%) may retain some neurological deficits permanently.
- **Epidemiology:** JE is endemic in several states such as Uttar Pradesh (Gorakhpur district), Assam, Manipur, etc. which account for the largest burden of cases
- **Laboratory diagnosis:** Diagnosis of JE is made by:
  - IgM antibody capture (MAC) ELISA detecting IgM antibodies
  - Real-time RT-PCR has been developed to detect JE virus-specific envelope (E) gene in blood.
- **Treatment:** Only by supportive measures; no specific antiviral drugs are available
- **Vaccine:** Live attenuated using SA 14-14-2 strain of JE virus is available
  - *Under the national immunization program*, it is given to children (1–15 years) in specific endemic districts of states such as—UP, Bihar, Assam, West Bengal, and Karnataka
  - *Schedule:* Two doses (subcutaneously); 1st at 9–12 months of age and 2nd at 16–24 months.

WEST NILE ENCEPHALITIS

West Nile virus (WNV) is another Arbovirus related to JE virus. It is mainly transmitted by *Culex* mosquito.

- **Clinical manifestations:** It causes West Nile fever and West Nile encephalitis
- **India:** WNV is highly prevalent in India in various states and has caused several outbreaks in the past, such as in Kerala (2011) and Assam (2006)
- **Diagnosis:** IgM antibody capture ELISA detecting IgM antibodies in serum and CSF is available.

YELLOW FEVER

Yellow fever is an acute, febrile illness; affecting the liver to cause jaundice (hence the name yellow fever), hemorrhage, with high mortality.

- **Vector:** Humans get the infection by the bite of *Aedes aegypti* or the tiger mosquito
- **Geographical distribution:** Yellow fever is endemic in West Africa and Central South America. It is not found in the rest of the World including India. But India has the vector (*A. aegypti*) widely distributed and therefore has the risk of getting cases in future
- **Clinical manifestations:** The incubation period is about **3–6 days**. The disease is characterized by:
  - Febrile illness: occurs in the early stage
  - Hemorrhagic manifestations
  - Platelet dysfunction
  - Features of liver involvement (hepatitis) such as jaundice.
- **Laboratory diagnosis:** Diagnosis of yellow fever is made by:
  - Antibody detection: IgM ELISA can be done after 3 days of onset of symptoms
  - RT-PCR detecting specific viral RNA (NS5 region) in blood.
- **Treatment:** Only by symptomatic care, no antiviral drugs are available. Preventive measures include vaccination and mosquito control
- **Yellow fever 17D vaccine:** It is a live attenuated vaccine
  - A strict cold chain has to be maintained during the transport (–30°C to +5°C)
  - Dosage: Single-dose, given subcutaneously

- A certificate of vaccination is issued after 10 days of vaccination and renewed (i.e. re-immunization) every 10 years. This is the recommendation followed for international travel.

ZIKA VIRUS DISEASE

Zika virus (ZIKV) has recently gained attention due to the large outbreak that occurred in 2015–16 worldwide.

- **Transmission:** ZIKV is primarily transmitted by the *Aedes aegypti* mosquito. Other modes include—mother-to-child transmission (common in the first trimester) and rarely through sexual contact
- **Epidemiology:** The largest explosive epidemic reported was in **Brazil** (2015–2016) and then subsequently spread to other countries in America, the Caribbean, Europe, and Australia. In India, only a few cases are reported so far
- **The clinical manifestations:** The incubation period ranges from a few days to 1 week. Various clinical presentations include:
  - The majority (>80%) of infections are asymptomatic
  - Zika fever with minor symptoms
  - Congenital Zika syndrome: Characterized by microcephaly and other neurological features
  - Neurological complications.
- **Laboratory diagnosis:** The laboratory tests for confirmation of ZIKV disease include:
  - *RT-PCR* has been the investigation of choice. It can detect Zika virus RNA in blood and urine up to 7 days after onset of symptoms
  - *IgM antibody detection* by enzyme immunoassays and immunofluorescence assays.
- **Treatment:** No effective treatment and vaccine are available so far. Cases are managed only with symptomatic treatment.

EXPECTED QUESTIONS

I. **Write an essay on:**
  1. List the arboviruses that are prevalent in India. Discuss the pathogenesis, clinical presentation, and laboratory diagnosis of dengue.

II. **Write short notes on:**
  1. Chikungunya virus.
  2. Kyasanur forest disease virus.
  3. Japanese B encephalitis.
  4. Yellow fever virus.
  5. Zika virus.

III. **Multiple Choice Questions (MCQs):**
  1. Dengue is transmitted by___?
     a. *Aedes aegypti*
     b. *Culex*
     c. Tick
     d. *Anopheles*
  2. Japanese B encephalitis is transmitted by___?
     a. *Anopheles*
     b. *Aedes aegypti*
     c. *Culex*
     d. Tick
  3. Kyasanur forest disease is transmitted by___?
     a. *Aedes aegypti*
     b. *Culex*
     c. Tick
     d. *Anopheles*
  4. 17 D vaccine is given for___?
     a. Yellow fever
     b. Dengue
     c. Japanese encephalitis
     d. Zika virus disease

Answers
1. a   2. c   3. c   4. a

CHAPTER 23: Rabies and Polio

CHAPTER PREVIEW

- Rabies
- Poliomyelitis

This chapter covers two important viral infections of the central nervous system (CNS): rabies and polio.

RABIES

Rabies virus causes a rapidly progressive, acute infectious disease of the CNS in humans and animals, transmitted from another rabid animal. It is considered a major public health problem because it is almost always fatal.

Morphology

Rabies virus is bullet-shaped and comprises a nucleocapsid (with helical symmetry), surrounded by an envelope. Rabies virus has two major antigens **(Fig. 23.1)**.
1. **Glycoprotein-G:** It is the envelope proteins embedded into the lipid part of the envelope. It is the major antigen responsible for pathogenesis (by binding to acetylcholine receptors in neural tissues). Antibodies to Glycoprotein-G are protective in nature
2. **Nucleoprotein:** It is the nucleocapsid protein. It has a diagnostic role. The direct-immunofluorescence (DIF) test detects the nucleoprotein antigens in the patient's serum.

Pathogenesis

The pathogenesis of rabies involves the following sequential steps.
- ❖ **Transmission:** Rabies virus is usually transmitted to humans by the **bite of rabid dogs**, bats, and other wild animals such as foxes, jackals, etc. Rarely, it can also be transmitted by various non-bite exposures, e.g.—
  - Direct contact with the saliva of infected animals with mucosa or fresh skin wounds
  - Inhalation of virus-containing aerosols (important for laboratory workers)
  - Cornea or other organ transplantation.
  Transmission by human bite is not documented yet.
- ❖ **Spread to CNS:** The virus multiplies locally and spreads via the peripheral motor nerves to reach to CNS, where it affects mainly the hippocampus and cerebellum

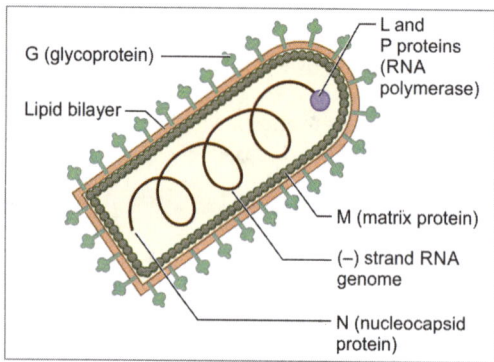

Fig. 23.1: Rabies virus (schematic diagram).

- ❖ **Centrifugal spread:** From CNS, the virus spreads along the sensory and autonomic nerves to various tissues such as salivary glands, cornea, and others. Shedding of the virus in the saliva of rabid animals acts as the source of infection.

Clinical Manifestations

The incubation period is prolonged and variable (20-90 days). It can be shorter if the traveling distance to reach CNS is less such as for children, bites on the head/neck/upper limbs, and for short people. The clinical spectrum is divided into 3 phases as follows.

Prodromal Phase

It lasts for 2-10 days, characterized by non-specific symptoms such as fever, malaise, nausea, photophobia, etc.

Acute Neurologic Phase

This may be either encephalitic type or paralytic type.
- ❖ **Encephalitic or furious rabies:** It is the most common type (80%), lasts for 2-7 days, and is characterized by:
  - *Hyperexcitability*: Anxiety, agitation, hyperactivity
  - *Autonomic (sympathetic) dysfunction* features may be seen such as ↑lacrimation, and ↑salivation (which leads to *foaming* at the mouth)
  - *Hydrophobia* (fear of water) or *aerophobia* (fear of air)—the act of swallowing precipitates an involuntary, painful spasm of the respiratory muscles.
- ❖ **Paralytic or dumb rabies:** This occurs in 20% of cases, especially in people who are partially vaccinated. It is characterized by flaccid paralysis of limbs. However, hydrophobia and other features of encephalitic rabies are typically absent.

Coma and Death

Following the acute neurological phase, the patient develops coma that eventually leads to death within 14 days. Death may get delayed up to 30 days in case of paralytic rabies.

Laboratory Diagnosis

- ❖ **Rabies antigen detection:** Direct fluorescent antibody (DFA) test can be performed to detect rabies nucleoprotein antigens in specimens such as hair follicle of the nape of the neck (most sensitive, best specimen) and corneal impression smear
- ❖ **Virus isolation** can be performed using suckling mice (intracerebral inoculation) or cell lines such as mouse neuroblastoma cell lines
- ❖ **Antibody detection:** Detection of CSF antibodies is more significant than serum antibodies, as the serum antibodies appear late and can also be present after vaccination. Several formats are available such as:
  - Mouse neutralization test (MNT)
  - Rapid fluorescent focus inhibition test (RFFIT)
  - Fluorescent antibody virus neutralization test (FAVN)
  - Indirect fluorescence assay (IFA).
- ❖ **Virus RNA detection:** Reverse transcription-PCR (RT-PCR) can be used to amplify specific genes (e.g. nucleoprotein gene). It is the most sensitive and specific assay available
- ❖ **Negri body detection:** It is useful to confirm the postmortem diagnosis of rabies **(Fig. 23.2)**

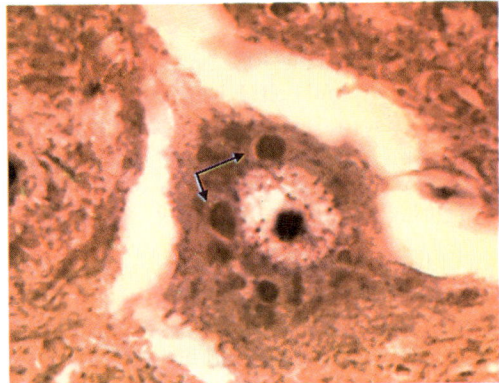

Fig. 23.2: Negri bodies in brain biopsy by H and E stain (*arrows showing*).

Source: Public Health Image Library, ID# 3377//Dr. Daniel P. Perl/Centers for Disease Control and Prevention (CDC), Atlanta (*with permission*).

- It is an intracytoplasmic eosinophilic inclusion body, composed of rabies virus proteins and viral RNA
- Commonly observed in cerebellum and hippocampus
- Negri body detection is pathognomonic of rabies: But may not be detected in 20% of cases.

> **TREATMENT** — Rabies
>
> There is no specific treatment for rabies. Symptomatic treatment may prolong life, but the outcome is almost always fatal.
> - Isolation of the patient
> - Sedatives and anti-anxiety drugs
> - Maintenance of hydration and urination.

Prevention of Human Rabies

There are three strategies available for the prevention of rabies.

Local Wound Care

Involves *physical cleansing* of all bite wounds and scratches with soap and water, followed by applying antiseptics. *Suturing should be strictly avoided* as it causes local tissue damage, which may help in the spreading of the virus.

Rabies Vaccine

Cell line-derived non-neural vaccines are recommended.
1. Purified chick embryo cell (PCEC) vaccine
2. Purified Vero cell (PVC) vaccine
3. Human diploid cell (HDC) vaccine.

Note: The neural vaccines derived from the brain of infected animals are no longer used.

(3) Rabies Immunoglobulin (RIG)

It neutralizes the virus at the wound site within a few hours.
- RIG should be administered as soon as possible and not beyond day 7
- It is available in two forms; human RIG (hRIG) and equine RIG (eRIG)
- Recommended dose: 20 IU (for hRIG) or 40 IU (for eRIG) per kg body weight.

WHO Guideline of Post-exposure Prophylaxis

WHO has provided a guideline (2018) for post-exposure prophylaxis (PEP) for rabies. The components included in PEP depend upon the type of exposure categories **(Table 23.1)**.
- **For category I exposures:** Require only wound care. Vaccines or RIG are not required
- **For category II exposures:** Require local wound care and rabies vaccine. RIG is not required except for immunodeficient individuals who need RIG in addition
- **For category III exposures:** All three components are required—local wound care, vaccine, and RIG.

Schedule: Rabies vaccine can be administered by intradermal (ID) or intramuscular (IM). The ID regimens are cost-effective and therefore are preferred over IM regimens

Table 23.1: Risk categorization and recommended anti-rabies prophylaxis (WHO, 2018)

Category of risk	Type of exposure	Recommended prophylaxis **
Category I (No risk)	• Touching, or feeding of animal • Licks on intact skin	No treatment is needed if history is reliable
Category II (Minor risk)	Minor scratches or abrasions without bleeding or nibbling of uncovered skin	• Wound management • Rabies vaccine • Observe the dog for 10 days
Category III (Major risk)	• Single or multiple transdermal bites with oozing of blood • Licks on broken skin (fresh wounds) or mucous membrane • Direct contact with bats or wild animals	• Wound management • Rabies immunoglobulin • Rabies vaccine • Observe the dog for 10 days*

*Vaccine may be discontinued if the animal (dogs and cats) is healthy after 10 days of the bite.
**In India post-exposure prophylaxis is indicated following exposure to any animal bite except rodents and bat bite.

- **ID PEP regimen (2-2-2):** 2-site ID vaccine is given on days 0, 3 and 7 (total 6 doses, 0.1 mL/dose)
- **IM PEP regimens:** A total of four doses are given (entire vial/dose). Two schedules are available
  1. 1-site IM vaccine given on days 0, 3, 7, and the fourth dose between days 14 to 28 or
  2. 2-site IM vaccine given on day 0 and 1-site IM on days 7 and 21.

PEP for Individuals Previously Vaccinated

The individuals who previously received the rabies vaccine do not need RIG regardless of exposure category. They need local wound care and an accelerated vaccine regimen (with a reduced number of doses).

Pre-exposure Prophylaxis (PrEP)

It is recommended for—individuals at higher occupational risk (e.g. animal handlers) or for people in remote endemic areas. The PrEP regimen is given in any of the schedules:
- 2-site ID vaccine given on days 0 and 7
- 1-site IM vaccine given on days 0 and 7.

POLIOMYELITIS

Polioviruses cause a highly infectious childhood disease called polio (or poliomyelitis)—acute flaccid paralysis due to the involvement of the nervous system. Polio is on the verge of eradication globally.

Antigenic Types

Wild polioviruses (WPV) cause natural cases of poliomyelitis. Based on the viral protein (VP1) present on the capsid, there are three types of wild strains (WPV 1-3)
- All three strains are identical, produce similar manifestations and severity of illness
- However, they are antigenically distinct. The antibody response is type-specific and not cross-protective. Therefore, each strain needs to be eradicated individually
- Currently, all the natural cases are caused by WPV1. It has also been the common serotype to cause poliomyelitis till now

- Both WPV2 and WPV3 are globally eradicated, in the years 1999 and 2019 respectively.

Vaccine-derived poliovirus (VDPV): They are the vaccine strains of poliovirus that have regained neurovirulence and are capable of producing disease in man (described subsequently in this chapter).

Pathogenesis

Polioviruses are transmitted by the feco-oral route.
- **Spread:** They multiple locally in GIT and then spread to CNS by:
  - Hematogenous route (most common), or
  - Rarely by direct neural route: This occurs especially following tonsillectomy.
- **Site of action:** The final target site for poliovirus is the motor nerve ending, i.e. anterior horn cells of the spinal cord which leads to muscle weakness and flaccid paralysis
- **Neuron degeneration:** Virus-infected neurons undergo degeneration. The earliest change in the neuron is the degeneration of the Nissl body (aggregates of ribosomes)
- **Pathological changes** are always more extensive than the distribution of paralysis.

Clinical Manifestations

The incubation period is usually 7-14 days. The manifestations may range from asymptomatic stage to the most severe paralytic stage.
- **Inapparent infection:** Following infection, the majority (91–96%) of cases are asymptomatic
- **Abortive infection:** About 5% of patients develop minor symptoms (e.g. fever, malaise, sore throat, etc.)
- **Nonparalytic poliomyelitis:** It is seen in 1% of patients, and presented as aseptic meningitis
- **Paralytic poliomyelitis** is the least common form (<1%), characterized by descending asymmetric acute flaccid paralysis (AFP) **(Figs. 23.3A and B)**
- **Risk factors:** Paralytic disease is more common among: (1) older children and adults, (2) pregnant women, (3) following

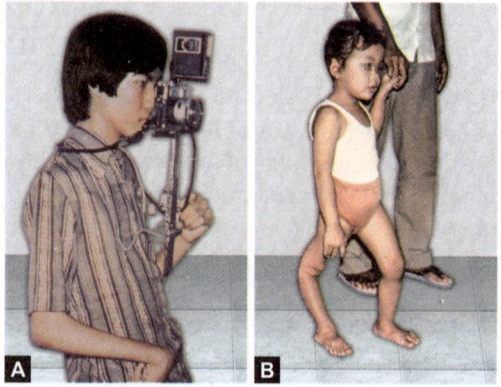

Figs. 23.3A and B: Deformities seen in poliomyelitis.
Source: Public Health Image Library, **A.** ID#: 5579; **B.** ID#: 5578, Centers for Disease Control and Prevention (CDC), Atlanta (*with permission*).

heavy muscular exercise, (4) tonsillectomy, (5) IM injections.

Laboratory Diagnosis

Useful specimens are stool, rectal swabs, and throat swabs.
- **Virus isolation** in primary monkey kidney cell line from specimens—viral growth is detected by demonstration of cytopathic effect (crenation and degeneration of the entire cell sheet), or detection of viral antigen or viral gene in cell line
- **Antibody detection**—by neutralization test
- **Real-time multiplex reverse-transcriptase PCR** has been developed using primers from VP1 region, which can detect and differentiate between various types of wild and vaccine polioviruses (Vaccine-associated paralytic poliomyelitis and Vaccine-derived poliovirus strains) directly from the stool specimen.

Vaccine

Both inactivated and live-attenuated polio vaccines are available; both have their unique useful properties as well as drawbacks **(Table 23.2)**.
- **Under the national immunization schedule** (India), both IPV and bivalent OPV are given
  - IPV: The fractional-dose of IPV is given by the intradermal route. It contains all three serotypes
  - Bivalent OPV is given orally. It contains serotypes 1 and 3.

Table 23.2: Differences between injectable and oral polio vaccines.		
Polio vaccine	**Injectable polio vaccine (Salk)**	**Oral polio vaccine (Sabin)**
Developed by	Jonas Salk, in 1952	Albert Sabin, 1955
Formulations	IPV contains three serotypes 1, 2 and 3. It can be given in two doses: • Full dose IPV (0.5mL): given by IM route • Fractional-dose (0.1mL): given by ID route	OPV is available as: (given as 2 drops/dose, oral route) • Trivalent OPV (serotypes 1, 2 and 3) • Bivalent OPV (serotypes 1 and 3) • Monovalent OPV (any one serotype)
National immunization schedule (India, 2022)	Two fractional doses (intra-dermal route at the upper arm, 0.1 mL/dose): Given at 6th and 14th weeks of age along with bivalent OPV	Total five doses of bivalent OPV (serotype 1 and 3): • Zero dose—given at birth • 1st, 2nd, and 3rd dose —given at 6th, 10th, 14th week of age; booster dose is given at 16–24 months
Safety	Relatively safer than OPV	Safe except in immunocompromised patients, pregnancy, old age
Efficacy	A full course of IPV: produce 80–90% efficacy The immune response is developed at a slower rate than OPV	90–100% efficacy is achieved even by 1 or 2 doses of OPV efficacy decreases by: • Interference by other enteroviruses • Diarrheal diseases and breastfeeding
Economy	Relatively expensive	Economical

Contd...

Contd...

Polio vaccine	Injectable polio vaccine (Salk)	Oral polio vaccine (Sabin)
Duration of protection	Short, need booster doses periodically	Long-lasting
In epidemics	Can precipitate paralysis	Can be used safely
Herd immunity	Not provided	Provided due to feco-oral spread of vaccine virus
Local immunity	Weakly stimulated	Strongly stimulated (due to IgA antibody)
Storage condition	Relatively stable Does not require a stringent condition	Should be stored at (−20°C) Stabilized in $MgCl_2$ pH<7
VAPP and VDPV	Zero chance	Relatively more chance

Abbreviations: VAPP, vaccine-associated paralytic poliomyelitis; VDPV, vaccine-derived polioviruses.

❖ In OPV, the live-attenuated vaccine virus can undergo genetic change to regain neurovirulence and such strains are capable of causing poliomyelitis. Two types of vaccine-induced poliomyelitis have been reported
  1. **Vaccine-associated paralytic poliomyelitis (VAPP):** Caused by OPV-like strain which has a minor genetic difference (<1%) than OPV strain. They are not capable of circulating in the community and do not cause secondary cases or outbreaks
  2. **Vaccine-derived polioviruses (VDPV):** They have a genetic difference from OPV strain by >1%. They are capable of circulating in the community and therefore have a higher risk of causing outbreaks.

Epidemiology

Polio is on the verge of eradication globally.

Pulse Polio Immunization (PPI) was initiated globally to eradicate poliomyelitis. In India, it is in operation since 1995–96.
❖ **World:** Currently, wild polio is endemic only in two countries—Pakistan, and Afghanistan. However, vaccine-derived polio cases are still occurring in a few other countries of the world
❖ **India** became polio-free in 2014. No natural case has been reported since 2011.

EXPECTED QUESTIONS

I. **Write short notes on:**
   1. Pathogenesis of rabies.
   2. Laboratory diagnosis of rabies.
   3. Post-exposure prophylaxis of rabies.
   4. Polio vaccines.

II. **Multiple Choice Questions (MCQs):**
   1. **Rabies is transmitted by all,** *except?*
      a. Dog bite
      b. Ingestion
      c. Bat bite
      d. Inhalation
   2. **Negri bodies are pathognomonic for___?**
      a. Rabies   b. Polio
      c. Dengue   d. HIV
   3. **Currently, all the wild polio cases are caused by___?**
      a. WPV-1   b. WPV-2
      c. WPV-3   d. All of the above
   4. **National immunization schedule of India recommends___?**
      a. OPV only   b. OPV + IPV
      c. IPV only
      d. Polio vaccines are not required
   5. **Not true about salk vaccine:**
      a. Expensive than OPV
      b. Not useful in epidemics
      c. Provides herd immunity
      d. Booster doses are required

Answers
1. b   2. a   3. a   4. b   5. c

CHAPTER 24: HIV/AIDS

CHAPTER PREVIEW
- Morphology
- Pathogenesis
- Clinical Diagnosis
- Epidemiology
- Laboratory Diagnosis
- Post-exposure Prophylaxis

MORPHOLOGY

Human immunodeficiency virus (HIV) is the etiologic agent of Acquired Immunodeficiency Syndrome (AIDS)—the biggest threat to mankind in the last three decades.

- HIV belongs to retroviruses—a group of RNA viruses that possesses a unique enzyme called **reverse transcriptase** which converts the viral RNA into DNA inside the host cell **(Fig. 24.1)**
- It has a nucleocapsid surrounded by an envelope
- **Nucleocapsid** has icosahedral in symmetry, comprises of a capsid enclosing two copies of ssRNA
- **Envelope** comprises of a lipid membrane into which the two types of protein spikes are embedded:
  - Glycoprotein 120 (gp 120): They are projected as knob-like spikes on the surface, and
  - Glycoprotein 41 (gp 41): They form anchoring transmembrane pedicles.

HIV Genome

HIV contains three structural genes—*gag, pol,* and *env*

- The *gag* gene codes for the core and shell of the virus

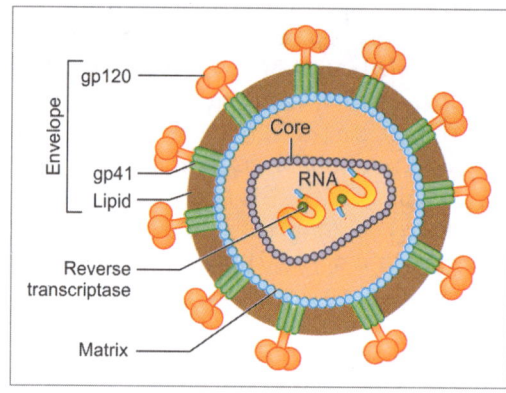

Fig. 24.1: Structure of HIV.

- The *pol* gene codes for viral enzymes such as reverse transcriptase, protease, and integrase
- The *env* gene codes for the envelope glycoproteins such as gp 120 and gp 41. Frequent mutations in the *env* gene account for antigenic diversity seen in HIV. This is the main reason which explains why:
  - HIV evades the host's immune response
  - Vaccination against HIV is extremely difficult.

HIV Serotyping

Based on sequence differences in the *env* gene, HIV comprises of two serotypes HIV-1 and 2.

- HIV-1 comprises of three distinct groups (M, N, O)
- 'M' is the dominant group worldwide. It comprises of eleven **subtypes** or "clades" (A-K)
- **Geographical distribution:** The serotypes vary from each other in geographic distribution
  - Subtype A is common in West Africa
  - Subtype B is predominant in Europe, America, Japan, and Australia
  - Subtype C is the most common form worldwide.

PATHOGENESIS

Mode of Transmission

HIV is transmitted through the following modes:
- **Sexual mode:** It is the most common mode (75%). The heterosexual route is more common, whereas anal sex has a higher risk of transmission
- **Blood transfusion** although is a less common mode (5%), the risk of transmission is maximum (90–95%)
- **Percutaneous/mucosal** transmission such as needle stick injury, splash injury on eyes, injection drug abuse, and sharing razors or tattooing
- **Mother-to-baby transmission:** Risk is maximum during delivery although transmission may occur at any time during pregnancy and breastfeeding
- **Viral load** is maximum in blood, genital secretions, and CSF; variable in breast milk and saliva; zero to minimal in other body fluids or urine.

Replication

The replication of HIV inside the host cell involves the following sequential steps.
- **Virus entry:** For the virus to enter into the host cell, the following receptor interaction is essential
  - *Main receptor:* HIV enters into the target cells by binding its gp120 to the CD4 receptor on the host cell surface (such as helper T cells and macrophages)
  - *Second co-receptor:* CXCR4 molecules of helper T cells or CCR5 molecules of macrophages.
- **Fusion:** Following receptor attachment, fusion of HIV to host cell takes place; mediated by the fusion protein gp41
- **Reverse transcription:** Inside the host cytoplasm, the ssRNA of HIV gets reversed transcribed into dsDNA
- **Integration:** The dsDNA (called proviral DNA) subsequently gets integrated into the host chromosome, mediated by viral integrase
- **Latency:** In the integrated state, HIV establishes a latent infection, which lasts for a variable period.

CLINICAL STAGES (DISEASE PROGRESSION)

The clinical course of HIV infection includes the following five stages.
1. **Acute HIV disease or acute retroviral syndrome:** Initially, HIV destroys the infected T cells and spills into the bloodstream to cause primary viremia, which coincides with an initial flu-like illness that occurs in many patients (50–75%); 3–6 weeks after the primary infection. There is a significant drop in the number of circulating CD4 T cells at this stage
2. **Asymptomatic stage** (clinical latency): Restoration of adequate immune response develops within 1 month in most of the patients. It is a state of *clinical latency*, but *not microbiological latency*
3. **Persistent generalized lymphadenopathy (PGL):** It occurs as a result of HIV replication in lymph nodes
4. **Symptomatic HIV infection (AIDS-related complex):** After a variable period of clinical latency, the CD4 T cell level starts falling. Eventually, patients develop constitutional symptoms such as:
   - Unexplained diarrhea, lasting for more than 1 month
   - Weight loss (>10%), malaise, and night sweat
   - Mild opportunistic infections such as oral thrush.

5. **AIDS**: It is an advanced end-stage of HIV infection; characterized by:
   - Rapid fall in CD4 T cell count (usually <200 cells/μL)
   - High viral load
   - Lymphoid tissue is totally destroyed and replaced by fibrous tissue
   - Opportunistic infections set in secondary to profound immune suppression **(Table 24.1)**
   - Development of neoplasia **(Table 24.1)**
   - Development of direct HIV-induced manifestations such as HIV encephalopathy **(Table 24.1)**.

EPIDEMIOLOGY

HIV has a **global prevalence** of 0.7% in adults, whereas, in India, the prevalence is much lower (0.22%).

Table 24.1: Opportunistic infections and neoplasia associated with HIV/AIDS.

Bacterial opportunistic infections:
- Recurrent severe bacterial infections
- Extrapulmonary tuberculosis
- Disseminated non-tubercular mycobacterial infection
- Recurrent septicemia (including non-typhoidal salmonellosis)

Viral opportunistic infections:
- Chronic HSV infection
- Progressive multifocal leukoencephalopathy
- CMV (retinitis, or infection of other organs)

Fungal opportunistic infections:
- *Pneumocystis jirovecii* pneumonia
- Esophageal candidiasis
- Extrapulmonary cryptococcosis (meningitis)
- Disseminated mycoses (histoplasmosis and coccidioidomycoses)

Parasitic opportunistic infections:
- *Toxoplasma* encephalitis
- Chronic intestinal cystoisosporiasis (>1 month)
- Atypical disseminated leishmaniasis

Neoplasia:
- Kaposi's sarcoma
- Invasive cervical cancer
- Lymphoma (cerebral, B cell, and non-Hodgkin)

Other conditions (direct HIV induced):
- HIV encephalopathy
- Symptomatic HIV-associated nephropathy or cardiomyopathy

- **Sub-Saharan Africa** remains the most severely affected region
- **In India,** northeast states such as Mizoram, Manipur, and Nagaland have the highest prevalence. Whereas in terms of the absolute number of cases, Maharashtra is the worst affected state followed by Andhra Pradesh, Karnataka, and Telangana.

LABORATORY DIAGNOSIS

Diagnosis of HIV/AIDS is not like other infectious diseases. A number of moral, ethical, legal, and psychosocial issues are associated with a positive HIV status. The following care should be taken (3Cs) while performing the test for HIV.

- **Consent** in written format should be taken before the test is done. The patient should be explained about the nature of the test is performed
- **Confidentiality** of a positive test result is a must. The patient's name or the word "HIV positive" should not be written on the report form.
- **Counseling** should be provided to motivate the individual to tell the spouse/family and induce behavioral change.

The tests employed for laboratory diagnosis of HIV/AIDS can be grouped into specific and non-specific tests **(Table 24.2)**.

Antibody Detection

Detection of anti-HIV antibodies is the mainstay of diagnosis of HIV. Tests to detect specific HIV antibodies can be classified into screening and supplemental tests.

Screening Antibody Detection Tests

Screening assays usually take less time and have high sensitivity and specificity (≥98–99%).
- **Antigens used** in most of the screening tests are:
  - HIV-1 specific antigens: p24, gp 120, gp41
  - HIV-2 specific gp36.
- **Formats** available for screening tests are:
  - ELISA: Takes 2–3 hours

Table 24.2: Laboratory diagnosis of HIV/AIDS.

Specific Tests for HIV Infection

- **Screening tests** (antibody detection):
  - ELISA (takes 2–3 hours)
  - Rapid/Simple test (takes <30 minutes)
- **Supplemental tests** (antibody detection):
  - Western blot assay
  - Line immunoassay (LIA)
- **Confirmatory tests**
  - p24 antigen detection (after 12–26 days of infection)
  - Viral culture—by co-cultivation technique
  - HIV RNA (best confirmatory method)—can be detected 10–14 days after infection
    - Reverse transcriptase PCR (RT-PCR)
    - Branched DNA assay
    - NASBA (nucleic acid sequence-based amplification)
    - Real time RT-PCR for estimating viral load
  - HIV DNA detection: Useful for diagnosis of pediatric HIV

Non–specific Immunological Methods

- Low CD4 T cell count
- Hypergammaglobulinemia:
  - Neopterin
  - β2-macroglobulin
- Altered CD4: CD8 T cell ratio

- Rapid/simple test: Takes less than 30 minutes. Various test formats available are:
  - Dot blot assays (or immunoconcentration or flow through method, e.g. Tridot test)
  - Immunochromatography (ICT)
  - Dip stick/Comb tests (Enzyme immune assay-based tests).
- **Should be confirmed:** Results of a single screening test should never be used as the final interpretation of HIV status as false-positive results or technical errors can occur. It is always subjected to confirmatory tests.

Supplemental Antibody Detection Tests

These assays are highly specific antibody detection methods; hence used for validation of positive results of screening tests. They are expensive, labor-intensive, need expertise to interpret, and may also give equivocal/indeterminate results. Examples include:

- Western blot assay
- Line immunoassay (LIA).

Confirmatory Tests

The following are confirmatory tests for diagnosis of HIV such as—detection of p24 antigens, HIV RNA and DNA detection, and virus isolation.

Detection of p24 Core Antigen

The p24 core antigen can be detected by various formats such as ELISA. This test is useful for:

- For confirmation of the diagnosis of HIV/AIDS
- Diagnosis of HIV during the window period
- Diagnosis of HIV in infants (not reliable)
- Monitoring the progress of HIV infection
- To resolve equivocal western blot results.

Viral RNA Detection

Detection of viral RNA is the **"gold standard"** method for confirmation of HIV diagnosis. Various formats are available targeting *pol* and *env* genes.

- Reverse transcriptase-polymerase chain reaction (RT-PCR)
- Real-time RT-PCR: For estimating viral load

Apart from the routine diagnosis of HIV, RNA detection has several other uses such as:

- It is the **most sensitive** and **specific** method and is the best method **for confirmation** of HIV
- It is the best tool for diagnosis of HIV during the **window period** and detects HIV earlier than all available methods (10–14 days post-exposure)
- **Viral load monitoring:** Real-time RT-PCR can quantify the viral load and is the most appropriate tool for monitoring the response to antiretroviral therapy
- **Typing:** To differentiate between HIV-1 and HIV-2 infections and also to determine the specific subtype
- Detection of **drug resistance** genes.

DNA PCR

PCR detecting proviral DNA is extremely useful for the diagnosis of pediatric HIV.

Non-specific Immunological Methods

Non-specific immunological methods are as follows:
- Low CD4 T cell count
- Altered CD4: CD8 T cell ratio
- Hypergammaglobulinemia, e.g. detection of neopterin and β2-macroglobulin.

NACO Strategy for HIV Diagnosis

For the resource-poor countries, it is impracticable to confirm the result of HIV screening tests by PCR or western blot as these assays are expensive and available only at limited centers.

NACO (National AIDS Control Organization, India) has formulated a strategic plan **(Fig. 24.2)** for HIV diagnosis. The guidelines are as follows:
- Depending on the situation/condition, for which the test is done, the positive result of the first screening test should be either considered as such or confirmed by another one or two screening tests
- The first screening test should be highly sensitive, whereas the second and third screening tests should have high specificity
- The three screening tests should use different principles or different antigens. The same kit should not be used again
- Supplemental or confirmatory tests should be used only when the screening test(s) results are equivocal/indeterminate.

There are four NACO Strategic Algorithms **(Fig. 24.2)**:
1. **Strategy I:** It is done for the screening of the blood donors in blood banks. Only one test

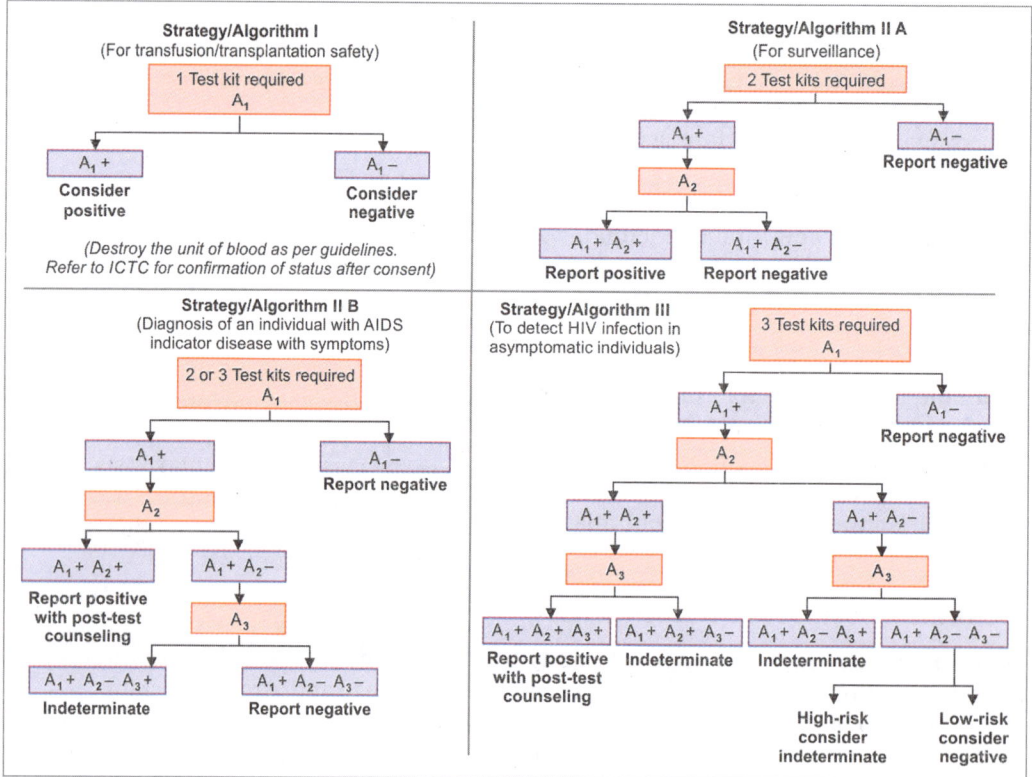

Fig. 24.2: NACO strategies/algorithms for diagnosing HIV infection.
Abbreviations: NACO, National AIDS Control Organization; ICTC, Integrated Counselling and Testing Centre.

should be done. If found reactive, then the unit of blood is destroyed
2. **Strategy IIa**: It is done for sentinel surveillance of HIV infection to estimate the prevalence of infection. Positive results of the first test should be confirmed by a second test. If the second test is negative, then it is reported as negative
3. **Strategy IIb:** It is followed for the diagnosis of HIV/AIDS in symptomatic patients. A positive result of the first test should be confirmed by a second test. If the second test is negative, then a third test is done for confirmation
4. **Strategy III**: It is done for the diagnosis of asymptomatic HIV patients, antenatal screening, and screening of patients awaiting surgeries
   - **Three tests format:** All positive results in the first test should be confirmed by the second and third tests. A positive report is sent only if all three test results are found reactive
   - For indeterminate results of strategies IIB and III, (i.e. first test positive but second or third test negative), a repeat test is done after 14–28 days and the sample should be sent to the reference center for confirmation by western blot or RT-PCR.

Prognosis/Monitoring of HIV

Various tools available for monitoring the response to antiretroviral therapy include:
- CD4 T cell count: Most commonly used
- HIV RNA load: Most consistent and best tool
- p24 antigen detection
- Neopterin and β2 macroglobulin level.

Note: Viral antibody levels are inconsistent and variable during the late stage due to immune collapse; hence not reliable for prognosis.

Diagnosis of Pediatric HIV Infection

The routine screening methods (ELISA or rapid/simple tests) detect IgG antibodies.
- They cannot differentiate between a baby's IgG or maternally transferred IgG, hence cannot be used for the diagnosis of pediatric HIV
- As all maternal antibodies would disappear by 18 months; therefore IgG assays can be performed after 18 months of birth.

Pediatric HIV can be reliably diagnosed by methods such as:
- **HIV DNA PCR:** This is the most recommended method for the diagnosis of pediatric HIV
- **Other tests include:** HIV RNA detection and p24 antigen detection.

Diagnosis of HIV in Window Period

The window period refers to the initial time interval between the exposure and appearance of detectable levels of antibodies in the serum.
- The antibodies appear in blood within 2–8 weeks after infection but usually become detectable after 3 weeks to 12 weeks with the assays available presently. It can be as low as 22 days; when the newer third-generation antibody detection kits with high sensitivity are used
- **p24 antigen detection:** It can be detected by 12–26 days after infection
- **HIV RNA detection** (by RT-PCR) is the best method—it detects HIV RNA around 10–14 days after infection.

TREATMENT	HIV infection

Antiretroviral therapy (ART) Guideline, NACO 2021

Indication to start ART: TREAT ALL; i.e., antiretroviral therapy (ART) has to be started in all patients irrespective of CD4 count, clinical stage, age, population, or associated opportunistic infections (OIs).

HAART: Highly active antiretroviral therapy (HAART) refers to the use of a combination of at least three antiretroviral drugs to maximally suppress HIV and stop the progression of the disease.

TLD regimen: Tenofovir + Lamivudine + Dolutegravir is the preferred first-line ART regimen for all HIV patients (HIV-1 and/or -2) in adults including pregnant women.
- It is given as as fixed dose combination in a single pill once a day
- It is also the regimen of choice for is used for post-exposure prophylaxis for healthcare workers (Chapter 43)

SECTION 4 ♦ Viral Infections

▶ EXPECTED QUESTIONS ◀

I. Write an essay on:
1. Discuss the pathogenesis, clinical stages, and laboratory diagnosis of HIV infection.

II. Write short notes on:
1. Morphology of HIV.
2. NACO strategy for HIV diagnosis.
3. Tests for monitoring response to treatment in AIDS patients.
4. Tests for diagnosis of HIV in the window period.

III. Multiple Choice Questions (MCQs):

1. **HIV transmission: Maximum risk is associated with___?**
   a. Sexual transmission
   b. Mother-to-child
   c. Needlestick injury
   d. Blood transfusion

2. **The most common mode of HIV transmission is___?**
   a. Sexual transmission
   b. Mother-to-child
   c. Needlestick injury
   d. Blood transfusion

3. **Tests for monitoring response to treatment in HIV include all, *except*?**
   a. ELISA for IgG antibody detection
   b. P24 antigen detection
   c. HIV RNA detection
   d. HIV DNA detection

4. **Tests for diagnosis of HIV in the window period include all, *except*?**
   a. ELISA for IgG antibody detection
   b. P24 antigen detection
   c. HIV RNA detection
   d. HIV DNA detection

Answers
1. d   2. a   3. a   4. a

CHAPTER 25

Viral Hepatitis

CHAPTER PREVIEW

- Hepatitis A
- Hepatitis B
- Hepatitis C
- Hepatitis D
- Hepatitis E

Hepatitis viruses are a diverse group of viruses, having a common feature of being hepatotropic, and causing hepatitis. There are five major types of hepatitis viruses—A to E. Recently hepatitis G has also been detected. There is no hepatitis F virus.

All hepatitis viruses are RNA viruses, except for hepatitis B which is a DNA virus. The features of hepatitis viruses have been depicted in **Table 25.1**.

- ❖ Hepatitis A virus (HAV) and hepatitis E virus (HEV) have similarities in various aspects such as transmission (feco-oral route), etc.
- ❖ Similarly, hepatitis B virus (HBV), hepatitis C virus (HCV), and hepatitis D virus (HDV) resemble in many properties—e.g. transmitted by blood, sexual and vertical routes.

HEPATITIS A

Hepatitis A virus (HAV) is a non-enveloped RNA virus, that belongs to picornaviruses (Enterovirus 72).

Clinical Manifestation

HAV has an incubation period of about 15–45 days. Onset is relatively abrupt (subacute).

- ❖ **Clinically,** HAV infection is indistinguishable from other hepatitis viruses; characterized by:
  - Pre-icteric phase (mainly gastrointestinal symptoms like nausea) followed by;
  - Icteric phase or jaundice (dark urine, yellowish sclera, and mucus membrane).
- ❖ Complete recovery occurs in most (98%) cases
- ❖ There is no chronic or carriers state
- ❖ **Complications** may occur such as fulminant hepatitis; characterized by severe necrosis of hepatocytes.

Table 25.1: Features of hepatitis viruses.

HAV and HEV	HBV, HCV and HDV
Both HAV and HEV are RNA viruses	• HBV is a DNA virus • HCV and HDV are RNA viruses
Feco-oral transmission	Blood (common), sexual, and vertical
Incubation period: 15–50 days, onset-abrupt	Incubation period: 30–180 days, insidious onset
No carriers	Carriers seen
No chronicity	Chronicity seen
Not oncogenic	Oncogenic
Fulminant: Rare (<1%); except HEV in pregnancy (10–20%)	Fulminant: Rare (1–2%) except HDV (10–20%)
Non-enveloped; icosahedron symmetry	Enveloped; spherical symmetry

Epidemiology

HAV is the most common cause of acute viral hepatitis in children.
- ❖ Children and adolescents are commonly affected
- ❖ **Risk factors:** Poor personal hygiene and overcrowding are the most important risk factors.

Laboratory Diagnosis

The HAV infection is diagnosed by the following modalities.
- ❖ **Anti-HAV antibody detection** (by ELISA): IgM positive–indicates the presence of acute HAV infection, whereas IgG antibody detection indicates past infection or recovery. There is no chronic stage
- ❖ **Detection of HAV particles:** HAV appears in stool from −2 to +2 weeks of jaundice, and can be detected by electron microscopy
- ❖ **HAV antigen detection:** ELISA format is available to detect HAV antigen from a stool sample from −2 to +2 weeks of jaundice
- ❖ **Non-specific findings:** Such as elevated liver enzymes and serum bilirubin levels.

Prevention

- ❖ **Vaccines:** The indications to administer the HAV vaccine include: all children of >1 year age, travelers to endemic countries, and patients with chronic liver disease. Two types of vaccines are available
  1. Formaldehyde inactivated vaccine
  2. Live attenuated vaccine.
- ❖ **Human immunoglobulin (HAV-Ig):** It is useful for post-exposure prophylaxis of **intimate contacts** of persons with hepatitis A or **travelers**.

> **TREATMENT** — Hepatitis A
> There is no specific antiviral drug is available.

HEPATITIS B

Hepatitis B virus (HBV) is the most widespread and the most important agent among hepatitis viruses. It is the only hepatitis virus to be a DNA virus and belongs to hepadnaviruses.

Morphology

HBV exists in three morphologic forms (**Figs. 25.1A and B**)—spherical and tubular forms are incomplete forms, exclusively made up of hepatitis B surface antigen (HBsAg) and a third form is a complete form called Dane particles.

Dane particles are spherical; comprise of three antigens:
- ❖ **Outer surface envelope:** made up of hepatitis B surface antigen or HBsAg (also called Australia antigen)

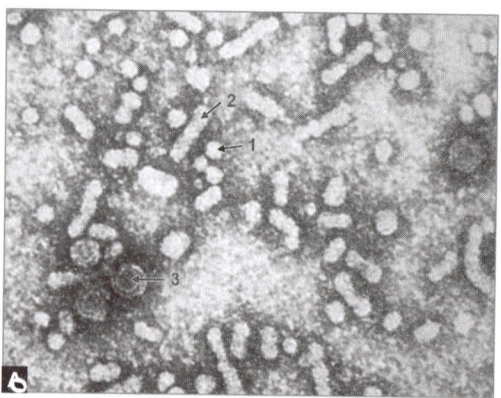
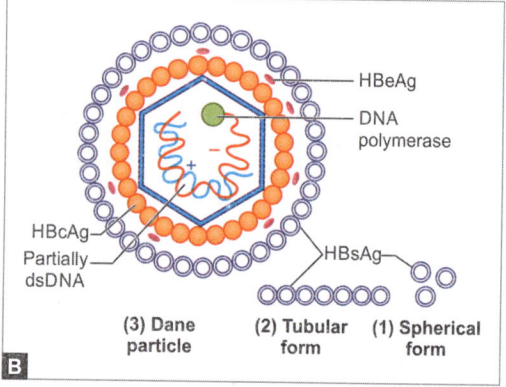

Figs. 25.1 A and B: A. Electron microscopic appearance of hepatitis B virus, showing 1-spherical form, 2-tubular form, and 3-Dane particle; **B.** Schematic diagram of hepatitis B virus.
Source: **A.** ID# 5631/Public Health Image Library/Centers for Disease Control and Prevention (CDC), Atlanta (*with permission*).

- **Inner nucleocapsid:** It consists of core antigen (HBcAg) and pre-core antigen (HBeAg) and partially double-stranded DNA.

Transmission

The transmission of HBV occurs via multiple routes.
- **Parenteral route** via blood and blood products transfusion and needle prick injuries. It is considered as the most common mode in developing countries
- **Sexual transmission** is found to be the most common route in most developed countries; particularly homosexual males being at higher risk
- **Vertical (perinatal) transmission:** Transmission occurs at any stage such as in-utero, during delivery (maximum risk), and during breastfeeding. The risk of transmission is maximum if the mother is HBeAg positive
- **Direct skin contact** with infected open skin lesions may transmit the virus, e.g. impetigo (especially in children).

High-risk groups which are more prone to acquire HBV infection are:
- Surgeons, technicians, phlebotomists
- Paramedical workers
- Sex workers especially homosexual males
- Recipients of blood transfusion and organ transplantation
- Drug addicts.

Clinical Manifestations

Hepatitis B has an incubation period of about 30–180 days. The onset of infection is slow and insidious.
- Patients may present with subclinical infection, acute or chronic hepatitis
- **Acute hepatitis:** Clinical presentation of HBV infection is as discussed for HAV; characterized by: pre-icteric phase and icteric phase or jaundice
- **The clinical outcome** of acute HBV infection may be either complete recovery (90-95%) or development of carrier state (5%) or chronic infection (5%)
- **Carriers:** There are two types of carriers:
  1. *Simple carriers*: They are capable of low infectivity (negative for HBeAg and HBV DNA). This stage is also called as chronic inactive HBV infection
  2. *Supercarriers:* Here, the virus is actively multiplying and capable of high infectivity (positive for HBeAg and HBV DNA). This stage is also called as immunotolerant chronic HBV infection.
- **Chronic hepatitis:** This can also occur in two stages:
  1. Chronic inactive hepatitis: Capable of low infectivity (negative for HBeAg and HBV DNA)
  2. Immunoreactive (chronic active) hepatitis: Here, the virus is actively multiplying and capable of high infectivity (positive for HBeAg and HBV DNA).
- **Hepatic complications:** Rarely, it may proceed to complications such as fulminant hepatitis or cirrhosis, or hepatocellular carcinoma
- **Extrahepatic complications:** May develop in some cases due to immune complex deposition. It is characterized by arthritis, rash, angioedema, etc.

Epidemiology

Hepatitis B virus infection occurs throughout the world; usually sporadic, but occasional outbreaks can occur in hospitals.
- **Reservoir of infection:** Humans are the only reservoir of infection, who can be either cases or carriers
- **Carriers** can also be grouped into:
  - **Simple carriers:** They are of low infectivity, and transmit the virus at a lower rate. They possess a low level of HBsAg and no HBeAg
  - **Super carriers:** They are highly infectious and transmit the virus efficiently. They possess higher levels of HBsAg and HBeAg, DNA polymerase, and HBV DNA.
- **HBV prevalence:** There are three epidemiological patterns observed among various countries:
  1. *Low endemicity:* The carrier rate is less than 2%

2. *Intermediate endemicity:* The carrier rate is between 2 and 8%. It is observed in India, China, and many countries in Eastern Mediterranean and Southeast Asian regions
3. *High endemicity:* The carrier rate is more than 8%.

Laboratory Diagnosis of Hepatitis B

A definitive diagnosis of hepatitis B depends on the serological demonstration of the viral markers, which can be classified as:
- **Antigen markers:** HBsAg and HBeAg
- **Antibody markers:** Anti-HBs, anti-HBe, and anti-HBc
- **Molecular markers:** HBV DNA
- **Nonspecific markers:** Elevated liver enzymes and serum bilirubin.

Test Methods Employed

- **HBV antigens and antibodies:** The most common method employed is ELISA; although various rapid test formats (such as ICT) and chemiluminescence immunoassay (CLIA) are also available
- **Viral DNA** can be detected by polymerase chain reaction (PCR). Real-time PCR is very useful for the quantification of HBV DNA
- HBV does not grow in any conventional culture system.

HBsAg (Hepatitis B Surface Antigen)

It is the first marker to be elevated following infection; becomes positive within 8–12 weeks.
- It appears during the incubation period
- The presence of HBsAg indicates the onset of infectivity
- It remains elevated for the entire duration of acute hepatitis. However, it can rarely persist beyond 6 months, if the disease progresses to chronic hepatitis or in a carrier state
- It is used as an epidemiological marker of hepatitis B infection.

HBeAg (Pre-core Antigen) and HBV DNA

They appear concurrently with or shortly after the appearance of HBsAg in serum. They are the markers of active viral replication and high viral infectivity. HBV DNA load is used to monitor the response to treatment.

HBcAg (Hepatitis B Core Antigen)

Hepatitis B core antigen (HBcAg) is a hidden antigen, nonsecretory in nature; hence, it cannot be detected in the blood. However, can be detected in hepatocytes by immunofluorescence.

Anti-HBc IgM (Hepatitis B Core Antibody)

Anti-HBc IgM is the first antibody to elevate following infection:
- It appears within the first 1–2 weeks after the appearance of HBsAg and lasts for 3–6 months
- Its presence indicates acute HBV infection.

Anti-HBc IgG (Hepatitis B Core Antibody)

Anti-HBc IgG appears in the late acute stage and remains positive indefinitely whether the patient proceeds to—the chronic stage or carrier state or recovery. It can also be used as an epidemiological marker of HBV infection.

Anti-HBe Ab (Anti-hepatitis B Precore Antibody)

Anti-HBe antibodies appear after the clearance of HBeAg and their presence signifies diminished viral replication and decreased infectivity.

Anti-HBs Ab (Anti-hepatitis B Surface Antibody)

Anti-HBs antibody appears after the clearance of HBsAg and remains elevated indefinitely.
- Its presence indicates recovery, immunity, and noninfectivity (i.e., stoppage of transmission)
- It is also the marker of vaccination; if the rest of all markers are negative **(Fig. 25.2)**.

Various outcomes following HBV infection and markers for diagnosis is depicted in **Figure 25.2**.

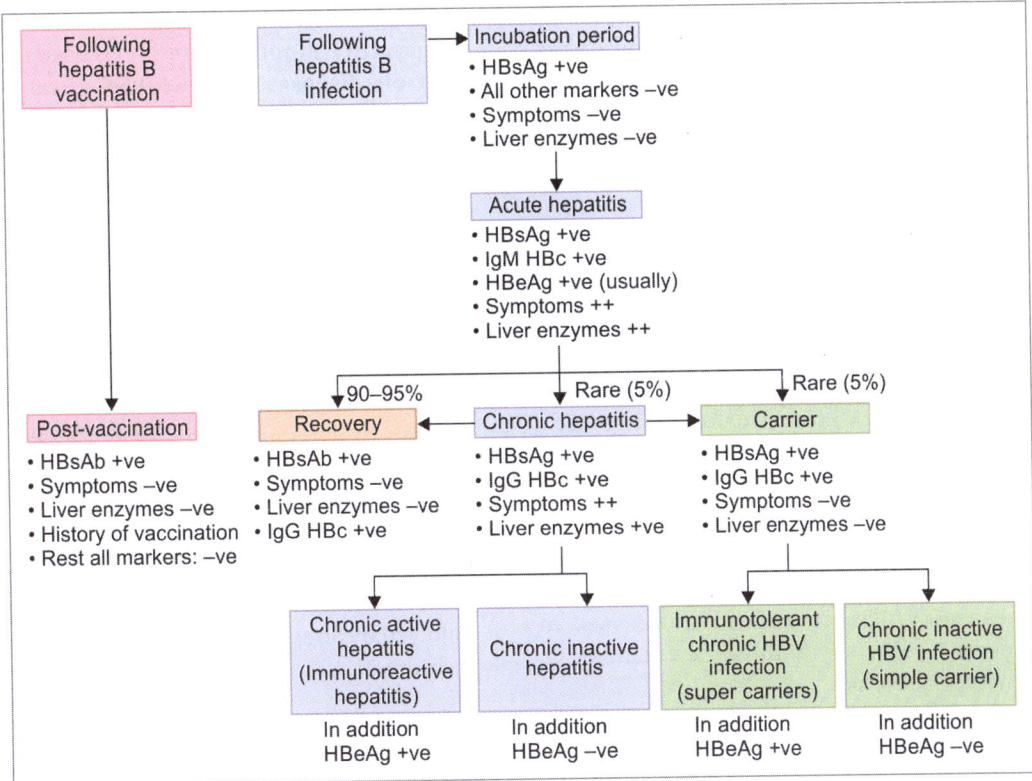

Fig. 25.2: Various outcomes following hepatitis B infection and markers for diagnosis.

| TREATMENT | Hepatitis B |

Treatment is indicated for chronic hepatitis, supercarriers, and associated cirrhosis. Antiviral agents include:
- **Antiviral agents**: Nucleoside analogs such as tenofovir and telbivudine are the agent of choice currently
- **Pegylated interferon alfa**: Was used previously; now not in use because of adverse effects.

Prevention (HBV)

Hepatitis B Vaccine (Active Immunization)

Hepatitis B vaccine is a recombinant subunit vaccine, made up of **HBsAg**, prepared in Baker's yeast by DNA recombinant technology.
- **Route:** Administered by intramuscular route over deltoid (in infant—anterolateral thigh)
- **Schedule:** Three doses are given at 0, 1, and 6 months. Under the National Immunization Schedule, it is given at 6, 10, and 14 weeks (along with the DPT vaccine)
- **Marker of protection:** Recipients are said to be protected if the anti-HBsAg antibody titer is above 10 mIU/mL.

Hepatitis B Immunoglobulin

Hepatitis B immunoglobulin (HBIG) is used in the following situations where an immediate protection is warranted; given at a dose of 0.06 mL/kg or 10–12 IU/kg.
- Acutely exposed to HBsAg positive blood, e.g., surgeons, nurses, laboratory workers
- Sexual partners of acute hepatitis B patients
- Neonates borne to hepatitis B carrier mothers
- Post-liver transplant patients who need protection against HBV infection
- Following accidental exposure.

The post-exposure prophylaxis for HBV is discussed in Chapter 43.

General Prophylactic Measures

- Screening of blood bags, semen, and organ donors

- Following safe sex practices (e.g. using condoms, avoiding multiple sex partners)
- Following safe injection practices—use of the disposable syringes and needles
- Following safe aseptic surgical practices
- Health education.

HEPATITIS C

Hepatitis C virus (HCV) is a common cause of post-transfusion hepatitis in developing countries. Among hepatitis viruses, HCV has the maximum risk of developing into a chronic infection. It is a RNA virus, comprises of a nucleocapsid, surrounded by an envelope.

Genetic Diversity of HCV

Similar to HIV, the hepatitis C virus displays diversity in the RNA genome that occurs because of high rates of mutations seen in the virus, especially in the gene encoding E2 envelope protein.
- **Genotypes:** HCV is divided into six major genotypes
- **Subtypes:** Genotypes are further divided into more than 100 subtypes
- The genotypes also vary from each other in their—epidemiological distribution and also in susceptibility to antiviral drugs.

Transmission

Various modes of transmission of HCV are as follows:
- **Parenteral:** Blood transfusions, blood products or organ transplantations, needle stick and splash injury, injection drug users
- **Vertical transmission** from infected mother to fetus
- **Sexual transmission** (rare).

Clinical Manifestations

The incubation period is about 15–160 days. Following infection with HCV:
- **Asymptomatic infection:** Seen in about >75% of cases
- **Acute hepatitis:** About 20% of people develop acute hepatitis. In about 5–15% of infections, the virus gets cleared spontaneously within 12 weeks. Rest progress to chronic disease
- **Chronic disease:** About 75–85% of cases develop the chronic disease; which subsequently progresses into either—(i) chronic hepatitis, (ii) cirrhosis, or (iii) hepatocellular carcinoma
- **Extrahepatic manifestations:** Due to deposition of circulating immune complexes in extrahepatic sites. Various manifestations can set in such as:
  - Mixed cryoglobulinemia
  - Glomerulonephritis
  - Arthritis and joint pain.

Epidemiology

Hepatitis C virus infection occurs worldwide.
- Higher population prevalence rates have been documented in Africa (up to 10%) followed by South America and Asia
- In India, the prevalence of HCV is about 1%.

Laboratory Diagnosis

The diagnostic modalities available for HCV infections are as follows:
- **HCV antibody detection assay:** ELISA is the most common platform used; followed by rapid test and chemiluminescence (CLIA) formats
  - *Third generation ELISA:* This has been the standard method for HCV serology. It employs antigens from the NS5 region in addition to core, NS3, and NS4 regions
  - *Advantages* include: (i) increased sensitivity and specificity (>99%), (ii) becomes positive within 5 weeks of infection
  - *Disadvantages*: These assays detect IgG antibodies to HCV, hence, they do not discriminate between active or past infection; for which HCV RNA test is required.
- **HCV core antigen assay:** Automated quantitative test detecting core antigen has been available recently
  - This test is less expensive and less time consuming than HCV RNA PCR

- *Advantages:* Used for (i) diagnosis of active/ current infection, (ii) monitoring response to treatment
- *Disadvantage:* Less sensitive than RT-PCR; hence not recommended for blood screening purposes.
- **Real-time RT-PCR** detecting HCV RNA has been the gold standard method. It is useful for:
  - Confirmation of active infection: HCV RNA can be detected in blood as early as 2–3 weeks after infection
  - Quantification of HCV RNA, which helps in monitoring the response to treatment
  - For determining HCV genotype and subtype.

TREATMENT — Hepatitis C

Treatment of HCV infection aims to achieve a sustainable viral response (i.e. undetectable HCV RNA in the blood). This is achieved by the use of the agents, as given below.
- **Interferon alfa plus ribavirin:** Earlier, pegylated-interferon (PEG-IFN) alpha plus ribavirin (RBV) was used for the treatment of HCV infection. But this was associated with high adverse effects.
- **Direct-acting antiviral agents** (DAAs): They are now the treatment of choice for HCV infection. **Three classes of DAAs** are available:
  - NS3/4A (proteases) inhibitors: e.g. grazoprevir
  - NS5B (polymerases) inhibitors: e.g. sofosbuvir
  - NS5A inhibitors: e.g. daclatasvir
- **Combination therapy:** Currently, the treatment regimen for HCV includes combinations of different DAAs with or without PEG-IFN and ribavirin. The regimens are genotype-specific, given for a duration of 12 or 24 weeks.

HEPATITIS D

Hepatitis D virus (HDV) is a defective virus; cannot replicate by itself; depends on the hepatitis B virus for its survival, which forms the envelope (HBsAg) of HDV. The association of HDV with HBV is of two types.
- **Co-infection:** It occurs when a person is exposed simultaneously to both HDV and HBV
- **Super-infection:** It occurs when a chronic carrier of HBV is exposed to serum-containing HDV. It has a higher risk of development of complications such as fulminant disease, chronic hepatitis, and cirrhosis
- **Epidemiology:** Hepatitis D virus infection occurs worldwide, but the prevalence varies greatly. Surprisingly, HDV is not prevalent in Southeast Asia including India; where HBV carriers are maximum
- **Laboratory diagnosis:** Both co-infection and super-infection have a rise of IgM-HDV and HBsAg, but can be differentiated by anti-HBc
  - In co-infection, HBV usually occurs as an acute infection (positive for IgM anti-HBc), whereas
  - In super-infection, HBV is present as a chronic infection (positive for IgG anti-HBc).

TREATMENT — Hepatitis D

Patients with HDV infection can be treated with IFN-α. Treatment for HBV should be continued as described earlier.

HEPATITIS E

Hepatitis E virus (HEV) causes an enterically transmitted (feco-oral mode) hepatitis primarily affects young adults and can cause epidemics in developing countries.

Clinical Manifestations

The incubation period is about 14–60 days.
- **Acute hepatitis:** Most of the patients present as self-limiting acute hepatitis lasting for several weeks followed by complete recovery
- **Fulminant hepatitis** may occur in 1–2% of cases; except for the **pregnant women** where the risk is higher (20%)
- There is no chronic infection or carrier state.

Epidemiology

Hepatitis E virus is a zoonotic pathogen affecting various animals such as monkeys, cats, pigs and dogs.

- **Transmission:** It is fecal-orally transmitted via sewage contamination of drinking water or food
- **Epidemics** of HEV infections have been reported primarily from Asia, Africa and Central America; HEV is the most common cause of acute hepatitis in this zone
- **In India,** HEV infection accounts for maximum (30–60%) cases of sporadic acute hepatitis and epidemic hepatitis.

Laboratory Diagnosis

The diagnostic modalities available for HEV infections are as follows:
- **HEV RNA** (by reverse transcriptase PCR) and **HEV virions** (by electron microscopy) can be detected in stool and serum even before the onset of clinical illness
- **Serum antibody** detection by ELISA:
  - **IgM anti-HEV** appears in serum simultaneously with the increased levels of liver enzymes; indicates acute infection
  - **IgG anti-HEV** replaces IgM in 2 to 4 weeks (once the symptoms resolve) and persists for years; indicates recovery or past infection.

TREATMENT — Hepatitis E

There is no specific antiviral drug available.

EXPECTED QUESTIONS

I. **Write an essay on:**
1. Clinical manifestations, and laboratory diagnosis of HBV infection.

II. **Write short notes on:**
1. Prevention of HBV infection.
2. Hepatitis A virus infection.
3. Hepatitis C virus infection.
4. Hepatitis D virus infection.
5. Hepatitis E virus infection.

III. **Multiple Choice Questions (MCQs):**
1. Which is transmitted by feco-oral mode?
   a. HBV
   b. HCV
   c. HDV
   d. HEV
2. Which is a defective virus?
   a. HBV
   b. HCV
   c. HDV
   d. HEV
3. Which is a DNA virus?
   a. HBV
   b. HCV
   c. HDV
   d. HEV
4. Which hepatitis virus has the maximum risk of chronicity?
   a. HBV
   b. HCV
   c. HDV
   d. HEV

Answers
1. d 2. c 3. a 4. b

CHAPTER 26

Miscellaneous RNA Virus Infections

CHAPTER PREVIEW

- Viral Gastroenteritis
- Ebola
- Rodent-Borne Viral Infections
- Oncogenic Viruses
- Slow Virus Infection

VIRAL GASTROENTERITIS

Viral etiology accounts for the majority of the acute infectious gastroenteritis worldwide **(Table 26.1)**.

- ❖ Viral gastroenteritis most commonly occurs among children. However, persons of all ages can be affected
- ❖ Several enteric viruses can cause acute gastroenteritis in humans, the most common being rotavirus.

Rotavirus Diarrhea

Rotaviruses are the most common cause of diarrheal illness in children.

- ❖ It has a segmented double-stranded RNA, surrounded by a triple-layered, wheel-shaped capsid
- ❖ It is typed into several serotypes and genotypes
- ❖ The **most common type** seen in the world as well as in India is **G1P[8]** type, which accounts for nearly 70% of total isolates.

Pathogenesis and Clinical Manifestations

Rotaviruses are transmitted by fecal–oral route, then they progress further to destroy enterocytes of the small intestine.

- ❖ They multiply in the cytoplasm of enterocytes and damage their transport mechanisms resulting in secretory diarrhea

Table 26.1: Viruses causing gastroenteritis.

Virus	Gastroenteritis features
Rotavirus*	**Group A:** Most common cause of severe endemic diarrheal illness in children worldwide **Group B:** Causes outbreaks of diarrhea in adults in China
Norwalk virus	Causes outbreaks of vomiting and diarrheal illness in all ages (especially in older children and adults)
Sapovirus Astrovirus	Causes sporadic cases and occasional outbreaks of diarrheal illness in infants, young children, and in elderly
Adenovirus* (type 40 and 41)	Second most common viral agent of endemic diarrheal illness of infants and young children worldwide

*Clinical severity is maximum.

- ❖ The incubation period is about 1–3 days. It has an abrupt onset, characterized by vomiting followed by watery diarrhea, fever, and abdominal pain
- ❖ Recovery usually occurs in the majority, but a few children may suffer from severe loss of electrolytes and fluids leading to dehydration.

Laboratory Diagnosis

Feces collected early in the illness is the most ideal specimen.

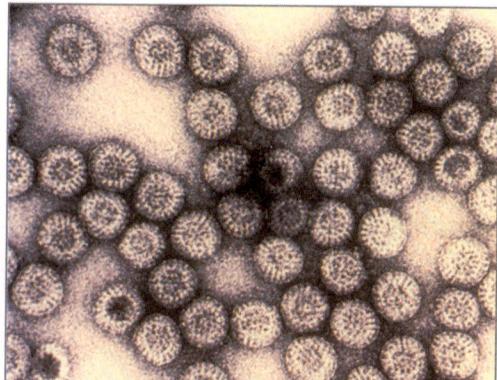

Fig. 26.1: Rotavirus (electron micrograph).
Source: Public Health Image Library, /ID# 15194/Dr Erskine L Palmer/Centers for Disease Control and Prevention (CDC), Atlanta (*with permission*).

- **Direct detection of virus:** Rotaviruses can be demonstrated in stool by **electron microscopy**. They have a sharp edged triple shelled capsid; look like the spokes grouped around the hub of a wheel **(Fig. 26.1)**
- **Isolation** of rotavirus is difficult. Rolling of tissue cultures may be attempted to enhance replication
- **Detection of viral antigen** in stool by ELISA and latex agglutination-based methods
- **RT-PCR** is the most sensitive detection method for detection of rotavirus from stool
- **Serologic tests** (ELISA) can be used to detect the rise of antibody titer. This may be useful for seroprevalence purposes.

TREATMENT	Viral gastroenteritis
Treatment is mainly supportive. Correct the loss of water and electrolytes such as oral or parenteral fluid replacement.	

Vaccine

Two brands of vaccine are available: Rotavac and Rotarix.

Rotavac is introduced under the National Immunization Schedule of India (2022), in selected states

- Three doses (5 drops/dose)
- Administered orally at 6, 10, and 14 weeks along with DPT and OPV.

General Preventive Measures

It includes—(1) measures to improve hygiene and sanitation in the community, and (2) contact precautions such as strict hand hygiene to prevent transmission from infected persons (Chapter 38).

EBOLA VIRUS DISEASE

Ebola and Marburg are filoviruses, known to cause hemorrhagic fever with high mortality. They have been reported from various countries in Western Africa.

The Ebola virus has become a global threat because of its explosive outbreak in 2014 in West Africa. It is named after the **Ebola River**, Africa.

- **Geographical distribution:** Most of the current Ebola outbreaks are largely seen in the Democratic Republic of the Congo and other African countries
    - *West African Epidemic (2014-16):* The largest outbreak occurred in 2014-16; reporting 28,616 cases with 11,310 deaths (40% mortality). Three primary countries affected were—Guinea, Liberia, and Sierra Leon
    - *India:* There is no confirmed case documented yet.
- **Transmission:** Ebola virus spreads among people via direct contact with blood, secretions of infected people, or indirect contact with infected surfaces and materials
- **Reservoir hosts:** Fruit bats or primates (apes and monkeys) are considered as the reservoir host
- **Risk group:** Health-care workers and close contacts/family members of infected individuals are at greater risk of contracting the infection
- **Clinical manifestations:** The incubation period is about 2–12 days. It mainly presents as hemorrhagic fever. The mortality rate is very high (50–90%)
- **Laboratory diagnosis:** Ebola virus disease is diagnosed by various modalities such as:
    - *Serum antibody detection* by ELISA: Detects both IgM and IgG separately by

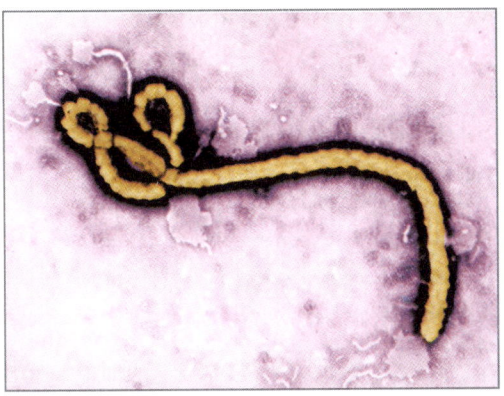

Fig. 26.2: Ebola virus, filamentous shaped (Electron micrograph).

Source: ID# 10815, Public Health Image Library, /Centers for Disease Control and Prevention (CDC), Atlanta (*with permission*).

   using recombinant nucleoprotein (NP) and glycoprotein (GP) antigens
  - *Serum antigen* is detected by capture ELISA. The target proteins are NP, VP40, and GP
  - *Molecular methods* such as RT-PCR and real-time RT-PCR assays are useful to detect specific RNA such as NP and GP gene
  - *Electron microscopy* of the specimen shows typical filamentous viruses (**Fig. 26.2**).
- **Treatment:** Supportive care such as rehydration and symptomatic treatment improves survival. No proven treatment or vaccine is available yet
- **Prevention:** Practice proper infection control and sterilization measures such as strict hand hygiene and personal protective equipment (PPE such as coverall and N95 respirator)
  - Isolate the patients with Ebola from other patients
  - If traveling to an Ebola outbreak area, should be monitored for 21 days after returning.

RODENT-BORNE VIRAL INFECTIONS

Rodent-borne viruses or roboviruses are transmitted from rodents to man by contact with infected body fluids or excretions. Major rodent-borne viruses include:

- **Hantaviruses:** They cause hemorrhagic fever with renal syndrome (HFRS) and hantavirus pulmonary syndrome (HPS)
- **Arenaviruses**: They are a group of segmented RNA viruses, divided into:
  - New world viruses (e.g. Junin, Machupo): They cause South American hemorrhagic fever
  - Old world viruses: e.g. Lassa viruses—cause hemorrhagic fever in Africa.

ONCOGENIC VIRUSES

Viruses account for 15% of all human malignancies. There are several oncogenic viruses found worldwide, which include the agents of two major vaccine-preventable malignancies—human papillomavirus causing carcinoma cervix and hepatitis B virus causing liver cancer (**Table 26.2**).

Table 26.2: Human oncogenic viruses and associated malignancies.

Virus Family	Human cancer
DNA oncogenic viruses	
Human papillomaviruses	• Cervical carcinoma • Other genital tract carcinomas: anal, vulval/vaginal, penile • Esophageal carcinoma • Laryngeal carcinoma • Oropharyngeal carcinoma
Epstein-Barr virus	• Burkitt's lymphoma • Hodgkin's disease • Nasopharyngeal carcinoma • B cell lymphoma
Human herpesvirus-8	• Kaposi's sarcoma • Castleman's disease • Primary effusion lymphoma
Hepatitis B virus	Hepatocellular carcinoma
RNA oncogenic viruses	
HTLV-I	Adult T cell leukemia/lymphoma
HIV	AIDS-related malignancies
Hepatitis C virus	Hepatocellular carcinoma

Abbreviation: HTLV, human T cell lymphotropic virus.

SLOW VIRUS INFECTIONS

Slow virus diseases and prion diseases are a group of neurodegenerative conditions affecting both humans and animals and characterized by:
* **The long incubation period**, ranging from months to years
* Predilection for CNS
* Invariably fatal
* Strong **genetic** predisposition
* **They lack antigenicity**; hence, there is a lack of immune response against viral proteins and a lack of associated inflammation
* Does not produce a cytopathic effect in vitro.

Slow Virus Disease

Slow virus diseases are caused by a number of conventional viruses **(Table 26.3)**. They produce a chronic form of encephalitis/encephalopathy—described as chronic, progressive demyelinating disease of the CNS.

Prion Disease

Prions are infectious protein particles that lack any nucleic acid. They are filterable like viruses; but are resistant to a wide range of chemical and physical agents of sterilization.
* **Examples:** There are several prion diseases of humans and animals; *Scrapie* being the prototype **(Table 26.3)**

Table 26.3: Slow virus and prion diseases.

Slow virus disease	Hosts
Progressive multifocal leukoencephalopathy (JC virus)	Human
Subacute sclerosing panencephalitis (Measles)	Human
Progressive rubella panencephalitis	Human
Visna virus encephalitis	Sheep
Maedi virus* progressive pneumonia	Sheep
Prion disease	**Hosts**
Kuru	Humans, monkeys chimpanzees
Creutzfeldt-Jakob disease	
Scrapie	Sheep, goats
Bovine spongiform encephalopathy	Cattle
Transmissible mink encephalopathy	Mink
Chronic wasting disease	Mule deer, elk

Abbreviation: JC, John Cunningham.
*Does not produce CNS disease, causes progressive pneumonia.

* **Mechanism of prion diseases:** Following infection, the infectious protein particles are carried to the brain, and induce misfolding of normal cellular prion proteins (**PrP^C**) to form its disease-causing isoform (**PrP^{Sc}**)
* **Human prion diseases:** The various human prion diseases are as follows: Kuru and Creutzfeldt-Jakob disease (CJD), etc.

EXPECTED QUESTIONS

I. Write short notes on:
1. Viral gastroenteritis.
2. Ebola virus disease.
3. Malignancies produced by oncogenic viruses.

II. Multiple Choice Questions (MCQs):
1. **The most common viral cause of gastroenteritis:**
   a. Rotavirus
   b. Norwalk virus
   c. Adenovirus 40,41
   d. Hepadnavirus

2. **Carcinoma cervix is caused by___?**
   a. Herpes simplex virus
   b. Human papillomavirus
   c. Enterovirus
   d. Parvovirus

3. **Viral gastroenteritis in adults is caused by __?**
   a. Rotavirus
   b. Norwalk virus
   c. Adenovirus 40,41
   d. Hepadnavirus

Answers
1 a   2. b   3. b

SECTION 5: Parasitic Infections

SECTION OUTLINE

27. Amoebae, *Giardia* and *Trichomonas* Infections
28. Hemoflagellates: *Leishmania* and *Trypanosoma*
29. *Plasmodium* (Malaria Parasite)
30. Opportunistic Coccidian Parasites and Others
31. Cestode Infections
32. Trematode Infections
33. Intestinal Nematode Infections
34. Tissue Nematode Infections

Prevention of Diarrhoeal Disease

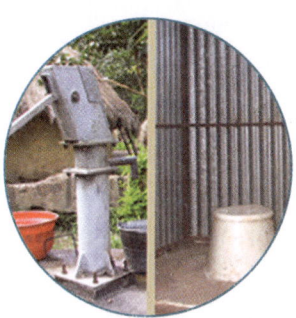

Safe water/ Adequate sanitation
Treat water before use and dispose of waste safety

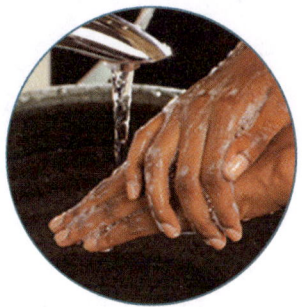

Improved hygiene
Wash hands when appropriate

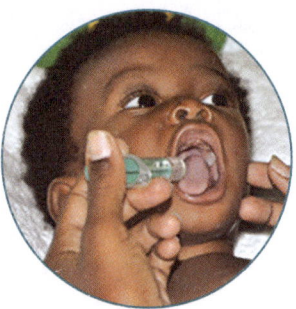

Routine vaccination
Provide rotavirus vaccine

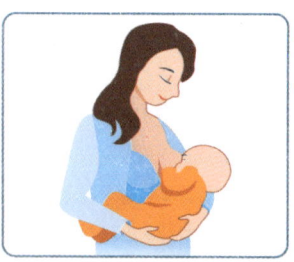

Exclusive breastfeeding for the first six months

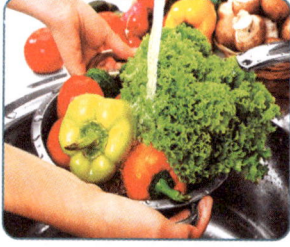

Good personal and food hygiene

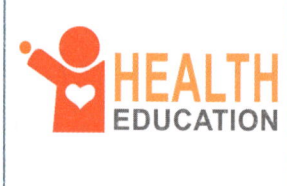

About how infections spread

Material is adapted from WHO

Chapter 27: Amoeba, Giardia and Trichomonas Infections

CHAPTER PREVIEW

- Entamoeba histolytica
- Free-living amoebae
- Giardia duodenalis
- Trichomonas vaginalis

AMOEBAE

Amoebae are classified into two groups. Based on the habitat they are of two types:

1. **Intestinal amoebae:** They reside in the human intestine. *Entamoeba histolytica* is the most important pathogenic intestinal amoeba. Most other species of *Entamoeba* are harmless commensals in the human intestine; e.g. *Entamoeba coli*
2. **Free-living amoebae:** They are small, freely living, and widely distributed in soil and water. They can cause opportunistic infections in humans, affecting the central nervous system. Important human pathogenic free-living amoebae are *Naegleria*, *Acanthamoeba*, and *Balamuthia*.

ENTAMOEBA HISTOLYTICA

Entamoeba histolytica causes amoebic dysentery and also extraintestinal amoebiasis affecting the liver (amoebic liver abscess). It is worldwide in distribution but more common in tropical and subtropical countries.

Morphology

E. histolytica exists in three morphological forms:

1. **Trophozoite:** It is the invasive form as well as the feeding and replicating form of the parasite found in the feces of patients with active disease
2. **Precyst:** It is the intermediate stage between trophozoite and cyst
3. **Cyst:** It is the diagnostic form of the parasite found in the feces of carriers as well as patients with active disease. It exists as immature forms (uni- and bi-nucleated) and mature cyst (quadrinucleated). Mature cysts are the infective form.

Life Cycle (Fig. 27.1)

Host: *E. histolytica* completes its life cycle in a single host, i.e. man.

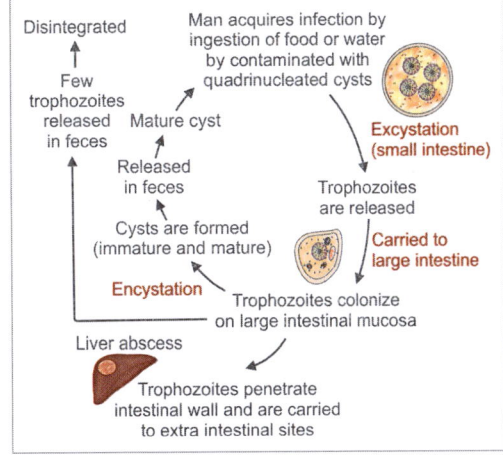

Fig. 27.1: Life cycle of *Entamoeba histolytica*.

Infective form: Mature quadrinucleated cyst is the infective form.

Mode of transmission: *E. histolytica* is transmitted by mainly by **feco-oral route** by ingestion of food or water contaminated with mature quadrinucleated cysts, which contaminate the food and water.

Development in Human Intestine

- **Small intestine:** Cysts bypass gastric juice and reach the small intestine, where they undergo **excystation**. The cyst wall gets lysed to release the trophozoites
- **Large intestine:** Trophozoites are carried to the large intestine, where they multiply actively, and then colonize on the intestinal mucosa
- After colonization, trophozoites show different courses depending on host susceptibility
    - **Asymptomatic cyst passers:** In the majority of individuals, trophozoites do not cause any lesion, transform into cysts, and are excreted in feces
    - **Amoebic dysentery:** In some individuals, trophozoites adhere to intestinal mucosa producing intestinal ulcers and dysentery
    - **Invasive amoebiasis**: Very rarely, trophozoites invade the intestinal mucosa, gain access to the portal veins and migrate to extraintestinal sites, the most common site being the liver where they cause an amoebic liver abscess.
- **Encystation:** The trophozoites transform into precysts then into cysts (immature and mature), which are then liberated in feces. Encystation occurs only in the large intestine
- **Cysts** released in feces can survive in the environment and become **infective form**. Trophozoites are also excreted but get disintegrated either in the environment or by gastric juice when ingested.

Pathogenesis

The pathogenesis of intestinal amoebiasis occurs through the following steps.

- **Colonization:** Trophozoites first colonize the large intestinal mucosa
- **Adhesion:** Then the trophozoites adhere to the large intestinal mucosa by amoebic lectin antigen
- **Flask-shaped ulcers:** Trophozoites produce characteristic flask-shaped ulcerative lesions in the large intestine
- **Invasion:** Amoebae then invade the large intestinal wall; migrate to extraintestinal sites (the most common site being liver). The invasion is facilitated by cysteine proteases and hydrolytic enzymes
- **Liver abscess:** The amoebic trophozoites occlude the hepatic venules; which leads to anoxic necrosis of the hepatocytes. Inflammatory response surrounding the hepatocytes leads to the formation of an abscess
- A liver abscess has a **thick wall** (made up of hepatocytes invaded with amoebic trophozoites) and thick chocolate brown colored pus called **anchovy sauce pus.**

Clinical Manifestations

Intestinal Amoebiasis

The incubation period varies from one to four weeks. The majority of infections (90%) result in asymptomatic cyst passers. The remaining (10%), develop intestinal amoebiasis; characterized by:

- **Amoebic dysentery:** Symptoms include bloody diarrhea (up to 10 times per day) with mucus and pus cells, colicky abdominal pain, and fever
- **Intestinal complications:** Rarely patients develop complications such as amoebic appendicitis, amoeboma (a palpable abdominal mass), and fulminant colitis.

Amoebic Liver Abscess (ALA)

About 2–8% of patients with intestinal amoebiasis develop extraintestinal amoebiasis.

- The liver is the most common site; followed by lungs, brain, genitourinary tract, and spleen
- **The most common hepatic site** affected is the posterior-superior surface of the right lobe of the liver

- **Presentation:** ALA presents with tender hepatomegaly and fever along with weight loss, sweating and weakness, very rarely jaundice, and cough
- **Complications:** Abscess may grow in various directions of the liver discharging the contents into the neighboring organs—leading to a subphrenic abscess, peritonitis, pericarditis, etc. Hematogenous spread can occur from the liver affecting brain, lungs, spleen and genitourinary organs, etc.

Laboratory Diagnosis of Intestinal Amoebiasis

The stool is the specimen of choice. A minimum of three stool samples should be collected on an alternate day (within 10 days) as amoebae are shed intermittently.

Stool Macroscopy

The amoebic stool is foul-smelling, copious in amount, dark red in color mixed with blood and mucus, and is not adherent to the container. It should be differentiated from bacillary dysentery, where the stool is bright red, odorless, and adherent to the container.

Stool Microscopy

Direct examination of stool by saline and iodine mount is performed to demonstrate trophozoites and cysts (see highlight box below).
- **Stool concentration:** The sensitivity can further be improved by examining the stool samples after concentration by the formalin ether sedimentation method
- **Permanent staining:** Stool can also be examined by staining with permanent stains like trichrome stain.

> **Trophozoites**
> Demonstration of trophozoite in stool is considered as the gold standard microscopic test for active infection (**Figs. 27.2A and 27.3A**). They are not found in the stool of asymptomatic carriers.
> - **Measures** 15–20 µm, has cytoplasm and single nucleus
>
> *Contd...*

Contd...
- **Motility:** They are actively motile, with finger-like pseudopodia
- **Ingested RBCs** in the cytoplasm may be found, which is a feature of *E. histolytica* (being invasive)
- **Nucleus:** It has a central karyosome and fine peripheral chromatin granules lining the nuclear membrane.
- Trophozoites are better appreciated in saline mount than in iodine mount as iodine kills the trophozoites and motility cannot be appreciated.

> **Quadrinucleated cysts**
> Cysts are found in stool specimens of both patients (with active infection) and carriers.
> - The internal structure of cysts is clearly appreciated by iodine mount than saline mount.
> - Cysts appear round, 12–15 µm in size containing 1–4 nuclei (**Figs. 27.2B and 27.3B**).
> - Both mature cysts (contain 4 nuclei) and immature cysts (contain 1 or 2 nuclei) are found in stool.

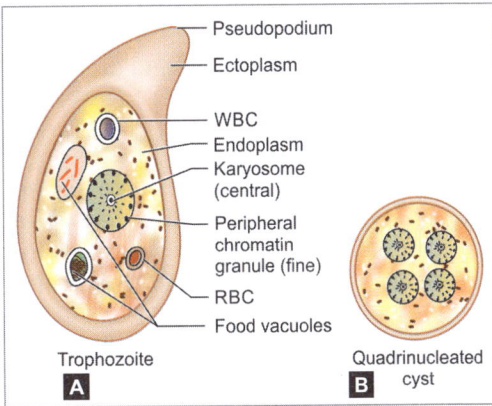

Figs. 27.2A and B: *Entamoeba histolytica* (schematic diagram): **A.** Trophozoite; **B.** Cyst.

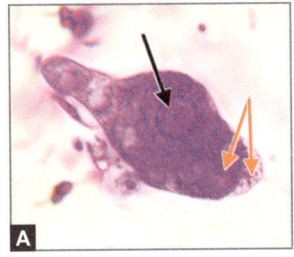
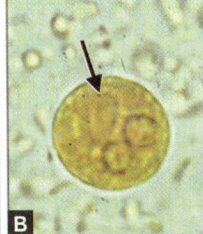

Figs. 27.3A and B: *Entamoeba histolytica*: **A.** Trophozoite (Trichrome stain); **B.** Cyst (Iodine mount).

Source: Swierczynski G, Milanesi B. Atlas of human intestinal protozoa microscopic diagnosis (*with permission*).

Histology

Trophozoites can be detected in sigmoidoscopy-guided biopsies collected from the colonic mucosa and stained with Periodic acid–Schiff (PAS) or H&E stains.

Stool Antigen Detection (Coproantigen)

Various tests used to detect antigens in stool are:
- **ELISA** detecting lectin antigen of *E. histolytica* in stool specimen
- **Immunochromatographic test (ICT):** It is a rapid diagnostic test that simultaneously detects three parasitic antigens in stool—*Giardia lamblia*, *E. histolytica/E. dispar*, and *Cryptosporidium parvum* (e.g. Triage Parasite Panel).

Serology

Amoebic Antigen

ELISA is available detecting lectin antigen of *E. histolytica* in serum. It is found only in patients with active infection and disappears after clinical cure.

Amoebic Antibody

ELISA is available detecting serum antibodies (IgG) against lectin antigen. Antibodies appear only in the later stages of intestinal amoebiasis and therefore are not much useful in diagnosis.

Molecular Diagnosis

Molecular methods have emerged as the gold standard test for the diagnosis of amoebiasis.
- **Nested multiplex PCR** is available targeting small-subunit rRNA genes. It can differentiate *E. histolytica* and *E. dispar* with good sensitivity and specificity
- **Real-time PCR** targeting the 18S rRNA gene can be used as an alternative to conventional PCR. It is more sensitive, can quantitate the parasite load, and takes less time than conventional PCR.

Other Nonspecific Findings

- **Imaging method:** Colonoscopy can be performed to detect flask-shaped amoebic ulcers
- **Charcot-Leyden crystals** in stool: They are diamond-shaped, eosinophilic breakdown products found in the stool in some cases
- **Moderate leukocytosis** in blood.

Laboratory Diagnosis of Amoebic Liver Abscess (ALA)

Laboratory diagnosis of ALA comprises of the following modalities.
- **Microscopy of liver pus:** It can detect trophozoites, but its sensitivity is very poor (<25%). Trophozoites may be found only in the last portion of the aspirated material from the abscess wall
- **Antigen detection** (in serum, liver pus, and saliva): ELISA can be performed to detect lectin antigen
- **Antibody detection:** ELISA can be performed to detect antibody to lectin antigen, It is much more useful in extraintestinal than intestinal amoebiasis.
- **Molecular diagnosis:** Nested multiplex PCR and real-time PCR can be performed on amebic liver pus detecting 18S rRNA
- **Radiologic examination** such as ultrasonography or CT scan or MRI can detect the site of the abscess and its extension.

> **TREATMENT** — Amoebiasis
>
> **Asymptomatic carriage:** Treatment helps in reducing the passage of cysts in stool and thereby preventing disease transmission. Luminal agents are used for treatment.
> - Iodoquinol (for 20 days) or
> - Paromomycin (for 10 days)
>
> **Amoebic dysentery or liver abscess:** Treatment consists of:
> - *Tissue agents:* Metronidazole (for 5–10 days) or tinidazole (for 3 days) *plus*
> - Luminal agents as above
>
> **Other measures** include fluid and electrolyte replacement and symptomatic treatment.

Nonpathogenic Amoebae

Many nonpathogenic amoebae may be found as harmless commensals in the human intestine.
- *Entamoeba dispar:* It is morphologically (both cyst and trophozoite) similar to that of *E. histolytica*. It can be differentiated

from *E. histolytica* by various methods such as:
- PCR amplifying small subunit rRNA gene
- Detection of lectin antigen in stool
- RBC inside trophozoites.

❖ *Entamoeba coli*: It is the most common nonpathogenic amoeba that colonizes the large intestine.
- It is frequently found in the stool samples of healthy individuals and should be differentiated from that of *E. histolytica*
- The cyst of *Entamoeba coli* is round, larger (15–25 µm), and contains 1–8 nuclei.

FREE-LIVING AMOEBA

They are small, freely living amoebae, widely distributed in soil and water; but can cause opportunistic infections in man.
❖ *Naegleria fowleri*: It affects CNS and causes primary amoebic meningoencephalitis (PAM)
❖ *Acanthamoeba* species: They cause two types of infections:
  1. In HIV individuals, it produces a CNS infection called granulomatous amoebic encephalitis (GAE)
  2. In contact lens users, it can cause corneal ulcers.
❖ *Balamuthia mandrillaris*: It can also cause granulomatous amoebic encephalitis (GAE), similar to that of *Acanthamoeba*.

INTESTINAL AND GENITAL FLAGELLATES

Giardia duodenalis is a protozoan intestinal flagellate, associated with diarrheal manifestations.
Trichomonas vaginalis is a genital flagellate causing sexually transmitted infection (STI), called trichomoniasis.

GIARDIA DUODENALIS

Giardia duodenalis (also known as *G. intestinalis* or *G. lamblia*) is an intestinal flagellate associated with diarrheal manifestations. It exists in two forms—trophozoite and cyst.
❖ **Trophozoite:** It is the pathogenic form of the parasite, found in the feces of patients with active disease. It bears flagella as the organ of locomotion
❖ **Cyst:** It is the diagnostic form of the parasite, found in the feces of carriers as well as patients with active disease. It is also the infective form.

Life Cycle

Man acquires infection by ingestion of food and water contaminated with mature cysts (infective form).
❖ The cysts transform into trophozoites in the duodenum. Trophozoites adhere to the duodenal mucosa, multiply and cause infection. Gradually, the trophozoites transform into cysts
❖ Both trophozoites and cysts are excreted in feces. The cyst can survive in the environment and are infective to man.

Clinical Features

Fatty diarrhea (steatorrhea): This is the typical presentation, that occurs due to the malabsorption of fat.
❖ Diarrhea is often foul-smelling with foul flatus
❖ Other symptoms include abdominal pain, bloating, belching, vomiting, and profound weight loss leading to growth retardation.

Laboratory Diagnosis

Stool microscopy is considered as the gold standard for the diagnosis of giardiasis, which detects cysts and trophozoites.
❖ To increase the chance of detection in the stool:
  - Repeated stool examination should be done
  - Stool concentration techniques are employed
❖ If stool examination is negative, then direct duodenal aspirates (obtained by **enterotest**) are examined for trophozoites
❖ Saline and iodine mount examination is performed first. Permanent stains such

as trichrome stain can be used for better visualization of internal structure.

> **Trophozoite (*Giardia duodenalis*)**
> The presence of trophozoites indicates the active stage of the disease **(Figs. 27.4A and 27.5A)**
> - **Measure** 10–20 μm in length and 5–15 μm in width
> - **Shape:** It is pear-shaped, and has a falling leaf-like **motility**
> - It is bilaterally symmetrical; bears the following structures:
>   ➢ One pair of nuclei
>   ➢ Adhesive or sucking disk (bilobed) at its ventral surface
>   ➢ Four pairs of flagella
>   ➢ Pair of axonemes (intracellular portion of flagella)
>
> **Cyst (*Giardia lamblia*)**
> *Giardia* cyst is oval-shaped, measures 11–14 μm in length and 7–10 μm in width **(Figs. 27.4B and 27.5B)**
> - It contains four nuclei and axonemes
> - Cysts cannot differentiate active disease from carriers, as they are passed in stool in both.

Other diagnostic modalities for diagnosis of giardiasis include:
- **Antigen detection** in the stool (copro-antigen) by ELISA and direct-IF test or rapid ICT (e.g. triage parasite panel)
- **Molecular methods:** Detection of *Giardia*-specific gene in stool by PCR is highly sensitive and specific.

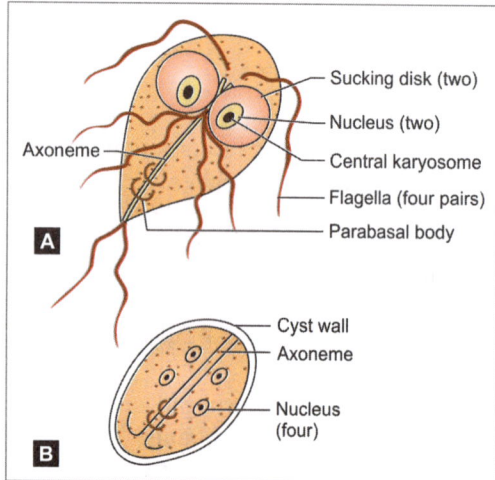

Figs. 27.4A and B: *Giardia duodenalis* (schematic diagram): **A.** Trophozoite; **B.** Cyst.

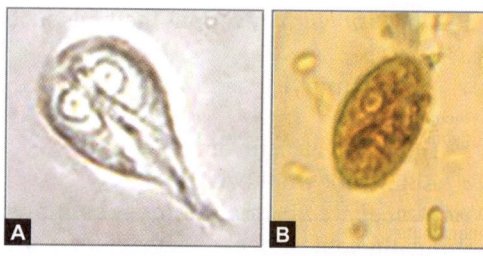

Figs. 27.5A and B: *Giardia duodenalis*: **A.** Trophozoite (saline mount); **B.** Cyst (iodine mount).

> **TREATMENT** — Giardiasis
> - Tinidazole is the drug of choice
> - Metronidazole or nitazoxanide is given alternatively.

TRICHOMONAS VAGINALIS

It is a flagellated protozoan of the genital tract and causes trichomoniasis—the most common parasitic sexually transmitted infection (STI).
- **Life cycle:** It has only trophozoite stage; there is no cyst stage. Trophozoites are the infective form, transmitted by sexual route. They multiply in the genital tract, cause infection, and are discharged in vaginal/urethral secretions
- **Clinical features:** It causes **vulvovaginitis** in females, characterized by thin profuse foul-smelling purulent vaginal discharge
  - Discharge may be frothy (10% of cases)
  - Strawberry appearance of vaginal mucosa (**colpitis macularis**) may be seen in some cases
  - In males, it presents as nongonococcal urethritis.
- **Laboratory diagnosis:** Wet (saline) mount of fresh vaginal discharge can demonstrate the trophozoites (**Fig. 27.6A**) and pus cells. Other methods include permanent stains (e.g. Giemsa, **Fig. 27.6B**), acridine orange stain, and direct-IF.

> Trophozoite is pear-shaped and measures 7–23 μm (**Fig. 27.6A**), and shows characteristic jerky or twitching motility. It bears five flagella—four anterior and one recurrent.

- **Treatment:** Metronidazole or tinidazole is the drug of choice, given to both sexual partners.

CHAPTER 27 ♦ Amoeba, Giardia and Trichomonas Infections

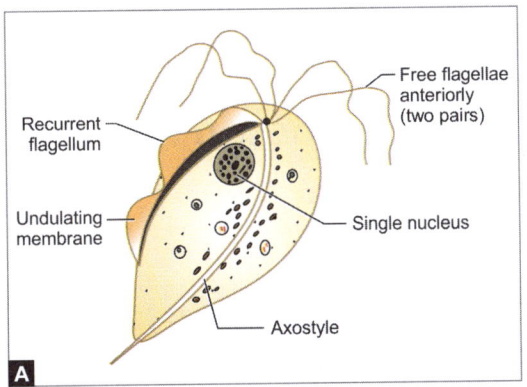
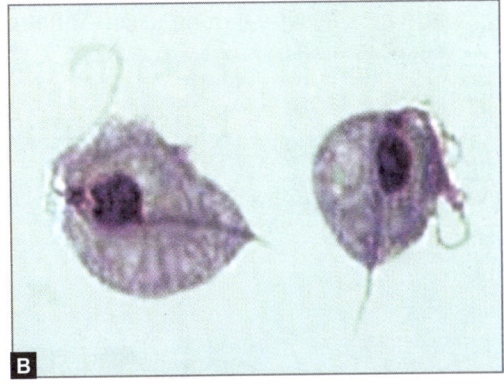

Figs. 27.6A and B: Trophozoite of *Trichomonas vaginalis*: **A.** Schematic diagram; **B.** Giemsa staining.
Source: **B.** DPDx Image Library, Centers for Disease Control and Prevention (CDC), Atlanta (*with permission*).

EXPECTED QUESTIONS

I. **Write an essay on:**
   1. Discuss the clinical manifestations and laboratory diagnosis of intestinal amoebiasis.

II. **Write short notes on:**
   1. Amoebic liver abscess.
   2. Free-living amoeba infections.
   3. Giardiasis.
   4. Trichomoniasis.

III. **Multiple Choice Questions (MCQs):**
   1. **Cyst of *E. histolytica*: All are true, *except*?**
      a. Infective form b. Diagnostic form
      c. Pathogenic form d. 1–4 nuclei
   2. **Trophozoite of *E. histolytica*: All are true, except?**
      a. Pathogenic form
      b. 1–4 nuclei
      c. Finger-like pseudopodia
      d. The saline mount is preferred over iodine
   3. **Primary amoebic meningoencephalitis is caused by __?**
      a. *Naegleria*
      b. *Acanthamoeba*
      c. *Balamuthia*
      d. *E. histolytica*
   4. **Enterotest is done for __?**
      a. *E. histolytica*
      b. *Trichomonas vaginalis*
      c. *Enterobius vermicularis*
      d. *Giardia duodenalis*

Answers
1. c   2. b   3. a   4. d

CHAPTER 28

Hemoflagellates: Leishmania and Trypanosoma

CHAPTER PREVIEW
- Leishmania
- Trypanosoma

Hemoflagellates are the flagellated protozoa that are found in peripheral blood circulation. Examples include *Leishmania* and *Trypanosoma*; both are transmitted by the bite of the insect vector.

LEISHMANIA

Leishmania is a flagellated protozoan that primarily affects the reticuloendothelial system of the host.

- ❖ **Vector:** It is transmitted by the bite of the female sandfly vector
- ❖ **Clinical forms:** Leishmaniasis presents in various clinical forms
  - *Visceral leishmaniasis* (VL) or kala-azar: It affects viscera such as spleen, liver, bone marrow, etc.
  - *PKDL* (post-kala-azar dermal leishmaniasis): It occurs a few months to years following VL
  - *Cutaneous forms:* Occurs in various forms such as cutaneous leishmaniasis (CL), diffuse cutaneous leishmaniasis (DCL), leishmaniasis recidivans (LR), and mucocutaneous leishmaniasis (MCL)
  - *Old and new world:* Depending upon the geographical distribution, leishmaniasis is classified into two groups (see highlight box).

Old World Leishmaniasis
It occurs in Asia, Africa, and less frequently in Europe; transmitted by sandfly of the genus *Phlebotomus*.
- *L. donovani*: causes VL and PKDL
- *L. infantum*: causes VL and PKDL
- *L. tropica* complex: causes CL

New World Leishmaniasis
It occurs in Central and South America; transmitted by sandfly of the genus *Lutzomyia*.
- *L. chagasi*: causes VL and CL
- *L. mexicana* complex: causes CL
- *L. braziliensis* complex: causes MCL and CL

Leishmania donovani

Leishmania donovani causes VL and also PKDL. It exists in two morphological forms (Figs. 28.1A and B):

- ❖ **Amastigote:** It is the diagnostic form, found in man. It does not have a flagellum

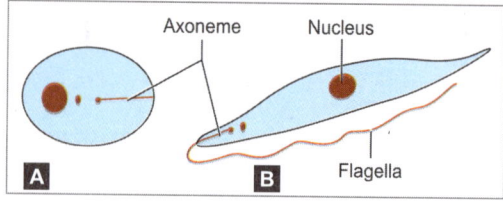

Figs. 28.1A and B: Various morphological forms of *Leishmania* (schematic diagrams): **A.** Amastigote; **B.** Promastigote.

but has only the intracellular portion of the flagellum, called axoneme
- **Promastigote:** It is the infective stage to man, found in the insect vector. It possesses a single flagellum, arises anterior to the nucleus.

Epidemiology of VL

- **World:** VL has mainly been reported from three regions—(i) South-East Asia: India, Bangladesh, and Nepal; (ii) East Africa: Ethiopia, Sudan, and Kenya; (iii) Brazil
- **India:** India is one of the worst affected countries. Maximum cases were reported from Bihar, followed by Jharkhand.

Life Cycle (Fig. 28.2)

L. donovani completes its life cycle in two hosts—(i) man, and (ii) female sandfly (*Phlebotomus argentipes*).
- **Infective form:** Promastigote forms found in the alimentary canal of female sandfly serve as the infective form
- **Mode of transmission:** By the bite of an infected female sandfly, discharging the promastigotes (infective form) into the skin of a man
- **In humans:** Promastigotes are phagocytosed by the skin macrophages, where they transform into amastigote forms
  - The amastigote forms multiply inside the macrophages, causing cell rupture and are released into the circulation
  - Amastigotes are carried out in the circulation to various organs like liver, spleen, and bone marrow and invade the reticuloendothelial cells like macrophages, endothelial cells, etc.
- **In sandfly:** During the blood meal, the amastigotes are ingested and transformed into promastigote forms in the insect gut, which multiply and then migrate to their foregut. The cycle continues when this sandfly bites a new host.

Clinical Features

Visceral leishmaniasis (VL) is also called kala-azar (a Hindi term meaning 'black fever'). The incubation period ranges from 2 to 6 months. VL is characterized by:
- **Fever:** Abrupt in onset, moderate to high grade, associated with chills and rigors
- **Splenomegaly:** It is the most consistent sign. The spleen becomes enlarged and nontender **(Fig. 28.3A)**
- **Hepatomegaly** (nontender)
- **Lymphadenopathy:** Common in most of the African endemic regions (rare in the Indian subcontinent)

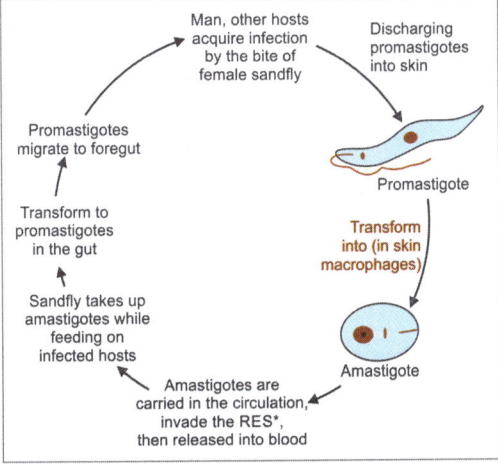

Fig. 28.2: Life cycle of *Leishmania donovani*.
*RES-Reticuloendothelial system.

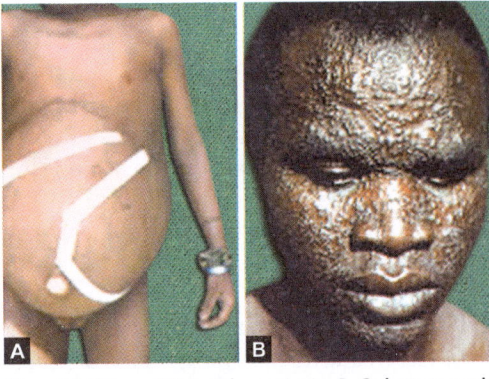

Figs. 28.3A and B: Leishmaniasis: **A.** Splenomegaly seen in visceral leishmaniasis; **B.** Extensive facial nodular lesions in PKDL.

Source: World Health Organization "Manual on visceral leishmaniasis control" Slide1/Desjeux; Slides 4 and 5/ El Hassan; Slide 6/ Bryceson (*with permission*).

- **Hyperpigmentation** is observed on the face, hands, feet, and abdomen; hence the name kala-azar or black fever. This is a characteristic feature of Indian VL
- **Bone marrow dysfunction** leading to pancytopenia and hypergammaglobulinemia
- Nodular skin lesions (in African cases).

Post-kala-azar Dermal Leishmaniasis (PKDL)

PKDL is a nonulcerative lesion of the skin that occurs in 2–50% of patients of VL following treatment with antimonials. It is aggravated by exposure to sunlight.
- Mainly seen in India and East African countries
- It develops as hypopigmented macule near the mouth which spreads to the face, arms and trunk and finally becomes nodules resembling leprosy **(Fig. 28.3B)**.

Laboratory Diagnosis

Diagnosis of VL includes the following modalities.

Microscopy

Demonstration of amastigotes inside the macrophages (also known as **Leishman-Donovan bodies** or **LD bodies**) is the gold standard method for the diagnosis of VL **(Figs. 28.4A and B)**. Smears should be stained with Leishman, Giemsa, or Wright stains. The various samples include:
- Splenic aspiration: Most sensitive specimen, but less preferred because of the risk of splenic puncture
- Bone marrow aspiration: Most common specimen
- Lymph node aspiration: Useful in African patients
- Liver biopsy
- Peripheral blood from buffy coat area (after blood is centrifuged): particularly useful in HIV patients.

Other Diagnostic Modalities

Other modalities for the diagnosis of VL include:
- **Culture:** Using media such as Novy-MacNeal-Nicolle (NNN) medium and Schneider's Drosophila insect medium. Amastigotes transform into **promastigotes** in the culture fluid which are detected by staining with Giemsa stain

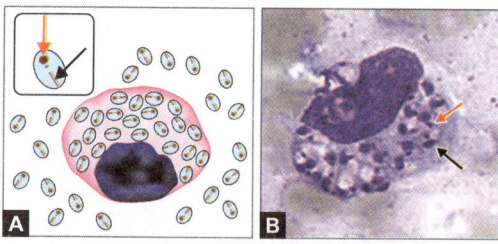

Figs. 28.4A and B: *L. donovani* amastigotes: showing a macrophage containing multiple *Leishmania* amastigotes: **A.** Schematic; **B.** In bone marrow smear stained with Giemsa. Note that each amastigote has a nucleus (red arrow) and a rod-shaped kinetoplast (black arrow).

Source: **B.** DPDx Image Library, Centers for Disease Control and Prevention (CDC), Atlanta (*with permission*).

- **Antibody detection in serum:** Sensitive, but less specific. Methods available are:
  - Direct agglutination test (DAT)
  - Others: ICT, ELISA, and indirect IF test.
- **Antigen detection:** A latex agglutination test has been available. It is more useful (i) in HIV-VL co-infection, (ii) as a prognostic marker, and (iii) in indicating active infection
- **Molecular methods:** Various formats such as PCR, nested PCR, and real-time PCR are available targeting specific kinetoplast (mitochondrial) DNA
- **Leishmanin test (Montenegro test):** It is a skin test to detect delayed hypersensitivity to *L. donovani* antigens
  - It is positive in people with good CMI: Asymptomatic individuals, cutaneous leishmaniasis, after recovery from VL
  - However, this test is negative when CMI is low: Such as in the case of active VL and diffuse CL.

> **TREATMENT** — Visceral leishmaniasis
>
> The various drugs used in the treatment of VL are:
> - **Liposomal amphotericin B:** It is the current drug of choice for leishmaniasis
> - **Pentavalent antimonials:** It has been the drug of choice in the past. However, currently, its use is restricted due to the emergence of resistance.
> - **Others:** Miltefosine and paromomycin.

Prevention of VL

National Vector Borne Disease Control Programme (NVBDCP) is a national program in India that works for the control of six common vector-borne diseases in India. It has launched the **accelerated plan for kala-azar elimination** in 2017.

Cutaneous Leishmaniasis

Leishmania species can produce various cutaneous manifestations—associated with several old world and new world species of *Leishmania*.

Old World Cutaneous Leishmaniasis (CL)

Old world CL is caused by *Leishmania* tropica complex, which in turn comprises of three species—*L. tropica, L. aethiopica,* and *L. major.*
- *L. tropica* causes a type of CL called **oriental sore**, affecting the face and hands. In India, it is seen in Rajasthan. It is transmitted by *Phlebotomus sergenti*
- *L. aethiopica* causes diffuse cutaneous leishmaniasis. It is transmitted by *Phlebotomus longipes.*

New World Cutaneous Leishmaniasis

New World cutaneous leishmaniasis is mainly caused by:
- *Leishmania mexicana* **complex:** They cause a specific form of CL called as **chiclero ulcer**; characterized by persistent ulcerations in pinna
- *Leishmania braziliensis* **complex:** They cause mucocutaneous leishmaniasis (MCL), called **espundia**—ulcerative lesions on the nose and oral cavity
- *Leishmania chagasi:* It causes atypical CL and American VL.

TRYPANOSOMA

Trypanosomes are the hemoflagellates, that cause two distinct types of diseases in man.
1. **Chagas' disease:** It is caused by *Trypanosoma cruzi,* seen in America. It is transmitted by the vector reduviid bug
   - It is characterized by a painful subcutaneous nodule (called chagoma) and unilateral painless edema of the eyelid (called Romana's sign)
   - Subsequently, the parasite multiples in the muscles (cardiac and GIT) producing dilated cardiomyopathy, megaesophagus, and megacolon.
2. **African sleeping sickness:** It is caused by *Trypanosoma brucei* complex; transmitted by the vector tsetse fly. It produces progressive chronic meningoencephalitis with characteristic daytime somnolence (hence called as 'sleeping sickness'), with restlessness and insomnia at night. It occurs in two forms
   i. West African sleeping sickness: It is caused by *T. brucei gambiense*
   ii. East African sleeping sickness: It is caused by *T. brucei rhodesiense.*

Diagnosis of trypanosomiasis involves peripheral blood smear examination, which demonstrates the characteristic trypomastigote form.

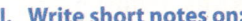

EXPECTED QUESTIONS

I. **Write short notes on:**
   1. Visceral leishmaniasis.
   2. Chagas' disease.

II. **Multiple Choice Questions (MCQs):**
   1. **Oriental sore is caused by___?**
      a. *Leishmania donovani*
      b. *Leishmania mexicana*
      c. *Leishmania major*
      d. *Leishmania tropica*
   2. **African sleeping sickness is caused by___?**
      a. *Leishmania donovani*
      b. *Trypanosoma cruzi*
      c. *Trypanosoma brucei*
      d. *Leishmania tropica*

Answers
1. d   2. c

CHAPTER 29

Plasmodium (Malaria Parasite)

CHAPTER PREVIEW

- Plasmodium
- Babesia

PLASMODIUM (MALARIA PARASITE)

Malaria is a mosquito-borne febrile illness, caused by *Plasmodium*. Four different species usually infect man—*P. vivax, P. falciparum, P. malariae* and *P. ovale*.

Life Cycle (Fig. 29.1)

Host: *Plasmodium* completes its life cycle in two hosts: definitive host—female *Anopheles* mosquito (sexual cycle takes place) and intermediate host—man (asexual cycle takes place).

Transmission to Man and Infective Form

- Man acquires infection by the bite of a female *Anopheles* mosquito, transmitting the infective form—sporozoites present in its salivary gland
- Rarely, it can also be transmitted by blood transfusion or transplacental transmission—here, trophozoites (or merozoites) act as the infective form.

Human Cycle

In humans, the asexual cycle takes place through three stages: (1) pre-erythrocytic schizogony, (2) erythrocytic schizogony, and (3) gametogony.

Pre-erythrocytic schizogony: Sporozoites leave the circulation and infect the liver.

- **Trophozoites:** Inside the hepatocyte, the sporozoites transform into trophozoites
- **Schizonts:** The trophozoites multiply actively and subsequently undergo several nuclear divisions and transform into schizonts
- **Schizogony:** The schizonts undergo schizogony to release merozoites which initiate the erythrocytic cycle
- **Hypnozoites:** Some sporozoites of *P. vivax* and *P. ovale* do not develop further and may remain in the liver as hypnozoites and cause a relapse of malaria after many years.

Erythrocytic schizogony: Hepatic merozoites after entering into the bloodstream, infect the RBCs.

- Inside the RBCs, the hepatic merozoites transform into trophozoites
- The early trophozoites are ring-shaped (called ring forms) multiply actively and subsequently transform into late trophozoites and then into schizonts
- The schizonts undergo schizogony to release merozoites which either infect fresh RBCs to continue the erythrocytic cycle or transform into gametocytes.

Gametogony: When intended to leave the infected person, the merozoites transform into gametocytes.

- Gametocytes are of two types—male and female
- They are the sexual form; and also the infective form to the mosquito.

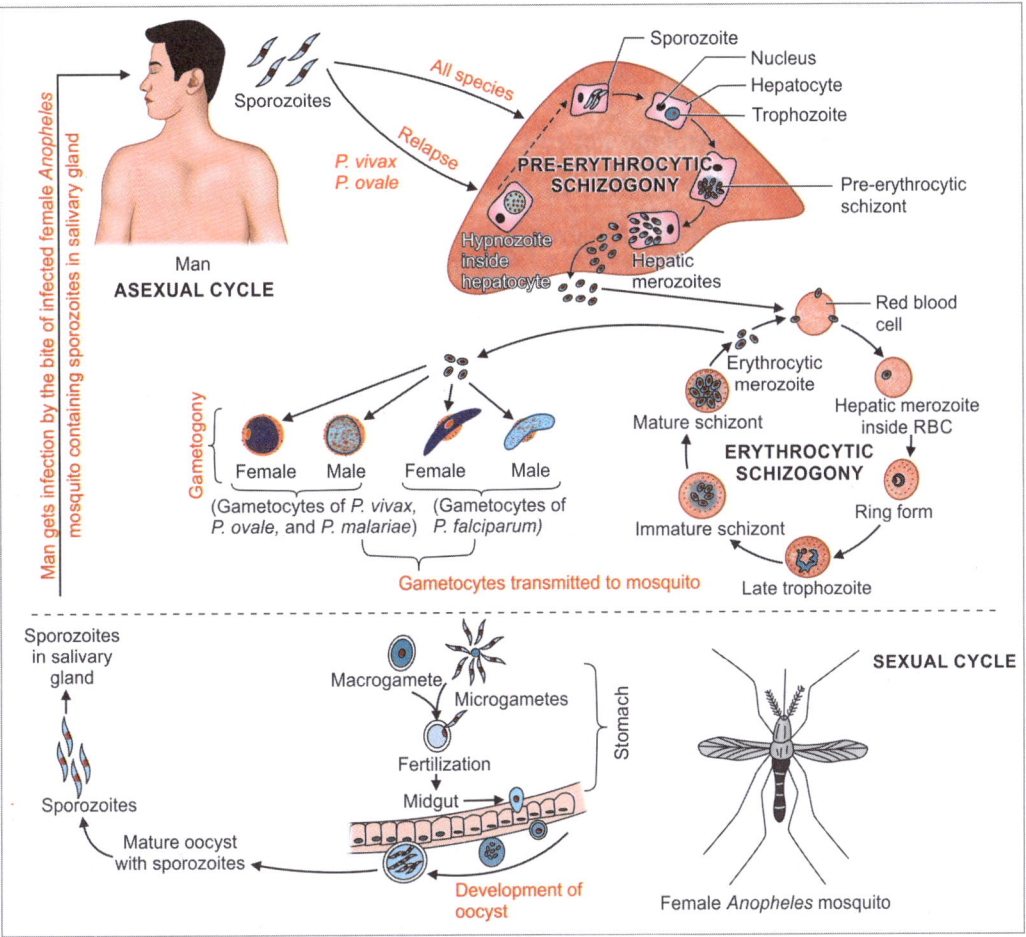

Fig. 29.1: Life cycle of the malaria parasite.

Mosquito Cycle

The gametocytes (male and female) are transmitted to the female *Anopheles* mosquito during the blood meal.

- **Gamete:** Inside the mosquito gut, each male gametocyte undergoes exflagellation and transforms into eight male gametes. Whereas the female gametocyte directly transforms into a single female gamete
- **Fertilization:** The male gamete fertilizes with the female gamete to form a **zygote**, which subsequently transforms into a motile form called **ookinete**
- **Oocyst:** The ookinete penetrates the stomach wall of the mosquito, where it transforms into oocysts
- **Sporogony:** Each oocyst undergoes sporogony to produce four spindle-shaped sporozoites
- **Sporozoites:** On rupture of the mature oocyst, the sporozoites are released and migrate to the salivary gland and the cycle is repeated.

Pathogenesis and Clinical Feature

Benign Malaria

Benign malaria is milder in nature and can be caused by all four species. It is characterized by a triad of febrile paroxysm, anemia, and splenomegaly.

- **Febrile paroxysm:** Fever comes intermittently depending on the species

- It occurs every fourth day (72-hour cycle for *P. malariae*) and every third day (48-hour cycle for other three species)
- Paroxysm corresponds to the release of the successive broods of merozoites into the bloodstream, at the end of the RBC cycle.
❖ **Anemia:** Results from lysis of RBC due to release of merozoites
  - Anemia is severe in most cases of *P. falciparum* as it infects RBCs of all age groups
  - *P. vivax* and *P. ovale* infect the young RBCs and reticulocytes, whereas *P. malariae* infects the old RBCs.
❖ **Splenomegaly** is due to the massive proliferation of macrophages inside the spleen to remove the parasitized RBCs.

Falciparum Malaria (Malignant Tertian Malaria)

The pathogenesis of *P. falciparum* is different from other species.

Sequestration of the Parasites

An important feature of the pathogenesis of *P. falciparum* is its ability to sequester (holding back) the parasites in the blood vessels of deep visceral organs like brain, kidneys, etc. This leads to blockage of vessels, congestion, and hypoxia of internal organs. Sequestration is mediated by:
❖ **Cytoadherence:** It refers to the binding of infected erythrocytes to endothelial cells
❖ It is mediated by a specialized antigen called as *P. falciparum* erythrocyte membrane protein-1 **(PfEMP-1)**, which binds to specific receptors present on the vascular endothelium of deep organs
❖ Since the parasites are sequestrated back in deep vessels, they can avoid frequent spleen passage, and hence can escape splenic clearance.

Complications

Complications of Falciparum Malaria

P. falciparum infection is more acute and severe with more complications than benign malaria.

❖ **Cerebral malaria:** This is the most serious complication seen in falciparum malaria. It results due to the plugging of brain capillaries by the sequestered parasitized RBCs
❖ **Pernicious malaria:** It is characterized by blackwater fever, algid malaria, and septicemic malaria
❖ **Blackwater fever:** This syndrome is characterized by sudden intravascular hemolysis followed by fever, hemoglobinuria, and dark urine
❖ **Algid malaria:** Characterized by cold clammy skin, hypotension, peripheral circulatory failure, and profound shock
❖ **Others:** Pulmonary edema and adult respiratory distress syndrome, hypoglycemia, renal failure, bleeding/disseminated intravascular coagulation, severe jaundice, severe normochromic and normocytic anemia.

Chronic Complications of Malaria

❖ **Tropical splenomegaly syndrome:** It results from an abnormal immunologic response to repeated malaria infections and is characterized by— elevated IgM and massive splenomegaly
❖ **Quartan malarial nephropathy:** It is seen with *P. malariae*, characterized by nephrotic syndrome due to immune complexes mediated injury of renal glomeruli
❖ **Promotes Burkitt's lymphoma:** Malaria-induced severe immunosuppression in African children provokes Epstein-Barr virus infection to develop Burkitt's lymphoma.

Epidemiology of Malaria

Malaria is the most lethal parasitic disease of humans.
❖ ***P. falciparum*** is the most common species worldwide; accounting for 99.7% of malaria cases in Africa, 50% in Southeast Asia including India
❖ In India, **Eastern Indian states** such as Odisha, Chhattisgarh, and Jharkhand account for the maximum cases
❖ **NVBDCP:** The malaria control in India has been operated through the National

Vector-borne Disease Control Programme (NVBDCP)
- The national framework for malaria elimination (NFME) has been in operation in India with the vision of malaria elimination by 2030.

Laboratory Diagnosis

The diagnostic tests for malaria can be divided into:
- **Microscopic test:** Peripheral blood smear, and QBC
- **Non-microscopic tests:** Rapid diagnostic test (antigen detection) and molecular test.

Peripheral Blood Smear

Peripheral smear study still remains the simple and gold standard confirmatory test for detection of malarial parasites.

Types of Peripheral Blood Smear

It is of two types—(1) Thin, and (2) Thick smears. Both the smears are made at the same time from capillary blood either on the same or different slides **(Fig. 29.2)**.
- **For thick smear**, a big drop of blood is spread over 1–2 cm square area on a clean glass slide
- **For thin smear**, a small drop of blood is taken on a corner of a slide. It is spread by another spreader slide at an angle of 45° and then is lowered to an angle of 30° and is pushed gently to the left, till the blood is exhausted

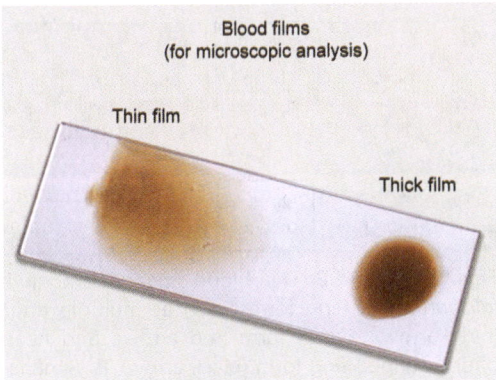

Fig. 29.2: Glass slide showing thin and thick blood smear.

- **Stains:** They are stained with one of the Romanowsky stains such as Leishman's, Giemsa and Field's, Wright's, or JSB (Jaswant Singh and Bhattacharya) stain
- **Examination:** Both the smears are examined under oil immersion objective (100x)
- **Advantages:** Peripheral smear is simple, rapid, and cheap
  - A thick smear is useful in— (1) Detecting the parasites: It is 40 times more sensitive than a thin smear (2) Quantification of parasitemia; (3) Demonstrating the malaria pigments
  - A thin smear is useful in the speciation of malaria parasites (see the highlight box).
- **Disadvantages:** It is labor-intensive and requires an experienced microscopist.

> **Speciation of Malaria Parasites**
>
> The speciation by thin smear is based on the detection of the ring forms, schizonts, gametocytes, type of pigments produced, and RBC size **(Fig. 29.3)**.
> - **Parasitized RBC size:** Differ among species
>   - Normal in size and shape for *P. falciparum* and *P. malariae*
>   - Enlarged in size for *P. vivax*, whereas
>   - Enlarged with fimbriated margin: for *P. ovale*
> - **Ring forms:** It is the most important form that helps in accurate speciation. It comprises of a vacuole in the center, a peripheral thin rim of blue cytoplasm, surrounding the red nucleus.
>   - *P. vivax*: Rings occupies 1/3rd of the RBC size **(Fig. 29.4A)**.
>   - *P. falciparum*: Rings are smaller and occur in three forms **(Fig. 29.5A)**:
>   - Multiple ring forms (inside the same RBC)
>   - Accole form: Ring form attached to RBC membrane
>   - Double dot/headphone shaped ring form: Ring form with a fragmented nucleus
>   - *P. ovale*: Ring forms are similar to that of *P. vivax*, but present inside oval-shaped RBC **(Fig. 29.3)**
>   - *P. malariae*: Early trophozoite is similar to that of *P. vivax*, but late trophozoite is band-shaped (called band forms) **(Fig. 29.3)**.
> - **Schizonts:** Speciation is made based on the number of merozoites present per schizont.

Contd...

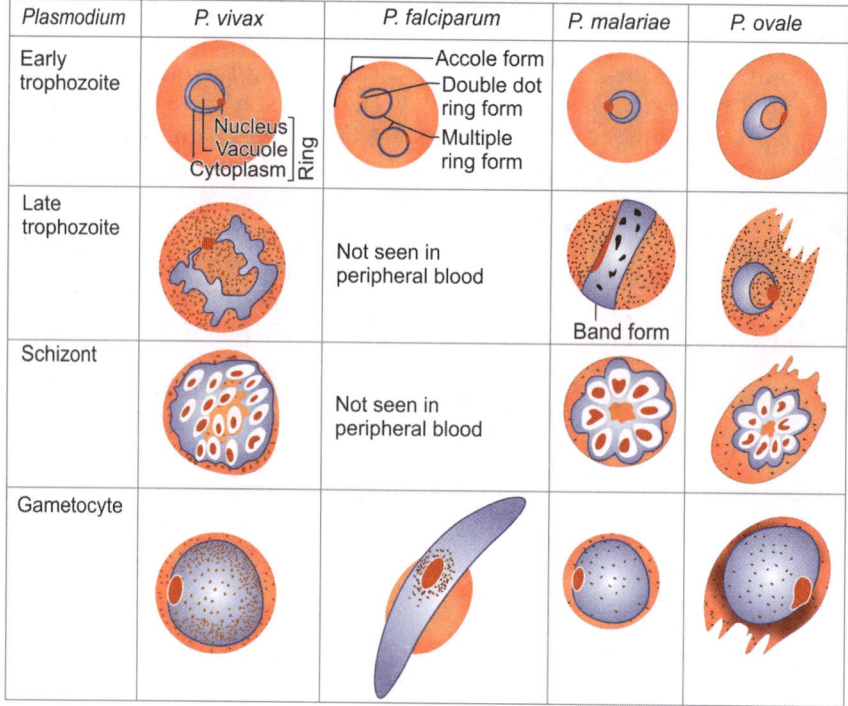

Fig. 29.3: Morphological forms of malaria parasites seen in the peripheral smear.

Contd...

> - Schizonts are not seen in the peripheral smear for *P. falciparum*
> - **Gametocytes:** In *P. falciparum*, the gametocyte is crescentic or banana-shaped and larger than RBCs, whereas, for other species, it is spherical and almost occupies the RBC **(Figs. 29.4B and 29.5B)**.

Quantitative Buffy Coat Examination

The quantitative buffy coat (QBC) is an advanced microscopic technique for malaria diagnosis.

It consists of following basic steps:

- ❖ **Procedure:** Blood is collected in a capillary tube coated internally with acridine orange **(Fig. 29.6A)** and then centrifuged. The capillary tube is then examined at the buffy coat region under an ultraviolet (UV) light source **(Figs. 29.6B and C)**
- ❖ **Interpretation:** Parasitized RBCs appear as brilliant green dots **(Figs. 29.6C)**

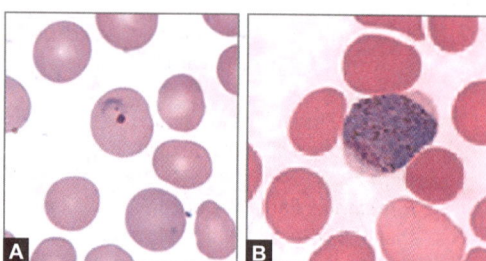

Figs. 29.4A and B: Thin blood smear *Plasmodium vivax*: **A.** Ring form; **B.** Gametocyte.

Source: DPDx Image Library, Centers for Disease Control and Prevention (CDC), Atlanta (*with permission*).

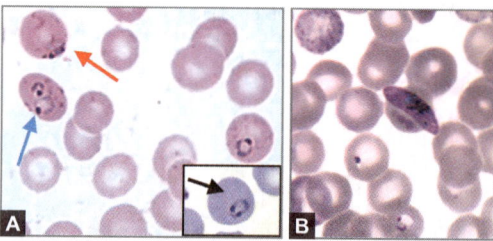

Figs. 29.5A and B: Thin blood smear *Plasmodium falciparum*: **A.** Ring forms such as multiple rings (blue arrow), accole form (red arrow), and head phone-shaped ring form (black arrow); **B.** Banana-shaped gametocyte

Source: DPDx Image Library, Centers for Disease Control and Prevention (CDC), Atlanta (*with permission*).

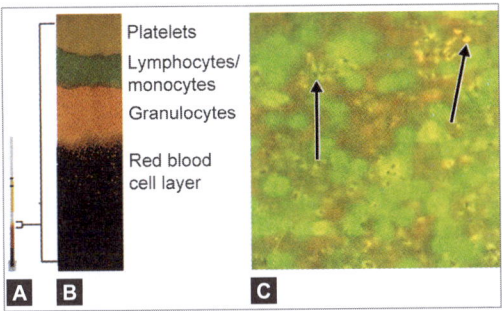

Figs. 29.6A to C: A. QBC capillary tube; **B.** Magnified view of QBC capillary tube after centrifugation; **C.** Crescent-shaped gametocyte of *Plasmodium falciparum*

Source: **C.** Department of Microbiology, Sri Siddhartha Medical College, Tumkur, Karnataka (*with permission*).

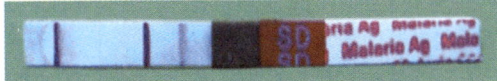

Fig. 29.7: Rapid diagnostic test kit positive for *Plasmodium falciparum*

Source: Department of Microbiology, Sri Siddhartha Medical College, Tumkur, Karnataka (*with permission*).

- ❖ **Advantage:** QBC is faster, more sensitive and quantification is possible
- ❖ **Disadvantage:** It is expensive, less specific and speciation is difficult.

Rapid Diagnostic Tests

Rapid diagnostic tests (RDTs) have revolutionized the diagnosis of malaria.
- ❖ **Principle:** Malaria RDT kits are based on the principle of immunochromatographic test (ICT)
- ❖ **Antigens:** Malaria RDT kits are designed to detect several antigens of *Plasmodium* species such as:
  - Lactate dehydrogenase (LDH) and aldolase: Produced by all *Plasmodium* species
  - Histidine rich protein-2 (HRP-II): It is produced only by *P. falciparum*.
- ❖ **Advantages:** RDTs are simple to perform, and do not need extra equipment or trained microscopist
- ❖ **Disadvantages:** RDTs cannot differentiate between the non-falciparum malaria species.

Molecular Methods

Various molecular tests have recently gained attention for malaria diagnosis.
- ❖ Nested multiplex PCR targeting 18S rDNA has been developed for speciation of malaria parasite
- ❖ PCR can also be used to detect drug-resistant genes
- ❖ Real-time PCR is useful for quantification.

TREATMENT — Malaria

The treatment regimen given for malaria is as per guidelines provided by NVBDCP, India.

Vivax malaria: Chloroquine (for three days) plus primaquine (for 14 days) is the regimen recommended

Falciparum malaria: State-specific regimens are recommended
- **Northeast states:** Artemether-lumefantrine (for 3 days) plus primaquine (single dose) is given
- **Other states:** Artesunate for 3 days plus sulfadoxine-pyrimethamine (single dose, on 1st day) plus primaquine (single dose, on the second day)

Severe malaria: The drug of choice includes IV artemisinin derivatives (such as artesunate, artemether, arteether) or IV quinine

Chloroquine resistance in *P. falciparum* has been reported in India, especially from the northeast states.

Prophylaxis against Malaria

Prophylaxis against malaria includes chemoprophylaxis, vector control strategies, and vaccine prophylaxis.
- ❖ **Chemoprophylaxis:** It is recommended for travelers going to highly endemic areas of malaria. Agents such as doxycycline or mefloquine are recommended
- ❖ **Vector control strategies:** Include spraying with insecticides like malathion, environmental sanitation, and improvement of the drainage system
- ❖ **Vaccination:** RTS, S/AS01 is the only vaccine candidate that has been approved by WHO, for use in children living in regions with moderate to high transmission (e.g. sub-Saharan Africa).

BABESIA

Babesia is another protozoan infecting the bloodstream, similar to the malaria parasite. **Hard tick** is the definitive host.

- **Clinical features** are similar to malaria, except that it is less severe, with no cerebral involvement
- **Diagnosis:** Peripheral blood smear examination reveals ring forms inside RBC arranged in pairs or tetrads (called *Maltese cross forms*)
- **Treatment:** Atovaquone plus azithromycin is given for treatment.

EXPECTED QUESTIONS

I. Write an essay on:
1. Discuss the pathogenesis and laboratory diagnosis of falciparum malaria.

II. Write short notes on:
1. The life cycle of malaria parasite.
2. Clinical stages of malaria.
3. Complications of falciparum malaria.
4. Laboratory diagnosis of vivax malaria.

III. Multiple Choice Questions (MCQs):

1. **Cerebral malaria is caused by___?**
   a. Plasmodium falciparum
   b. Plasmodium vivax
   c. Plasmodium ovale
   d. Plasmodium malariae

2. **Banana-shaped gametocyte is seen for___?**
   a. Plasmodium vivax
   b. Plasmodium falciparum
   c. Plasmodium ovale
   d. Plasmodium malariae

3. **Which of the laboratory diagnostic test is best for the speciation of malaria parasites?**
   a. Thick smear examination
   b. Thin smear examination
   c. Rapid diagnostic tests
   d. QBC

4. **Schizonts in peripheral blood can be seen in all, *except*?**
   a. Plasmodium vivax
   b. Plasmodium falciparum
   c. Plasmodium ovale
   d. Plasmodium malariae

5. **Band forms are seen for___?**
   a. Plasmodium vivax
   b. Plasmodium falciparum
   c. Plasmodium ovale
   d. Plasmodium malariae

Answers
1. a   2. b   3. b   4. b   5. d

CHAPTER 30

Opportunistic Coccidian Parasites and Others

CHAPTER PREVIEW

Opportunistic Coccidian Parasites
- *Toxoplasma gondii*
- *Cryptosporidium parvum*
- *Cyclospora cayetanensis*
- *Cystoisospora belli*

Others
- *Balantidium coli*
- *Blastocystis hominis*

Coccidian parasites can cause opportunistic infections in HIV-infected patients. They can be grouped into:
- ❖ *Toxoplasma gondii:* Can cause encephalitis in HIV infected patients and can also infect fetus to cause congenital infection
- ❖ **Intestinal coccidian parasites:** *Cryptosporidium, Cyclospora,* and *Cystoisospora*: can produce profuse watery diarrhea in HIV infected patients.

TOXOPLASMA GONDII

Toxoplasma gondii is an obligate intracellular parasite affecting a wide range of mammals and birds including humans.
- ❖ **Disease:** Though human infection is common; very few progress to disease, mostly restricting to immunocompromised persons such as with HIV/AIDS (developing encephalitis) and congenital infection in the fetus
- ❖ **Morphology:** It exists in three morphological forms—two asexual forms (tachyzoite and tissue cyst) and one sexual form (oocyst, containing bradyzoites).

Life Cycle (Fig. 30.1)

Host: The life cycle involves two hosts:

1. **Definitive hosts** are cats and other felines; where the sexual cycle takes place
2. **Intermediate hosts** are man and other mammals (e.g. rodents); where the asexual cycle takes place.

Human (Asexual) Cycle

- ❖ **Transmission:** *T. gondii* infection transmission to man occurs by:
    - Ingestion of tissue cyst from undercooked meat (most common route)
    - Ingestion of sporulated oocysts from contaminated soil, food, or water
    - Blood transfusion, organ transplantation; tachyzoites are the infective form
    - Mother-to-fetus; tachyzoites are the infective form.
- ❖ **Transform into tachyzoites:** In the intestine, sporozoites are released from sporulated oocyst, and bradyzoites are released from the tissue cyst. They invade the intestinal epithelium and transform into tachyzoites
- ❖ **Transform into tissue cyst:** Tachyzoites multiply actively in blood and spread to extraintestinal organs like brain, muscles, eye, liver, etc. where they transform into bradyzoites which subsequently encysted to form tissue cysts.

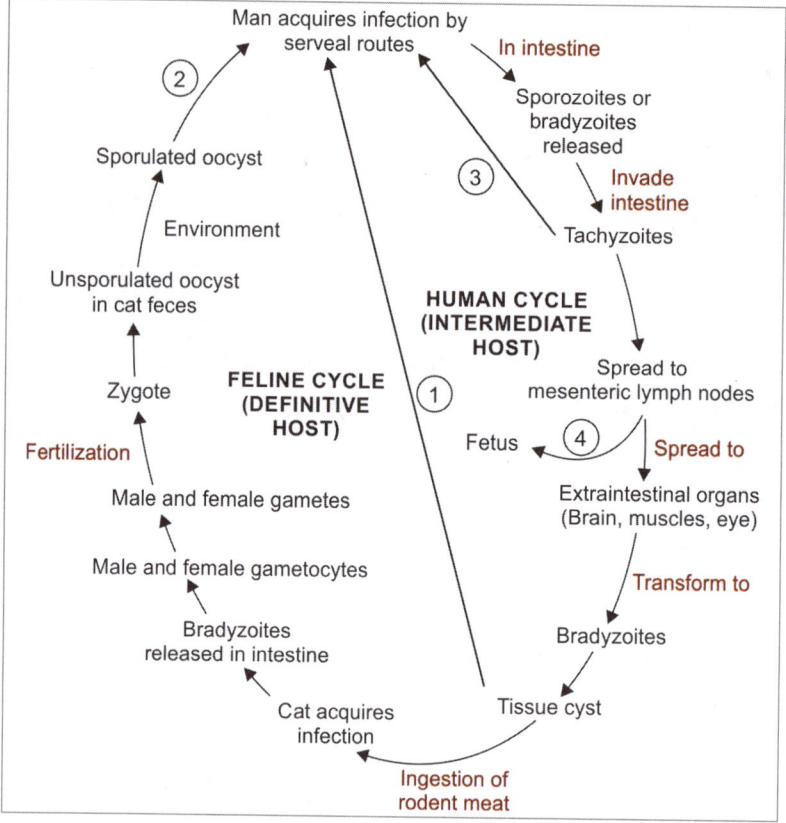

Fig. 30.1: Life cycle of *Toxoplasma gondii*.
Note: 1 to 4 are various modes of transmission of *Toxoplasma gondii* infection to man.

Cat (Sexual) Cycle

Cat and other felines (definitive host) acquire infection by ingestion of tissue cysts present in the rodent meat.

- Bradyzoites are released from the tissue cysts in the intestine, which transform into gametocytes and then into gametes
- The male and female gametes then fertilize to form zygotes, which subsequently transform into oocysts that are excreted in the cat's feces.

Clinical Manifestations

The clinical manifestations of toxoplasmosis can vary depending upon the patient population affected.

- **Immunocompetent host:** The infection usually remains asymptomatic and self-limited. Rarely progresses to acute toxoplasmosis, characterized by lymphadenopathy (e.g. cervical)
- **Immunocompromised hosts** such as patients infected with HIV, transplant recipients, and malignancies, the clinical manifestations are more severe. Encephalitis is the most common presentation
- **Congenital toxoplasmosis:** Mother-to-fetus transmission of *T. gondii* can occur any time during pregnancy, maximum being in the third trimester. But the risk of fetal damage is maximum in the first trimester, producing various congenital malformations such as chorioretinitis, hydrocephalus, and intracranial calcifications, etc.

Laboratory Diagnosis

Direct Microscopy

The specimens such as peripheral blood, bone marrow aspirate, and biopsy material from muscle and brain, etc. are stained with Giemsa, H & E, and PAS.

CHAPTER 30 ♦ Opportunistic Coccidian Parasites and Others

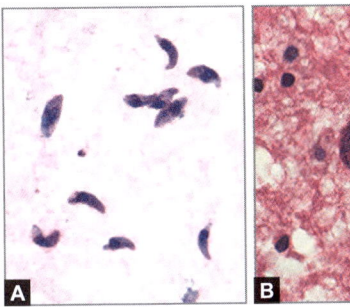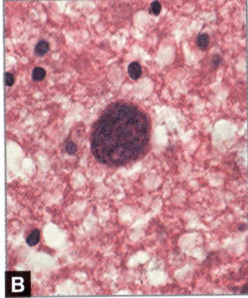

Figs. 30.2A and B: *Toxoplasma gondii:* **A.** Giemsa stain showing comma-shaped tachyzoites in the blood smear; **B.** Tissue cyst containing bradyzoites (section of brain).

Source: **A and B.** DPDx Image Library; Centers for Disease Control and Prevention (CDC), Atlanta (*with permission*).

- ❖ **Comma-shaped tachyzoites** are detected in the smear made from blood, body fluids, and tissue; their presence indicates acute infection **(Fig. 30.2A)**
- ❖ Tissue cysts containing strongly PAS-positive **bradyzoites** can be detected in various tissues like the brain or muscle **(Fig. 30.2B)**.

Antibody Detection

Antibody detection is useful in immunocompetent individuals. In immunocompromised patients, antibodies are produced at a very low level and therefore are not useful. Various methods available are:
- ❖ **Capture ELISA:** It can detect specific antibodies such as IgM, IgG, and IgA
    - Acute toxoplasmosis can be diagnosed by the presence of IgM or a four-fold rise of IgG
    - In congenital toxoplasmosis, detection of IgM or IgA is useful for diagnosis.
- ❖ **ISGA:** Immunosorbent agglutination assay
- ❖ **Sabin-Feldman Dye test:** It is the gold standard antibody detection method. But its use is limited to only the reference laboratories.

Molecular Diagnosis

Polymerase chain reaction (PCR) can be employed to detect *Toxoplasma*-specific DNA from various clinical samples like blood, CSF, or amniotic fluid.

> **TREATMENT** — Toxoplasmosis
> - Cotrimoxazole is the drug of choice.
> - It is given in AIDS patients, both for treatment and prophylaxis, as the disease may progress to encephalitis.

INTESTINAL COCCIDIAN PARASITES

The intestinal coccidian parasites can cause opportunistic infections in HIV-infected patients producing profuse watery diarrhea.
- ❖ **Agents:** The intestinal coccidian parasites are:
    - *Cryptosporidium parvum*
    - *Cyclospora cayetanensis*
    - *Cystoisospora belli.*
- ❖ **Transmission:** Man acquires infection by ingestion of food and water contaminated with feces with oocysts (infective form). In addition, the oocysts of *Cryptosporidium* are also transmitted by *autoinfection* through contaminated fingers
- ❖ **In the human intestine,** the oocysts undergo further development and are excreted in the feces
- ❖ **Clinical features:** The majority of infections remain asymptomatic. Some individuals develop self-limiting diarrhea
    - However, in immunocompromised hosts (e.g. AIDS), they produce **chronic persistent profuse diarrhea** (resembling cholera)
    - The disease is more severe in *Cryptosporidium*, due to repeated autoinfection.
- ❖ **Stool microscopy** demonstrates the characteristic acid-fast oocysts. Based on the oocyst morphology, the coccidian parasites can be differentiated
    - *Cryptosporidium:* Oocyst is round, measures 4–6 μm in size, and contains four sporozoites **(Figs. 30.3A and 30.4A)**
    - *Cyclospora:* Oocyst is round, measures 8–10 μm in size, and contains two sporocysts, each comprising two sporozoites **(Figs. 30.3B and 30.4B)**
    - *Cystoisospora:* Oocyst is oval and larger, measuring 20–33 μm in length; contains

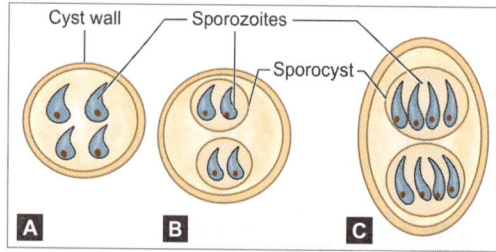

Figs. 30.3A to C: Sporulated oocysts (schematic diagram) of **A.** *Cryptosporidium;* **B.** *Cyclospora;* **C.** *Cystoisospora.*

two sporocysts, each comprising four sporozoites **(Figs. 30.3C and 30.4C)**.
- **Other diagnostic modalities** include—(i) antigen detection by ICT or ELISA, and (ii) molecular test by PCR or real-time PCR, which can differentiate between the coccidian parasites
- **Treatment:** Cryptosporidiosis is treated with nitazoxanide; whereas for cyclosporiasis and cystoisosporiasis cotrimoxazole is the drug of choice.

BALANTIDIUM COLI

Balantidium coli is a ciliated parasite, that resides in the large intestine, and produces **dysentery** similar to *E. histolytica*.
- Pigs are the primary hosts. Man is an accidental host
- Man gets infection by ingestion of food and water contaminated with cysts (infective form)
- Diagnosis is made by stool examination, which reveals characteristic ciliated trophozoite and cyst
- Tetracycline is the drug of choice.

BLASTOCYSTIS HOMINIS

Blastocystis hominis is a protozoan parasite that resides in the intestine of humans and many animals as commensal; however, recently its pathogenic role has been described. Few present with symptoms of irritable bowel syndrome.

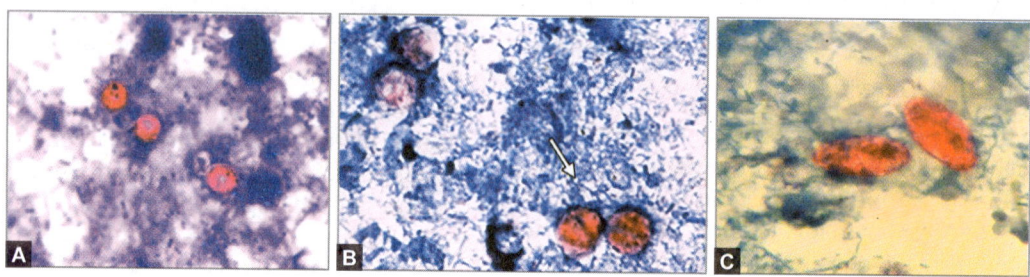

Figs. 30.4A to C: Modified acid-fast stain from diarrheal specimen demonstrating oocysts of: **A.** *Cryptosporidium;* **B.** *Cyclospora;* **C.** *Cystoisospora.*

Source: **A and B.** Swierczynski G, Milanesi B. Atlas of human intestinal protozoa microscopic diagnosis (*with permission*); **C.** Dr Anand Janagond, Department of Microbiology, S Nijalingappa Medical College, Bagalkot, Karnataka (*with permission*).

> ### EXPECTED QUESTIONS

I. Write short notes on:
1. Laboratory diagnosis of intestinal coccidian parasitic infections.
2. Congenital toxoplasmosis.

II. Multiple Choice Questions (MCQs):
1. **Autoinfection is seen with___?**
    a. *Cryptosporidium*
    b. *Cyclospora*
    c. *Cystoisospora*
    d. All of the above
2. **Most common infective form, for Toxoplasma___?**
    a. Oocyst
    b. Tissue cyst
    c. Tachyzoite
    d. All of the above

Answers
1. a   2. b

CHAPTER 31: Cestode Infections

CHAPTER PREVIEW
- *Taenia solium* and *Taenia saginata*
- *Echinococcus granulosus*
- *Hymenolepis nana*
- *Diphyllobothrium latum*

INTRODUCTION

Cestodes are long, segmented, flattened, tape-like worms, therefore also called tapeworms. Based on habitat, they are classified into two groups:

1. **Intestinal cestodes:** Here, the adult worms inhabit in human intestine. Examples include:
   - *Diphyllobothrium* species
   - *Taenia solium* and *Taenia saginata* causing intestinal taeniasis
   - *Hymenolepis nana*.
2. **Somatic/tissue cestodes:** Here, the larvae are found in the human muscles or organs. Examples include:
   - *Taenia solium*—causes cysticercosis affecting CNS, muscle, and eye
   - *Echinococcus granulosus* —the agent of hydatid disease affecting the liver.

Morphology

In general, cestodes exist in three morphological forms.
- ❖ **Adult worm:** It is long, segmented, and varies in length from a few mm to several meters. It consists of—the head (or scolex), neck, and body (strobila). The strobila further comprises of a number of segments (or proglottids) **(Fig. 31.1)**
- ❖ **Eggs:** They are formed following fertilization, fill the proglottids, and

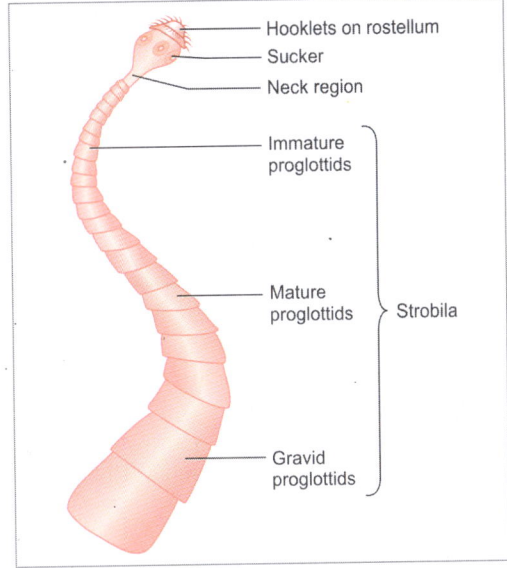

Fig. 31.1: Adult worm of cestode (schematic diagram).

are subsequently released in feces—considered as the diagnostic form
- ❖ **Larva:** Embryonated eggs undergo further development to form larvae. The larval form is called with different names for different cestodes
   - *Taenia saginata*: Cysticercus bovis
   - *Taenia solium* Cysticercus cellulosae
   - *Echinococcus*: Hydatid cyst
   - *Hymenolepis* species: Cysticercoid larva

Table 31.1: Life cycle of various cestodes.

Cestodes	Host Definitive	Host Intermediate	Mode of transmission	Infective form	Diagnostic form	Organs affected
Taenia saginata	Man	Cattle	Ingestion	Cysticercus bovis	Embryonated eggs	GIT
Taenia solium (intestinal taeniasis)	Man	Pig	Ingestion	Cysticercus cellulosae	Embryonated eggs	GIT
Taenia solium (cysticercosis)	Man	Man	Ingestion, autoinfection	Embryonated eggs	Cysticercus larvae	CNS, muscle, eye
Echinococcus granulosus	Dog	Man	Ingestion	Embryonated eggs	Hydatid cyst (larva)	Liver
Hymenolepis nana	Man	–	Ingestion, autoinfection	Embryonated eggs	Embryonated eggs	GIT
Diphyllobothrium latum	Man	1st- Cyclops, 2nd- Fish	Ingestion	Plerocercoid larvae	Operculated eggs	GIT

- *Diphyllobothrium* species: It has 3 larval stages— coracidium, procercoid, and plerocercoid.

The life cycle of cestodes pathogenic to man has been discussed in **Table 31.1**.

TAENIA SAGINATA AND T. SOLIUM

Taenia saginata and *T. solium* cause two types of manifestations in humans.
- **Intestinal taeniasis**—caused by both *T. saginata* and *T. solium*
- **Cysticercosis**—caused by only *T. solium*. It infects various tissues such as CNS, eyes, and muscles.

Intestinal Taeniasis

Life Cycle

The life cycle of *Taenia* passes through two hosts **(Fig. 31.2)**. Man is the definitive host; whereas the intermediate host is cattle for *T. saginata* (hence called beef tapeworm) and pigs for *T. solium* (hence called pork tapeworm).
- **Transmission:** Man acquires infection by ingestion of contaminated undercooked beef or pork containing the larvae (infective form)—i.e. cysticercus bovis (for *T. saginata*) or cysticercus cellulosae (for *T. solium*)

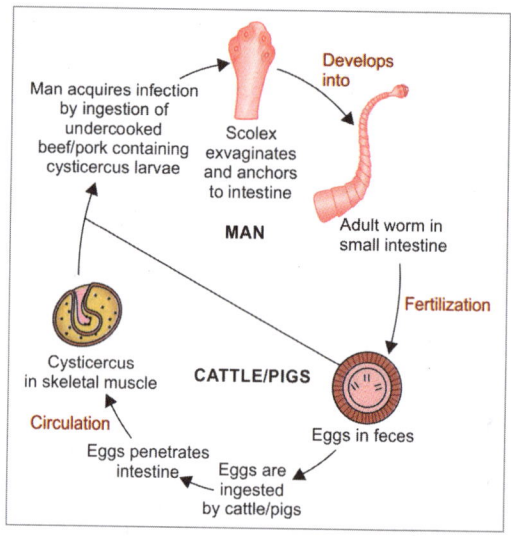

Fig. 31.2: Life cycle of *Taenia saginata* and *T. solium* causing intestinal taeniasis.

- **Human GIT:** The larvae develop into adult worms in the intestine, which undergo fertilization to produce eggs, that are released into feces (diagnostic form)
- **Intermediate hosts (cattle or pigs):** Eggs are ingested by cattle or pigs while grazing the field. Eggs penetrate the intestinal wall and migrate to skeletal muscles via blood, where they transform into larvae (cysticercus) that get encysted and deposited as cysts. This is the infective form to man and the cycle is repeated.

Note: T. solium has an additional part of the life cycle in man, which causes cysticercosis (discussed subsequently).

Clinical Manifestations

The majority of cases are asymptomatic. Common symptoms include mild abdominal pain, nausea, loss of appetite, and change in bowel habits and perianal pruritus may be felt (when proglottids are discharged).

Laboratory Diagnosis

Laboratory diagnosis of intestinal taeniasis includes:
- **Stool examination:** Wet mount (saline or iodine) examination of stool can demonstrate the characteristic eggs and less often proglottids of *Taenia* species
  - **Eggs:** Round (31–43 μm size) and consist of an embryo with six hooklets surrounded by an embryophore. Eggs are bile-stained; do not float in the saturated salt solution **(Fig. 31.3)**
  - **Proglottids** of *T. saginata* and *T. solium* can be differentiated by various features.
- **Antigen detection in stool:** Detection of *Taenia*-specific antigen (coproantigen) in the stool by ELISA
- **Molecular detection by** PCR; which can distinguish between *Taenia* species.

> **TREATMENT** — Intestinal taeniasis
>
> Praziquantel is the drug of choice for intestinal taeniasis.
> Niclosamide is also effective but is not widely available.

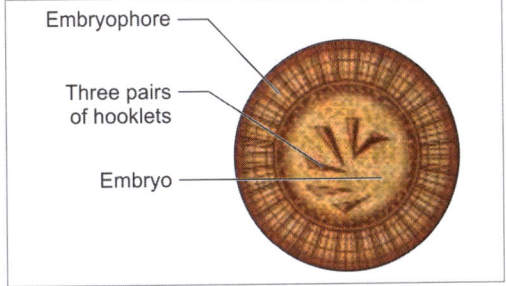

Fig. 31.3: Egg of *Taenia solium* or *T. saginata*.

Cysticercosis

Cysticercosis is caused by the larval stage of the tapeworm *Taenia solium*, affecting CNS, muscles, and the eye.
- It is a major public health problem, especially in the developing world
- In India, it is highly prevalent in the northern states such as Bihar, Odisha, Uttar Pradesh, Punjab, etc.

Life Cycle of Taenia solium Causing Cysticercosis

The life cycle of *T. solium* causing cysticercosis is different than its life cycle when it causes intestinal taeniasis.
- **Host:** Man acts as both definitive and intermediate host
- **Infective stage:** Eggs of *T. solium*
- **Mode of transmission:** Firstly man acquires the infection by—(1) ingestion of contaminated food or water containing eggs of *T. solium*, and (2) autoinfection, i.e. eggs excreted in the feces re-infect the same individual
- **Human cycle:** In the gut, the egg ruptures to release the embryo, which penetrates the intestine and enters the circulation to reach various organs like subcutaneous tissue, muscle, eye, and brain where it is transformed into the larval stage.

Clinical Manifestations (Cysticercosis)

Clinical spectra of the disease depend upon the localization of the cyst—common sites are CNS, subcutaneous tissue, skeletal muscle, and eyes.

Neurocysticercosis

Neurocysticercosis (NCC) is the most common form of cysticercosis; accounts for 60–90% of cases of cysticercosis.
- **Site:** NCC occurs most commonly in the brain parenchyma, followed by subarachnoid space
- **Clinical manifestations** include **seizure** (most common), hydrocephalus, increased intracranial pressure, chronic meningitis, etc.

- The clinical presentation is variable and depends on the number, location, and size of the cyst, and the host immune response
- **NCC and HIV:** Patients with HIV have a higher risk of NCC co-infection.

Other Forms of Cysticercosis

- **Subcutaneous cysticercosis:** It may manifest as palpable nodules
- **Muscular cysticercosis:** Manifest as muscular pain, weakness, or pseudohypertrophy
- **Ocular cysticercosis:** Can involve the eyelids, conjunctiva, and sclera.

Laboratory Diagnosis

Cysticercosis is diagnosed by the following modalities.
- **Radiodiagnosis:** CT scan and MRI are the two important imaging methods used to detect cysticerci in the brain. They are useful for detecting the number, location, size of the cysticerci, and stage of the disease **(Fig. 31.4)**
- **Antibody detection** in serum or CSF by ELISA or Western blot
- **Antigen detection** in serum or CSF by ELISA. Antigen disappears following treatment hence, can be used for monitoring
- **Histopathology** of muscles, eyes, subcutaneous tissues, or brain biopsies—can detect cysticerci
- **FNAC** of the cyst and then staining with Giemsa stain

- **Fundoscopy** of the eye: can detect larvae if present.

> **TREATMENT** — Cysticercosis
>
> - **Antiparasitic agents:** Albendazole or praziquantel are the drugs of choice
> - **Symptomatic treatment** is necessary for seizures or hydrocephalus, etc.
> - **Surgery:** Surgery is indicated for ocular, spinal and ventricular lesions.

ECHINOCOCCUS GRANULOSUS

Echinococcus granulosus is the causative agent of cystic echinococcosis, also known as hydatid disease.

Morphology

Echinococcus granulosus is a tissue cestode, exits in three morphological forms—adult, larva (called hydatid cyst), and egg.
- **Adult worm** resides in dog's intestine.
- **Larval form** is called as hydatid cyst. It is the pathogenic form, forms cystic lesions in liver and other viscera of man.
- **Eggs:** *E. granulosus* eggs are morphologically similar to *Taenia* eggs.

Life Cycle (Fig. 31.5)

Host: *E. granulosus* passes its life cycle through two hosts:
1. Definitive host: Dogs and other canine animals

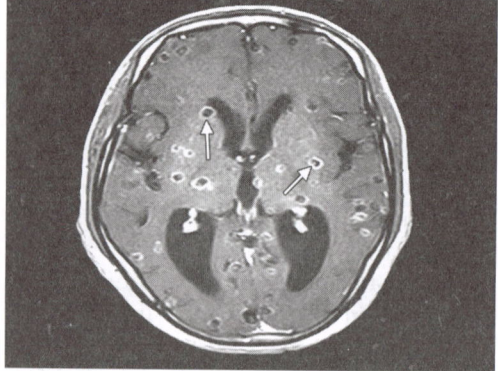

Fig. 31.4: CT scan of the brain showing multiple ring-enhancing lesions with eccentric scolex (neurocysticercosis).

Source: Dr A Subathra. Department of Radiodiagnosis, JIPMER, Puducherry (*with permission*).

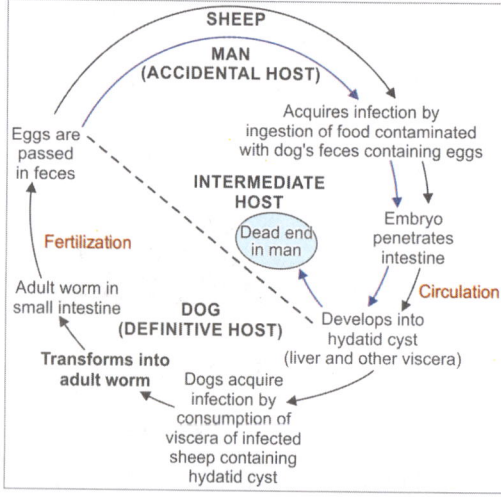

Fig. 31.5: Life cycle of *Echinococcus granulosus*.

2. **Intermediate hosts:** Sheep and other herbivores are the usual intermediate host. Man acts as an accidental intermediate host (dead end).

Infective form: Eggs are the infective form.

Mode of transmission: Man (and other intermediate hosts) acquires the infection by ingestion of food contaminated with dog's feces containing *E. granulosus* eggs.

Development in Man/Sheep

- In the duodenum, the embryo is released, which penetrates the intestinal wall, enters the portal circulation, and is carried to the liver or rarely to other organs
- The embryo develops into a fluid-filled bladder-like cyst called as **hydatid cyst**, which undergoes maturation and increases in size
- This stage is infective to dog and other definitive hosts
- Man is a dead end, as dogs do not feed on human viscera and therefore the cycle stops there.

Development in Dog

They acquire infection by consumption of the contaminated viscera of intermediate hosts (sheep) containing hydatid cysts.

- The hydatid cyst (larva) transforms into adult worm in the dog's intestine
- The adult worms sexually mature, and fertilize to produce eggs which are passed in feces and are infective to man.

Clinical Features

The manifestations are related to the deposition of the hydatid cysts in various organs—the most common site being the liver (60–70%, right lobe) or lung (20%), followed by other viscera.

- **Pressure effect of enlarging cyst:** Leads to palpable abdominal mass, hepatomegaly, abdominal tenderness, portal hypertension, and ascites
- **Obstruction:** Daughter cysts may erode into the biliary tree or a bronchus and enter into the lumen to cause cholestasis, cholangitis, and dyspnea

- **Secondary bacterial infection,** causing pyogenic abscess in the liver
- **Anaphylactic reactions** may occur due to cyst leakage or rupture.

> **Hydatid Cyst**
> It is a fluid-filled bladder-like cyst; the average size measures 5–8 cm **(Figs. 31.6 and 31.7)**.
> - **Cyst wall** consists of three layers: outer pericyst (host-derived), middle ectocyst, and inner endocyst
> - **Brood capsule:** The inner side of the endocyst gives rise to brood capsule which contains a number of protoscolices (future head)
> - **Hydatid fluid:** It is clear, pale yellow colored fluid, which is antigenic, and anaphylactic
> - **Hydatid sand** is formed by deposition of some of the brood capsules and protoscolices at the bottom
> - **Fate:** The hydatid cyst may undergo—(i) spontaneous resolution, or (ii) rupture of the cyst, which may lead to the formation of secondary cysts.

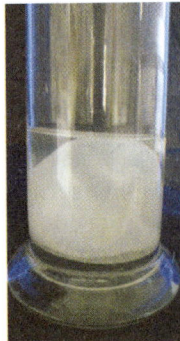

Fig. 31.6: Hydatid cyst, gross specimen.
Source: Head, Department of Microbiology, Sri Siddhartha Medical College, Tumkur, Karnataka (*with permission*).

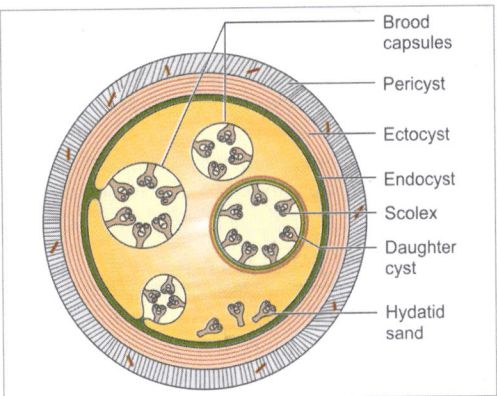

Fig. 31.7: Microscopy of hydatid cyst (schematic).

Laboratory Diagnosis

Hydatid disease is diagnosed by the following modalities.
- ❖ **Hydatid fluid microscopy**: Fluid aspirated from a surgically removed hydatid cyst can be subjected to direct mount—detects brood capsules and protoscolices
- ❖ **Histological examination**: Hematoxylin and eosin (H & E) staining demonstrates the three layers of the cyst wall and attached brood capsules
- ❖ **Antibody detection**: It is done by a screening test (ELISA or immunogold filtration assay) and confirmatory test by western blot
- ❖ **Imaging methods** such as X-ray, USG, CT scan, MRI, etc. can be performed. USG is the imaging method of choice for the diagnosis of hydatid disease
    - USG helps in determining the exact location of the cyst, size of cyst, number of cysts, activity (active or dormant)
    - The membranes may be detached; floating within the cyst cavity (known as the **water-lily sign**).
- ❖ **Molecular methods**: PCR targeting mitochondrial DNA has been developed
- ❖ **Skin test: Casoni test** is an immediate hypersensitivity reaction, that develops following injection of hydatid fluid antigens.

TREATMENT — Hydatid disease

The following are the treatment strategies for hydatid disease.
- **PAIR** (puncture, aspiration, injection, and re-aspiration): It is a semiconservative method, indicated for a single uncomplicated hepatic cyst
- **Surgical removal** of the cyst is indicated for an inaccessible cyst or extrahepatic cysts
- **Antiparasitic agents**: Albendazole is the drug of choice, given to prevent recurrence and to reduce the size of the cyst before surgery or PAIR.

HYMENOLEPIS NANA

Hymenolepis nana, which is the smallest cestode infecting man, hence also called as dwarf tapeworm.

- ❖ **Transmission**: Man is the only host. Eggs are the infective form. Man acquires the infection by ingestion of food and water contaminated with eggs or by autoinfection (with the eggs released in their small intestine)
- ❖ **Clinical manifestations**: Patients develop symptoms like anorexia, abdominal pain, headache, dizziness, and diarrhea with mucus
- ❖ **Laboratory diagnosis**: Stool microscopy detecting the characteristic eggs confirms the diagnosis **(Fig. 31.8A)**
    - The egg is round to oval in shape, 30–47 μm in size
    - It has two membranes that surround an embryo with six hooklets
    - Polar filaments at both the poles
    - Non-bile stained (colorless in saline mount)
    - Eggs are the infective form as well as the diagnostic form of the parasite.
- ❖ **Treatment**: Praziquantel is the treatment of choice.

DIPHYLLOBOTHRIUM LATUM

Diphyllobothrium latum, also known as fish tapeworm—is the largest known parasite found in the human intestine.
- ❖ **Manifestation**: The adult worm causes malabsorption of vitamin B12, which leads to vitamin B12 deficiency and **megaloblastic anemia**

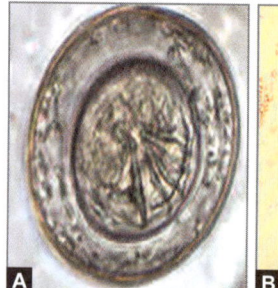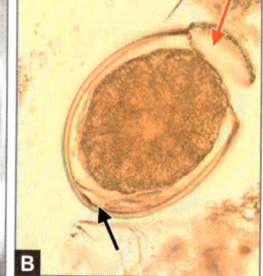

Figs. 31.8A and B: A. Egg of *Hymenolepis nana* (non-bile stained); **B.** Egg of *Diphyllobothrium latum*—note the operculum (red arrow).

Source: DPDx Image Library, Centers for Disease Control and Prevention (CDC), Atlanta (*with permission*).

- **Diagnosis** is made by detection of characteristic operculated eggs **(Fig. 31.8B)** in stool microscopy
- **Treatment:** Praziquantel is the treatment of choice. Vitamin B12 supplement needs to be given.

EXPECTED QUESTIONS

I. Write short notes on:
1. Discuss the clinical manifestations and laboratory diagnosis of cysticercosis.
2. Discuss the life cycle, clinical manifestations, and laboratory diagnosis of *Echinococcus granulosus*.

II. Write short notes on:
1. Intestinal taeniasis.
2. *Hymenolepis nana*.
3. *Diphyllobothrium latum*.

III. Multiple Choice Questions (MCQs):
1. Which is a somatic cestode?
   a. *Echinococcus granulosus*
   b. *Hymenolepis nana*
   c. *Diphyllobothrium latum*
   d. *Taenia saginata*
2. Which causes megaloblastic anemia?
   a. *Echinococcus granulosus*
   b. *Hymenolepis nana*
   c. *Diphyllobothrium latum*
   d. *Taenia saginata*
3. Which of the following produces non-bile stained egg?
   a. *Echinococcus granulosus*
   b. *Hymenolepis nana*
   c. *Diphyllobothrium latum*
   d. *Taenia saginata*
4. The causative agent of hydatid disease?
   a. *Echinococcus granulosus*
   b. *Hymenolepis nana*
   c. *Diphyllobothrium latum*
   d. *Taenia saginata*
5. Definitive host for Echinococcosis is:
   a. Man
   b. Dog
   c. Sheep
   d. Pig

Answers
1. a   2. c   3. b   4. a   5. b

CHAPTER 32: Trematode Infections

CHAPTER PREVIEW
- Schistosomes
- Fasciolopsis buski
- Liver flukes
- Paragonimus westermani

TREMATODE INFECTIONS

Trematodes (or flukes) are unsegmented, leaf-like, and flatworms. The various trematodes that infect man are:
- **Blood flukes**—e.g. *Schistosoma*
- **Intestinal flukes**—e.g. *Fasciolopsis buski*.
- **Hepatic flukes**—e.g. *Fasciola hepatica* in the liver, *Clonorchis*, and *Opisthorchis* in the bile duct
- **Lung flukes**—e.g. *Paragonimus westermani*.

Blood Flukes (Schistosoma)

Schistosomes reside in the venous plexus of various viscera. There are three species, that infect man—*S. haematobium*, and *S. mansoni* (both are prevalent in Africa), and *S. japonicum* (prevalent in Asia).
- **Hosts:** Humans are the definitive host. Snails are the only intermediate host, there is no second intermediate host
- **Transmission:** Man acquires infection by skin penetration of cercaria larvae (infective form), that are present freely in water
- **Life cycle:** The larvae penetrate the skin and travel via systemic circulation to reach the liver where they develop into adult worms. Adult worms migrate to their habitat, i.e.,
    - Venous plexuses of the urinary bladder—for *S. haematobium*
    - Venous plexuses of the intestine—for *S. mansoni* and *S. japonicum*.
- **Clinical features:** The clinical manifestations are:
    - *Cercarial dermatitis*—an itchy maculopapular rash develops at the site of skin perpetration of cercaria larvae (also called swimmer's itch)
    - *Katayama fever*— a serum sickness-like illness, due to the deposition of immune complexes
    - *Chronic schistosomiasis*—is due to the deposition of eggs trapped in the small venules in various organs causing egg granuloma
        - *S. mansoni* and *S. japonicum:* They cause intestinal followed by hepatosplenic disease
        - *S. haematobium:* Causes urogenital disease, characterized by dysuria, hematuria, obstructive uropathies, and squamous cell carcinoma of the bladder.
- **Microscopy:** Reveals large non-operculated oval eggs with a characteristic spine **(Figs. 32.1A to C)**
    - The egg of *S. haematobium* has a terminal spine (in urine microscopy)
    - The egg of *S. mansoni* has a lateral spine (in stool microscopy)
    - The egg of *S. japonicum* is more spherical and has a rudimentary lateral spine (in stool microscopy).

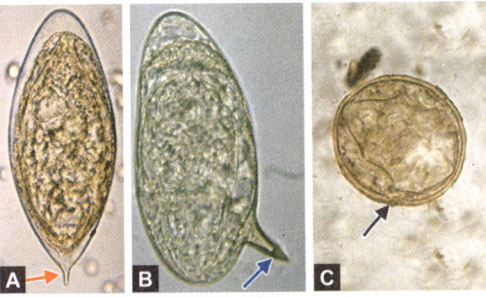

Figs. 32.1A to C: *Schistosoma* eggs: **A.** *S. haematobium*; **B.** *S. mansoni*; **C.** *S. japonicum*.
Source: **A.** ID# 4843, **B.** ID# 4841, **C.** ID#4842. Public Health Image Library, Centers for Disease Control and Prevention (CDC), Atlanta (*with permission*).

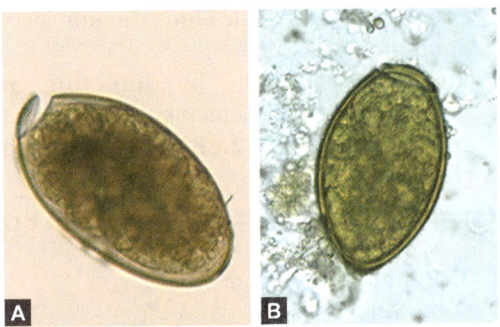

Figs. 32.2A and B: Operculated egg of **A.** *Fasciolopsis buski/Fasciola hepatica*; **B.** *Paragonimus westermani*.
Source: **A and B.** DPDx Image Library, Centers for Disease Control and Prevention (CDC), Atlanta (*with permission*).

- **Antigen detection:** ELISA or dipstick tests are available to detect antigens in the serum and urine
- **Treatment:** Praziquantel is the drug of choice.

Intestinal Flukes (Fasciolopsis buski)

Fasciolopsis buski resides in the intestine and may cause various GI symptoms.
- **Hosts:** Humans are the definitive host. Snails are the first intermediate host, whereas the aquatic plant is the second intermediate host
- **Transmission:** Man acquires infection by eating the aquatic plants, carrying the infective form, the metacercaria larvae
- **Clinical features** include malabsorption with profuse yellowish-green stool
- **Diagnosis** is made by detection of characteristic large operculated eggs in stool microscopy **(Fig. 32.2A)**
- **Treatment:** Praziquantel is the drug of choice.

Hepatic Flukes

Hepatic flukes include—(i) *Fasciola hepatica*, (ii) *Clonorchis sinensis*, and (iii) *Opisthorchis viverrini*
- **Hosts:** Humans are the definitive host. Snails are the first intermediate host, whereas the second intermediate host is aquatic plant (for *Fasciola*) or crayfish (for *Clonorchis,* and *Opisthorchis*)
- **Transmission:** Man acquires infection by eating the second intermediate host carrying the infective form (i.e. the metacercaria larvae)
- **Clinical features:** Vary depending on the species
  - *Fasciola hepatica* infects the liver and bile duct causing right upper quadrant pain, hepatomegaly, and biliary cirrhosis. It does not cause malignancies
  - *Clonorchis* and *Opisthorchis* infect the bile duct leading to cholangitis and bile duct carcinoma.
- **Diagnosis** is made by detection of characteristic operculated eggs in stool microscopy
  - In *Fasciola:* The eggs are large operculated eggs, similar to that of *Fasciolopsis buski* **(Fig. 32.2A)**
  - In *Clonorchis* and *Opisthorchis:* The eggs are small flask-shaped and operculated.
- **Treatment:** Praziquantel is the drug of choice for liver flukes, except for *F. hepatica* where triclabendazole is given.

Lung Flukes (Paragonimus westermani)

Paragonimus westermani is endemic in Northeast states of India like Manipur.
- **Hosts:** Humans are the definitive host. Intermediate hosts are snails (first), and crabs (second)
- **Transmission:** Man acquires infection by eating the crabs carrying the metacercaria larvae (infective form)
- **Clinical features:** The adult worm multiplies in the lungs to cause **endemic hemoptysis**—characterized by productive

cough with brownish blood-tinged rusty sputum

❖ **Diagnosis** is made by detection of characteristic operculated eggs in sputum microscopy **(Fig. 32.2B)**. ELISA is also available for antigen detection, which indicates active infection

❖ **Treatment:** Praziquantel is the drug of choice for the treatment of paragonimiasis.

EXPECTED QUESTIONS

I. Write short notes on:
1. Schistosomiasis.
2. Paragonimiasis.
3. Liver flukes.

II. Multiple Choice Questions (MCQs):
1. **Eggs with the terminal spine are produced by__?**
   a. *Schistosoma haematobium*
   b. *Schistosoma mansoni*
   c. *Schistosoma japonicum*
   d. *Fasciola hepatica*
2. **Operculated eggs are produced by__?**
   a. *Schistosoma haematobium*
   b. *Schistosoma mansoni*
   c. *Schistosoma japonicum*
   d. *Fasciola hepatica*
3. **Which of the following is transmitted by skin penetration?**
   a. *Schistosoma hematobium*
   b. *Paragonimus westermani*
   c. *Fasciola hepatica*
   d. *Fasciolopsis buski*
4. **The causative agent of swimmer's itch?**
   a. *Paragonimus westermani*
   b. *Fasciola hepatica*
   c. *Schistosoma mansoni*
   d. *Fasciolopsis buski*

Answers
1. a   2. d   3. a   4. c

CHAPTER 33

Intestinal Nematode Infections

CHAPTER PREVIEW

- *Trichuris trichiura*
- *Enterobius vermicularis*
- *Ascaris lumbricoides*
- Hookworm
- *Strongyloides stercoralis*

NEMATODES

Nematodes are developmentally higher helminths, probably the most widespread helminths occurring in the world.

Classification based on Habitat

Based on their habitat, nematodes infecting humans are classified into two groups.

Intestinal nematodes: Include five common parasites
- Small intestinal nematodes—*Ascaris*, hookworm, and *Strongyloides*
- Large intestinal nematodes—*Trichuris* and *Enterobius*.

Somatic or tissue nematodes: They reside in various tissues or organs.
- Filarial nematodes: They comprise of several vector-borne parasites
  - *Wuchereria bancrofti* and *Brugia malayi* cause lymphatic filariasis
  - *Loa loa, Onchocerca volvulus*, and *Mansonella* cause cutaneous filariasis.
- *Dracunculus medinensis*: Causes Guinea-worm disease; presents as painful cutaneous blisters
- *Trichinella spiralis*: Produces profuse watery diarrhea and myalgia.

Classification based on they Lay Egg or Larva

Nematodes can be classified into three groups based on whether they lay eggs or larvae after fertilization of male and female worms.
- **Oviparous:** Female worms lay eggs. Most of the intestinal nematodes are oviparous except for *Strongyloides*
- **Viviparous:** Female worms directly give birth to larvae; there is no egg stage. All somatic nematodes are viviparous
- **Ovoviviparous:** Female worms lay eggs, from which the larvae immediately hatch out—e.g. *Strongyloides* species.

TRICHURIS TRICHIURA

Trichuris trichiura is a soil-transmitted helminth, that commonly affects children. It is also called as **whipworm** (as the adult worm resembles a handle of a whip). *T. trichiura* resides in the large intestine of man (mainly cecum and appendix).
- **Life cycle (Fig. 33.1):** Humans are the only host, acquire infection by ingestion of contaminated food and water containing embryonated egg (infective form)
  - **In the large intestine**: Eggs hatch out to form larva, which further develops into

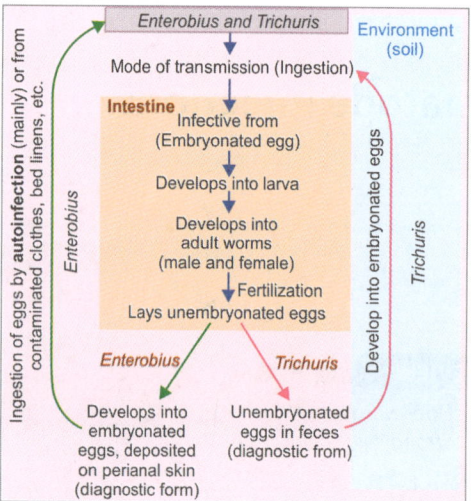

Fig. 33.1: Life cycles of *Trichuris* and *Enterobius*.

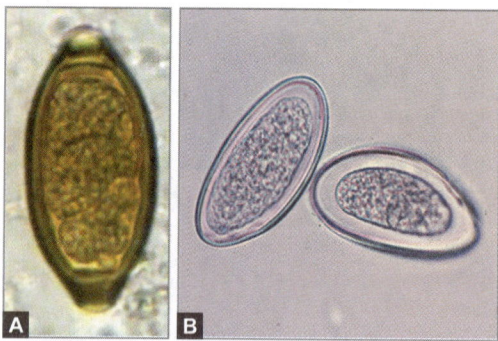

Figs. 33.2A and B: Saline mount of stool showing: **A.** Egg of *Trichuris trichiura* (bile stained); **B.** Egg of *Enterobius vermicularis* (non-bile stained).

Source: DPDx Image Library, Centers for Disease Control and Prevention (CDC), Atlanta (*with permission*).

an adult worm, which after fertilization produce eggs, which are excreted in feces
- **Environment:** The eggs become embryonated in the environment and the cycle continues.
- **Clinical manifestations:** Adult female worms get buried in the large intestinal mucosa, which leads to abdominal pain, dysentery, iron deficiency anemia, recurrent rectal prolapse, malnutrition leading to growth retardation
- **Laboratory diagnosis:** Stool microscopy reveals characteristic eggs—barrel-shaped with mucus plugs at the ends. Eggs measure 50×22 μm in size, are bile-stained, and float in saturated salt solution (Fig. 33.2A)
- **Treatment:** Mebendazole or albendazole are the drug of choice.

ENTEROBIUS VERMICULARIS

Enterobius vermicularis is a common large intestinal nematode affecting children. It is also called as **pinworm** or **threadworm**.

Life Cycle (Fig. 33.1)

Humans are the only host. Embryonated eggs are infective to man.
- **Transmission:** Infection occurs via: (i) autoinfection (contaminated fingers) or (ii) through ingestion of eggs in the environment (e.g. surfaces, clothes, etc.)
- Larvae hatch out from eggs in the cecum and then develop into adult worms
- After fertilization, the gravid female worms migrate to the large intestine and start laying eggs on the perianal skin
- The eggs are embryonated (carrying larvae) and are the infective stage to man.

Pathogenicity and Clinical Features

Children are commonly affected. The most cardinal symptom is **perianal pruritus,** which often gets worse at night as a result of the nocturnal migration of the female worm
- The worms may be found in undergarments and lying in the buttock area of infected children
- Repeated scratching is the main reason of contaminated fingers; which causes autoinfection.

Laboratory Diagnosis

Microscopy of the perianal skin samples is the test of choice which detects characteristic eggs.
- Specimen is collected by cellophane tape or by NIH swab. A series of 4–6 consecutive tapes may be necessary as the female worms migrate intermittently
- **Timing:** Samples should be collected when the chance of egg deposition is more such as in late evening or early morning.

Eggs of *Enterobius*

Eggs are plano-convex (one side is convex and the other side is flat), and measure 50–60 μm long **(Fig 33.2B)**
- Embryonated egg when freshly passed contains a tadpole-shaped larva inside
- Non-bile-stained, colorless in saline mount
- Floats in a saturated salt solution.

TREATMENT — Enterobiasis

The recommended drugs are mebendazole or albendazole or pyrantel pamoate.
- The same treatment should be repeated after 2 weeks
- Treatment of household members is advocated to eliminate asymptomatic reservoirs.

Prevention

Improving personal hygiene such as proper washing of bedclothes, keeping nails short and clean, and frequent hand washing are the key measures to contain the transmission.

ASCARIS LUMBRICOIDES

Ascaris lumbricoides is the largest nematode parasitizing the human intestine. It is commonly called as **roundworm**. It is a soil-transmitted helminth.

Morphology

Similar to other nematodes, *Ascaris* exists in three forms: adult worm, larvae (four stages—L_1 to L_4), and egg. The adult worm is cylindrical and measures 15–31 cm. The female worms liberate two types of eggs—(1) fertilized eggs, and (2) unfertilized eggs.

Life Cycle (Fig. 33.3)

Ascaris involves only one host (man). Embryonated eggs containing the L_2 larvae are the infective form.
- **Mode of transmission:** Ingestion of embryonated eggs from the contaminated soil, food, and water
- **Migratory phase:** Following ingestion, the eggs hatch out to liberate the L_2 larvae → molt once to form L_3 larvae → penetrate

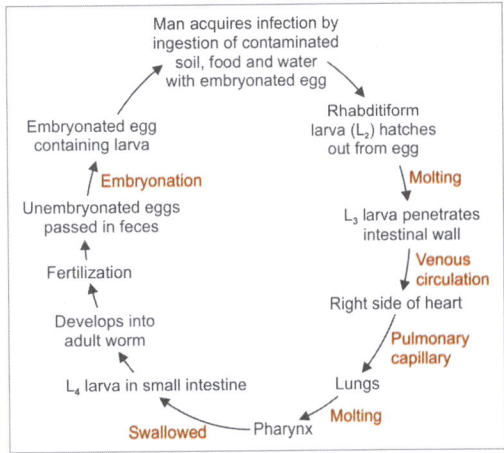

Fig. 33.3: Life cycle of *Ascaris lumbricoides*.

the intestine, reach the right side of the heart via portal circulation → then enter the lungs → molt once to form L_4 larvae in the lungs → migrate up to reach pharynx → finally are swallowed to re-enter the intestine
- **Intestinal phase:** The L_4 larvae undergo final molt to develop into adult worms in the small intestine. Following fertilization, the female worms start laying the fertilized eggs which are passed in the feces
- **Development in soil:** The fertilized eggs molt twice and become embryonated (carrying L_2 larvae), which is infective to man, and the life cycle continues. The unfertilized eggs cannot develop further, are not infective, and disintegrate in some time.

Pathogenesis and Clinical Feature

Clinical features occur in two stages.
- **Pulmonary phase:** It occurs due to migrating larvae in the lungs, which provoke an immune-mediated hypersensitivity response—called eosinophilic pneumonia **(Loeffler's syndrome)**
- **Intestinal phase:** It results due to the effect of adult worm in the intestine; characterized by:
  - *Malnutrition and growth retardation* robbing the nutrition from the host by the adult worm. It is often associated

with impairment of educational performance, language learning, etc.
- *Intestinal complications:* Intestinal obstruction by a large bolus of entangled worms causing perforation, intussusception, or volvulus.

Laboratory Diagnosis

Stool examination: Detecting both fertilized and unfertilized eggs in saline and iodine wet mount. Concentration techniques by sedimentation method should be done to improve the detection.

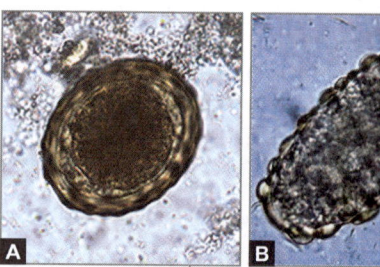

Figs. 33.5A to B: Eggs of *Ascaris lumbricoides*: **A.** Fertilized egg; **B.** Unfertilized egg.
Source: DPDx Image Library, Centers for Disease Control and Prevention (CDC), Atlanta (*with permission*).

> **Eggs of *Ascaris* (Figs. 33.4 and 33.5)**
> *Fertilized eggs* (Figs. 33.4A and 33.5A)
> Round to oval, measure 45–75 µm × 35–50 µm
> - Surrounded by a thick mamillated, albuminous coat
> - Contains a large unsegmented ovum with clear crescentic space at both the poles
> - Bile-stained, appear golden brown in saline mount
> - Floats in saturated salt solution
>
> *Unfertilized eggs* (Figs. 33.4B and 33.5B)
> Elongated, measure 85–95 µm × 43–47 µm
> - Albuminous coat is thin, distorted, and scanty
> - Contains an unsegmented, small atrophied ovum and no crescentic space at the poles
> - Bile-stained, appear golden brown in saline mount
> - Do not float in the saturated salt solution.

Other diagnostic modalities include:
- **Adult worms** may be detected occasionally in stool or sputum of the patients by naked eye or barium meal X-ray of the GIT

- **Larvae** can be found in sputum or gastric aspirates
- **Antibody detection** by ELISA and other formats
- **Molecular test** by PCR targeting *Ascaris*-specific genes in the stool
- **Eosinophilia** is prominent during the early lung stage.

> **TREATMENT** — Ascariasis
> Albendazole or mebendazole is the drug of choice. It effectively kills the adult worm.

HOOKWORM

Hookworm is a soil-transmitted helminth, one of the important causes of iron deficiency anemia.
- **Pathogens:** Two species are human pathogens; cause intestinal disease
  - *Ancylostoma duodenale*
  - *Necator americanus.*
- **Epidemiology:** Hookworm infection is widespread in the world and also in India. *Necator* infection is more common than *Ancylostoma*
- **Morphology:** Similar to other nematodes, hookworm exist as an adult worm, larvae (four stages—L_1 to L_4), and egg
  - The adult worm is small in size and has a bent in the anterior end (hence called as hookworm)
  - L_1 larva is called as rhabditiform larva whereas L_3 stage larva is called as filariform larva

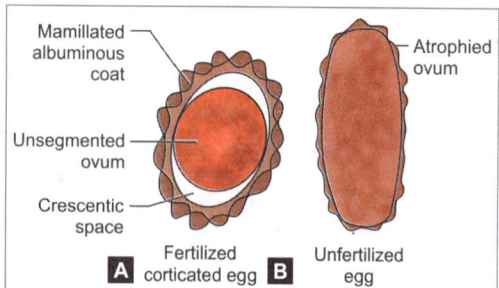

Figs. 33.4A and B: Eggs of *Ascaris lumbricoides*: **A.** Fertilized egg; **B.** Unfertilized egg (schematic diagram).

- *Ancylostoma* and *Necator* can be differentiated by the morphology of adult worm and third stage larva. Eggs of both are morphologically indistinguishable.

Life Cycle (Fig. 33.6)

Hookworm involves only one host (man). Third stage filariform (L_3) larva is the infective form.

- ❖ **Mode of transmission:** Through penetration of the skin by the L_3 larva; during walking barefoot in dampened soil
- ❖ **Migratory phase**: Following penetration, the L_3 larvae are carried to the lungs through venous circulation. From the lungs, they migrate up to the pharynx, and finally, by swallowing of sputum, they enter the GIT
- ❖ **Intestinal phase:** The L_3 larvae molt twice in the small intestine to develop into adult worms, which attach to the intestinal mucosa by their teeth in the buccal capsule. Following fertilization, female worms lay eggs, which are excreted in the feces

- ❖ **Development in soil:** Eggs released in feces become embryonated in soil and subsequently the L_1 (rhabditiform) larvae hatch out from eggs which molt twice to develop into L_3 larvae (infective form). Thus the life cycle is continued.

Clinical Features

Affect due to Migrating Larva

- ❖ Cutaneous lesions: (i) **Ground itch:** pruritic maculopapular rashes at the site of skin penetration; (ii) **serpiginous tracks** may be formed due to subcutaneous migration of the larva
- ❖ Mild transient pneumonitis due to passage of migrating larvae through the lungs.

Affect due to Adult Worm in Intestine

The clinical spectrum produced by adult hookworm depends upon the worm load.

- ❖ **Early intestinal phase (less worm load):** Infected persons may develop epigastric pain, inflammatory diarrhea, etc. accompanied by eosinophilia

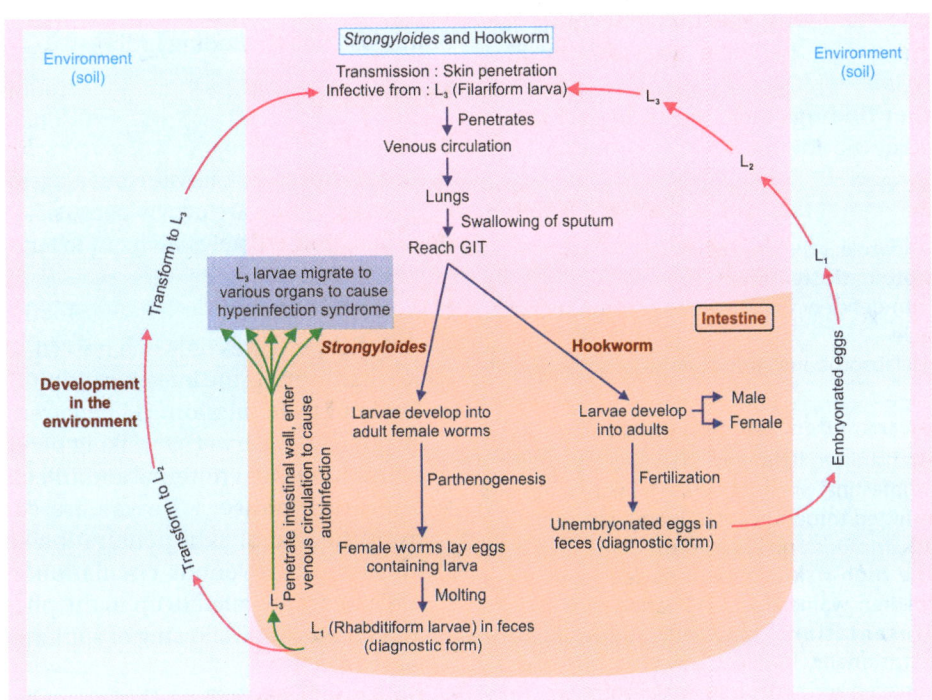

Fig. 33.6: Life cycles of Hookworm and *Strongyloides*.

- **Late intestinal phase** (chronic infection with heavy worm load): Patients develop iron deficiency anemia and protein-energy malnutrition resulting from blood loss.

Laboratory Diagnosis

Following tests are useful to establish the diagnosis:
- **Stool microscopy:** The diagnosis is established by finding characteristic eggs in the feces. Stool concentration procedures may be required to detect eggs in case of lighter infections **(Fig. 33.7)**.
  - Hookworm eggs are not bile stained, oval, measure 60×40 μm, surrounded by thin eggshell.
  - Ovum is segmented; comprises of four blastomeres
  - Presence of clear space between the eggshell and the embryo
  - Floats in saturated salt solution
  - Eggs of both *A. duodenale* and *N. americanus* are morphologically indistinguishable.
- **Molecular diagnosis:** By PCR-based assays targeting specific genes and can differentiate between *Ancylostoma* and *Necator*.
- **Other findings** include—(i) hypochromic microcytic anemia, and (ii) eosinophilia

> **TREATMENT** — Hookworm infections
>
> Albendazole is the drug of choice.
> **Symptomatic treatment**
> - Iron-deficiency anemia with oral iron and folic acid
> - Malabsorption warrants nutritional support.

> **Soil-transmitted Helminth Infections**
>
> Soil-transmitted helminth (STH) infections refer to the intestinal worms infecting humans that are transmitted through contaminated soil such as *Ascaris*, *Trichuris*, and hookworm.
> - **The high-risk groups** include school-age children, women of child-bearing age
> - **Presentation:** Infected children are nutritionally, intellectually, and physically impaired and suffer from malabsorption.
>
> *Contd...*

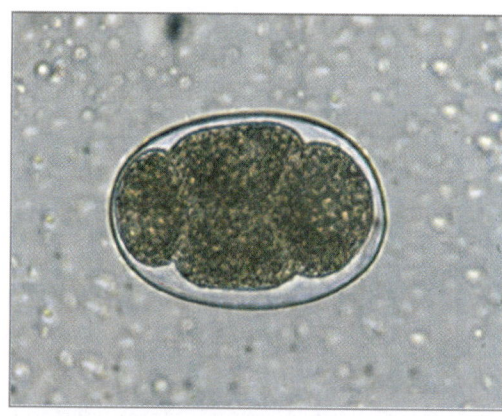

Fig. 33.7: Hookworm egg with four blastomeres.
Source: DPDx Image Library, Centers for Disease Control and Prevention (CDC), Atlanta (with permission).

Contd...

> - **Deworming:** Deworming should be done once or twice a year based on the prevalence of STH infection; single-dose albendazole is given to all children aged 1–19 years.

STRONGYLOIDES STERCORALIS

Strongyloides stercoralis is a small intestinal nematode and is the agent of strongyloidiasis. The disease is particularly common in Southeast Asia (including India).

Morphology

Similar to other nematodes, *S. stercoralis* exists in three forms: adult, larvae (four stages), and egg. *Strongyloides* are ovoviviparous, i.e. eggs once laid, immediately hatch out to larvae.

Life Cycle (Fig. 33.6)

S. stercoralis involves only one host (man). L_3 larva (filariform) is the infective form.
- **Mode of transmission:** (1) Penetration of skin by the L_3 larva (by walking barefoot); (2) Autoinfection (internal autoinfection)
- **Migratory phase:** L_3 larvae are carried from the site of skin penetration to the lungs through venous circulation. From the lungs, they migrate up to the pharynx, and finally, by swallowing of sputum, they enter the GIT
- **Intestinal phase:** The L_3 larvae molt twice in the small intestine to develop into adult

female worms, which are then buried in the intestinal mucosa. However, adult males are not found in the human intestine

- **Laying eggs:** The female worms can directly lay eggs without fertilization, by a process called as **parthenogenesis**
- Being ovoviviparous, eggs immediately hatch out liberating the rhabditiform (L_1) larvae into the intestinal lumen, which are passed in the feces (diagnostic form). Sometimes L_1 larvae are transformed into L_3 larvae and penetrate the intestinal wall to enter into venous circulation to cause autoinfection.
- **Development in the environment:** The L_1 larvae molt twice to form the L_3 larvae. This L_3 larvae are infective stage to man.

Pathogenesis and Clinical Feature

Effect due to Migrating Larva

- **Cutaneous larva migrans:** Migrating larvae may produce the pathognomonic serpiginous urticarial rash (commonly on the thigh) called as **larva currens**
- **Pulmonary symptoms** are uncommon compared to ascariasis and hookworm infection.

Effect due to Adult Worm and Filariform Larva

- **Mild to moderate worm load:** May produce epigastric pain, nausea, diarrhea, constipation, and blood loss
- **Heavy larva load:** Hyperinfection syndrome and disseminated strongyloidiasis are the important complications, observed in heavy larva load **(Table 33.1)**.

Laboratory Diagnosis

Following tests are useful to establish the diagnosis.

- **Stool microscopy:** Stool microscopy reveals the characteristic rhabditiform larvae (diagnostic form) **(Fig. 33.8)**. Repeated stool examination and concentration techniques can be performed to increase the yield.
- **Serology:** Antibody detection by ELISA using crude larval antigens; less sensitive.
- **Coproantigen detection** in stool by antigen capture ELISA.
- **Molecular diagnosis:** By PCR-based assays targeting specific genes in fecal sample is highly specific.

Table 33.1: Complications of strongyloidiasis.

Hyperinfection syndrome

The underlying cause is the repeated autoinfection cycles; which lead to the generation of a large number of filariform larvae.
- **Risk factors:** Impaired host immunity, e.g. glucocorticoid therapy, transplant recipients
- **Features:** Colitis, enteritis, or malabsorption, and in severe cases disseminated strongyloidiasis may develop

Disseminated strongyloidiasis

Larvae may invade the GIT and migrate to various organs.
- **CNS invasion:** Leads to brain abscess and meningitis
- **Passage of enteric flora** through disrupted mucosa leads to gram-negative bacterial sepsis/meningitis
- **The mortality rate** is very high if left untreated

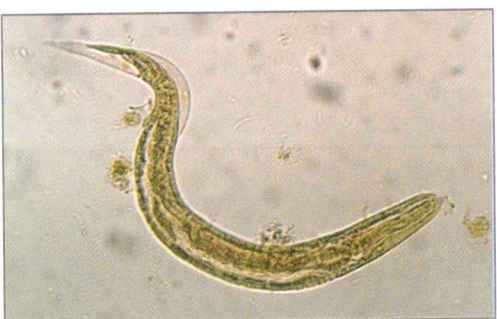

Fig. 33.8: Rhabditiform larva of *Strongyloides stercoralis* (Iodine mount).

Source: Department of Microbiology, Meenakshi Medical College, Chennai (*with permission*).

TREATMENT	Strongyloidiasis

Ivermectin is the drug of choice and is more effective than albendazole.

SECTION 5 ♦ Parasitic Infections

► EXPECTED QUESTIONS ◄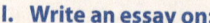

I. Write an essay on:
1. Discuss the life cycle, clinical manifestations and laboratory diagnosis of *Ascaris lumbricoides* infection.
2. Discuss the life cycle, clinical manifestations, and laboratory diagnosis of hookworm infection.

II. Write short notes on:
1. *Enterobius vermicularis* infection
2. *Trichuris trichiura* infection
3. *Strongyloides stercoralis* infection.

III. Multiple Choice Questions (MCQs):
1. **All of the following intestinal nematodes are oviparous, *except*:**
   a. Roundworm
   b. *Strongyloides*
   c. Hookworm
   d. *Enterobius*
2. **Barrel-shaped eggs are seen for:**
   a. Pinworm
   b. Roundworm
   c. Hookworm
   d. Whipworm
3. **Perianal pruritus is seen with infection of:**
   a. Pinworm
   b. Roundworm
   c. Hookworm
   d. Whipworm
4. **Hyperinfection syndrome is seen with infection of:**
   a. Roundworm
   b. *Strongyloides*
   c. Hookworm
   d. *Enterobius*
5. **Larva currens is caused by:**
   a. *Ascaris*
   b. *Enterobius*
   c. *Strongyloides*
   d. *Trichuris*

Answers
1. b   2. d   3. a   4. b   5. c

CHAPTER 34: Tissue Nematode Infections

CHAPTER PREVIEW
- Filarial nematodes
- *Dracunculus medinensis*
- *Trichinella spiralis*
- Larva Migrans

Somatic or tissue nematodes are the group of nematodes that reside in various tissues or organs. Examples include—filarial nematodes, *Dracunculus medinensis* and *Trichinella spiralis*.

FILARIAL NEMATODES

Filarial nematodes are vector-borne parasites that reside in the lymphatic system, skin, subcutaneous tissue, and rarely in body cavities. Accordingly, they cause various types of clinical manifestations in man.
- ❖ **Lymphatic filariasis:** Filarial worms reside in the lymphatics; produce chronic obstruction and fibrosis of lymphatics. Agents include—*Wuchereria bancrofti* and *Brugia malayi*
- ❖ **Cutaneous and ocular filariasis:** The agents include *Loa loa*, *Onchocerca volvulus*, and *Mansonella* species. They reside in the skin, subcutaneous tissues, and some in the eyes and serous cavity. They produce various cutaneous and ocular manifestations.

Morphology

Filarial nematodes are viviparous; exist in two morphological forms: adult worm and larvae (four stages). There is no egg stage.
- ❖ **Filariform larva:** It is the third stage larva; which is the infective form to man
- ❖ **Microfilariae:** They are the first-stage larvae and also the diagnostic form in the blood. They usually reside in pulmonary blood vessels and occasionally come to the peripheral blood at a specific time, according to the '*periodicity of the parasite*'
  - **Nocturnal:** Peak at night (9 pm to 4 am), e.g. *Wuchereria* and *Brugia*
  - **Diurnal:** Peaks at mid-day (12 noon–2.00 pm), e.g. *Loa loa*
  - **Non-periodic:** No periodicity is noticed, e.g. *Onchocerca* and *Mansonella*.

WUCHERERIA BANCROFTI

W. bancrofti is the most widely distributed filarial parasite of humans; accounts for >90% of cases of lymphatic filariasis.

Life Cycle (Fig. 34.1)

W. bancrofti completes its life cycle in two hosts—(i) man (definitive host), and (ii) intermediate hosts are the mosquitoes such as *Culex quinquefasciatus* (principle vector) or rarely *Anopheles* or *Aedes*.

Human Cycle

L_3 filariform larvae (infective form) get deposited in the skin by the mosquito bite.
- ❖ **Develop into adults:** Larvae penetrate the skin, enter into lymphatic vessels and

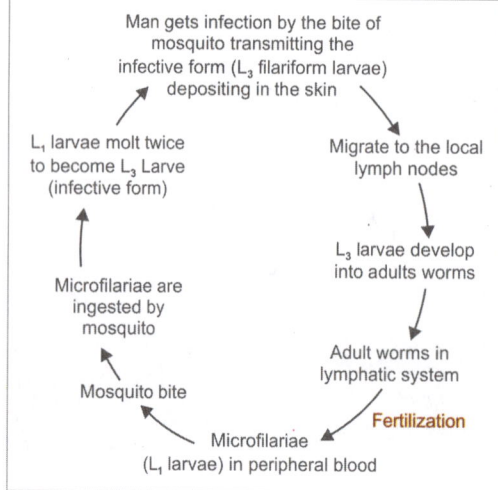

Fig. 34.1: Life cycle of *Wuchereria bancrofti*.

migrate to the local lymph nodes where they molt twice to develop into adult worms
- **Adults lay L_1 larvae:** Adult worms reside in the lymphatics or lymph nodes where undergo fertilization to produce L_1 larvae (**microfilariae**).

Mosquito Cycle

When the mosquito bites an infected man, the microfilariae are ingested. *Culex* bites at night, whereas *Aedes* bites in the daytime. Inside the mosquito, the microfilariae molt twice to develop into L_3 larvae (infective stage to man).

Clinical Features

The incubation period is about 8–16 months. Clinical manifestations can be categorized into: (1) lymphatic filariasis, and (2) tropical pulmonary eosinophilia.

Lymphatic Filariasis

Lymphatic filariasis can occur in two stages.
- **Acute filariasis** (acute adenolymphangitis): It is characterized by recurrent episodes of:
  - Filarial fever (high-grade fever)
  - Lymphatic inflammation (lymphangitis and lymphadenitis)
  - Early pitting edema
  - Dermatolymphangitis: Plaque like lesion is formed over the affected skin with fever, chill, and lymphatic inflammation.
- **Chronic filariasis:** It develops 10–15 years after infection. It results from fibrosis of the lymph vessels leading to severe lymphatic obstruction and pedal edema. The common manifestations are:
  - Elephantiasis: Swelling of lower limb or less commonly arm, vulva, or breast (**Fig. 34.2A**)
  - Hydrocele: Fluid collection in testes (**Fig. 34.2B**)
  - Chronic funiculitis and epididymitis
  - Chyluria: Excretion of a milky white fluid (chyle) in urine, due to rupture of lymph vessels into the urinary system.

Tropical Pulmonary Eosinophilia (TPE)

TPE is also called as occult filariasis, represents a hypersensitivity reaction to microfilaria antigen in lungs.
- **Common features** include nocturnal paroxysmal cough and wheezing weight loss, low-grade fever
- **Diagnosis** is made by eosinophilia, diffuse infiltration (chest X-ray), and elevated serum IgE levels. However, microfilariae are not detected in the peripheral blood
- **Treatment:** It responds well to diethylcarbamazine (DEC).

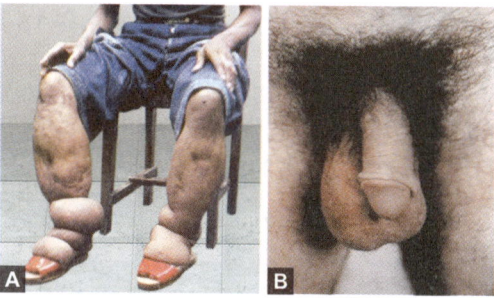

Figs. 34.2A and B: Clinical features of filariasis: **A.** Elephantiasis; **B.** Hydrocele of scrotum.

Source: **A.** ID#-373; **B.** ID# 354, Public Health Image Library, Centers for Disease Control and Prevention (CDC), Atlanta (*with permission*).

Laboratory Diagnosis

Microscopy (To Detect Microfilariae)

Microfilariae can be found in blood, and occasionally in hydrocele fluid, urine, or other body fluids.
- **Methods:** Include (i) direct wet mount, (ii) peripheral blood smear (thick and thin), and (iii) quantitative buffy coat examination (QBC)
- **Collection time:** Should be as per the periodicity of the microfilariae—e.g. for nocturnal periodicity, blood should be collected between 9 pm and 4 am
- **DEC provocation test:** This test is done to collect the blood in the daytime.

Microfilaria (*W. bancrofti*)

Detection of microfilariae in peripheral blood is diagnostic of filariasis **(Figs. 34.4A and B)**.
- It measures 260 µm long, covered by a long hyaline sheath
- The head end is blunt while the tail end is pointed
- The nuclei are large, coarse, and well-separated and present throughout the body except near the tail end
- It differs from the microfilaria of *Brugia malayi* in the head and tail region **(Figs. 34.3 and 34.4)**.

Antigen Detection

Circulating antigens of *W. bancrofti* can be detected by by methods like ELISA and ICT
- **Advantages:** (i) more sensitive than microscopy, (ii) can be detected in the daytime, and (iii) can differentiate the current from past infection
- Not useful for detecting *Brugia* infection.

Antibody Detection

They are useful only for epidemiologic purposes as they cannot differentiate active infection and exposure—e.g. flow-through assay.

Molecular Methods

Molecular methods such as PCR and real-time PCR are available which provide several advantages.
- Can detect low level of parasitemia
- Can differentiate past from present infection
- Useful for monitoring treatment response.

Other Methods

- **Ultrasound:** Serpentine movement of adult worms within the lymphatic vessels of the scrotum, called **filarial dance sign**

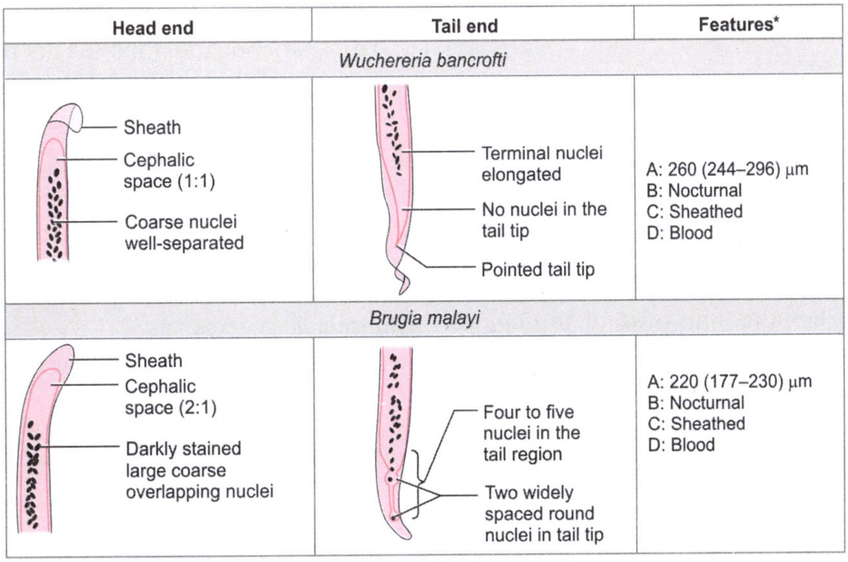

Head end	Tail end	Features*
Wuchereria bancrofti		
Sheath; Cephalic space (1:1); Coarse nuclei well-separated	Terminal nuclei elongated; No nuclei in the tail tip; Pointed tail tip	A: 260 (244–296) µm B: Nocturnal C: Sheathed D: Blood
Brugia malayi		
Sheath; Cephalic space (2:1); Darkly stained large coarse overlapping nuclei	Four to five nuclei in the tail region; Two widely spaced round nuclei in tail tip	A: 220 (177–230) µm B: Nocturnal C: Sheathed D: Blood

*A, Size; B, Periodicity; C, Sheath; D, Habitat

Fig. 34.3: Differences between the microfilaria of *Wuchereria bancrofti* and *Brugia malayi*.

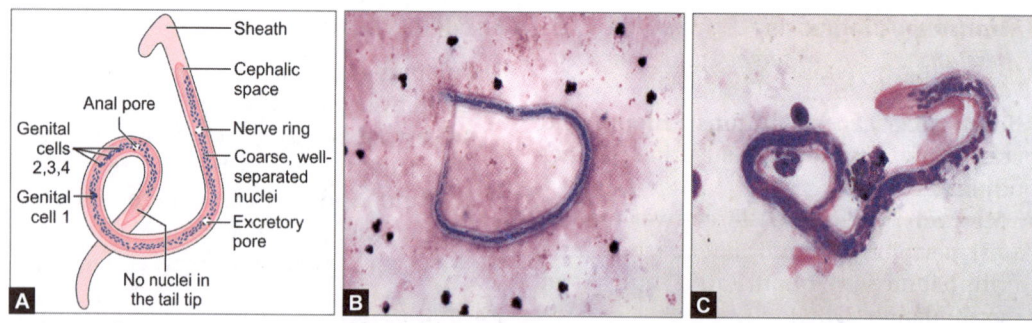

Figs. 34.4A to C: A. Microfilaria of *Wuchereria bancrofti* (schematic); **B and C.** Thick blood smear stained with Giemsa stain showing microfilariae of (B) *Wuchereria bancrofti*; (C) *Brugia* species

Source: **B.** ID# 3009/; **C.** ID# 3003; Dr. Mae Melvin, Public Health Image Library, Centers for Disease Control and Prevention (CDC), Atlanta (*with permission*).

- Eosinophilia and elevated serum IgE
- Urine examination reveals microscopic hematuria and proteinuria.

BRUGIA MALAYI

Brugia malayi accounts for 10% of lymphatic filariasis.
- It occurs primarily in Eastern India and Kerala
- The life cycle of *B. malayi* is similar to *W. bancrofti* except that *Mansonia* is the main vector followed by *Anopheles* and *Aedes*
- **Clinical features** are similar to bancroftian filariasis except:
  - Genital involvement and chyluria are not seen
  - Elephantiasis is limited to the leg below the knee.
- **Detection of microfilaria** of *B. malayi* in peripheral blood confirms the diagnosis. (Figs. 34.3 and 34.4C)
  - Sheathed, measures 220 µm long
  - Nuclei are large, coarse, darkly stained, overlapping, and present throughout the body, extending till the tail region
  - The tail tip is blunt and contains two widely spaced nuclei.

TREATMENT	Lymphatic filariasis

- Diethylcarbamazine (DEC) and albendazole are recommended in Indian cases
- Ivermectin is used only in Africa, but not in India.

- **Antibody detection methods:** ELISA and ICT methods are used under the filariasis control program.

Elimination of Lymphatic Filariasis (ELF)

It is a global program to eliminate lymphatic filariasis by the year 2020. However, till date, only 16 countries achieved the LF elimination status.
- **MDA strategy:** WHO recommends mass drug administration (MDA) once a year to all people at-risk in the endemic areas for five years
- **MDA regimen:** Single dose of DEC (6 mg/kg) + albendazole (400 mg) is the MDA regimen of choice.

CUTANEOUS FILARIASIS

There are many other filarial nematodes which reside in skin and subcutaneous tissue producing several cutaneous manifestations—*Loa loa, Onchocerca volvulus*, and *Mansonella* species.
- ***Loa loa:*** It is also called an African eye worm. *Chrysops* species (deer flies) are the vectors. It produces subcutaneous swelling of the knee or wrist (called **Calabar swelling**)
- ***Onchocerca volvulus:*** It is transmitted by the bite of *Simulium* (black flies). It affects skin (dermatitis) and eyes (river blindness)

- **Mansonella:** Important species are— *M. perstans*, *M. streptocerca*, and *M. ozzardi*. *Culicoides* (midges) are the main vector. They produce skin lesions like pruritic rashes, swelling, etc.

Diagnosis of cutaneous filariasis is made by detection of characteristic microfilariae in skin snip smear or blood. DEC or ivermectin are given for treatment.

DRACUNCULUS MEDINENSIS

Dracunculus medinensis causes **Guinea worm disease** or **dracunculiasis**, characterized by cutaneous painful blisters in the lower legs. It is on the verge of eradication, currently endemic only to 3-4 countries in sub-Saharan Africa (e.g. Chad).

TRICHINELLA SPIRALIS

Trichinella spiralis is a zoonotic infection of pigs.
- **Transmission:** Man is an accidental host, acquires infection by ingestion of uncooked pork containing infective form L_1 larvae
- **Clinical features:** Ingested L_1 larvae are released from pig meat in the intestine and are carried to skeletal muscles, where they become encysted (*muscle encystment*). Common symptoms are myositis, muscle edema, and weakness (myalgia)
- **Diagnosis** is made by the demonstration of larvae in muscle biopsy (e.g. gastrocnemius, deltoid)
- **Treatment:** Mebendazole or albendazole is given.

LARVA MIGRANS

Larva migrans refer to the lesions produced by nematodes of lower animals when they accidentally infect man.

Arrested Life Cycle and Pathogenesis

There are a number of nematodes of lower animals for which humans are an abnormal accidental host.
- Larvae of these nematodes when accidentally infect man, and their life cycle gets arrested. The larvae wander aimlessly in the body. This is called as larva migrans (LM)
- It occurs in two forms—cutaneous and visceral.

Cutaneous Larva Migrans

Also called as **creeping eruption**. Larva migration occurs in the skin and subcutaneous tissue, following which the life cycle gets arrested.
- It is mainly caused by nonhuman hookworm species such as *Ancylostoma brasiliensis*, *A. caninum*, and *A. ceylanicum*
- Rarely, can be caused by human nematodes such as *Strongyloides stercoralis* (larva currens), *Ancylostoma duodenale*, and *Necator americanus* (ground itch).

Visceral Larva Migrans

Larva migrates to viscera, following which the life cycle gets arrested. It is caused by various nematodes of lower animals such as:
- *Toxocara canis*: Infects liver (hepatomegaly) and other organs. It can also infect eyes (ocular larva migrans)
- *Angiostrongylus cantonensis:* Infects CNS and causes eosinophilic meningitis.

EXPECTED QUESTIONS

I. **Write short notes on:**
  1. Lymphatic filariasis.
  2. Larva migrans.

II. **Multiple Choice Questions (MCQs):**
  1. **Lymphatic filariasis is caused by:**
     a. *Loa loa*
     b. *Wuchereria*
     c. *Onchocerca*
     d. *Mansonella*
  2. **Causative agent of Calabar swelling is:**
     a. *Loa loa*
     b. *Wuchereria*
     c. *Onchocerca*
     d. *Mansonella*

Answers
1. b   2. a

Deworming infants, children and women for better health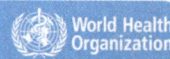

Intestinal parasitic worms (soil-transmitted helminths) are spread through soil, contaminated by human faeces.

Worm infections interfere with children's nutritional uptake and can result in malnourishment, anaemia, and stunted growth.

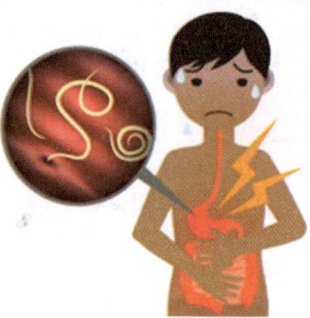

Periodic treatment of at-risk populations reduces the intensity of infection. No individual diagnosis is needed.

Treatment with what?
Free deworming medicines such as albendazole or mebendazole

Why treat everyone?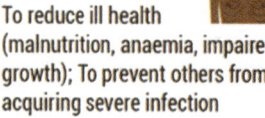
To reduce ill health (malnutrition, anaemia, impaired growth); To prevent others from acquiring severe infection

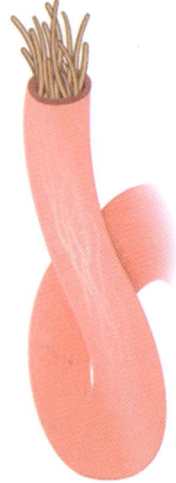

Who should be treated?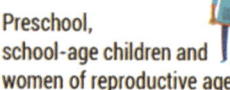
Preschool, school-age children and women of reproductive age

Where can treatment be sought?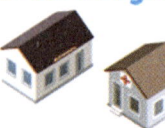
Schools and community health centres

Global target: To reach 75% of children in need of treatment by 2020

SECTION 6: Fungal Infections

SECTION OUTLINE

35. Medical Mycology

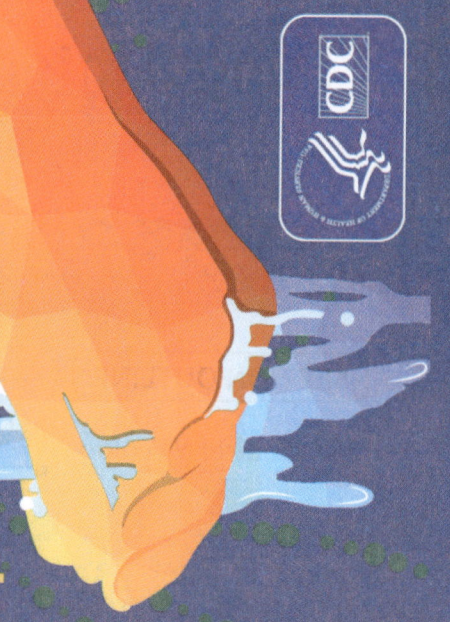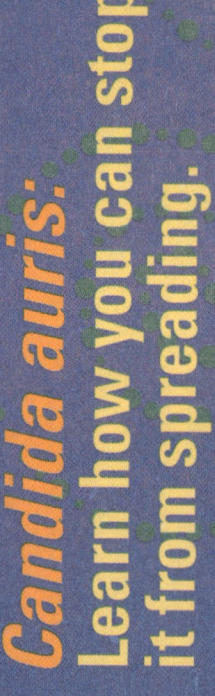

CHAPTER 35

Medical Mycology

CHAPTER PREVIEW

- Superficial Mycoses
- Subcutaneous Mycoses
- Systemic (Deep) Mycoses
- Opportunistic Mycoses

Fungal infections can be classified into four groups based on the organ/system involved and clinical manifestations produced: superficial mycoses, subcutaneous mycoses, systemic (deep) mycoses, and opportunistic mycoses.

SUPERFICIAL MYCOSES

These are fungal infections involving the skin, hair, nail, and mucosa. Examples include—tinea versicolor, tinea nigra, piedra, and dermatophytosis.

Tinea Versicolor

It is a chronic recurrent condition involving the superficial layer of skin, caused by *Malassezia furfur*.

- **Clinical feature:** Manifests as scaly patches of non-pruritic hypopigmented lesions on the skin **(Fig. 35.1)**. It also causes *dandruff* in adults (erythematous pruritic scaly lesions of the scalp)
- **Direct microscopy:** Skin scrapings are examined microscopically after treating with 10% KOH. A mixture of budding yeasts and short septate hyphae are seen, described as **spaghetti and meatballs** appearance
- **Culture:** On Sabouraud dextrose agar (SDA), *Malassezia furfur* typically produces '**fried egg**' colonies

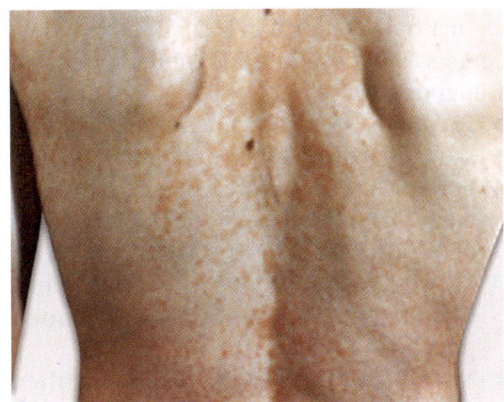

Fig. 35.1: Tinea versicolor (hypopigmented patches).

- **Treatment:** Topical lotions like selenium sulfide shampoo, ketoconazole shampoo or cream, and terbinafine cream should be used for 2 weeks.

Tinea Nigra

It is characterized by painless, black, non-scaly patches present on the palm and sole. It is caused by *Hortaea werneckii*. It is a black-colored yeast-like fungus.

Piedra

Piedra is characterized by nodule formation on the hair shaft, which may be either black or white in color. Accordingly, piedra is of two types.

- White piedra: Caused by *Trichosporon beigelii*
- Black piedra: Caused by *Piedraia hortae*.

Dermatophytoses

Dermatophytoses (or tinea or ringworm) is the most common superficial mycoses affecting skin, hair, and nail; caused by a group of related fungi called **dermatophytes**. These include:

- *Trichophyton* species: Infect skin, hair, and nail
- *Microsporum* species: Infect skin and hair
- *Epidermophyton* species: Infect skin and nail.

Pathogenesis and Clinical Types

Dermatophyte infection is acquired by direct contact with soil, animals, or humans infected with fungal spores.

- **Predisposing factors** include moist humid skin and tight ill-fitting underclothing
- **Spread:** The spores are carried to different areas (skin, hair, or nail) due to scratching of the inoculated site
- **Skin:** Dermatophytes produce well-demarcated annular- or ring-shaped pruritic scaly skin lesions
- **Nails:** They invade the nails and then spread throughout the nails
- **Hair shafts:** They can invade within the hair shaft (called endothrix) or may be found surrounding it (called ectothrix). Hair becomes brittle and areas of alopecia may appear
- **Clinical types:** Depending on the site of involvement, various clinical types of ringworm infections are produced (**Table 35.1**). The incubation period is about 1–2 weeks.

Laboratory Diagnosis

Specimen Collection

Skin scrapings, hair pluckings, and nail clippings are obtained from the active margin of the lesions and are kept in folded black paper. Hair should be plucked, but not cut.

Table 35.1: Clinical types of dermatophytoses.

Clinical types	Area involved
Tinea capitis (Fig. 35.2A)	Infection of the scalp, producing scaly patches on the scalp, and broken hair shafts (alopecia)
Tinea faciei	Infection of the non-bearded area of the face (Fig. 35.2B)
Tinea pedis	Infection of the web space between the toes (also called athlete's foot) (Fig. 35.2C)
Tinea corporis	Infection of the non-hairy skin of the body (trunk and limbs) (Fig. 35.2D)
Tinea cruris	Infection of the groin area (called jock itch)
Tinea barbae	Infection of the beard area of the face
Tinea unguium	Infection of nail beds

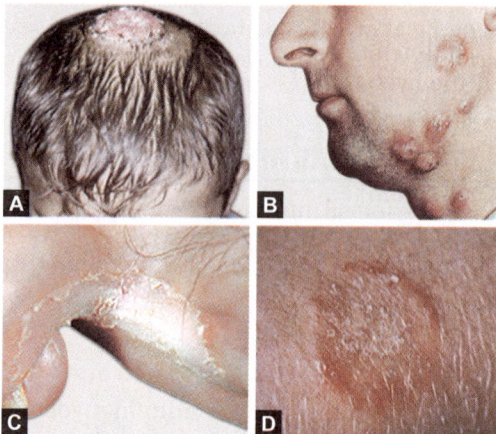

Figs. 35.2A to D: Ring worm infections (tinea): **A.** Tinea capitis; **B.** Tinea faciei; **C.** Tinea pedis; **D.** Tinea corporis.

Source: Public Health Image Library: **A.** ID#: 2936; **B.** ID#: 4807; **C.** ID#: 2939; **D.** ID#: 2938 Centers for Disease Control and Prevention (CDC), Atlanta (*with permission*).

Culture

Specimens should be inoculated onto SDA and incubated at 26–28°C for 4 weeks. Identification is made by:

- Macroscopic appearance of the colonies
- Microscopic appearance: The colonies are teased and subjected to lactophenol

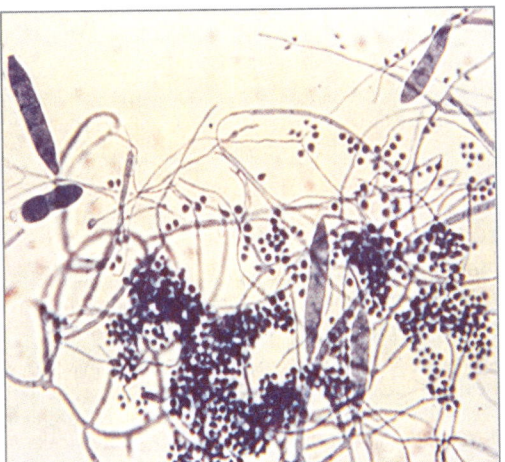

Fig. 35.3: Microscopic appearance (LPCB mount) of *Trichophyton* species demonstrating macroconidia and macroconidia.

Source: Public Health Image Library/ID#: 15105; Centers for Disease Control and Prevention (CDC), Atlanta (*with permission*).

cotton blue (LPCB) mount to demonstrate the hyphae and spores. Spores are of two types—macroconidia and macroconidia, which help in identification **(Fig. 35.3)**.

Other Methods of Diagnosis

Apart from culture, there are several other methods available for the identification of dermatophytes such as:
- Hair perforation test
- Urease test
- Dermatophyte test medium
- Dermatophyte identification medium
- Molecular methods such as polymerase chain reaction (PCR)
- Woods lamp examination.

> **TREATMENT** — Dermatophytoses
> - **Oral terbinafine or itraconazole** are the drugs of choice for the treatment of dermatophytosis
> - Alternative: Oral griseofulvin and ketoconazole
> - Topical lotion such as Whitfield ointment or tolnaftate can be applied.

SUBCUTANEOUS MYCOSES

The agents of subcutaneous mycoses usually inhabit the soil. They enter the skin by traumatic inoculation with contaminated material.

Mycetoma

Mycetoma is a chronic, slowly progressive granulomatous infection of the skin and subcutaneous tissues.
- Mycetoma is also known as **Maduramycosis** or **Madura foot,** as it was first described in Madurai
- **Types**: Mycetoma can be classified into two types, based on the etiological agent and color of granules
  - **Eumycetoma:** Caused by fungal agents such as *Madurella mycetomatis* (produces black granules)
  - **Actinomycetoma:** Caused by bacteria such as *Nocardia* species (produces white granules).

Clinical Features

It manifests as a triad of painless subcutaneous swelling, discharging sinuses, and discharge oozing from the sinuses containing granules.
- Eumycetoma produces single swelling with serous discharge and whereas in actinomycetoma the swellings are multiple with purulent discharge
- Feet are the most common site affected, although any site can be involved **(Fig. 35.4)**

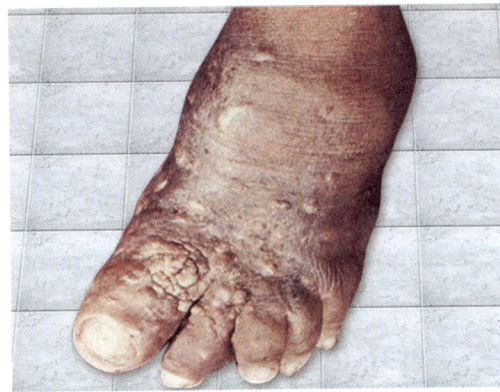

Fig. 35.4: Mycetoma of the foot.

Source: Public Health Image Library/ID#: 14816/Centers for Disease Control and Prevention (CDC), Atlanta (*with permission*).

- Can invade underlying fascia and bones, producing osteolytic or osteosclerotic bony lesions.

Laboratory Diagnosis

- **Specimen collection:** The lesions should be cleaned with antiseptics and the grains should be collected on sterile gauze by pressing the sinuses from the periphery or by using a loop
- **Direct examination:** Granules are thoroughly washed in sterile saline; crushed between the slides and examined
- **For suspected eumycetoma:** The black granules are subjected to KOH mount, which reveals thin septate hyphae of 2–6 μm width
- **If actinomycetoma is suspected:** The white granules are subjected to—(1) Gram staining which reveals filamentous gram-positive bacilli; or (2) modified acid-fast stain (*Nocardia* is partially acid-fast)
- **Culture:** Granules obtained from deep biopsies are the best specimen for culture as they contain live organisms. Both fungal (e.g. SDA) and bacteriological media (such as Lowenstein-Jensen media) should be included in the panel.

> **TREATMENT** — **Mycetoma**
>
> Consists of surgical removal of the lesion followed by use of:
> - For eumycetoma: Antifungal agents such as itraconazole or amphotericin B or
> - For actinomycetoma: Antibiotics such as Welsh regimen (amikacin plus cotrimoxazole).

Sporotrichosis

Sporotrichosis or Rose Gardner's disease is presented as a subcutaneous granulomatous disease; caused by *Sporothrix schenckii*.

- **Transmission:** Spores are introduced into the skin following minor trauma such as thorn prick, etc.
- **Clinical features:** It presents as noduloulcerative lesions (painless), which spread along the lymphatics
- **Diagnosis:** *S. schenckii* is a dimorphic fungus, that presents in two forms **(Figs. 35.5A and B):**

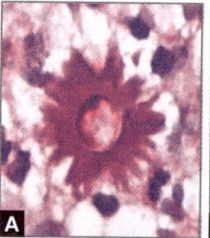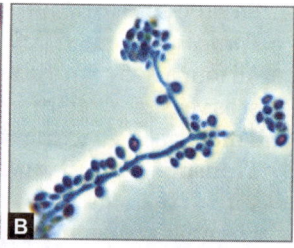

Figs. 35.5A and B: *Sporothrix schenckii:* **A.** Yeast form (asteroid body); **B.** Mold form showing thin septate hyphae with flower-like sporulation.

Source: **A.** Dr Manoj Singh and Dr M Ramam, AIIMS, New Delhi; **B.** Public Health Image Library/Dr Libero Ajello B. ID#: 4208/Centers for Disease Control and Prevention (CDC), Atlanta (*with permission*).

- Yeast form at 37°C: Described as cigar-shaped asteroid bodies in tissue sections stained by histopathological stains
- Mold form at 25°C: LPCB mount of SDA culture shows thin septate hyphae with flower-like sporulation.
- **Treatment:** Itraconazole is the drug of choice, except for the disseminated form where amphotericin B is recommended.

Rhinosporidiosis

It is characterized by large friable polyps in the nose.

- Caused by *Rhinosporidium seeberi*
- Stagnant water is the main source of infection
- **Diagnosis** is made by histopathology of the polyps that demonstrates **spherules** (large sporangia containing numerous endospores). It is not cultivable and does not grow in culture
- **Treatment:** Radical surgery with cauterization is the mainstay of treatment.

SYSTEMIC (DEEP) MYCOSES

Systemic mycoses include the four important fungal diseases that involve multiple organs.
1. Histoplasmosis, caused by *Histoplasma capsulatum*
2. Blastomycosis, caused by *Blastomyces dermatitidis*
3. Coccidioidomycosis, caused by *Coccidioides immitis*

4. Paracoccidioidomycosis, caused by *Paracoccidioides braziliensis*.

All four agents are **dimorphic fungi**, which exist as yeast at 37°C (inside the human body) and mold at 25°C (in the environment).

- **Transmission:** They are saprophytic fungi, spread by inhalation of spores leading to pulmonary infection
- **Spread:** In the lungs, the mold form transforms into the yeast form. Then the yeasts form disseminate to cause various systemic manifestations.

Histoplasmosis

Histoplasma capsulatum is widely prevalent, but particularly endemic in USA.

- **Clinical manifestations:** Various clinical forms are:
  - Pulmonary histoplasmosis: It is the most common form
  - Mucocutaneous histoplasmosis: Skin and oral mucosal lesions
  - Disseminated histoplasmosis may occur in patients with low immunity. The common sites are bone marrow, spleen, liver, eyes, etc.
- **Laboratory diagnosis:** Useful specimens include sputum, bone marrow aspirate, blood, etc.
  - Histopathological staining of the specimens reveals tiny oval yeast cells (2–4 μm size) with narrow-based budding
  - Culture on SDA yields mycelial forms at 25°C (described as tuberculate macroconidia) and yeast form (creamy white colonies) at 37°C.
- **Treatment:** Amphotericin B is the drug of choice.

Blastomycosis

Blastomycosis is also endemic in North America, caused by *Blastomyces dermatitidis*.

- **Clinical manifestations:** Acute pulmonary blastomycosis is the most common form. Other sites involved are skin, bone (osteomyelitis), CNS (brain abscess)
- **Histopathological staining** of the tissue biopsy specimens reveals thick-walled round yeast cells of 8–15 μm size with single broad-based budding (Figure of 8 appearance)
- **Culture media** such as SDA, yields are mycelial form at 25°C and yeast at 37°C (dimorphic fungi)
- **Treatment:** Amphotericin B is the drug of choice.

Coccidioidomycosis

It is also called desert rheumatism or Valley fever, caused by a dimorphic fungus, *Coccidioides immitis*.

- **Clinical manifestations:** Pulmonary infection is the most common form. Rarely disseminated form may be seen involving skin, bone, joints, soft tissues, and meninges
- **Histopathological staining** of sputum or tissue biopsy specimens demonstrates **spherules** which are large sac-like structures (20–80 μm size), filled with endospores
- **Cultures** on SDA produce mycelial growth, described as fragmented hyphae consisting of **barrel-shaped arthrospores**
- **Treatment:** Azoles such as itraconazole are the drug of choice to treat most cases.

Paracoccidioidomycosis

It is a systemic disease caused by the dimorphic fungus—*Paracoccidioides brasiliensis*. It is endemic in South America.

- **Clinical manifestations:** It occurs in two major forms—disseminated infection in young adults or pulmonary infection in older men
- **Histopathological staining** of pus, tissue biopsies, or sputum reveals round thick-walled yeasts, with multiple narrow-necked buds attached circumferentially giving rise to **Mickey mouse or pilot wheel** appearance
- **Culture** on SDA yields mycelial form at 25°C which converts into yeast phase at 37°C when grown in BHI agar supplemented with blood and glutamine
- **Treatment:** Amphotericin B is the drug of choice.

OPPORTUNISTIC MYCOSES

Opportunistic mycoses include the fungal infections which usually occur in immunocompromised patients, such as:
- Candidiasis
- Cryptococcal meningitis
- Zygomycoses
- Aspergillosis
- Penicillosis
- *Pneumocystis jirovecii* pneumonia.

Candidiasis

Candidiasis is the most common fungal disease in humans; caused by *Candida*, a yeast-like fungus that produces pseudohyphae. Various species of *Candida* include:
- *Candida albicans:* It is the most pathogenic species of *Candida* infecting humans
- Other *Candida* species that can also cause infection are *C. tropicalis* (the most common species), *C. glabrata*, *C. krusei*, *C. parapsilosis*, and *C. auris*.

Predisposing Factors

Predisposing factors that are associated with increased risk of infection with *Candida* include:
- **Physiological state:** Extremes of age (infancy, old age), pregnancy
- **Low immunity:** Patients on steroid or immunosuppressive drugs, post-transplantation, malignancy, HIV-infected people
- Patients on **broad-spectrum antibiotics**—suppress the normal flora
- **Others:** Diabetes mellitus, febrile neutropenia, and zinc or iron deficiency.

Clinical Manifestations

Candida species produce a spectrum of infections ranging from skin and mucosal infections to invasive infections.
- **Invasive candidiasis:** It results from the hematogenous or local spread of the fungi. Various forms are:
    - Urinary tract infection
    - Pulmonary candidiasis
    - Septicemia and meningitis
    - Arthritis and osteomyelitis
    - Ocular—keratoconjunctivitis and endophthalmitis
    - Disseminated candidiasis
    - Nosocomial candidiasis (*C. auris* and *C. glabrata*).
- **Mucosal candidiasis:** The various mucosal manifestations include:
    - Oropharyngeal candidiasis (oral thrush): It presents as white, adherent, painless patches in the mouth **(Fig. 35.6A)**
    - Vulvovaginitis: It is characterized by pruritus, pain, and vaginal discharge that is usually thin, but may become whitish curd like in severe cases
    - Esophageal candidiasis: Common in HIV-infected persons.
- **Cutaneous candidiasis:** The cutaneous manifestations seen in candidiasis are intertrigo (pustules in the skin folds) and nail infections such as paronychia and onychomycosis **(Fig. 35.6B)**.

Laboratory Diagnosis

- **Direct microscopy:** Gram-positive oval budding yeast cells with pseudohyphae **(Fig. 35.7A)**
- **Culture on SDA:** Produces creamy white and pasty colonies **(Fig. 35.7B)**
- **Tests for species identification:**
    - Germ tube test (positive for *C. albicans*)
    - Dalmau plate culture for chlamydospore production
    - CHROMagar: Different *Candida* species produce different colored colonies on CHROMagar
    - Growth at 45°C (positive for *C. albicans*)

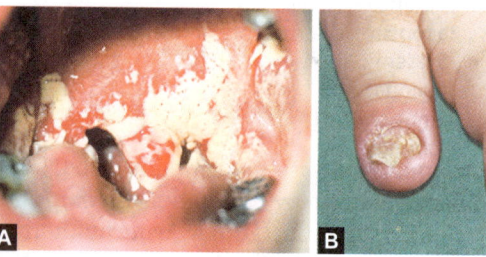

Figs. 35.6A and B: Candidiasis: **A.** Oral thrush; **B.** Onychomycosis.

Source: Public Health Image Library/**A.** ID#: 1217; **B.** Mr Gust, ID#: 15669/Centers for Disease Control and Prevention (CDC), Atlanta (*with permission*).

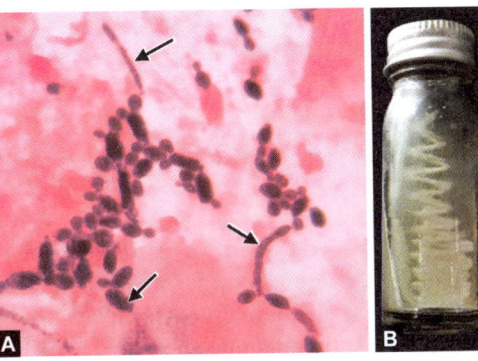

Figs. 35.7A and B: A. *Candida albicans*—gram-positive oval budding yeast cells with pseudohyphae; **B.** SDA shows creamy white colonies.
Source: Department of Microbiology, Pondicherry Institute of Medical Sciences, Puducherry (*with permission*).

- Carbohydrate assimilation and fermentation tests
- Automated identification systems, e.g. MALDI-TOF and VITEK
- Molecular methods such as PCR detecting genes specific to various *Candida* species.
❖ **Immunodiagnosis:**
  - Antibody detection against cell wall mannan antigen
  - Antigen detection such as cell wall mannan antigen
  - Enzyme detection, e.g. enolase
  - β-D-glucan assay: It is a marker of invasive fungal infections and can be used for monitoring treatment response.

TREATMENT — Candidiasis

The antifungal drugs given depend upon the type of infection.
- Cutaneous candidiasis: The drug of choice is a topical azole
- Systemic candidiasis: Drugs given are oral fluconazole, voriconazole or caspofungin or amphotericin B

C. glabrata, C. krusei and *C. auris* exhibit resistance to azoles; therefore, should be treated with caspofungin or amphotericin B.

Cryptococcal Meningitis

Cryptococcal meningitis is potentially fatal meningitis, caused by a capsulated yeast called *Cryptococcus neoformans*.

Pathogenesis

Infection is acquired by inhalation of yeast cells.
❖ **Spread:** First, it infects the lungs and subsequently disseminates through the blood to various organs such as CNS, bones, and skin
❖ **Virulence factor:** Polysaccharide capsule is the principal virulence factor of the fungus. It is anti-phagocytic in nature
❖ **Risk factors:** Individuals at high risk for cryptococcosis include:
  - Patients with advanced HIV infection
  - Patients with hematologic malignancies
  - Transplant recipients
  - Patients on immunosuppressive or steroid therapy.

Clinical Manifestations

Various clinical manifestations of cryptococcosis include:
❖ Pulmonary cryptococcosis: It is the first and the most common presentation
❖ Cryptococcal meningitis: It presents as chronic meningitis, with headache, fever, sensory and memory loss, cranial nerve paresis, and loss of vision (due to optic nerve involvement)
❖ Others: Skin lesions and osteolytic bone lesions.

Laboratory Diagnosis

Specimens such as CSF, blood, or skin scrapings can be collected.
❖ **Negative staining:** Modified India ink stain is used to demonstrate the capsule, which appears as refractile delineated clear space surrounding the round budding yeast cells against a black background (**Fig. 35.8A**)
❖ **Gram staining** may show gram-positive round budding yeast cells
❖ **Antigen detection:** The capsular antigens can be detected from CSF or serum by latex agglutination test. It is a rapid and sensitive and specific method
❖ **Culture:** CSF is inoculated onto SDA, blood agar, or chocolate agar and incubated at 37°C. Blood culture is also performed

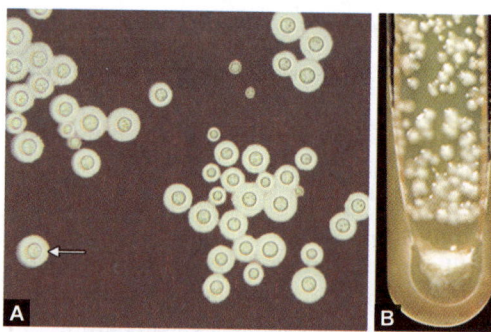

Figs. 35.8A and B: *Cryptococcus neoformans:* **A.** India ink staining shows clear refractile capsules surrounding round budding yeast cells (arrow showing); **B.** Growth on SDA at 37°C—shows creamy white mucoid colonies.

Source: Public Health Image Library/**A.** Dr Leanor Haley, ID#:3771 **B.** Dr William Kaplan, ID#:3199/Centers for Disease Control and Prevention (CDC), Atlanta (*with permission*).

in addition. Colonies appear as mucoid creamy white and yeast-like **(Fig. 35.8B)**.

> **TREATMENT** — **Cryptococcosis**
>
> Treatment depends upon the type of cryptococcosis.
> - Cryptococcosis without CNS involvement: Fluconazole is the drug of choice
> - HIV-infected patients with CNS involvement: The regimen is an induction phase (amphotericin B ± flucytosine) followed by oral fluconazole therapy.

Zygomycosis

Zygomycosis (or mucormycosis) is a life-threatening infection caused by a group of aseptate fungi called Zygomycetes. Common agents are *Rhizopus* and *Mucor*.

Pathogenesis

Zygomycetes are found ubiquitously in the environment. Transmission to man occurs via inhalation or inoculation of spores.
- **Spread**: Spores develop into a mycelial form containing wide aseptate hyphae. The hyphae are angioinvasive resulting in the spread of infection
- **Predisposing factors:** Common conditions that increase the risk of mucormycosis include **diabetic ketoacidosis** (most common), end-stage renal disease, and patients taking iron therapy, etc.

Clinical Manifestations

Mucormycosis manifest in various clinical forms.
- **Rhinocerebral mucormycosis**: It is the most common form; presents as orbital cellulitis, proptosis, and vision loss
- **Pulmonary mucormycosis**: It occurs in patients with leukemia
- **Other forms:** Cutaneous, gastrointestinal, and disseminated mucormycosis.

Laboratory Diagnosis

- **Histopathological staining** of tissue biopsies shows broad aseptate hyaline hyphae
- **Culture on SDA at 25°C:** Reveals characteristic white cottony woolly colonies which become brown-black later, due to sporulation giving rise to **salt and pepper** appearance **(Fig. 35.9A)**
- **Microscopic appearance:** LPCB mount of the colonies reveals broad aseptate hyaline hyphae, sporangiophore ending at sporangium, and a root-like growth arising from hyphae, called rhizoids **(Fig. 35.9B)**. In *Mucor*, rhizoids are absent.

> **TREATMENT** — **Zygomycosis**
>
> Amphotericin B remains the drug of choice for mucormycosis. Posaconazole or isavuconazole can be given alternatively.

Aspergillosis

Aspergillosis is a group of invasive fungal diseases caused by a hyaline mold named *Aspergillus*. The important pathogens are— *A. fumigatus, A. flavus* and *A. niger*.

Pathogenesis

Aspergillus is widely distributed in nature. Transmission to man occurs by inhalation of airborne conidia. Risk factors for invasive aspergillosis are:
- Glucocorticoid use (the most important risk factor)

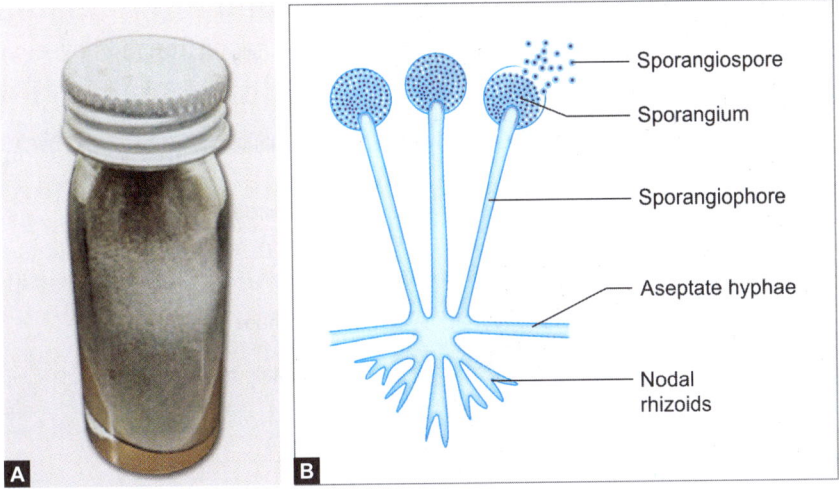

Figs. 35.9A and B: *Rhizopus:* **A.** Colonies on SDA show white cottony woolly colonies with black spores (salt and pepper appearance); **B.** Microscopic schematic diagram.
Source: **A.** Department of Microbiology, Pondicherry Institute of Medical Sciences, Puducherry (*with permission*).

- Profound neutropenia
- Neutrophil dysfunction
- Underlying pneumonia, chronic obstructive pulmonary disease, tuberculosis or sarcoidosis
- Transplant recipients.

Clinical Manifestations

Depending upon the site of involvement, *Aspergillus* produces various clinical manifestations such as:
- **Pulmonary aspergillosis:** It is the most common form of aspergillosis; includes various manifestations like:
  - Allergic bronchopulmonary aspergillosis (ABPA)
  - Severe bronchial asthma
  - Aspergilloma (fungal ball) in lungs
  - Invasive pulmonary aspergillosis.
- **Other forms** of aspergillosis include:
  - Invasive sinusitis
  - Systemic infection: Endocarditis, brain abscess
  - Ocular infection: Keratitis and endophthalmitis
  - Ear infection: Otitis externa
  - Cutaneous aspergillosis
  - Nail bed infection: Onychomycosis
  - Mycotoxicosis: Various *Aspergillus* species produce several fungal toxins, e.g. *A. flavus* produces aflatoxin, which causes liver carcinoma.

Laboratory Diagnosis

Useful specimens such as sputum and tissue biopsies, etc.
- **Direct microscopy:** KOH (10%) mount (**Figs. 5.2A**, Chapter 5) or histopathological staining of specimens reveals characteristic narrow septate hyaline hyphae with acute angle branching
- **Culture:** Specimens are inoculated onto SDA and incubated at 25°C. Species identification is done based on the macroscopic and microscopic (LPCB mount) appearance of the colonies. For example, *Aspergillus fumigatus* shows the following features:
  - *Colonies on SDA*: Produces smoky green, velvety to powdery colonies (**Fig. 35.10A**)
  - *LPCB mount:* Shows a conical-shaped vesicle, single row of phialides and conidia arise from the upper third of the vesicle (**Fig. 35.10B**).
- **Antigen detection:** Enzyme immunoassays are available to detect antigens such as:
  - β-D-glucan antigen assay: Raised in any invasive fungal infections including aspergillosis
  - Galactomannan antigen: Specific for *Aspergillus*.

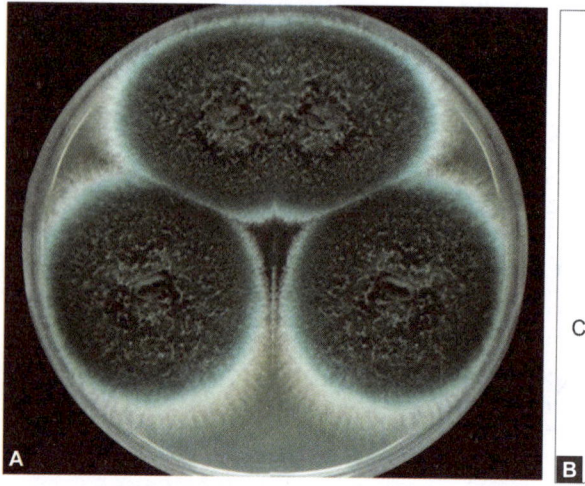
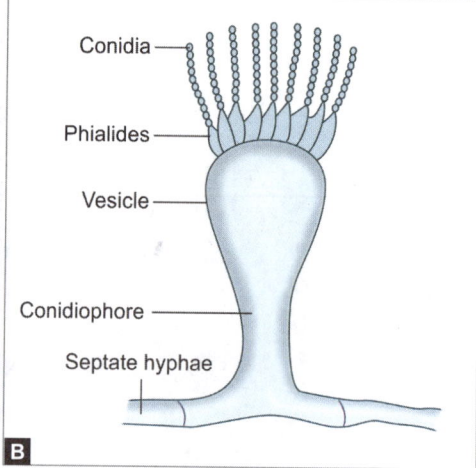

Figs. 35.10A and B: *Aspergillus fumigatus:* **A.** Smoky green, velvety to powdery colonies on SDA; **B.** Schematic microscopic picture.
Source: Department of Microbiology, Pondicherry Institute of Medical Sciences, Puducherry (*with permission*).

> **TREATMENT** — **Aspergillosis**
>
> Following are the first-line treatment recommended in different forms of aspergillosis.
> - For invasive aspergillosis—voriconazole is the drug of choice
> - For ABPA—itraconazole is the drug of choice.

Penicilliosis

Penicilliosis denotes the group of infections caused by pathogenic *Penicillium* species.
- *Penicillium marneffei*: It is a dimorphic fungus, that produces wart-like skin lesions (discussed below)
- Other *Penicillium* species are usually found in the environment. Rarely they are associated with human diseases such as otomycosis, keratitis, and allergic disease like asthma.

Laboratory Diagnosis

Except for *P. marneffei* which is a dimorphic fungus, all other *Penicillium* species occur only as molds, and can grow easily on SDA at 25°C.
- **Colonies** are rapidly growing, flat with velvety to powdery texture, and greenish in color **(Fig. 35.11A)**
- **Microscopic appearance:** LPCB mount of the colonies reveals hyaline thin septate hyphae, and the vesicles are absent. The conidiophore and its branches give rise to elongated metulae, from which flask-shaped phialides originate which bear a chain of conidia. Such an arrangement is called as **brush border appearance (Fig. 35.11B)**.

Penicillium Marneffei Infection

Penicillium marneffei (new name *Talaromyces marneffei*) is a dimorphic fungus that causes opportunistic infection in HIV-infected patients.
- **Clinical features:** It produces both systemic infection and skin lesions (described as warty lesions mimicking molluscum contagiosum)
- **Histopathological staining** of tissue sections and skin scrapings shows oval yeast cells with central septation
- **Culture:** *P. marneffei* being dimorphic; produces yeast-like colonies at 37°C and mold form at 25°C. The mold form has a characteristic **brick red pigment**
- **Treatment:** AIDS patients with severe penicilliosis are treated with amphotericin B.

PNEUMOCYSTIS PNEUMONIA

Pneumocystis pneumonia has been increasingly reported after the discovery of HIV/AIDS.

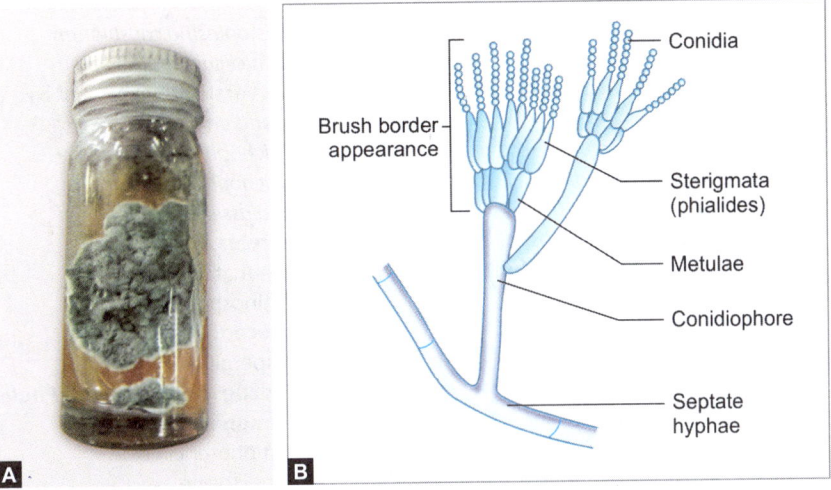

Figs. 35.11 A and B: *Penicillium* species: **A.** Colonies on SDA; **B.** Schematic microscopic picture.
Source: A. Department of Microbiology, Pondicherry Institute of Medical Sciences, Puducherry (*with permission*).

- **Taxonomy:** It exists in cyst and trophozoite forms like protozoa and therefore was previously thought to be a protozoan. But based on molecular studies, it is now classified under fungus
- **Pathogenesis:** Once inhaled, the cysts are carried to the lungs where they transform into the trophozoite stage. The trophozoites induce an inflammatory response that leads to the recruitment of plasma cells. The plasma cells induce a **frothy exudate** filling the alveoli. Hence, this condition is also called **plasma cell pneumonia**
- **Laboratory diagnosis:** Useful specimens include bronchoalveolar lavage (BAL), or open lung biopsy, etc.
  - Gomori's methenamine silver (GMS) staining is the method of choice to demonstrate the cysts of *P. jirovecii*. The cysts resemble black colored **crushed ping-pong balls**, against the green background
  - *Pneumocystis* is not cultivable and there is no serological test available
  - PCR assay has been developed for the detection of *P. jirovecii* specific genes
  - Detection of 1, 3 β-D-glucan in serum.
- **Radiology:** Chest X-ray depicts the classical finding of bilateral diffuse infiltrates. CT of the lung may reveal **ground-glass opacities.**

> **TREATMENT** — Pneumocystis pneumonia
>
> Cotrimoxazole is the drug of choice, given for treatment and prophylaxis of *Pneumocystis* pneumonia in patients with HIV.

EXPECTED QUESTIONS

I. Write short notes on:
1. Clinical manifestations of dermatophytosis.
2. Laboratory diagnosis of candidiasis.
3. Aspergillosis.
4. Cryptococcal meningitis.
5. Mucormycosis.
6. Mycetoma.

II. Multiple Choice Questions (MCQs):
1. Asteroid bodies are seen in___?
   a. *Sporothrix*   b. *Rhinosporidium*
   c. *Candida*   d. *Aspergillus*
2. Germ tube test is positive for___?
   a. *Candida auris*
   b. *Candida parapsilosis*

c. *Candida albicans*
d. *Cryptococcus*
3. Broad-based budding yeast cells are seen for __?
   a. *Histoplasma capsulatum*
   b. *Blastomyces dermatitidis*
   c. *Coccidioides immitis*
   d. *Paracoccidioides braziliensis*
4. The most important risk factor for mucormycosis is___?
   a. HIV
   b. Glucocorticoid therapy
   c. Diabetic ketoacidosis
   d. Transplant recipients
5. Organism that does not affect nail:
   a. *Trichophyton*   b. *Epidermophyton*
   c. *Microsporum*   d. *Candida albicans*
6. Which of the following organism is not been isolated in artificial culture media?
   a. *Cryptococcus neoforman*
   b. *Rhinosporidium seeberi*

c. *Histoplasma capsulatum*
d. *Penicillium marneffei*
7. Tinea versicolor is caused by:
   a. *Candida albicans*
   b. *Trichophyton rubrum*
   c. *Trichophyton violaceum*
   d. *Malassezia furfur*
8. Spherules are seen in:
   a. Dermatophytes
   b. Rhinosporidiosis
   c. Mucormycosis
   d. Aspergillosis
9. The drug of choice for *Pneumocystis* pneumonia is:
   a. Amphotericin B
   b. Flucytosine
   c. Cotrimoxazole
   d. Voriconazole
10. *Candida* species resistant to azoles is:
    a. *C. albicans*   b. *C. krusei*
    c. *C. tropicalis*   d. *C. dubliniensis*

Answers
1. a   2. c   3. b   4. c   5. c   6. b   7. d   8. b   9. c   10. b

SECTION 7: Hospital Infection Control

SECTION OUTLINE

36. Healthcare-associated Infections
37. Standard Precautions: Hand Hygiene and PPE
38. Transmission-based Precautions
39. Major Healthcare-associated Infection Types
40. HAI Surveillance and Hospital Infection Control Committee
41. Sterilization and Disinfection (Including CSSD)
42. Biomedical Waste Management
43. Needle Stick Injury (Occupational Exposure)
44. Environmental Surveillance (Bacteriology of Water, Air and Surface)
45. Laundry Management
46. Immunization of Healthcare Workers
47. Antimicrobial Stewardship

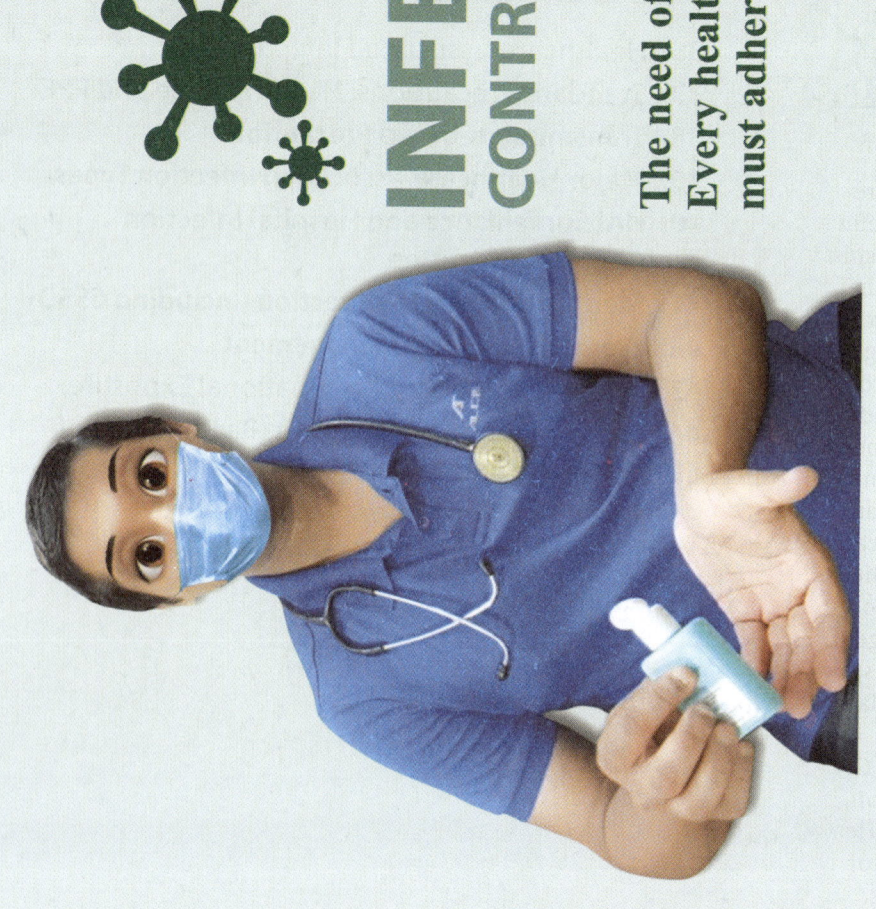

INFECTION
CONTROL

The need of the hour, Every healthcare personnel must adhere to.

CHAPTER 36

Healthcare-associated Infections

CHAPTER PREVIEW

- Healthcare-associated Infections
- Major HAI Types
- Prevention of HAI

HEALTHCARE-ASSOCIATED INFECTIONS

Definition

Healthcare-associated infections (HAIs) can be defined as—(i) infections acquired in the hospital by a patient admitted for a reason other than the infection in context, (ii) infection should not be present or incubating at the time of admission, and (iii) the symptoms should appear at least after 48 hours of admission. This also includes:

- Infections that are acquired in the hospital but symptoms appear after discharge
- Occupational infections among staff of the healthcare facility (e.g. needle stick injury transmitted infections)
- Infection in a neonate that results while passage through the birth canal (in contrast to congenital infection due to transplacental transmission, which is not HAI).

CDC (Centers for Disease Control and Prevention, Atlanta) has established the National Healthcare Safety Network (NHSN) to monitor the incidence of nosocomial infections.

As the site of healthcare facility has increasingly shifted from inpatient hospital care-based service to the ambulatory setting, the relevance of traditional terminologies such as "hospital-associated or nosocomial" infections has diminished.

Burden of HAI

HAIs are one of the most common adverse events in the care delivery system. According to World Health Organization (WHO), on average at any given time 7% of patients in developed and 10% in developing countries acquire at least one HAI. Mortality from HAI occurs in about 10% of affected patients. Treatment of these HAIs adds a huge economic burden to the hospital.

Factors Affecting HAIs

The principal factors that determine the likelihood that a given patient would acquire a HAI are:

- **Immune status:** Most admitted patients have impaired immunity either as a part of their preexisting disease or in some instances, due to the treatment they have received in the hospital
- **Hospital environment:** The hospital environment harbors a greater magnitude of microorganisms than that of the community. Transmission of these organisms to the patients can cause nosocomial outbreaks of infection
- **Hospital organisms:** Most of the organisms present in the hospital environment are

multidrug-resistant. This is because of the increased antibiotic usage in the hospital. The minor population of resistant organisms present, initially flourish in presence of constant antibiotic pressure and slowly replace the susceptible strains in the hospital
- **Diagnostic or therapeutic interventions** such as insertion of a central line or urinary catheters, or endotracheal tube, may introduce infection in susceptible patients; most of which are due to the patient's endogenous flora
- **Transfusion:** Blood, blood products, and intravenous fluids used for transfusion, if not properly screened, can transmit many blood-borne infections (BBI) such as HIV, hepatitis B, and C viruses
- **Poor hospital administration:** Strong administrative support is essential to control the HAIs; failing of which promotes the spread of HAIs.

Source of Infection

The source of infection in a healthcare setting can be either endogenous or exogenous.

Endogenous Source

The majority of nosocomial infections are endogenous in origin, i.e. they involve patient's own microbial flora which may invade the patient's body during some surgical or instrumental manipulations.

Exogenous Source

Exogenous sources are from the hospital environment, healthcare workers (HCW), or patients.
- **Environmental sources** include inanimate objects, air, water, and food in the hospital. Inanimate objects in the hospital are medical equipment (endoscopes, catheters, etc.), bedpans, surfaces contaminated by patients' excretions, blood and body fluids
- **Healthcare workers** may be potential carriers, harboring many organisms; which may be multidrug-resistant, e.g. nasal carriers of Methicillin-resistant *Staphylococcus aureus* (MRSA)
- **Other patients** in the hospital may also be the source of infection.

Microorganisms implicated in HAIs

HAIs can be caused by almost any microorganism, but those which survive in the hospital environment for long periods and develop resistance to antimicrobials and disinfectants are particularly important.

The ESKAPE pathogens: They are responsible for a substantial percentage of nosocomial infections in the modern era and represent the vast majority of multidrug-resistant isolates present in a hospital.
- *Enterococcus faecium*
- *Staphylococcus aureus*
- *Klebsiella pneumoniae*
- *Acinetobacter baumannii*
- *Pseudomonas aeruginosa*
- *Enterobacter* species.

Other infections that can spread in hospitals include:
- *Escherichia coli*
- SARS-CoV-2 (COVID-19)
- Nosocomially-acquired *Mycobacterium tuberculosis*
- *Legionella pneumophila*
- *Candida albicans*
- *Clostridioides difficile* diarrhea
- Blood-borne infections transmitted through needle prick injury or muco-cutaneous exposure of blood include HIV, hepatitis B and C viral infections.

Modes of Transmission

Microorganisms spread in the hospital through several modes such as contact, droplet, and airborne transmissions. They are discussed subsequently in Chapter 38 under transmission-based precautions.

MAJOR HAI TYPES

Though several types of HAIs exist, there are four most common types (listed below) which are often monitored to estimate the burden of HAI in a hospital. Out of these, the first three are together called as device-associated infections (DAIs).

1. Catheter-associated urinary tract infection (CAUTI)
2. Central line-associated bloodstream infection (CLABSI)
3. Ventilator-associated pneumonia (VAP)
4. Surgical site infection (SSI).

These major HAI types have been discussed in detail in Chapter 39.

PREVENTION OF HAI

The preventive measures for HAIs can be broadly categorized into:

1. **Standard precautions** (discussed in Chapter 37): They are indicated while handling all patients, specimens and sharps, e.g. hand hygiene
2. **Transmission-based or specific precautions** (Chapter 38): These are additional infection control practices that need to be taken only when a specific transmission risk is anticipated, e.g. N95 respirator for tuberculosis.

EXPECTED QUESTIONS

I. **Write short notes on:**
   1. Factors affecting healthcare-associated infections.
   2. ESKAPE pathogens.

II. **Multiple Choice Questions (MCQs):**
   1. **All the following statements are true regarding healthcare-associated infections, *except*:**
      a. The infections acquired in the hospital by a patient admitted for a reason other than the infection in context.
      b. The symptoms should appear at least after 48 hours of admission.
      c. The infection should be present at the time of admission.
      d. Infections that are acquired in the hospital but symptoms appear after discharge.
   2. **All of the following are the ESKAPE pathogens *except*:**
      a. *Enterococcus faecium*
      b. *Streptococcus pyogenes*
      c. *Klebsiella pneumoniae*
      d. *Acinetobacter baumannii*
   3. **All of the following are called as device-associated infections, *except*:**
      a. Catheter-associated urinary tract infection
      b. Central line-associated bloodstream infection
      c. Ventilator-associated pneumonia
      d. Surgical site infection

Answers
1. c   2. b   3. d

CHAPTER 37

Standard Precautions: Hand Hygiene and PPE

CHAPTER PREVIEW

- Standard Precautions
- Hand Hygiene
- Personal Protective Equipment (PPE)

The preventive measures for healthcare-associated infections (HAIs) can be broadly categorized into:

- ❖ **Standard precautions** (discussed below): Include the precautions which need to be taken all the time, e.g. hand hygiene
- ❖ **Transmission-based or specific precautions** (refer Chapter 38): These are additional infection control practices that need to be taken only when a specific transmission risk is anticipated, e.g. N95 respirator for tuberculosis.

STANDARD PRECAUTIONS

Standard precautions are a set of infection control practices (see highlight box below) used to prevent the transmission of diseases that can be acquired by contact with blood, body fluids, non-intact skin (including rashes), and mucous membranes. These measures should be followed when providing care to or handling:

- ❖ All individuals, whether they appear infectious/symptomatic or not
- ❖ All specimens (blood or body fluids) whether they appear infectious or not
- ❖ All needles and sharps whether they appear infectious or not.

Note: **Universal precaution** was a term used in the past to refer to the infection control practices to avoid contact with a patient's blood and other potentially infectious materials, by means of wearing nonporous articles such as medical gloves, goggles, and face shields. Now it is replaced by the word "standard precaution" which in addition includes contact with all body fluids regardless of whether blood is present.

Standard precautions

They are indicated while handling all patients, specimens, and sharps. Components of standard precautions include:

- **Hand hygiene:** (discussed in this chapter)
  - Wash hands promptly after contact with infective material
  - Use no-touch technique wherever possible.
- **Personal protective equipment:** Discussed in this chapter
- **Respiratory hygiene and cough etiquette** (Chapter 38)
- **Disinfection of patient-care items:** Ensure that all patient-care items such as instruments, devices, and linens are disinfected before reuse (Chapter 41)
- **Environmental cleaning** of surface and floor (Chapter 44)
- **Biomedical waste (BMW):** All BMW including sharps should be segregated and disposed of appropriately (Chapter 42)
- **Spillage cleaning:** Clean up spills of infective material promptly (Chapter 42)
- **Sharp:** Safe use and disposal of sharps (Chapters 42 and 43)

HAND HYGIENE

The hands of the healthcare workers (HCWs) are the main source of transmission of infections in healthcare facilities. Hand hygiene is therefore the most important measure to avoid the transmission of harmful microbes and prevent HAIs.

Types of Hand Hygiene Methods

Hand Rub

Alcohol-based (70–80% ethyl alcohol) and chlorhexidine (0.5–4%) based hand rubs are available. The duration of contact has to be at least for 20–30 seconds.
- **Advantage:** After a period of contact, it gets evaporated on its own, hence drying of hands is not required separately
- **Indications:** Hand rub is indicated during routine patient care activities or taking rounds in the wards or ICUs—whenever the opportunity for hand hygiene arises, except when the hands are visibly soiled with blood or other specimens.

Hand Wash

Antimicrobial soaps (liquid, gel, or bars) are available containing 4% chlorhexidine. If facilities are not available, then even ordinary soap and water can also be used. The duration of contact has to be at least for 40–60 seconds. Hand washing is indicated in the following situations:
- When the hands are visibly soiled with blood, excreta, pus, etc.
- Before and after eating
- After going to the toilet
- Before and after a shift of the duty
- When giving care to a patient with diarrhea.

Surgical Hand Scrub/Disinfection

Surgical hand scrub is indicated before any surgical procedure and also in between the cases; using 4% chlorhexidine hand wash. Alternatively, an alcohol-based hand rub can also be used for surgical hand disinfection. The duration of contact has to be at least for 3–5 minutes.

Indications (Five Moments for Hand Hygiene)

The WHO has published standard guidelines describing the situations or opportunities when hand hygiene is indicated in healthcare sectors **(Fig. 37.1)**—known as "My Five Moments for Hand Hygiene"; which include:
1. Before touching a patient
2. Before clean/aseptic procedures
3. After body fluid exposure/risk
4. After touching a patient
5. After touching patient's surroundings.

Steps of Hand Rubbing and Hand Washing

The WHO has also laid down the guidelines describing the appropriate steps involved for effective hand rubbing and handwashing **(Fig. 37.2)**. The steps of surgical hand disinfection have been depicted in **Figure 37.3**.

PERSONAL PROTECTIVE EQUIPMENT (PPE)

Personal protective equipment are used to protect the skin and mucous membranes of HCWs from exposure to blood and/or body

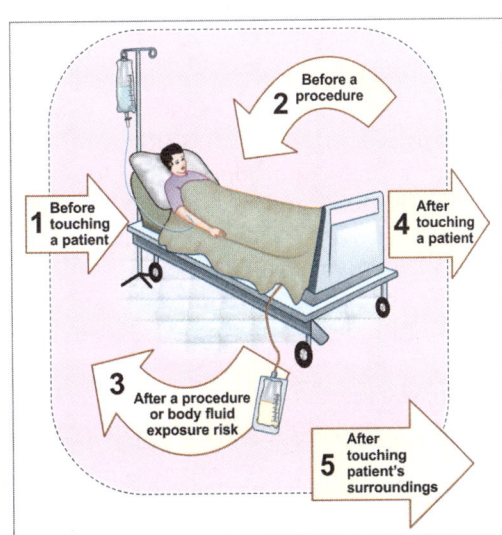

Fig. 37.1: My five moments for hand hygiene.
Source: World Health Organization (*with permission*).

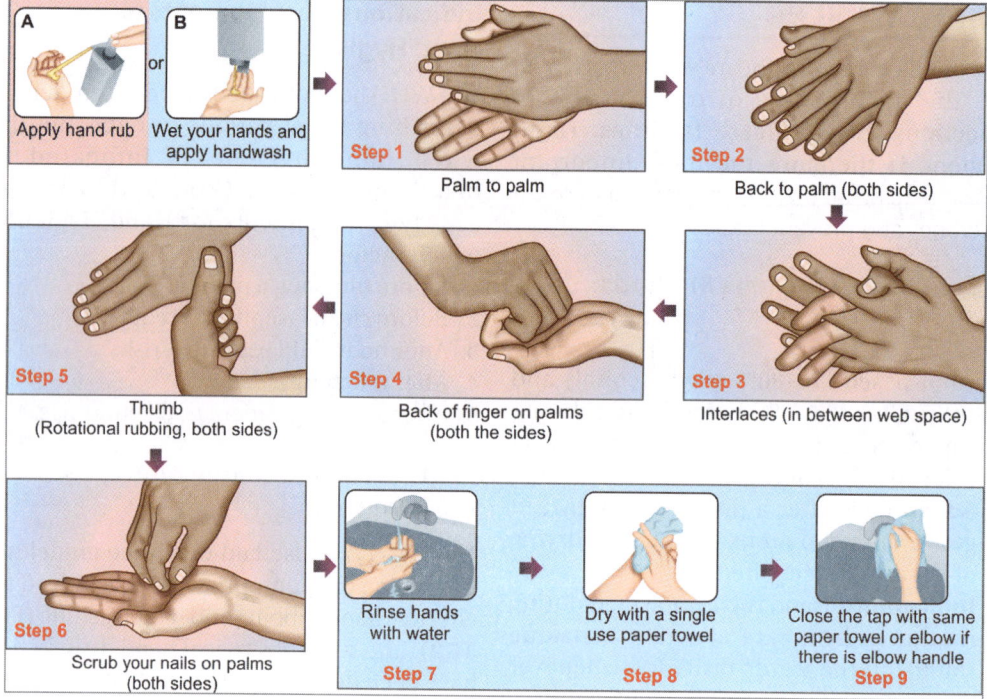

Fig. 37.2: Steps of hand rubbing and handwashing (WHO): Hand rub step 1 to 6 (20–30 seconds); Hand wash step 1 to 9 (40–60 seconds).

fluids and from the HCW to the patient during sterile and invasive procedures.
- The various PPE used in healthcare settings are gloves, mask/respirator, gown/plastic apron/coverall, goggles or face shield, shoe cover, and head cover **(Figs. 37.4A to N)**
- Selection of appropriate PPE is based on:
  - The level of risk associated with contamination of skin, mucous membranes, and clothing by blood and body fluids during a specific patient care activity or intervention (as a part of standard precaution)
  - Route of transmission of suspected organisms—contact, droplet and inhalation (as a part of transmission-based precaution).
- Though most PPE are used as a part of transmission-based precautions; there are few indications where some PPE are used as a part of standard precaution
- The PPE must be removed immediately following the indication for which it was used.

Gloves (37.4A)

Gloves can protect both patients and HCWs from exposure to microorganisms that have colonized their hands. It is used as part of standard, contact and droplet precautions. Gloves should be worn only when there is an indication **(Table 37.1)**. The use of gloves in situations when their use is not indicated represents a waste of resources and gives a false sense of security. Therefore, gloves should not be used when not clinically indicated **(Table 37.1)**.

Hand Hygiene and Glove Use

The glove is not a substitute for hand hygiene. In no way does the glove use modify hand hygiene indications or replace hand hygiene. The following measures should be adapted during gloves use.
- **Hand hygiene before gloves use:** This is to prevent possible cross-contamination of gloves with HCW's flora
- **Hand wash after glove use:** To prevent cross-contamination, hands must be

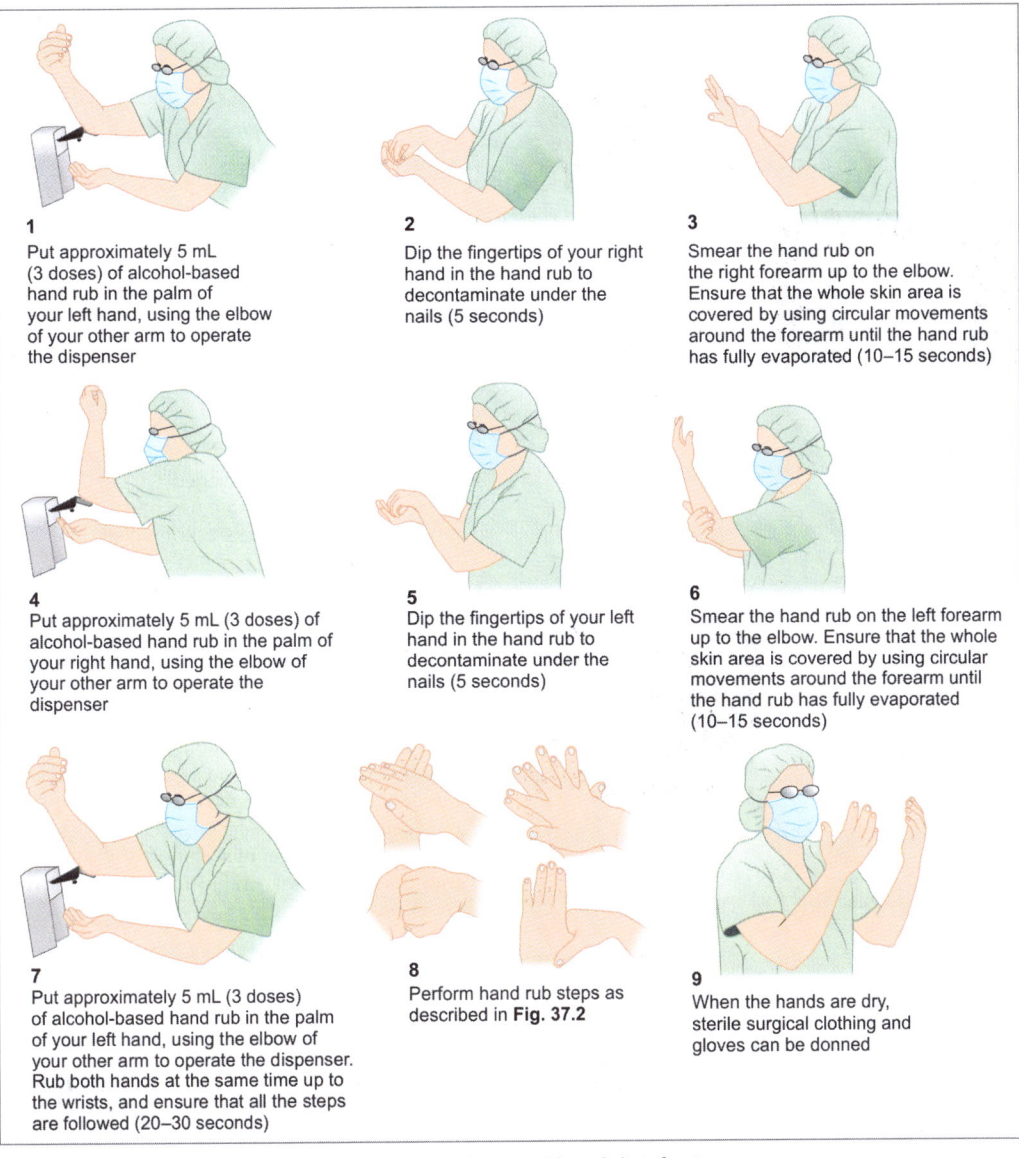

Fig. 37.3: Steps of surgical hand disinfection.

washed immediately after the removal of gloves as it creates a moist, warm, and occlusive environment between the skin and the glove which is a 'safe haven' for organisms to grow. Furthermore, micro-tears can occur in gloves during use, which may lead to transmission of organism if the HCW has had prior contact with blood or body fluid

❖ **Change:** Gloves should be worn for a single patient care activity and not beyond. Gloves must be changed between patient contacts and between separate procedures on the same patient
❖ **No hand hygiene over the gloved hand:** Gloved hands should neither be wiped with any form of hand rub nor washed with soap and water.

The technique for donning and doffing of gloves has been depicted in **Figures 37.5 and 37.6**.

Surgical (3-ply) Mask and Respirators

Respiratory protection is essential when there is a risk of transmission of droplets and

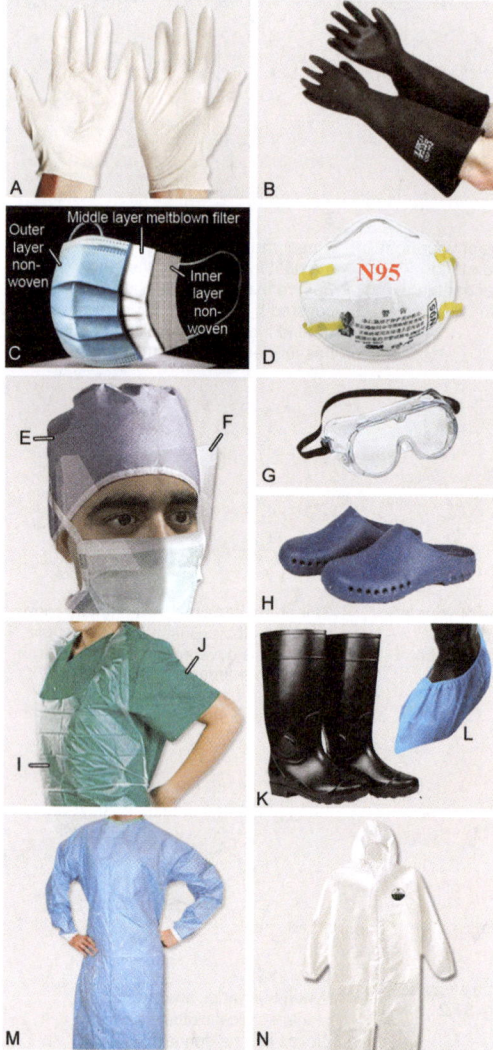

Figs. 37.4A to N: Personal protective equipment:
A. Gloves; **B.** heavy-duty gloves; **C.** Surgical mask; **D.** N95 respirator; **E.** Cap; **F.** Face shield; **G.** Goggles; **H.** Shoes; **I.** Plastic apron; **J.** Linen gown; **K.** Gumboot; **L.** Shoe cover; **M.** Disposable gown; **N.** Coverall.

Table 37.1: Indications for appropriate use of glove use.
Indications for glove use

• As a part of standard precautions
   ➢ Before a sterile procedure
   ➢ Anticipation of contact with blood or body fluid, regardless of the existence of sterile conditions and including contact with non-intact skin and mucous membrane
• As a part of contact precautions: Contact with a patient (and his/her immediate surroundings)
• Heavy duty gloves: To protect from sharp injuries, mainly used by biomedical waste handlers **(Fig. 37.4B)**

Indications for glove removal
• As soon as gloves are damaged • Gloves are meant for single-use, must be changed in-between patients or patient care activities • When there is an indication for hand hygiene
Clinical situations where use of gloves is not recommended
• For routine patient care activities if there is no anticipated risk to blood/body fluid or no indication for contact precautions • Examples: Measuring blood pressure, temperature, and pulse, while administering medications (oral or injections), during maintenance of IV cannula, during dressing and transporting patient, writing in the patient's case sheet, etc.

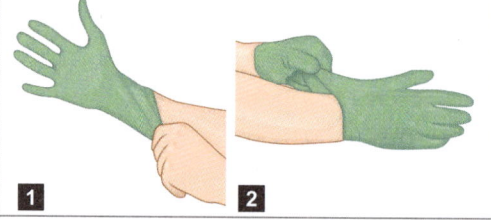

Fig. 37.5: Steps of gloves donning (wearing).
1. Donning of the first glove: Wear by touching and pulling only the edge of the cuff.
2. Donning of the second glove: Avoid touching the forearm skin by pulling external surface of second glove by the finger of gloved hand.

aerosols. There are two types of PPE available for respiratory protection; surgical mask and respirators.

Surgical Mask (3-ply Mask)

Surgical masks (also called as a medical mask or 3-ply mask) are loose-fitting, single-use items that cover the nose and mouth.
❖ They are used as part of standard precautions to prevent splashes or sprays from reaching the mouth and nose of the person wearing them
❖ They also provide some protection from respiratory secretions and are worn when caring for patients on droplet precautions.

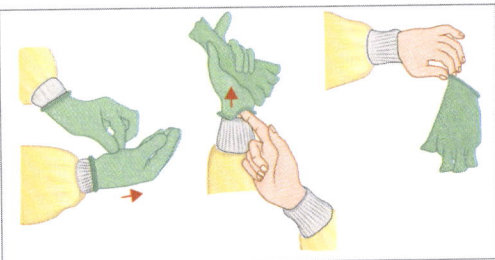

Fig. 37.6: Steps of gloves removal (doffing). Do not touch the outside of the gloves (contaminated)
- Using a gloved hand, grasp the palm area of the other gloved hand and peel off the first glove.
- Hold removed glove in gloved hand slide fingers of unglloved hand under the other glove at wrist and peel off the second glove over the first glove.
- The first glove will remain inside the pouch of the second glove.
- Perform hand hygiene after removal.

Composition

3-ply mask has three layers **(Fig. 37.4C)**:
1. **Outer fluid repellent layer**: Hydrophobic layer that can repel water, blood and body fluids
2. **Middle filter layer:** It is made up of melt-blown material; filters bacteria/viruses and also filters out the water droplets. In contrast to N95 respirator, the filter pore size of a surgical mask is not standardized
3. **Inner hydrophilic layer**: Absorbs water, sweat, and spit; made up of non-woven fabric.

Note: 2-ply masks may look similar to 3-ply mask in appearance. However, they have only two layers (outer and inner), but no middle filter layer. They should be used for hygienic and sanitation purposes—in restaurants, spa centers, food industry; but not in the hospitals.

Instructions

When using a surgical mask, the following measures should be considered:
- **Shelf-life:** Disposable (single-use); should be discarded or changed after 4–6 hours of use or earlier if it becomes soiled or wet
- **Donning:** Place the mask carefully, ensuring it covers the mouth and nose, adjust it to the nose bridge, and tie it securely to minimize any gaps between the face and the mask

- **Hanging mask syndrome:** Masks should not be left dangling around the neck, a common practice observed among doctors, doing so may contaminate the inner side of the mask
- Touching the **front of the mask** while wearing should be avoided
- Mask should not be worn with beard or unshaven face
- Hand hygiene should be performed before donning the mask, upon touching or discarding a used mask.

The technique of donning and doffing of surgical mask has been depicted in **Figures 37.7 and 37.8**.

Respirator (N95 Respirator) (Fig. 37.4D)

A respirator is a device designed to protect the wearer from airborne microorganisms (e.g. *M. tuberculosis*). There are many types of respirators. The most common respirator used in hospital settings is N95 respirator.

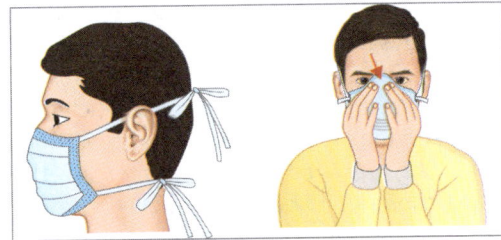

Fig. 37.7: Steps of mask donning (wearing).
- Pull the straps tight and pull the mask to below chin and then apply knots.
- Press on the nasal bridge part of the mask to seal tightly and for N95 respirator, perform fit check.

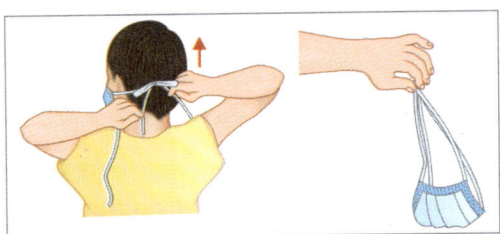

Fig. 37.8: Steps of mask removal (doffing).
- Do not touch front part of the mask.
- Untie the lower knot first, then the upper knot and remove the mask by holding its straps, without touching the front; hand wash after removal.

- N95 refers to 'not resistance to oil and ability to filter off 95% of airborne particles'
- **Composition:** The N95 respirator is comprised of four layers of material: an outer and inner layers of spun-bond polypropylene and middle two layers of cellulose/polyester, melt-blown polypropylene filter
- **Negative pressure:** N95 respirators are described as "negative pressure" because the pressure inside the respirator is negative during inhalation compared to the pressure outside the respirator
- **Removal:** N95 respirator should be removed or changed once in 8 hours or earlier if it gets clogged, wet or dirty on the inside, deformed, or torn
- **Single-use:** N95 respirator is for single-use only, should not be reused as it cannot be cleaned or disinfected
- **Fit checking:** After wearing the N95 respirator, the HCW must perform a fit check to ensure that it is properly fitted. No clinical activity should be undertaken until a satisfactory fit check has been achieved. It includes the following steps **(Fig. 37.13B)**:
  - *Sealing:* The respirator is compressed to ensure a seal across the face, cheeks, and the nasal bridge
  - *The positive pressure seal* of the respirator is checked by gently exhaling. If air escapes, the respirator needs to be adjusted
  - *The negative pressure seal* of the respirator is checked by gently inhaling. If the respirator is not drawn in towards the face, or air leaks around the face seal, the respirator is readjusted.
- **Fit testing:** Fit testing is done to identify which size and style of N95 respirator are suitable for an individual and to train the HCW on how to don and doff the N95 respirator. It should be done at the time of joining and thereafter annually.

Protective Body Clothing

Laboratory coats, plastic aprons, disposable gowns, and coverall (full body cover) are examples of protective body wears used in hospitals. They are worn when there is a risk that clothing may become exposed to blood or body fluids:

- **Laboratory coats:** They are used as a part of a standard precaution by all laboratory staff which protect their clothing and skin from the splash of blood or body fluid; however, they are not fluid resistant
- **Plastic aprons:** Worn when there is a low risk of contamination with blood/body fluid. They are fluid-resistant and for single-use only, i.e. used for one procedure or one patient care activity **(Fig. 37.4I)**
- **Disposable gowns:** They are long-sleeved, fluid-resistant; indicated when there is a moderate risk of contamination with blood/body fluid **(Fig. 37.4M)**
- **Coverall:** It comprises of a gown with pant and hood, which covers the whole body including the head. Coverall should be used in the following situations **(Fig. 37.4N)**:
  - Anticipated risk of splashing with a large volume blood/body fluid (e.g. cardiac surgeries)
  - Anticipated risk of extensive skin to skin contact with a patient known to harbor organisms of contact transmission (e.g. lifting a patient with uncontrolled diarrhea)
  - Handling patients infected with pathogens of high mortality (e.g. Nipah or Ebola) or in the laboratory while handling their specimens.
- **Donning:** Gown should be fully covered, torso from neck to knees, arms to end of the wrist and then wrapped around the neck. It should be fastened to the back of the neck and waist **(Fig. 37.9)**
- **Doffing:** Once the task is performed, the gown must be removed immediately after use by unfastening the gown ties taking care that sleeves should not contact the body while reaching for the ties **(Fig. 37.10)**.

Protective Eye/Face Wear

Protective eyewear (goggles, or face-shields) are used to protect the mucous membranes of the eyes, nose, and mouth

- Prevents exposure to blood and/or body fluids that may be splashed, sprayed, or

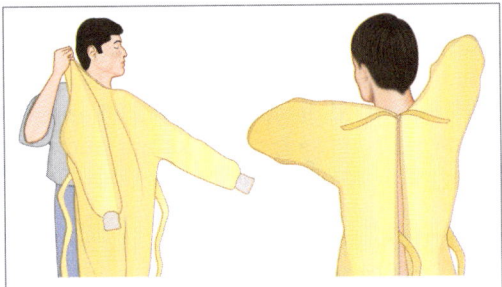

Fig. 37.9: Steps of gown donning (wearing).
- Fully cover torso from neck to knees, arms to the end of wrists, and wrap around the back.
- Fasten it on the back of the neck and waist.

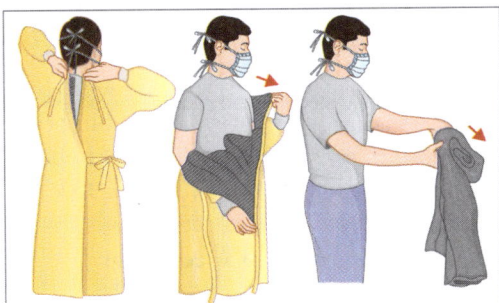

Fig. 37.10: Steps of gown removal (doffing). Do not touch front part of the gown.
- Unfasten gown ties, taking care that sleeves don't touch the body when reaching for ties.
- Pull the gown away from neck and shoulders, touching inside of gown only.
- Turn gown inside out and roll into a bundle and discard.
- Perform hand hygiene after removal.

splattered into the face during clinical procedures
❖ Eyewear must be worn during procedures that are likely to generate droplets or aerosols of blood and/or high-risk body fluids **(Figs. 37.4F and G)**.

Head Cover and Shoe Cover

❖ **Head cover or cap (Fig. 37.4E)** is used when spillage of blood is suspected, e.g. during major cardiac surgeries, etc.
❖ **Shoe covers** include: (1) Surgical shoes (slippers) and shoe covers **(Figs. 37.4H and L)**: Used mainly in ICUs and operation theaters to protect HCWs from organisms present on the floor and (2) Gumboots:

Used for anticipated risk of sharp injuries (e.g. for BMW handlers, laundry staff and housekeeping staff) **(Fig. 37.4K)**.

Donning and Doffing

To minimize the risk of transmission of infection, donning (wearing) and doffing (removing) of PPE must be performed in a particular sequence.

1. **Essential PPE:** If intended to use only the essential PPE (i.e. gown, mask, goggles, and gloves), then the sequence of donning and doffing to be followed is as below. Essential PPE is sufficient when giving care to patients with COVID-19, influenza or tuberculosis

   > **Donning (wearing):** Gown first → Mask or respirator → Goggles or face shield → Gloves
   > **Doffing (removing):** Gloves first → Gown → Face shield or goggles → Mask or respirator.

2. **Extended PPE:** If intended to use the extended set of PPE (i.e. gown, mask, goggles, and 2 pairs of gloves, cap, shoe cover), then the sequence of donning and doffing to be followed should be as depicted in **Figure 37.11**. An extended set of PPE may be necessary when giving care to any patient with an emerging life-threatening infection (e.g. Ebola).

Doffing

Doffing is extremely important as even a minor breach in the doffing procedure would subject the HCW to a huge risk of acquiring the infection. This could be a potential reason why many HCWs got infected during COVID-19 pandemic.
❖ All PPE should be removed just before exiting the patient room **except the respirator/mask**, which should be removed after leaving the patient room and closing the door
❖ **Segregation:** Discard into appropriate BMW bins:
  - *Yellow bag:* Gown/coverall, mask/respirator, shoe cover, and cap
  - *Red bag:* Plastic apron, goggles/face shield, gloves.

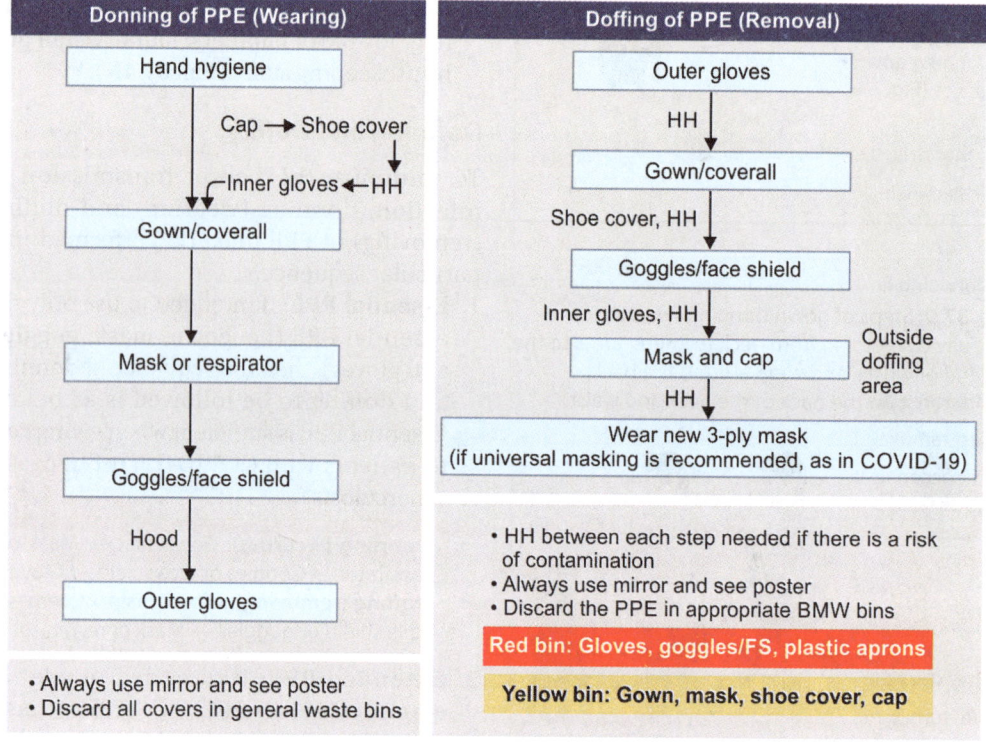

Fig. 37.11: Donning and doffing of the extended set of PPEs.
Abbreviations: BMW, biomedical waste; PPE, personal protective equipment; FS, face shield; HH, hand hygiene.

The common errors/breaches which can occur during donning and doffing have been enlisted in **Table 37.2**. HCWs should put efforts to minimize these errors as much as possible.

Table 37.2: Common breaches while donning and doffing and their corrective action and/or recommendations.	
Common breaches while donning	**Corrective action or recommendations**
Wrong selection of mask	
N95 respirator in COVID ward without aerosol risk	A 3-ply mask is recommended in the COVID ward
3-ply mask in COVID ICU (with aerosol risk)	N95 respirator is recommended in COVID ICU
Cloth mask in the nursing station	Cloth mask is not recommended in any area of the hospital
Double masks (3-ply and N95)	Double masks are not recommended
Wrong sequence of donning	
Donning the hood of the coverall first, followed by goggles **(Fig. 37.12A)**	Goggles should be donned first, followed by hood of the coverall so that it will help during doffing to remove the goggles, after the removal of the coverall
Donning goggles first, followed by a mask **(Fig. 37.12B)**	Mask should be donned first, followed by goggles to prevent any air leak around the nose
Donning 3-ply mask first, followed by N95 **(Fig. 37.12C)**	Double masking is not recommended. If intended to wear, N95 respirator (inner) should be donned first, followed by a 3-ply mask (outer)

Contd...

Contd...

Donning gown sleeve → inner gloves → outer gloves **(Fig. 37.12D)**	If double gloves are worn, then gown sleeve should be placed in-between outer and inner gloves; i.e. inner gloves → gown sleeve → outer gloves
Other breaches during donning	
Criss-crossing the straps of a 3-ply mask	Straps of the 3-ply mask should not be worn criss-cross. The upper strap is tied up and the lower strap is tied below **(Fig. 37.13A)**
Not doing fit check when donning N95 respirator	Fit check is mandatory when donning N95 **(Fig. 37.13B)**
Not wearing eye protection in COVID OPD	Eye protection is a must in any area of COVID area
Common breaches while doffing	
Breaches during gloves removal (Fig. 37.14A)	
Fast removal	Gloves should be doffed slowly
The second glove is removed by touching the outer surface	The second glove is removed by sliding the fingers of the ungloved hand under the second glove at the wrist and peeling off the second glove over the first glove. • First glove will remain inside the pouch of the second glove. • Care must be taken not to touch the outer surface of the second glove while removal
Breaches during gown removal (Fig. 37.14B)	
Not turning the gown inside out	The gown should be removed slowly by turning inside out and rolling into a bundle and discarded, without touching the outer surface
Touched the outer surface	
Not rolled into a bundle	
Breaches during goggles removal (Fig. 37.14C)	
Fast removal	Goggles should be removed slowly to prevent droplet splash
Overhead removal	Goggles should never be removed overhead
Not bending/more bending forward while removing	Slight bending forward is recommended Standing straight has a risk of falling droplets in the eyes More bending forward has a risk of touching the goggles to the neck area or shirt while removing
Not closing eyes	Eyes should be closed while doffing the goggles to prevent falling of droplets on the eyes
Breaches during mask removal (Fig. 37.14D)	
Mask removed inside the doffing area	Mask should be removed outside the doffing area
Removing mask in doffing area	Mask should be removed slowly
Overhead removal	Mask should never be removed overhead
Not bending/more bending forward while removing	Slight bending forward is recommended Standing straight has a risk of falling droplets in the eyes More bending forward has a risk of touching the mask to the neck area or shirt while removing
Not closing eyes	Eyes should be closed while doffing the mask to prevent falling of droplets on the eyes
Removing the upper elastic (strap) of the N95 respirator first, followed by the lower elastic **(Fig. 37.14D)**	Lower elastic has to be removed first, followed by upper elastic

Contd...

Contd...

Touched the outer surface	Mask should be removed by holding it at the edges, without touching the outer surface
Not washing hands	Hand hygiene is a mandate after mask removal
Wrong sequences in doffing	
Gown removed earlier gloves	The gown should be removed after gloves removal
Goggles doffed earlier to gown	Gloves → gown → goggles → mask
Mask doffed earlier	Mask should be doffed at the last
Inner gloves doffed earlier to gown	If double gloving is done, then the sequence of doffing is: Outer gloves → gown → goggles → inner gloves → mask

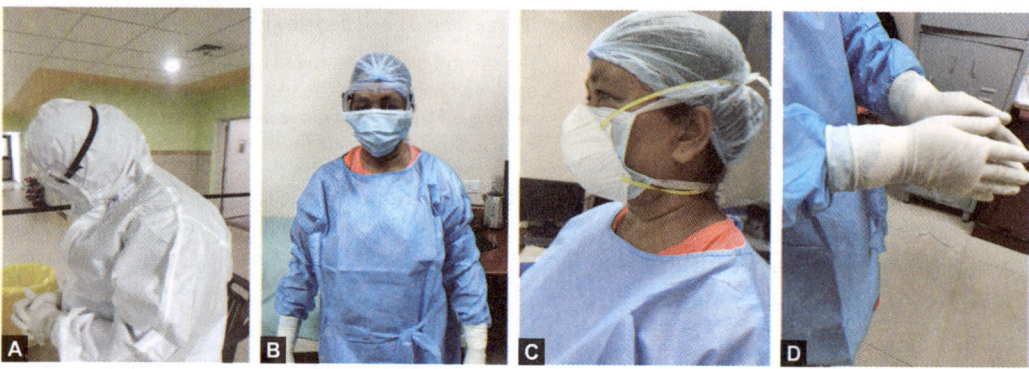

Figs. 37.12A to D: Common breaches during donning: **A.** Donning hood of the coverall first, followed by goggles; **B.** Donning goggles first, followed by mask; **C.** Donning 3-ply mask first, followed by N95; **D.** Donning gown sleeve → then inner gloves → then outer gloves.

Source: Hospital Infection Control and Prevention Unit, JIPMER, Puducherry (*with permission*).

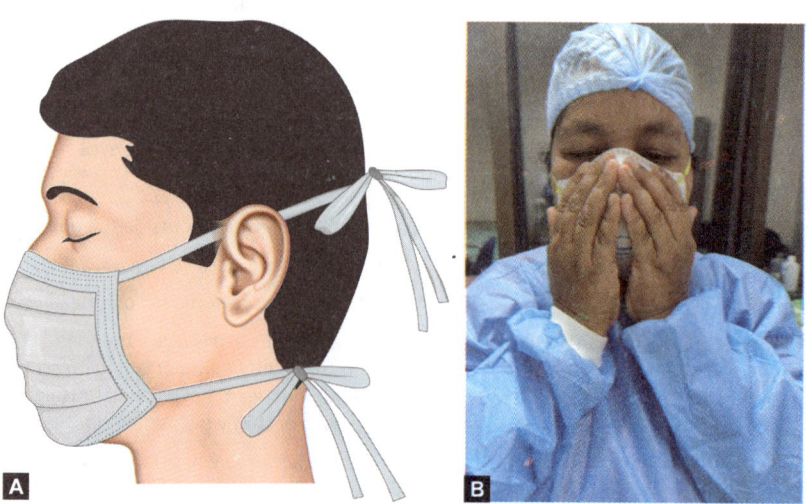

Figs. 37.13A and B: Correct method of mask use: **A.** Upper strap is tied up and lower strap is tied below; **B.** Fit check of N95 respirator.

Source: Hospital Infection Control and Prevention Unit, JIPMER, Puducherry (*with permission*).

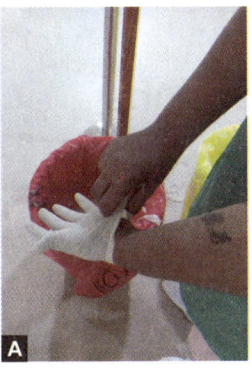 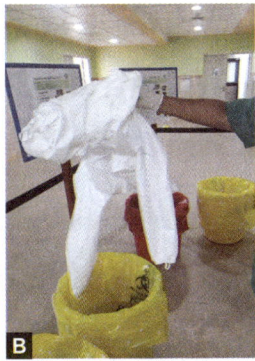 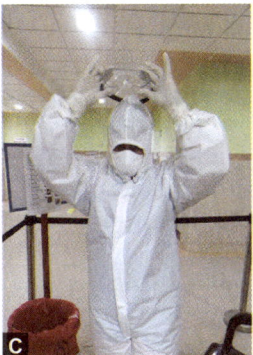 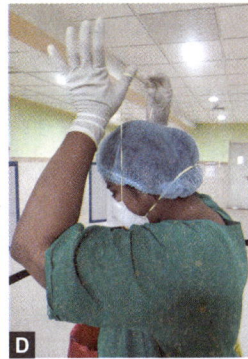

Figs. 37.14A to D: Common breaches during doffing: **A.** Second glove removed by touching the outer surface; **B.** Gown not turning the gown inside out and not rolled into a bundle; **C.** Goggles overhead removal, not bending forward and not closing eyes; **D.** N95 respirator, removing the upper elastic first.
Source: Hospital Infection Control and Prevention Unit, JIPMER, Puducherry (*with permission*).

EXPECTED QUESTIONS

I. Write short notes on:
1. Hand hygiene.
2. Standard precautions.
3. Donning and doffing of PPEs.

II. Multiple Choice Questions (MCQs):
1. Hand rub should not be used in which condition?
   a. Before touching patient
   b. After touching patient
   c. After touching patient's surrounding
   d. Hands are visibly soiled
2. How many moments of hand hygiene have been laid down by WHO?
   a. 5
   b. 6
   c. 7
   d. 8
3. Hand rub should be performed for a minimum of how much duration?
   a. 20 seconds
   b. 40 seconds
   c. 60 seconds
   d. 2 minutes
4. Hand wash should be performed for a minimum of how much duration?
   a. 20 seconds
   b. 40 seconds
   c. 60 seconds
   d. 2 minutes
5. Which of the following is not a component of standard precautions?
   a. N95 respirator for TB patient
   b. Gloves during surgery
   c. Hand hygiene
   d. Wearing gloves during phlebotomy
6. All of the following are the common breeches during donning of PPE, *except*:
   a. Donning hood of the coverall first, followed by goggles
   b. Donning goggles first, followed by mask
   c. Donning 3-ply mask first, followed by N95
   d. Performing fit check for N95 respirator
7. All of the following are the common breeches during doffing of PPE, *except*:
   a. Second glove removed by touching the outer surface
   b. Not turning the gown inside out and not rolled into a bundle
   c. Bending forward and closing eyes while goggles removal
   d. N95 respirator, removing the upper elastic first

Answers
1. d **2.** a **3.** a **4.** b **5.** a **6.** d **7.** c

CHAPTER 38

Transmission-based Precautions

CHAPTER PREVIEW
- Definition
- Contact Precautions
- Droplet Precautions
- Airborne Precautions

DEFINITION

Transmission-based precautions (TBPs), also called specific precautions are a set of infection control practices that should be followed over and above the standard precautions.
- TBPs should be practiced when giving care to the patients who are infected with infectious agents having specific modes of transmission such as contact, droplet, and airborne
- Accordingly, there are three types of TBPs—contact precautions, droplet precautions, and airborne precautions
- TBPs should be followed even when the specific infections are suspected and may be discontinued later when the diagnosis is ruled out.

CONTACT PRECAUTIONS

Contact precaution should be followed when there is definitive or suspected evidence of certain infectious agents that are transmitted by direct or indirect contact during patient care.
- **Direct transmission** occurs when infectious agents are transferred from one person to another person without a contaminated intermediate object or person. For example, direct contact through contaminated hands (the most common mode of transmission of the organism in healthcare settings) or direct contact with blood or body fluids from an infectious person
- **Indirect transmission** involves the transfer of an infectious agent through a contaminated intermediate object (clothes, patient-care devices, environmental surfaces, fomite) or person.

Agents transmitted through contact
- MRSA (Methicillin-resistant *S. aureus*)
- CRE (Carbapenem-resistant Enterobacteriaceae)
- VRE (vancomycin-resistant enterococci)
- MDR nonfermenting gram-negative bacilli such as *Acinetobacter, Pseudomonas*, etc.
- Agents of conjunctivitis (e.g. adenovirus, gonococcus, *Chlamydia*)
- Agents of diarrhea such as rotavirus, cholera, *Clostridioides difficile*
- Enterically-transmitted hepatitis viruses (HAV and HEV).

Infection Control Measures (Contact)

The following infection control measures should be applied in addition to other standard precaution measures:
- **Hand hygiene:** Strict adherence to hand hygiene is an absolute requirement of contact precaution as transmission via contaminated hands accounts for the majority of contact transmission
- **Personal protective equipment (PPE):** Gloves and gowns are the essential PPE

that the HCW should wear upon entry to the patient-care area and must be removed before leaving the patient-care area. A surgical mask and protective eyewear are optional PPE, needed if there is a risk of exposure to splashes or sprays of blood and body substances on the face and eyes
- **Equipment**: Single-use patient-dedicated equipment (e.g. blood pressure cuffs, stethoscopes, thermometers) must be used. If not possible, then the equipment should be cleaned and allowed to dry before use on another patient
- **Patient placement: Single isolation room** with a bathroom facility is preferred. If not available, then cohorting is recommended. **Cohorting** may be carried out in various ways
  - Patients with similar infections requiring contact precautions can be placed together either in the same isolation room or in the same cubicle or corner of a ward or
  - The spatial separation of a minimum of **3 feet distance** between the beds with privacy curtains.
- **Transfer of patients:** Patient movement should be limited only to medically-necessary purposes. When transport is necessary, the HCW must wear PPE before transport and the infected areas of the patient's body should be covered to contain the infection
- **Disinfection of the rooms:** Patient rooms must be frequently cleaned and disinfected adequately (e.g., at least daily and before use by another patient) focusing on frequently-touched surfaces and equipment in the immediate vicinity of the patient.

DROPLET PRECAUTIONS

Droplet precautions when used in addition to standard precautions are intended to prevent the spread of infectious agents that are transmitted through respiratory droplets via close respiratory or mucous membrane contact with respiratory secretions.
- Respiratory droplets are large particles (>5 μm in size) that are generated by a patient who is coughing, sneezing, or talking
- Transmission via large droplets requires close contact (<3 feet) as droplets do not remain suspended in the air and generally, only travel shorter distances
- Some infectious agents transmitted by the droplet route can also be significantly transmitted by contact mode. This is because the larger droplets settle on the surfaces and inanimate objects within a one meter distance, which subsequently spread to other individuals when they touch the contaminated surfaces and then touch their eyes, nose, or mouth.

Agents transmitted through droplets
- Diphtheria (pharyngeal)
- *Haemophilus influenzae* type b
- Pertussis (whooping cough)
- Pneumonic plague
- *Mycoplasma* pneumonia
- Streptococcal (group A) pharyngitis
- Influenza viruses, seasonal
- SARS-CoV2 (COVID-19)
- Viral hemorrhagic fevers (e.g. Ebola)
- Other viruses: Mumps, Parvovirus B19, Rhinovirus, Rubella, Adenovirus

Infection Control Measures (Droplet)

The following infection control measures should be applied in addition to standard precautions:

1. Hand Hygiene

Droplet transmission is also associated with contact transmission (as discussed earlier). Therefore, hand hygiene is an important component of droplet precautions.

2. PPE

HCWs should wear a **surgical mask** when close contact (<3 feet) with the patient is anticipated and also upon room entry.
- Patients should wear a surgical mask (all the time)
- HCWs should wear protective eyewear if there is a risk of splashes or spray to the eye/face. Gown and gloves should also be worn to prevent contact transmission
- The primary function of a surgical mask is for '**source control**'; which prevents the

transmission of droplets from the wearer to the environment. N95 respirator does not provide additional environmental protection and therefore, should not be used for this purpose
- The secondary function of the surgical mask is to protect the person wearing it from larger droplets in the environment
- **AGPs:** For certain diseases like seasonal influenza, viral hemorrhagic fever, or COVID 19, the HCWs should wear N95 respirator during aerosol-generating procedures (AGPs), described subsequently in this chapter.

3. Respiratory Hygiene/Cough Etiquette

The following measures are recommended for all individuals with respiratory symptoms **(Fig. 38.1)**:
- Directly coughing or sneezing on hands or rubbing of the nose should be strictly avoided
- The mouth and nose should be covered with tissue when coughing or sneezing. Tissues should be disposed into the yellow waste bins after use
- If no tissues are available, coughing or sneezing can be done into the inner elbow (sleeves), turning away from other patients

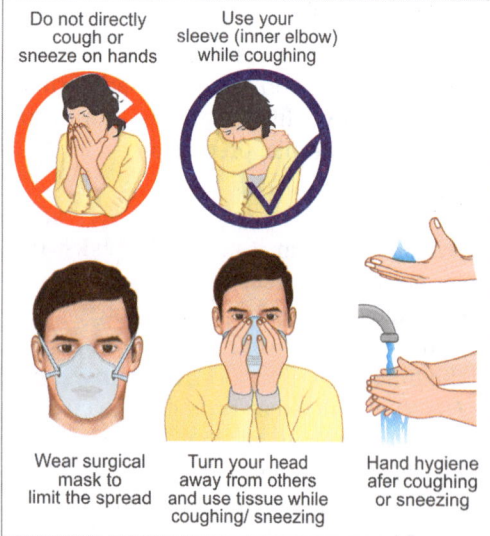

Fig. 38.1: Respiratory hygiene/cough etiquette.

- Hand hygiene should be performed after having contact with respiratory secretions
- Contaminated hands should be kept away from the mucous membranes of the eyes
- In outpatient settings, patients with respiratory symptoms should be segregated separately, provided with masks, and attending the cases must be fast-tracked
- **Social distancing:** Individuals with respiratory symptoms should always maintain a distance of at least 1 meter from others.

4. Patient Placement

A single room is preferred for patients who require droplet precautions. If it is not available, alternative placement options can be looked for similar to contact precautions such as cohorting, spatial separation of >3 feet, and drawing the curtain between patient beds.

5. Transfer of Patients

Transfer of patients on droplet precautions should be limited as there is a high risk of transmission. If unavoidable, then the following precautions should be undertaken:
- Patients should wear a surgical mask while they are being transferred
- Patients should follow respiratory hygiene and cough etiquette
- HCW transporting the patient should wear a surgical mask, gloves, gown, and protective eyewear.

6. Disinfection of the Rooms

Patient-care items, bedside equipment, frequently touched surfaces area, and environmental surfaces should be cleaned daily with appropriate disinfectants according to the hospital policy.

AIRBORNE PRECAUTIONS

Airborne precautions when used in addition to standard precautions are intended to prevent the spread of infectious agents that are transmitted through respiratory aerosols.

Aerosols are small particles (<5 μm) generated by an infectious person during coughing, sneezing, talking, or performing certain aerosol-generating procedures (e.g. intubation). These smaller droplets remain suspended in the air for long periods and may disperse to a distant place along with the air current.

Agents transmitted through Aerosols
- *Mycobacterium tuberculosis*
- Measles virus
- Varicella (chickenpox and zoster)
- Smallpox (variola) and monkeypox virus
- *Aspergillus* (pulmonary aspergillosis)

Aerosol-generating Procedures (AGPs)

AGPs are procedures that can generate much higher concentrations of aerosols as compared to coughing, sneezing, or speaking and are associated with a higher risk of pathogen transmission.
- ❖ Therefore, it is recommended to follow airborne precautions such as isolating the patient in a negative pressure room and wearing appropriate PPE like N95 respirator
- ❖ Examples of AGPs include: Endotracheal intubation, open respiratory and airway suctioning, tracheostomy care, cardiopulmonary resuscitation, sputum induction, and bronchoscopy.

Airborne Infection Control Measures

A prudent approach is to implement infection control measures at the earliest based on clinical suspicion and discontinue them later if the patient is subsequently diagnosed with a disease that does not require airborne precautions.

1. PPE

While giving care to a patient with airborne precaution, the HCWs must wear N95 or higher level respirator. The HCW must perform *fit checking* every time before donning the N95 respirator to ensure it is properly applied. Gloves, gowns, and protective eyewear may be needed if there is exposure risk.

2. Patient Placement

Patients should be placed in an airborne infection isolation room (AIIR). The components of AIIR include: adequate ventilation, ultraviolet germicidal irradiation (UVGI), and filtration.

3. Ventilation

Ventilation can reduce the risk of infection through dilution and removal of room air containing infectious aerosols by the introduction of clean or fresh air into the room, either by natural or mechanical ventilation.

Natural Ventilation

Natural ventilation refers to the fresh air that enters and leaves a room through openings such as windows or doors.
- ❖ The effect of natural ventilation is maximized when the door and windows are placed opposite to each other and are kept open to maintain airflow at all times
- ❖ In a consultation room with natural ventilation, the seating arrangement for patient and doctor should be made such that doctor should sit away from the direction of natural airflow, thus has a lesser risk of exposure **(Figs. 38.2A and B)**
- ❖ In ward set-up, the beds should be placed away from airflow (door-window direction) **(Fig. 38.3)**.

Mechanical Ventilation (Negative-pressure)

Negative-pressure room includes a mechanical ventilation system that maintains the pressure of the room slightly lesser than the pressure of the entry area (i.e. creating a "negative pressure"), so that it allows air to flow into the isolation room but not escape from the room, as air naturally flows from areas with higher pressure to the areas with lower pressure, thereby preventing contaminated air from escaping the room. The negative pressure room should have the following properties:
- ❖ **Air changes per hour** (ACH): Minimum of 12 ACH should take place in the high-risk area, compared to 6 ACH per hour in a low-risk area for airborne transmission. High-

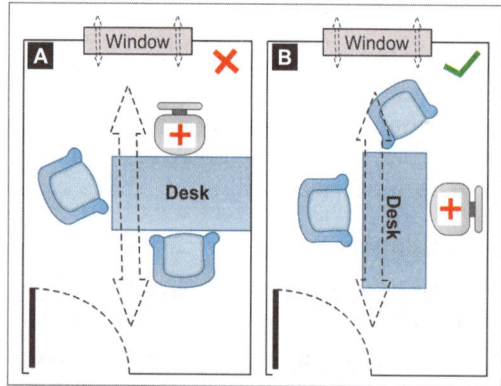

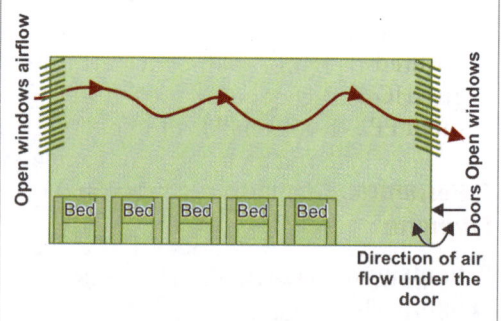

Fig. 38.3: Schematic diagram of a room with natural ventilation.

Figs. 38.2A and B: Schematic diagram showing seating directions of patient and doctor in a consultation room.
- In-room (A), the seating arrangement is along with direction of natural ventilation of airflow, so that the doctor has a higher risk of exposure to the potentially infected air.
- In room (B), the doctor is sitting away from the direction of natural airflow, thus has a lesser risk of exposure.

risk areas include TB/chest department (outpatient and inpatient), bronchoscopy procedure rooms, MDR-TB wards, and clinics, airborne precaution rooms
- **Negative pressure differential** between airflow from adjacent spaces to the patient room should be >2.5 Pascal
- **The door** should be kept closed at all times
- **Anteroom:** The negative pressure room should be preceded by an anteroom (a small outer waiting room that proceeds to the patient room).

4. Ultraviolet Germicidal Irradiation (UVGI)

If adequate ventilation is not possible, ultraviolet germicidal irradiation (UVGI) devices can be used as in addition to negative pressure ventilation. UVGI kills the organisms by irradiating. **UVGI** can be wall-mounted and should be installed at a higher level (>8 feet from the floor), so that it will not directly irradiate patients **(Fig. 38.4)**.

5. Filtration

The room air is directly exhausted to the outside through an exhaust fan or through

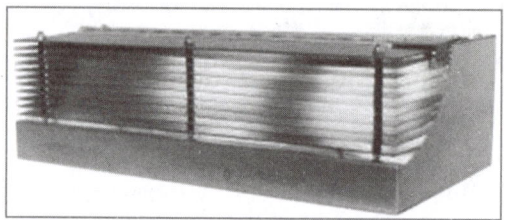

Fig. 38.4: Wall-mounted ultraviolet germicidal irradiation.

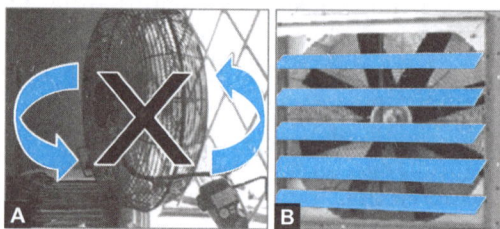

Figs. 38.5A and B: Exhaust fan: **A.** Poorly installed in an open window space; **B.** Well-installed, closely fitted.

HEPA (high-efficiency particulate air) filtration. Exhaust fans must be properly installed closely fitting to the window **(Figs. 38.5A and B)**.

6. Transfer of Patients

The patient on airborne precaution should be transferred outside the negative pressure room only when it is absolutely necessary. In such a case, the following measures should be undertaken:
- The patient should wear a surgical mask and follow respiratory hygiene and cough etiquette

- Any skin lesions associated with the condition (e.g. chickenpox) should be covered
- The HCW must wear N95 respirator and other PPE as indicated.

7. Respiratory Hygiene and Cough Etiquette

Patients must be explained in detail about cough hygiene as described under droplet precautions and **Figure 38.1**.

8. Visitors and Staff

Entry of the visitors and staff should be absolutely restricted or they should wear PPE before entry into the room. The staff who are immune to the specific airborne disease (e.g. chickenpox) should preferably be posted to the airborne precaution room.

The infection control measures that need to be taken for various standard and transmission-based precautions have been summarized in **Table 38.1**.

Table 38.1: Measures to be followed during standard and transmission-based precautions.

Type	Isolation room or cohorting	Hand hygiene	Gloves	Apron or gown	Mask	Eye protection	Handling of equipment	Visitors
Standard	Not required	Yes	As required*	If soiling likely#	As required$	As required$	Single use or reprocessed	No additional precautions
Contact	Essential	Yes	Essential	Essential	As required$	As required$	Same as standard	Same precautions as for HCWs
Droplet	Essential	Yes	As required*	If soiling likely#	Surgical mask is essential	As required$	Same as standard	Restricted. Same precautions as for HCWs
Airborne	Essential (negative pressure)	Yes	As required*	If soiling likely#	N95 respirator is essential	As required$	Same as contact	Same as for droplet

*Gloves are used when there is likely exposure to blood, body fluids, and contaminated items.
$Mask or eye protection is required during procedures likely to generate droplets or an anticipated splash of specimens on the face respectively.
#Soiling is likely to occur during procedures that are expected to generate contamination from blood and body fluids. Environmental cleaning with an appropriate disinfectant is required for all types of precautions.

EXPECTED QUESTIONS

I. **Write short notes on:**
  1. Contact precautions.
  2. Droplet precautions.
  3. Airborne precautions.

II. **Multiple Choice Questions (MCQs):**
  1. What are the PPE recommended for contact precautions?
     a. Gloves and mask
     b. Gown and mask
     c. Gloves and gown
     d. Gown and goggles
  2. All of the following are components of droplet precautions, *except*:
     a. N95 respirator
     b. Isolation room
     c. Respiratory hygiene/cough etiquette
     d. Distance of > 3 feet
  3. Which of the following is component of airborne precautions?
     a. N95 respirator
     b. Negative pressure room
     c. UVGI
     d. All of the above

Answers
1. c   2. a   3. d

CHAPTER 39

Major Healthcare-associated Infection Types

CHAPTER PREVIEW

- Catheter-associated Urinary Tract Infection
- Catheter-related Bloodstream Infection
- Ventilator-associated Pneumonia
- Surgical Site Infection
- Prevention of Device-associated Infections

INTRODUCTION

Theoretically, any infection developing in a patient after two days of hospitalization can be labelled as healthcare-associated infection (HAI). Among them, there are four major types which are commonly encountered and therefore need to be discussed in detail. These are also the HAIs for which surveillance is recommended.

1. Catheter-associated urinary tract infection (CAUTI)
2. Catheter-related bloodstream infection (CRBSI)
3. Ventilator-associated pneumonia (VAP)
4. Surgical site infection (SSI).

Out of these, the first three (CAUTI, CRBSI, VAP) are together called as device associated infections (DAIs).

CATHETER-ASSOCIATED URINARY TRACT INFECTION (CAUTI)

CAUTI is considered as the most common HAI worldwide, accounting for up to 40% of nosocomial infections. About 70–80% of healthcare–associated UTI are attributable to the presence of an indwelling urinary catheter.

Definitions

Catheter-associated bacteriuria (CA-bacteriuria) has been defined as the presence of significant bacteriuria in a catheterized patient. It can be classified as:

- Catheter-associated UTI (CAUTI): CA-bacteriuria with symptoms or signs referable to the urinary tract
- Catheter-associated asymptomatic bacteriuria (CA-ASB): CA-bacteriuria without symptoms or signs referable to the urinary tract.

Epidemiology

Approximately 15–25% of hospitalized patients require urinary catheterization at some time during their hospital stay.

- The risk of developing CA-bacteriuria increases with time with an average risk of 3–10% per catheter day, which may rise up to 25% at end of one week to nearly all cases (100%) in one month. However, only a fraction (less than a quarter) of these cases progress to CAUTI
- The CAUTI rate varies from 0 to 5 per 1000 catheterized patients depending upon the hospital location (ward vs ICU).

Microbiology

A broad range of bacteria can cause CAUTI, most of which are multidrug-resistant.

In short-term catheterized patients: Most CAUTI are caused by the monomicrobial

pathogens such as gram-negative bacilli or enterococci.
- ❖ *E. coli* is the predominant agent, although it is not as prevalent as in community-associated UTI
- ❖ Other gram-negative bacilli such as *Klebsiella*, *Pseudomonas* and *Acinetobacter* and gram-positive cocci such as *Enterococcus* account for most of the other infections.

In long-term catheterized patients, CAUTI is usually polymicrobial. In addition to the pathogens of short-term catheterization, other organisms such as *Proteus*, *Providencia* and *Morganella* are also encountered.

Pathogenesis

There are four main entry points through which the microorganism may reach the bladder in a catheterized patient **(Fig. 39.1)**.

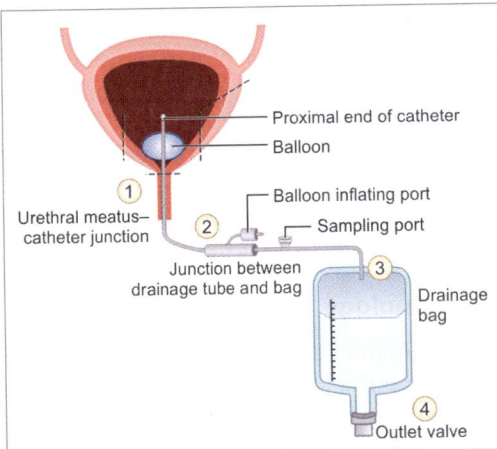

Fig. 39.1: Entry points through which the microorganism may reach the bladder in a catheterized patient.

The risk factors for the development of CAUTI is depicted in **Table 39.1**. Microorganisms may ascend to the urinary tract by either extraluminal or intraluminal surface of the catheter.

- ❖ **Extraluminal spread**: This accounts for two-thirds of cases
  - The source of the infection in catheterized patients may include patients' endogenous flora, hands of health care personnel, or inanimate objects
  - If asepsis is not maintained at the time of insertion or during maintenance of the catheter, there is always a risk of extraluminal migration of bacteria from one of these sources into the bladder
  - When a urinary catheter is inserted, the mechanism by which the urethral flora is constantly flushed out is interrupted. This helps in extraluminal migration of urethral and perineal flora into the bladder causing colonization and subsequent infection.
- ❖ **Intraluminal spread**: If the drainage bag is open type or when the closed drainage system is breached, there is a risk of reflux of contaminated urine from the drainage bag. This accounts for one-third of cases.

> **Why Indwelling Catheter is a Risk for UTI?**
> The presence of an urinary catheter is the single most important risk factor. The risk of developing CAUTI is directly proportional to the duration of catheterization.
> - **Urethral pressure:** An indwelling catheter exerts lateral urethral pressure causing decreased mucosal blood flow, urothelial mucosal disruption and impaired mucin secretion; all together predispose to infection
>
> *Contd...*

Table 39.1: Risk factors for CAUTI.		
Device-related risk factors	*Patient-related risk factors*	*Caregiver-related risk factors*
• **Duration:** Long-term (≥30 days) catheterization has a higher risk than short-term (<30 days) • **Type of catheter material:** Latex catheter has higher CAUTI risk (causes more urethritis, stricture formation, and obstruction) than silicone catheters	• Female gender • Fatal underlying illness • Older age (>50 years) • Diabetes mellitus • Poor personal hygiene • Incomplete emptying of bladder • Fecal incontinence	• Failure in adherence to aseptic technique (and other care bundle components) both during insertion and maintenance of catheter • Emergency catheter insertion outside the operating room

Contd...

- **Incomplete emptying:** In catheterized patients, bladder is often incompletely emptied because of pressure differentials created by patient movement or catheter manipulation. A small amount of urine always pools around the balloon which serves as a nidus for infection.

Laboratory Diagnosis

Urine should be collected through the catheter port using aseptic technique or, if a port is not present, by puncturing the catheter tubing with a needle and syringe. Urine should never be collected from the urobag.

The clinical diagnosis of CAUTI is based on the following three criteria.

1. **Catheter criteria:** Catheterized or history of recent catheterization within 48 hours
2. **Clinical criteria:** Presence of at least one sign or symptom of UTI such as fever, suprapubic tenderness, costovertebral angle pain, urinary urgency, frequency or dysuria (pain during micturition)
3. **Urine culture criteria:** Presence of significant bacteriuria, defined as colony count exceeding:
   - $\geq 10^3$ CFU/mL: in symptomatic patients
   - $\geq 10^5$ CFU/mL: in asymptomatic patients.

TREATMENT — CAUTI

Management of CAUTI includes removal of catheter and institution of appropriate antimicrobial therapy based on the susceptibility pattern of the organism isolated.

Treatment of asymptomatic bacteriuria (CA-ASB) is not recommended except when:
- Bacteriuria persists for >48 hours after removal of the catheter
- In pregnancy, as there is 20–30 fold increased risk of developing pyelonephritis and risk of premature delivery with low birth weight
- Prior to traumatic urological procedures such as transurethral resection of prostate where mucosal bleeding is anticipated which may cause bacteremia.

Prevention of CAUTI is discussed later in this chapter along with other major HAIs, under care bundle approach.

CATHETER-RELATED BLOODSTREAM INFECTION (CRBSI)

CRBSI refers to the development of bloodstream infections (BSI) in hospitalized patients which are attributed to the presence of a central line as a source of infection and is not associated with any other secondary cause of BSI. There is another related terminology called **CLABSI** (central line-associated bloodstream infection), which is strictly used only for surveillance purpose.

Central Line or Central Venous Catheter

A central line (CL) is an intravascular device that terminates in the great vessels. It is needed for various purposes such as central venous pressure monitoring and administration of drugs, total parenteral nutrition, etc. and for hemodialysis access (hemodialysis catheters).

Central line can be classified in various ways depending up on:
- Its intended life span, e.g. temporary or short-term (<72 hrs) versus permanent or long-term (≥72 hrs)
- Its site of insertion (e.g. subclavian, femoral, internal jugular and peripheral veins)
- Its pathway from skin to great vessel (e.g. tunneled versus non-tunneled).

Epidemiology

Approximately <3% of hospitalized patients require central line at some time during their stay, out of which 3–8% develop CLABSI. The CLABSI rate varies from 0% to 2.9% depending up on the location (wards or ICUs).

Pathogenesis

There are several routes by which the organisms gain access to the extraluminal or intraluminal surface of the CVC as given below in the decreasing order of frequency **(Fig. 39.2)**.

1. Migration of patient's skin flora along the surface of the catheter with colonization of catheter tip
2. Direct contamination of the catheter or its hub through the hands of healthcare workers (HCWs)

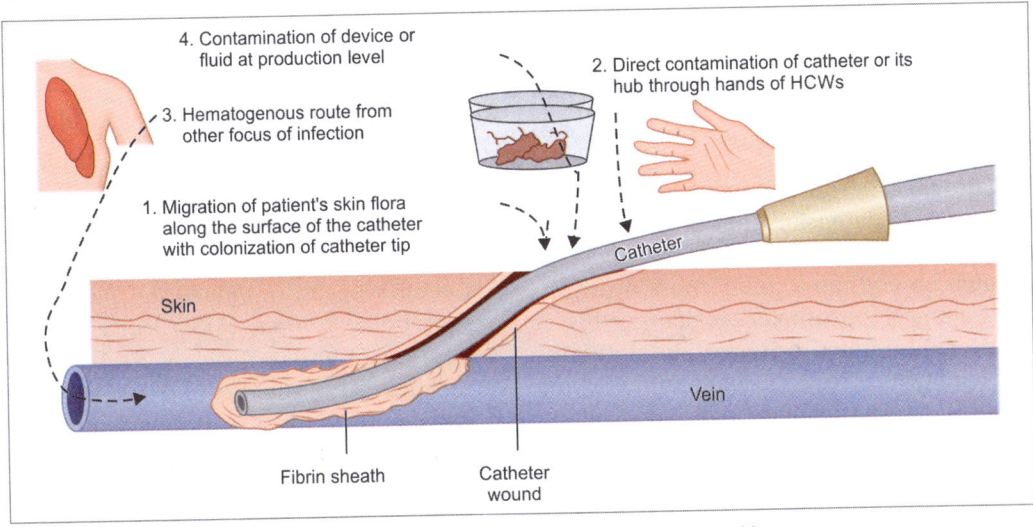

Fig. 39.2: Routes of access of organisms to central line.

3. Hematogenous route from other focus of infection
4. Contamination of the device or fluid at the production level.

There are various risk factors associated with pathogenesis of CRBSI, described in **Table 39.2**. The source of infection may be intraluminal (contamination occurs during device or fluid production) or extraluminal (contamination at the time of insertion) **(Table 39.3)**. Following events take place after the entry of the organism into the CL.

* Foreign body reaction, around the catheter insertion site
* **Colonization** of the organism by microbial adherence
* **Biofilm formation on catheter surface:** This is observed with many organisms such as coagulase-negative staphylococci, S. aureus, Pseudomonas aeruginosa, and Candida species.

Table 39.3: Intrinsic and extrinsic contamination of central line.

Intrinsic contamination (intraluminal source)	Extrinsic contamination (extraluminal source)
Contamination during device or fluid production	Contamination at the time of insertion
Due to defect during manufacture May cause outbreaks	Poor sterile precautions during drug or IV fluid admixture
Most common causative agents include *Klebsiella, Enterobacter* or *Pseudomonas*	Most common causative agents include skin commensals like CoNS and *S. aureus*

Abbreviation: CoNS, coagulase negative staphylococci.

Table 39.2: Risk factors for CRBSI.

Device-related	Patient-related	Caregiver-related
• Duration of central line (CL): Longer duration (≥72 hrs) has a higher risk than shorter duration (<72 hrs) • Site: Femoral vein CL has higher risk than jugular vein and subclavian vein • Catheter type: Non-tunneled catheters have higher risk than tunneled catheters • Number of lumens: Multi-lumen CLs have a higher risk than single-lumen • Insertion circumstances: Emergency insertion has a higher risk than elective insertion	• Immunodeficiency • Severe underlying illness • Hematologic malignancy • Loss of skin integrity (e.g. burns, psoriasis) • Presence of distant infection • Alteration in the patient's cutaneous microflora	• Poor hand hygiene • Lack of infection control practices (e.g. care bundle) • Skin antisepsis: Use of alcohol has a higher risk than chlorhexidine

Diagnosis of CRBSI

The diagnosis of CRBSI is established when a patient on CL meets the clinical criteria and microbiological criteria; in the absence of evidence of other sources of BSI.

- ❖ **Clinical criteria:** Presence of fever, chills, rigor or hypotension after the insertion of CL and/or signs of catheter site infection such as erythema, tenderness, warmth, swelling at the catheter exit site
- ❖ **Microbiological criteria:** Simultaneous blood culture from CL and peripheral line (PL) is carried out and the CL blood culture bottle flags ≥2 hrs earlier to peripheral line blood culture (i.e. differential time to positivity ≥2 hrs).

TREATMENT — CRBSI

Treatment of CRBSI consists of institution of appropriate systematic antimicrobial therapy and removal of the central line.
- **Systematic antimicrobial therapy (SAT):** The empirical therapy should be started as soon as the clinical suspicion is made, which should be modified later based on susceptibility report
- **Antibiotic lock therapy (ALT):** In situations where salvage of the catheter is considered (e.g. infection with CoNS, those with limited venous access and a history of recurrent CLABSIs), ALT is given along with SAT. It involves instillation of a highly concentrated antibiotic solution into the CL lumen and is left to dwell within the lumen for a short period.

Prevention of CRBSI is discussed later in this chapter along with other major HAIs, under care bundle approach.

VENTILATOR-ASSOCIATED PNEUMONIA

Ventilator-associated pneumonia (VAP) is the second most common nosocomial infection (after CAUTI) and accounts for 15–20% of the total HAIs.
- ❖ It is the most common cause of death among HAIs, with a mortality rate of up to 40% and is the primary cause of death in ICUs
- ❖ The VAP rate varies from 1.0 to 46.0 per 1000 mechanical ventilation (MV) days, depending up on the ICU facility and the hospital.

Microbiology

VAP can be divided into early- and late-onset.
- ❖ **Early-onset VAP:** It occurs during the first 4 days of mechanical ventilation. It is caused by typical community organisms such as pneumococcus, *H. influenzae,* methicillin susceptible *S. aureus* (MSSA), etc.
- ❖ **Late-onset VAP:** It develops ≥5 days after mechanical ventilation and is commonly caused by typical multidrug resistant hospital pathogens—*P. aeruginosa, Acinetobacter baumannii, E.coli, Klebsiella* and methicillin resistant *S. aureus* (MRSA). It is associated with high attributable mortality. Here, the source of infection may be:
    - **Endogenous,** i.e. patient's own oropharyngeal microbial flora transmitted to lungs by aspiration
    - **Exogenous,** e.g. hospital environmental sources like air, water, reusable equipment, nebulized medication, etc. contaminated with environmental organisms.

Pathogenesis and Risk Factors

The pathogenesis of VAP involves a complex interplay between various risk factors **(Table 39.4)**.
- ❖ **Colonization:** Following hospitalization of critically-ill patients, the normal oropharyngeal flora (e.g. viridans streptococci, *Haemophilus,* anaerobes) rapidly shifts toward "hospital-associated" pathogens such as *Pseudomonas, Acinetobacter* species, etc.
- ❖ **Endotracheal (ET) intubation** is the most important risk factor. It disrupts normal ciliary clearance of bronchial secretions, inhibits the cough reflex, damages the respiratory epithelium, and helps oropharyngeal bacteria to gain access directly into the lower respiratory tract
- ❖ **Biofilm:** The organism begins to form biofilm both inside and outside the endotracheal tube within a day of placement, which acts as a reservoir of infection,

Table 39.4: Risk factors for the development of VAP.

Device- or intervention-related	Patient-related	Healthcare personnel-related
Device-related • Duration of ventilation • Nasogastric tube • Frequent changes of ventilator circuit • Failed subglottic aspiration • Intra-cuff pressure <20 cm of H_2O **Intervention-related** • Use of antibiotics or sedatives • Stress ulcer prophylaxis • Tracheostomy	• Advanced age (>60 years) • Prior hospitalization • Patient position: Supine position • Critically-ill with comorbidities • Underlying condition such as COPD, ARDS, head trauma • Patients with coma • Immobilization • Thermal injury (burns)	• Improper adherence to aseptic techniques specially hand washing • Contaminated environmental sources

Abbreviations: COPD, chronic obstructive pulmonary disease; ARDS, adult respiratory distress syndrome.

preventing the entry of antimicrobials and the host immune system
- **Subglottic secretions**: Secretions pool on and above the ET tube cuff and intermittently seep (*microaspiration*) to the lower respiratory tract, particularly if the cuff is underinflated or gets shifted during patient movement **(Fig. 39.3)**. This can be prevented by:
    - Maintaining the cuff pressure at 20–30 cm of H_2O
    - Subglottic suctioning should be done regularly to remove the pooling of secretion above the cuff.
- **Sedation:** Sedation, coma or unconsciousness inhibits the natural ability to clear secretions and thereby increases the risk of aspiration

- **Supine position** facilitates microaspiration. Therefore, patients should be put on a semi-recumbent position (30–45°)
- **Nasogastric tubes:** Ventilated patients are very often kept on nasogastric tubes, which disrupt the lower esophageal sphincter and increase the risk of aspiration of gastric contents
- **Critical illness with comorbidities**, poor nutrition and immobilization may increase patients' susceptibility to infection
- **Stress ulcer prophylaxis:** Intubated patients are at high-risk for stress ulcers, which may lead to upper gastrointestinal hemorrhage. Therefore, stress ulcer prophylaxis is a common practice in ventilated patients. However, this itself is a risk factor for aspiration pneumonia. The only acceptable prophylaxis is by sucralfate, which is associated with lower risk of VAP.

Diagnosis

The diagnosis of VAP is based on a combination of clinical, radiological, and microbiological criteria.

Till date, there is no gold standard criteria available which can define VAP accurately. The most popular and widely used criteria is CPIS system.

Clinical pulmonary infection score (CPIS) system is a scoring system, based on six parameters (clinical, radiological and microbiological) with each parameter given a score scale ranging from 0 to 2 **(Table 39.5)**.

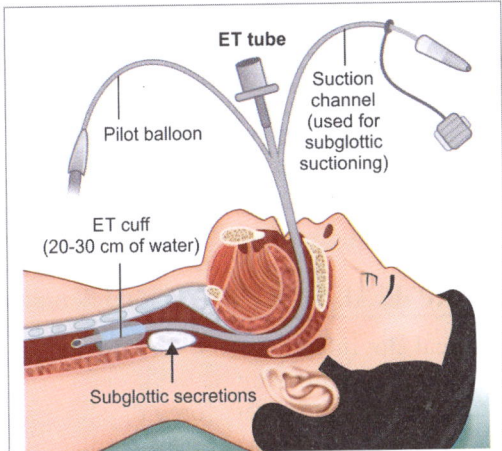

Fig. 39.3: Endotracheal (ET) tube with suction.

Table 39.5: Modified Clinical Pulmonary Infection Score (CPIS) used for ventilator-associated pneumonia.

CPIS points	0	1	2
Temperature (°C)	≥36.5°C and ≤38.4°C	≥38.5°C and ≤38.9°C	≥39°C or ≤36°C
Leukocyte count (per mm^3)	4,000–11,000	<4,000 or >11,000	<4,000 or >11,000 + band forms ≥50%
Tracheal secretions	Rare	Nonpurulent	Abundant + purulent
Oxygenation PaO$_2$/FiO$_2$ mm Hg	>240 with ARDS	-	≤240 and no ARDS
Chest radiograph	No infiltrate	Diffuse or patchy infiltrate	Localized infiltrate
Tracheal aspirate culture report	Light growth or no growth	Moderate or heavy growth of pathogenic bacteria	Moderate or heavy growth of bacteria and presence of bacteria with similar morphology on Gram stain

Abbreviations: ARDS, acute respiratory distress syndrome; FiO$_2$, fraction of inspired oxygen; PaO$_2$, arterial partial pressure of oxygen.

- The maximum score that can be obtained is 12 and a score >6 is diagnostic of VAP
- CPIS score is prone to significant inter-observer variability, mainly in the interpretation of the tracheal secretions and the chest X-ray.

Microbiological Criteria

The specimens for VAP include endotracheal aspirate (most common), bronchoalveolar lavage (BAL), protected specimen brush (PSB) or lung biopsy. Specimens should be processed immediately. Delay of no more than 2 hours is permissible.

- **Gram staining:** Gram stain should be performed from the mucopurulent part. The diagnosis of VAP is likely if Gram staining demonstrates—higher numbers of bacteria, intracellular bacteria or presence of fibrin strands. A negative Gram stain result suggests that VAP is unlikely
- **Culture:** The specimens are subjected to either quantitative or semi-quantitative culture
    - Quantitative culture: Considered significant if the colony count exceeds ≥10^5 CFU/mL for endotracheal aspirate, ≥10^4 CFU/mL for BAL and ≥10^3/mL for PSB
    - Semi-quantitative culture: Moderate to heavy growth is suggestive of colony count of ≥10^5 CFU/mL.

Radiological Criteria

Radiological diagnosis of VAP is highly subjective as many other clinical conditions may show similar findings. In general, the most accepted radiological criteria is chest X-ray or CT scan showing one of the following—infiltrate, consolidation or cavitation, in the absence of underlying pulmonary or cardiac disease.

TREATMENT — VAP

Treatment of VAP consists of institution of empirical antimicrobial therapy once the clinical diagnosis of VAP is made, which can be modified subsequently based on antimicrobial susceptibility report.
- Empirical regimen should include a combination of antimicrobial agents active against *S. aureus*, *Pseudomonas* and other gram-negative bacilli
- The choice of empirical regimen should be based on local antimicrobial resistance pattern of the hospital.

Prevention of VAP is discussed later in this chapter along with other major HAIs, under care bundle approach.

SURGICAL SITE INFECTION

Surgical site infections (SSI) are defined as infections that develop at the surgical site within 30 days of surgery (or within 90 days for some surgeries such as breast, cardiac and joint surgeries including implants).

- SSIs can cause significant morbidity and mortality as well as economic burden if left untreated
- SSI affects up to one third of patients who have undergone a surgical procedure, incidence is higher following abdominal operations
- In India, several studies reported SSI rate ranging from 4 to 11 per 100 surgeries.

Microbiology

The type of etiological agents implicated in SSI depends upon the site of surgical procedure and the source of infection from which they are acquired.

- **Endogenous source** such as the patient's own flora present on
  - **Skin:** *S. aureus* (the most common organism causing SSI), coagulase negative staphylococci (CoNS)
  - **Mucosa** (from opened viscus such as GIT, respiratory or genitourinary): Consists of predominantly aerobic gram-negative bacilli (*E.coli, Klebsiella*), gram-positive cocci (*Enterococcus*) and anaerobes such *Bacteroides*, and others.
- **Exogenous source** from contact with the operative room personnel or instruments or environment: *S. aureus* and gram-negative bacilli including nonfermenters such as *Pseudomonas* and *Acinetobacter*.

The inoculum load and the virulence of the microorganism can determine the risk of SSI

- **Inoculum of bacteria:** Surgical procedures involving the sites (e.g. bowel, vagina) which are heavily colonized with bacteria have a higher risk of developing SSI as large inoculum of bacteria lodge into the wound during surgery
- **Virulence of bacteria:** Higher is the virulence of infecting organism, more is the risk of development of SSI.

Pathogenesis and Risk Factors

In most patients, infection does not develop at surgical site due to the presence of strong host innate immunity eliminating microbial contaminants at the surgical site.

Table 39.6: Risk factors for development of SSI.

Patient-related	Procedure-related
Age >60 years	Improper surgical scrub
Malnutrition, diabetes	Inadequate skin antisepsis
Immunosuppression	Prolonged operative time
Skin colonization at the time of surgery (e.g. MRSA carrier)	Inadequate antimicrobial prophylaxis
Duration of hospital stay	Poor perioperative glycemic control
Smoking, obesity	Emergency procedures
Higher wound class	Preoperative shaving
Organism-related	**Environmental-related**
Inoculum size (e.g. bowel surgery)	Presence of blood/clot, suture material and foreign bodies at the surgical site
Bacterial virulence	Inadequate ventilation
Ability to form biofilm	Contaminated medications

However, when host defense mechanisms fail to eliminate the microbial contamination, compounded by the greater load and higher virulence of the invading microbes, all together pave path to the development of SSI.

The **risk factors** leading to the development of SSIs can be classified into patient-related, procedure-related, organism-related and environmental-related risk factors (**Table 39.6**); out of which the type of wound class is the most important, discussed below.

Wound Class Type

Depending up on the degree of microbial contamination, wounds are classified as clean, clean-contaminated, contaminated, or dirty/infected. The contaminated and dirty wound classes have a higher risk of developing SSI.

Class I, Clean Wound

It is an uninfected operative wound in which no inflammation is encountered and the hollow viscus such as respiratory, alimentary, genital, or urinary tract is not entered. SSI rate is usually less than 2% in clean operated wounds.

Class II, Clean-contaminated Wound

It is an operative wound in which the hollow viscus such as respiratory, alimentary, genital, or urinary tracts are entered under controlled conditions and without unusual contamination.
- Surgeries included in this category involve the biliary tract, appendix, vagina, and oropharynx; provided that no evidence of infection or major breach in the technique is encountered
- SSI rate is about 3% to 11% in clean-contaminated wounds.

Class III, Contaminated Wound

Contaminated wound includes the following:
- Open, fresh, accidental wounds
- Operations with major breaks in the sterile technique (e.g. open cardiac massage) or
- Operations with gross spillage from the gastrointestinal tract (colonic surgeries)
- Entry into biliary or genitourinary tract in the presence of infected bile or urine
- Incisions in which acute, nonpurulent inflammation is encountered including necrotic tissue without evidence of purulent drainage (for example, dry gangrene).

SSI rate is >10% in contaminated wounds even with administration of surgical antimicrobial prophylaxis.

Class IV, Dirty/Infected Wound

Surgical procedures performed when active infection is already present are considered dirty wounds. Examples include:
- Abdominal exploration for acute bacterial peritonitis or perforated viscera
- Intra-abdominal abscess
- Old traumatic wounds with retained devitalized tissue.

In dirty wound, the SSI rate can exceed 20–40%.

Classification and Diagnosis of SSI

SSIs are classified based on the level where infection developed into three types:
- **Superficial SSI**—develops at the level of superficial incisional site (skin and subcutaneous level) within 30 days regardless of the type of surgery
- **Deep SSI**—develops at the level of deep incisional site (muscle and facial level) within 30 days for all surgeries except for breast, cardiac and implant surgeries (90 days)
- **Organ space SSI**—develops at the level of organ space site within 30 days for all surgeries except breast, cardiac and implant surgeries (90 days).

The criteria for diagnosis of above mentioned three types of SSIs have been discussed in detail under surveillance of SSI, subsequently in this chapter.

> **TREATMENT** — SSI
>
> Treatment of SSI includes suture removal plus incision and drainage with adjunctive systemic antimicrobial therapy.

Prevention of SSI

Preventive measures of SSI can be categorized into preoperative, perioperative and postoperative measures. Both WHO and CDC recently published the guidelines for prevention of SSI which has been summarized in **Table 39.7**.

PREVENTION OF DEVICE-ASSOCIATED INFECTIONS

The majority of device-associated infections (DAIs) encountered in hospital are CAUTI, CLABSI and VAP.
- Presence of device itself is a major risk factor for developing such infection. This is because of various reasons:
  - Risk of introduction of patients own flora
  - Risk of introduction of HCW's hand flora due to improper handling during insertion or daily maintenance of the device
  - Ability of the invading organism to produce biofilm over the device.
- Strict aseptic techniques must be followed while insertion and daily maintenance of the devices

Table 39.7: Prevention of surgical site infections (SSIs).

Preoperative measures

1. **Preoperative bathing:** It should be performed using a plain soap or an antimicrobial soap to reduce the bacterial load, especially at the site of incision
2. **For MRSA carriers:** Decolonization with mupirocin ointment must be done for patients undergoing surgery who are nasal carriers of MRSA
3. **Hair removal:** For patients undergoing any surgical procedure, hair removal should not be done or, if absolutely necessary, it should be removed only with a clipper. Shaving is strongly discouraged at all times

Intraoperative measures

1. **SAP:** Surgical antimicrobial prophylaxis (SAP) must be provided for all except for clean surgeries.
   - *Timing*—SAP must be administered within 60–120 minutes before incision, which usually coincides with the induction of anesthesia
   - *Choice*—It depends upon local antibiotic policy. Cefazolin or cefuroxime are usually preferred
   - *Frequency*—SAP is usually given as a single dose. Repeat dose may be required only for:
     - Duration of surgery exceeds 4 hours
     - Cardiac surgeries
     - Drugs with lower half-lives (redosing required if duration of surgery exceeds 2 half-lives)
     - Extensive blood loss during surgery
   - *For ESBL prevalent area*—SAP should not be modified. ESBL screening for patients is not routinely recommended.
2. **Surgical hand disinfection-** Scrubbing with either antimicrobial soap (chlorhexidine) or with alcohol-based hand rub must be performed before donning sterile gloves, before surgery and in between surgeries
3. **Surgical site preparation** should be performed with alcohol-based chlorhexidine antiseptic solution before the commencement of surgery
4. **Perioperative maintenance** of oxygenation (target FiO_2 80%), temperature (normothermia), blood glucose level (target level of <200 mg/dL), adequate circulating volume (normovolemia) and nutritional support are necessary during the surgery and immediate 4–6 hours postoperative period

Postoperative measures

1. **Wound dressing**—Daily dressing of surgical site and removal of any discharge present at the site must be performed. Perform hand hygiene and use gloves before dressing
2. **OT disinfection**—Thorough postoperative disinfection of operation theater must be performed with a high level disinfectant in between cases and after the last case (terminal disinfection)
3. **Periodic monitoring of the air quality of operation theater** for various parameters must be performed such as no. of air exchanges, temperature, humidity, pressure and microbial contamination
4. **SAP prolongation is not recommended** in any situations (e.g. presence of a wound drain) for the purpose of preventing SSI as it promotes development of antimicrobial resistance

Source: Adapted from WHO's Global guidelines on the prevention of surgical site infection, 2016 and CDC's Guideline for the prevention of surgical site infection, 2017.
Abbreviation: ESBL, extended spectrum beta lactamase.

- The preventive measures for each of the DAIs are grouped as care bundle approach (described below).

Care Bundle Approach

Healthcare facilities must adhere to care bundle approach for the prevention of DAIs.
- Care bundle comprises of 3 to 5 evidence-based elements with strong clinician agreement; each of the component must be followed during the insertion or maintenance of the device
- Compliance to the care bundle is calculated as all-or-none way, i.e. failure of compliance to any of the component leads to non-compliance to the whole bundle
- The components of care bundle approach for prevention of DAIs have been described in **Table 39.8**.

Table 39.8: Care bundle approach for prevention of device-associated infections (DAIs).

Care bundle for urinary catheter

Insertion bundle	Maintenance bundle
1. Catheter should be inserted only when appropriate indication is present (e.g. acute urinary retention) 2. Only the sterile items are used for insertion of catheter 3. Catheter is inserted by non-touch technique with strict asepsis 4. Closed drainage system must be used 5. Catheter of appropriate size must be used 6. Catheter must be properly secured after placement (by plaster-tube-plaster technique)	1. Daily catheter care (vaginal or meatal care) must be given regularly and by strict aseptic measures such as hand hygiene and single use gloves 2. Catheter is properly secured all the time 3. Drainage bag must be always above the floor and below the bladder level 4. Closed drainage system is used all the time 5. While collection of urine from bag, the following steps must be followed—Hand hygiene, change of gloves between patients; use of separate jug for each bag, use of alcohol swabs for disinfection of outlet 6. Daily assessment of readiness for removal of catheter must be documented

Care bundle for central line

Insertion bundle	Maintenance bundle

1. Hand hygiene before and after insertion of central line
2. Use maximum sterile PPE: gloves, gown, drapes, cap and mask
3. Site of insertion—Subclavian preferred, avoid femoral
4. Skin preparation—by antiseptics such as chlorhexidine
5. Skin must be completely dry after use of antiseptics
6. Use semi-permeable dressing
7. Document data and time of insertion
	1. Daily aseptic central line care during handling:
	   ➤ Hand hygiene must be performed
	   ➤ Hub decontamination by alcohol
	2. Daily documentation of local signs of infection
	3. Change of dressing with 2% chlorhexidine
	4. Daily assessment of readiness for removal of central line must be documented

Maintenance care bundle for mechanical ventilator

1. Adherence to hand hygiene
2. Elevation of the head of the bed to 30–45°—this is to prevent oropharyngeal aspiration to respiratory tract
3. Daily oral care with chlorhexidine 2% solution
4. Need of PUD (peptic ulcer disease) prophylaxis should be assessed daily; if needed only sucralfate should be used
5. DVT (deep vein thrombosis) prophylaxis should be provided if needed
6. Daily assessment of readiness to remove mechanical ventilator must be documented

EXPECTED QUESTIONS

I. Write short notes on:
1. Care bundle approach for prevention of device-associated infections.
2. Catheter-associated urinary tract infection.
3. Central line-associated bloodstream infection.
4. Ventilator-associated pneumonia.
5. Prevention of surgical site infection.

II. Multiple Choice Questions (MCQs):
1. **Which is not a device-associated infection?**
   a. CAUTI (catheter-associated urinary tract infection)
   b. CLABSI (central line-associated bloodstream infection)
   c. VAP (ventilator-associated pneumonia)
   d. Surgical site infection

2. For device-associated infection, the device should be present in place at least for how many calendar days?
   a. 1
   b. 2
   c. 3
   d. 4
3. Repeat dose of surgical antimicrobial prophylaxis may be required for all of the following, *except*?
   a. Duration of surgery exceeds 4 hours
   b. Cardiac surgeries
   c. Extensive blood loss during surgery
   d. Thyroid surgery
4. The most common organism responsible for catheter-associated urinary tract infection (CAUTI) is:
   a. *Escherichia coli*
   b. *Klebsiella pneumoniae*
   c. *Enterococcus* species
   d. *Acinetobacter* species
5. The most important risk factors for catheter-associated urinary tract infection (CAUTI) is:
   a. Female gender
   b. Duration of catheterization
   c. Failure in adherence to aseptic technique during insertion and maintenance of catheter
   d. Type of catheter material
6. Early-onset ventilator associated pneumonia (VAP) occurs during the first ___ days of mechanical ventilation?
   a. 2 days
   b. 3 days
   c. 4 days
   d. 7 days
7. Late-onset ventilator associated pneumonia (VAP) is typical caused by all the following organisms, *except*:
   a. *Acinetobacter baumannii*
   b. *Klebsiella*
   c. *Haemophilus influenzae*
   d. *Pseudomonas aeruginosa*
8. Which of the following is the most common specimen collected for culture diagnosis of ventilator associated pneumonia (VAP)?
   a. Endotracheal aspirate
   b. Bronchoalveolar lavage (BAL)
   c. Protected specimen brush (PSB)
   d. Lung biopsy
9. Surgical site infections (SSI) are defined as infections that develop at the surgical site within ___ days of surgery.
   a. 30 days
   b. 60 days
   c. 90 days
   d. 1 year
10. Surgical antimicrobial prophylaxis (SAP) must be provided for all type of surgeries, *except*:
    a. Clean wound
    b. Clean contaminate wound
    c. Contaminate wound
    d. Dirty wound

Answers
1. d   2. b   3. d   4. a   5. c   6. c   7. c   8. a   9. a   10. a

CHAPTER 40: HAI Surveillance and HICC

CHAPTER PREVIEW
- HAI Surveillance
- Hospital Infection Control Committee (HICC)

HAI SURVEILLANCE

Healthcare-associated infections (HAIs) surveillance is a system that monitors the HAIs in a hospital. The main objectives of HAI surveillance include:
- Provides endemic or baseline HAI rate and information on the type of HAIs in the hospital
- Helps in comparing HAI rates within and between hospitals
- Identifies the problem area; based on which root cause analysis can be conducted to find out the breakdowns in infection control measures and then the appropriate corrective measures are implemented
- Provides timely feedback to the clinicians; thus, reinforcing them to adopt best practices.

Targeted Surveillance

The National Healthcare Safety Network (NHSN) division of CDC (Centers for Disease Control and Prevention) provides guidelines for the surveillance of HAIs.
- **Where to conduct:** HAI surveillance should be conducted only in high-risk locations such as intensive care units (ICUs)
- **What type of HAIs to be monitored:** As technically difficult, only the major types of HAIs can be monitored such as CAUTI, CLABSI, VAP, and SSI
- **Who will conduct:** The infection control nurses (ICNs) under the supervision of the officer-in-charge of HICC will conduct HAI surveillance
- **HAI surveillance diagnostic criteria:** The NHSN has provided the diagnostic criteria for four major types of HAIs **(Tables 40.1 to 40.4)**
    - These criteria are made very objective to maintain the uniformity of data collection between hospitals which helps in accurate comparison of HAI rates between hospitals of the same and different nations
    - The surveillance criteria are different from clinical and diagnostic criteria, and therefore these should strictly be used only for surveillance purposes, not for clinical diagnosis and treatment.

Table 40.1: NHSN surveillance diagnostic criteria for catheter-associated urinary tract infection.

Device criteria	Presence of a urinary catheter for >2 days
Clinical criteria	Presence of any one symptom of UTI such as fever, suprapubic tenderness, urgency, frequency, or dysuria
Culture criteria	Isolation of significant count ($\geq 10^5$/mL) of a UTI pathogen from urine

Abbreviations: NHSN, National Healthcare Safety Network; UTI, urinary tract infection.

Table 40.2: The NHSN surveillance diagnostic criteria for CLABSI (Central line-associated bloodstream infection).

		Blood culture criteria		
	Age	Organism isolated	No. of cultures positive	Clinical criteria
LCBI-1	Any age	LCBI pathogen[1]	1	Symptoms not required
LCBI-2	<1 year	LCBI commensal[2]	2	Any one symptom[3]
LCBI-3	<1 year	LCBI commensal[2]	2	Any one symptom[4]

Device criteria = catheter present for > two calendar days

LCBI *plus* catheter criteria met = called as CLABSI
LCBI *without* catheter criteria met = called as non-CLABSI

Abbreviation: LCBI, laboratory-confirmed bloodstream infection.
[1]LCBI pathogen, e.g. common healthcare-associated pathogens.
[2]LCBI commensal, e.g. coagulase-negative staphylococci.
[3]LCBI-2 symptoms—fever, chills, hypotension.
[4]LCBI-3 symptoms—fever, hypothermia, bradycardia, apnea.

Table 40.3: The NHSN surveillance diagnostic criteria for ventilator-associated events (VAE).

Stage-1: VAC (ventilator-associated condition)

Device criteria	Presence of a mechanical ventilator at least for 2 calendar days
Worsening oxygenation criteria	• Baseline period during which the daily minimum FiO$_2$ and PEEP values are stable or decreasing for 2 days followed by • Period of worsening of oxygenation—increased FiO$_2$ (by ≥20%) or PEEP (≥3 cm water) for at least two consecutive days

Stage-2: IVAC (infection-related ventilator-associated complications): VAC plus the following criteria

Clinical criteria	*Any one of the following:* Fever or hypothermia or leukocytosis or leukopenia
Antibiotic criteria	The new antimicrobial agent started and continued for ≥4 days

Stage-3: PVAP (Possible ventilator-associated pneumonia): IVAC plus the culture criteria

Culture criteria	Isolation of significant count of a pneumonia pathogen from respiratory specimens such as endotracheal aspirate, bronchoalveolar lavage, etc.

Abbreviations: FiO$_2$, fraction of inspired oxygen; PEEP, positive end-expiratory pressure.

Table 40.4: The NHSN surveillance diagnostic criteria for surgical site infection (SSI).

Definition and types of SSIs

Definition: SSIs are defined as infections that develop at the surgical site within 30 days of surgery (within 90 days for breast, cardiac and joint surgeries)

SSIs are classified based on the level where the infection is developed:
- *Superficial SSI:* Develops at the level of superficial incisional site (skin and subcutaneous level) within 30 days regardless of the type of surgery
- *Deep SSI:* Develops at the level of deep incisional site (muscle and fascial level) within 30 days for all surgeries except breast, cardiac, and implant surgeries (90 days)
- *Organ space SSI:* Develops at the level of organ space site within 30 days for all surgeries except breast, cardiac, and implant surgeries (90 days)

One among the following must be met:

Clinical criteria	1. Presence of purulent pus from the corresponding level of the surgical site or 2. Presence of local signs of infections (pain/ tenderness, swelling, erythema, heat, etc.)
Culture criteria	A positive culture from the discharge was collected at the corresponding level of the surgical site
Other evidence	1. For superficial SSI—Surgeon's diagnosis is taken as diagnostic criteria 2. For deep or organ space SSI—histopathological, imaging or gross anatomical evidence of abscess should be present

Method of Conducting *HAI* Surveillance

The HAI surveillance cycle consists of data collection → data analysis → data interpretation → data dissemination.

- ❖ **Data collection:** The ICNs visit daily to the high-risk areas (ICUs) and collect the clinical data of patients on devices (urinary catheter, central line, ventilator) and also patients admitted following surgeries. They also prospectively check the laboratory investigations to confirm a diagnosis
- ❖ **Data analysis:** The four types of HAIs are diagnosed according to HAI surveillance criteria of NHSN/CDC **(Tables 40.1 to 40.4)**

Table 40.5: Formulae of HAI infection rates.

HAI infection rates formulae	
CAUTI rate	No. of CAUTI cases/total no. of urinary catheter days × 1,000
CLABSI rate	No. of CLABSI cases/total no. of central line days × 1,000
VAE rate	No. of VAE cases/total no. of ventilator days × 1,000
SSI rate	No. of SSI/No. of surgeries done × 100

- Then the HAI rates are calculated as per the formulae given in **Table 40.5**
- Then the monthly report of location-wise HAI rates of the hospital is generated.

❖ **Data interpretation:** HAI rates are compared:
  - For the same location across different time frames
  - Between different locations of the same or different hospital during the same time frame.

❖ **Data dissemination:** The monthly HAI surveillance report should be shared with all clinical departments and administrators. It is also presented during HICC meetings. Accordingly, the appropriate corrective actions are planned in the problem areas.

HOSPITAL INFECTION CONTROL COMMITTEE (HICC)

The hospital infection control program is organized and run by the Medical Superintendent (MS), who he/she constitutes the Hospital infection control committee.

The HICC provides a forum for multidisciplinary input and cooperation, and information sharing, required for hospital infection control and prevention. The HICC is advisory to the MS and makes its recommendations to the MS.

Hospital Infection Control Committee constitution

The HICC should include wide representations from relevant departments/health sectors as follows:
- Chairperson, usually the Medical Superintendent

Contd...

Contd...

- Secretary, mostly the head of the department of microbiology
- Hospital Infection Control Officer (HICO), generally a representative from the department of microbiology
- Hospital Infection Control Nurses (HICN)
- Head of all the clinical (all medical and surgical) departments
- Nursing Superintendent
- Head of the staff clinic
- Operation Room Supervisor
- In-charge of Central Sterile Supplies Department (CSSD)
- In charge of biomedical waste management
- In charge of pharmacy
- In charge of hospital linen and laundry
- In charge of hospital kitchen
- Epidemiologist
- In charge of the engineering department of the hospital

Functions of HICC

The HICC supervises the implementation of the hospital infection control program. The various functions of the committee include:

❖ **HAI surveillance:** Maintains surveillance of hospital-acquired infections. The four key parameters used for HAI surveillance are as follows (discussed above):
  1. CAUTI (Catheter-associated urinary tract infection)
  2. CLABSI (Central line-associated bloodstream infection)
  3. VAP (Ventilator-associated pneumonia)
  4. SSI (Surgical site infection).

❖ **Develops a system** for identifying, reporting, analyzing, investigating and controlling healthcare-associated infections

❖ **Antimicrobial stewardship program (AMSP):** Develops antibiotic policies, monitors the antibiotic usage, advises the MS on matters related to the proper use of antibiotics, and also recommends remedial measures when antibiotic-resistant strains are detected

❖ **Policies:** Reviews and updates on the hospital infection control policies and guidelines from time to time

❖ **Education:** Conducts teaching sessions for healthcare workers regarding matters related to HAIs

- **Staff health:** Monitors employee health activities regarding matters related to HAIs such as needle stick injury prevention, hepatitis B vaccination, etc.
- **Outbreak management:** Develops strategies to identify infectious outbreaks, and their source and implements preventive and corrective measures
- **Other departments:** Communicates and cooperates with other departments of the hospital with common interests such as:
  - Pharmacy
  - Central Sterile Supplies Department (CSSD)
  - Linen and Laundry Department(s)
  - Antimicrobial Usage Committee
  - Biomedical Safety Committee
  - Blood Transfusion Committee.
- **Reviews** risk associated with new technologies, and monitor infectious risks of new devices and products, prior to their approval for use
- **HICC meetings:** HICC shall meet regularly not less than once a month and as often as required. However, in an emergency (such as an outbreak), this committee must be able to meet promptly as and when required.

Responsibility of Different Stakeholders of HICC

Hospital Administration

The hospital administration has a major role in implementing infection control program. They must provide leadership in initiating. Their responsibilities include:
- Establish a multidisciplinary HICC
- Provide adequate resources (financial and human) and support to HICC so that the infection prevention program can be implemented effectively
- Ensure availability of hand hygiene products, personal protective equipment (PPE), disinfectants, and vaccines for HCWs, etc.
- Approve and review policies and guidelines for infection control practices formulated by the HICC.

Infection Control Officer (ICO)

The ICO is either a clinical microbiologist or an infectious disease physician or any physician working full-time in infection control. In small hospitals where only one clinical microbiologist is available, he can act as both member secretary and ICO. He takes the overall responsibility for the activities of HICC and reports directly to the member secretary and chairman of HICC.

Duties of Infection Control Officer
- Involves in meticulous planning and implementation of infection control measures such as hand hygiene, care bundle, appropriate use of PPE, etc.
- Supervises the HAI surveillance activities- both data collection and analysis
- Plays an active role in the investigation of the outbreak with consultation from clinical and microbiology department
- Conducts research activities related to infection control practices
- Supervises the activities of department of Biomedical waste
- Acts as the nodal officer for management of needle stick injury and other occupational exposures
- Ensures implementation of safe work practices in all healthcare service sectors
- Ensures immunization of all HCWs (hepatitis B, influenza) as recommended by institutional policy
- Formulate and implement guidelines for sterilization of equipment and instruments (CSSD policy), disinfection policy including housekeeping policy, and then updates periodically
- Involves in drawing up annual plans, policies, and long-term programs including educational and surveillance activities for the prevention of HAIs
- Prepares the annual budget of HICC and involves in annual purchase activities
- Conducts regular surveys and surprise visits to objectively monitor ongoing implementation of all infection control measures
- Performs AMR surveillance and disseminates annual hospital location/department specific antibiogram

- Actively participate in implementing antimicrobial stewardship program and also coordinates formulation of antibiotic policy
- Review and revision of infection control manual.

Infection Control Nurse

An infection control nurse (ICN) is a registered nurse with an additional academic education and practical training in infection control, clinical and diagnostic microbiology, epidemiology and computer technology.

- They should undergo competency assessment tests at the beginning and then periodically to continually expand on their existing knowledge, understanding, and skills
- **Requirement:** It is recommended that at least 0.8–1.0 dedicated fulltime ICN is required per 100 beds in acute-care centers and one per 150–250 beds in long-term-care facilities.

Duties of Infection Control Nurse

The ICN is the bridge between the HICC and the hospital wards and ICUs. He/she goes on rounds and visits all hospital locations and monitors the compliance of HCWs to infection control measures in the hospital; identifies problems associated and implements the appropriate measures after discussing with ICO.
- Carry out data collection for HAI surveillance, hand hygiene audit, care bundle audit, PPE audit, etc. by performing daily visits to ICUs and wards
- Oversee the implementation of transmission based precautions wherever necessary
- Monitors the implementation of disinfection policy at the hospital
- Identifies the high risk areas for conducting environmental surveillance
- Involves in education of healthcare workers and patients
- Provides post-exposure prophylaxis for needle stick injury cases. They also maintain registers and data on needle stick injuries
- Conducts or oversees staff vaccination program for hepatitis B, influenza, etc.
- In a certain healthcare facility, ICNs are also involved in conducting antimicrobial stewardship activities.

Infection Control Links Nurse

If adequate ICNs are not available, then the existing nursing staff working in ICUs can be trained so that they can be part-time engaged in monitoring infection control activities of their concerned ICUs.

- It has been shown that competent infection control link nurses can motivate ward staff by enabling more effective practice
- This practice can be very much useful, provided the link nurses are adequately trained and backed up by a strong infection control team
- However, lack of adequate training, frequent turnover of nurses, lack of recognition of their role, are the problem areas that need to be addressed while implementing the link nurses program.

EXPECTED QUESTIONS

I. Write short notes on:
1. Ventilator-associated events surveillance criteria.
2. Surveillance criteria for surgical site infection.
3. Hospital infection control committee.
4. Role of infection control nurse.

II. Multiple Choice Questions (MCQs):
1. Which parameter is not included in HAI surveillance?
   a. CAUTI b. CLABSI
   c. VAP
   d. Open wound infections
2. Among the following VAE, which requires a culture to be positive?
   a. VAC b. IVAC
   c. PVAP  d. All of the above

Answers
1. d   2. c

CHAPTER 41: Sterilization and Disinfection

CHAPTER PREVIEW
- Sterilants
- High-level Disinfectants
- Intermediate-level Disinfectants
- Low-level Disinfectants
- Cleaning Agents
- Environmental Cleaning
- Methods to Test Efficacy of Sterilant/Disinfectant

INTRODUCTION

The sterilization and disinfection practices in a hospital is of paramount importance in preventing transmission of healthcare-associated infections.

Definitions

Sterilization, disinfection and cleaning are three separate but interrelated terminologies, all aiming at removing or destroying the microorganisms from materials or from body surfaces. However, they vary in their efficacy of destroying the microorganisms **(Table 41.1)**.

Sterilization

Sterilization is a process by which all living microorganisms including viable spores, are either destroyed or removed from an article, surface or medium. The agents which achieve sterilization are called as sterilants **(Table 41.2)**.

Disinfection

It refers to a process that destroys or removes most if not all pathogenic organisms but may or may not destroy bacterial spores. They are normally used only on inanimate objects, not on body surfaces. The agents which achieve disinfection are called as disinfectants **(Table 41.2)**.

Type of Disinfectants

Depending upon their efficacy, the disinfectants are further classified into three categories.
1. High-level disinfectants (HLD)
2. Intermediate-level disinfectants (ILD)
3. Low-level disinfectants (LLD).

All these categories of disinfectants are discussed in detail, subsequently in this chapter.

Note: **Antiseptics** are a type of disinfectants which are safe to apply on body surfaces (skin

Table 41.1: Level of sterilant/disinfectants according to their microbicidal action.

Level of disinfectant/sterilant	Bacterial spores	Tubercle bacilli	Non-enveloped viruses	Fungi	Vegetative bacteria	Enveloped viruses
Sterilant	Yes	Yes	Yes	Yes	Yes	Yes
Disinfectant						
High level	+/–	Yes	Yes	Yes	Yes	Yes
Intermediate level	No	Yes	Yes	Yes	Yes	Yes
Low level	No	No	+/–	+/–	Yes	Yes

Table 41.2: Agents used in the hospital for achieving sterilization, disinfection and cleaning.

Agents	Physical methods	Chemical methods
Sterilants		

Agents of sterilization	• Heat-based methods (>100°C):
	  1. Steam sterilizer (autoclave),
	  2. Dry heat sterilizer (hot air oven)
	• Filtration
	• Radiation: Ionizing and non-ionizing (infrared)
	• Others: Incineration, microwave
		• Ethylene oxide (ETO) sterilizer
		• Plasma sterilizer

Disinfectants		
High-level disinfectants	No physical methods in this category	• Aldehydes—glutaraldehyde, ortho-phthaldehyde, formaldehyde • Peracetic acid • Hydrogen peroxide
Intermediate-level disinfectants	• Heat-based methods: <100°C (pasteurization) and at 100°C (boiling, steaming) • Radiation: Non-ionizing (ultraviolet)	• Alcohols—ethyl alcohol and isopropyl alcohol • Phenolics—phenol, cresol, lysol • Halogens—iodine and chlorine
Low-level disinfectants	No physical methods in this category	• Quaternary ammonium compound (QAC) • Chlorhexidine
Cleaning		
Agents of cleaning	Automated washers such as ultrasonic washers, washer-disinfector and automated cart washers	• Enzymatic solution • Detergent • Soap (antimicrobial or plain soap)

and mucosa) resulting in the destruction of organisms present on the body surfaces. This type of disinfection is termed as **asepsis**.

Cleaning (Decontamination)

Cleaning refers to the reduction in the pathogenic microbial population to a level at which items are considered as safe without protective attire. Achieved by manual cleaning by soap and detergents to eliminate debris or organic matter from the medical devices or surfaces **(Table 41.2)**.

In a healthcare facility, most of the sterilization practices for surgical instrument and other critical care items are carried out in Central Sterile Supply Department (CSSD). Therefore, it is important to understand the workflow of CSSD.

Central Sterile Supply Department (CSSD)
CSSD is an integrated place in hospitals that performs sterilization of medical devices, equipment and consumables; that are used in

Contd...

Contd...

the operating theater (OT) of the hospital and also for other aseptic procedures.

The processing area of CSSD consists of four unidirectional zones starting from an unsterile area to a sterile area separated by a physical barrier **(Fig. 41.1)**.

Decontamination area → Packaging area → Sterilization area → Sterile storage area

1. **Decontamination area:** The items are collected and then decontaminated/cleaned by either manual wash or by automated machines (ultrasonic washer and washer-disinfector)
2. **Packaging area:** Here, the items (medical devices) are enclosed in materials or a container designed to allow the penetration and removal of the sterilant during sterilization and then to protect the device from contamination and other damage following sterilization and until the time of use
3. **Sterilization area:** The packed medical devices received from the packaging area are subjected to sterilization process by steam sterilizer, ethylene oxide sterilizer (ETO) or plasma sterilizer

Contd...

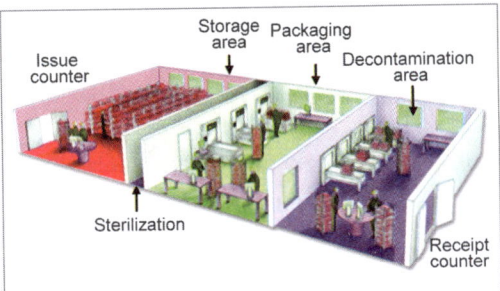

Fig. 41.1: Central Sterile Services Department (CSSD).

Contd...

> 4. **Sterile storage area:** After sterilization the sterilized items are stored in this area. It has an issue counter to supply the items to OTs and various other areas of the hospital.

Factors Influencing Efficacy of Sterilant/Disinfectant

The efficiency of a sterilant/disinfectant is affected by various factors.

- **Organism load:** As the bioburden increases, the contact time of the disinfectant also needs to be increased
- **Nature of organisms:** Organisms vary greatly in their resistance to disinfectants and sterilants

> The decreasing order of resistance of microorganisms to various agents used for sterilization or disinfection is as follows:
> Prions > bacterial spores > coccidian oocyst > mycobacteria > non-enveloped viruses > fungi > vegetative bacteria > enveloped viruses

- **Concentration:** The agents should be used at their optimal concentration to produce the desired antimicrobial action
- **Contact time:** It refers to the time period, a disinfectant is in direct contact with the surface or item to be disinfected. Lower exposure time does not achieve effective killing
- **Temperature:** The activity of most agents increases as the temperature increases. However, inappropriate higher temperatures may degrade the agent
- **Stability:** Some agents are unstable at in-use concentration, e.g. hypochlorite, and should be freshly prepared each day
- **Local pH:** The pH influences the antimicrobial activity
- **Relative humidity** is an important factor influencing the activity of gaseous disinfectant such as ethylene oxide (ETO)
- **Organic matter** such as pus, serum, blood, and stool can interfere with the antimicrobial activity of some disinfectants (e.g. hypochlorites and QAC)
  - This can be overcome by—(i) mechanically cleaning the instrument or surface/floor before it is subjected for disinfection/sterilization and (ii) increase in exposure time or concentration of the agent
  - However, few other disinfectants such as phenolics or glutaraldehyde retain their efficacy in the presence of organic matter.
- **Biofilm:** Formation of biofilm is another mechanism which prevents the entry of disinfectant/sterilant to act on the microorganisms which are embedded inside the biofilm.

Property of an Ideal Sterilant/Disinfectant

An ideal disinfectant/sterilant should have various properties—(i) broader microbicidal activity, (ii) fast acting, (iii) not affected by environmental factors such as organic matter, (iv) nontoxic, (v) compatible with surfaces/materials to which it is used, (vi) odorless or pleasant odor, (vii) economical and (viii) environmental friendly.

Spaulding's Classification of Medical Devices

Earle H Spaulding in 1971 devised a rational approach to classify the medical devices into three categories according to the degree of risk for infection involved in use of the items **(Table 41.3)**. This classification categorizes the medical devices according to their intended use and the subsequent level of reprocessing required to render the devices safe for reuse.

The various agents used in the hospital for achieving sterilization, disinfection and

Table 41.3: Spaulding's classification of medical devices.

Risk category	Definition	Recommended method	Medical equipment or surfaces
Critical device (high risk)	Items that enter a normally sterile site	Sterilization	Surgical instruments, implants/prosthesis, rigid endoscopes, syringes, needles
Semi-critical device (intermediate risk)	Items in contact with mucous membranes or body fluids	Disinfection (HLD)	Respiratory equipment, noninvasive flexible endoscopes, bedpans, urine bottles
Non-critical (low-risk)	Items in contact with intact skin	Disinfection (ILD or LLD)	Non-critical patient items[1] Non-critical environmental surfaces[2]

[1]**Non-critical patient items**—examples include blood pressure cuffs, ECG electrodes, thermometer and stethoscopes
[2]**Non-critical environmental surfaces**—medical equipment, computers, bedrails, food utensils, bedside tables, patient furniture and floor
Abbreviations: HLD, high-level disinfectant; ILD, intermediate-level disinfectant; LLD, low-level disinfectant.

cleaning are enlisted in **Table 41.2** and are discussed below.

STERILANTS

Steam Sterilizer (Autoclave)

Principle

Steam sterilizer functions similar to a pressure cooker and follows the general laws of gas.
- Water boils when its vapor pressure equals that of the surrounding atmosphere
- When the atmospheric pressure is raised, the boiling temperature is also raised
- At normal pressure, water boils at 100°C but when the pressure inside a closed vessel increases, the temperature at which water boils also increases.

Mechanism of action: Moist heat destroys microorganisms by irreversible coagulation, denaturation of enzymes and structural proteins.

Components of Steam Sterilizer (Autoclave)

Steam sterilizer is a pressure chamber; consists of a cylinder, a lid and an electrical heater.
- **Pressure chamber:** It consists of:
    - A large **cylinder** (vertical or horizontal) made up of gunmetal or stainless steel, in which the materials to be sterilized are placed
    - A **steam jacket** (water compartment).
- **Lid:** It bears the following:
    - A discharge tap for the passage of air and steam
    - A pressure gauge (sets the pressure at a particular level)
    - A safety valve (to remove the excess steam).
- **Electrical heater:** It is attached to the jacket; that heats the water to produce steam.

Procedure

The materials to be sterilized are placed inside the cylinder. The steam jacket is filled with sufficient water, lid is closed and the electrical heater is put on. The sterilization process can be divided into three phases.
- **Conditioning phase:** After the water boils, the air in the chamber is completely displaced by the steam produced. The steam pressure rises inside and when it reaches the desired set level (15 pounds per square inch), the safety valve opens and excess steam escapes out
- **Exposure phase:** The holding period is counted from this point of time, which is about 15 minutes in most cases
- **Exhaust phase:** After the holding period, the electrical heater is switched off and the steam sterilizer is allowed to cool till it reaches atmospheric pressure.

> **Sterilization Conditions**
> The steam sterilizer can be set to provide higher temperatures by adjusting the pressure provided to the vessel.
> - Cycle duration varies (3–18 min) depending on the sterilization temperature (121–135°C)
> - The most commonly used sterilization condition is 121°C for 15 min at a pressure of 15 pounds (lbs) per square inch (psi).

Uses of Steam Sterilizer (Autoclave)

Steam sterilizer is the most commonly used sterilization method in the hospital. It is used for:
- All critical and semi-critical items that are heat and moisture resistant: surgical instruments, anesthetic equipment, dental instruments, implanted medical devices and surgical drapes and linens
- Culture media preparation
- Biomedical waste treatment of waste and sharps.

Precautions

- It should not be used for sterilizing waterproof materials such as oil and grease or dry materials such as glove powder
- The chamber should not be overfilled and the material should not touch the sides or top of the chamber
- Separate steam sterilizers should be used for treatment of biomedical waste.

Types of Steam Sterilizer

Steam sterilizers are available in various sizes and dimensions.
- **Horizontal type** (large volume capacity) (**Figs. 41.2A and B**): It is used in CSSD, large-size laboratories and for biomedical waste treatment
- **Vertical type** (small volume capacity) (**Fig. 41.2C**): It is used for small-size laboratories.

Advantages

Steam sterilizer has the following advantages:
- It is low cost than ETO and plasma sterilizers
- Sterilization cycles are fast compared to ETO sterilizers
- It is nontoxic and leaves no by-product behind (unlike ETO).

Disadvantages

Disadvantages of steam sterilizer include:
- Heat can damage acrylics and styrene, PVC material and corrode some metals
- Higher temperature for a prolonged time can harm or shorten the life of instruments

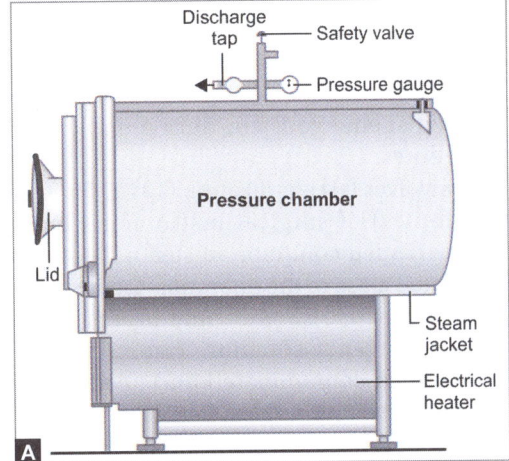
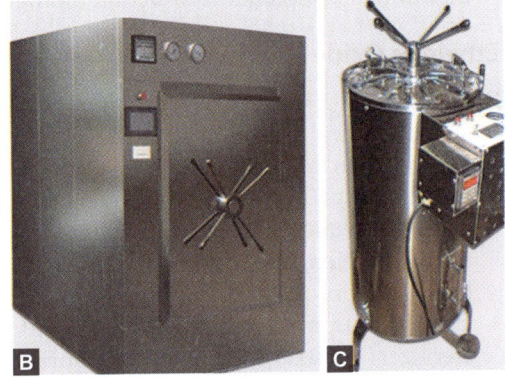

Figs. 41.2A to C: Steam sterilizer (autoclave): **A.** Schematic diagram; **B.** Horizontal autoclave; **C.** Vertical autoclave.

- Moisture also can adversely affect electronics and can cloud the sensitive materials or leave watermark stains on them.

Sterilization Control

The effectiveness of the sterilization achieved by steam sterilizer can be monitored by:
- **Biological indicator:** Spores of *Geobacillus stearothermophilus* are the best indicator. Their spores are killed in 12 minutes at 121°C
- **Chemical indicators**
  - External pack control, e.g. autoclave tape
  - Bowie-Dick test
  - Internal pack control.
- **Physical indicators**: For example, digital displays on the equipment displaying temperature, time and pressure.

Flash Sterilization

Flash sterilization is a modification of conventional steam sterilization, designed to be used at emergency or during unplanned procedures.

- It involves fast sterilization (134°C for 3–10 minutes) of surgical instruments in an unwrapped condition in steam sterilizers located close to the operation theater
- This practice should only be restricted for emergency situation, e.g. instrument has been contaminated and needs to be replaced in the surgical field immediately
- It is not suitable for porous and cannulated instruments, implants and suction tubing

Ethylene Oxide (ETO) Sterilizer

Ethylene oxide (ETO) is one of the widely used gaseous chemical sterilants in CSSD.

- **Mechanism of action:** ETO has broad microbicidal action including spores; causes alkylation of cell components such as cell proteins, DNA and RNA
- **Sterilization cycle:** It is carried out in a special equipment called ethylene oxide sterilizer (**Fig. 41.3**). The process comprises of three stages:
    - *Preconditioning:* At first, air is removed from the chamber and vacuum is created. Then the physical conditions (temperature, pressure and humidity) for sterilization are set in the chamber
    - *Sterilization:* ETO is allowed to enter the chamber. The four essential parameters that influence the effectiveness of ETO sterilization are—gas concentration, temperature, relative humidity and exposure time.
    At ETO concentration of 700 mg/liter and 40–80% relative humidity, sterilization is achieved in 4–5 hours at 38°C or 1 hour at 55°C
    - *Aeration (degassing):* The ETO residues left on surgical instruments and tubing may be toxic to the patients and staff. Therefore, extensive aeration of the sterilized materials for 8–12 hours is necessary to remove residual ETO.
- **Uses:** ETO is used by CSSD to sterilize critical items (and sometimes semicritical items) that are moisture or heat sensitive and cannot be sterilized by steam sterilization. Examples include:
    - Heart-lung machine components
    - Sutures, catheters and stents
    - Respirators and dental equipment
    - Devices with electronic components
    - Assembled complex devices
    - Multi-lumen tubings, etc.
- **Advantages of ETO:** (i) Large chamber capacity than plasma sterilization, (ii) suitable for heat sensitive items, (iii) high penetration power- ETO is highly diffusible, penetrates areas that cannot be reached by steam, (iv) non-corrosive to plastic, metal and rubber materials
- **Disadvantages:** (i) ETO is highly inflammable, irritant, explosive and carcinogenic, (ii) long duration of cycle (12–14 hours), (iii) high cost of instrument and consumables
- **Sterilization control:** Spores of *Bacillus atrophaeus* is used as biological indicator. Physical and chemical indicators are same as discussed for autoclave.

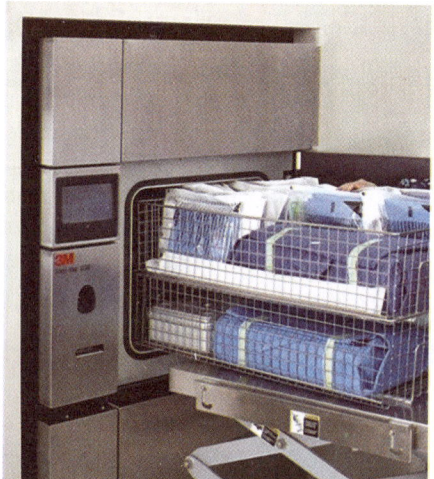

Fig. 41.3: Ethylene oxide sterilizer.
Source: 3M India Pvt. Ltd.

Plasma Sterilization

Plasma refers to a gaseous state consisting of ions, photons, free electrons and free radicals

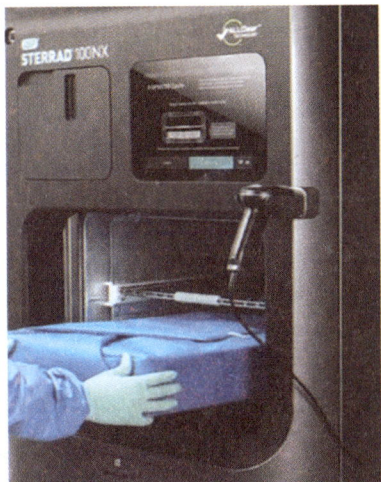

Fig. 41.4: Plasma sterilizer (Sterrad).
Source: Johnson & Johnson Pvt. Ltd.

(such as O and OH). Plasma sterilizer is a special device used to create the plasma state (commercial brands, such as *Sterrad*). It has the following steps **(Fig. 41.4)**:

- **Vacuum:** First, the chamber is evacuated to create a vacuum
- **Chemical sterilant:** Next step is injection of chemical sterilant hydrogen peroxide (H_2O_2) solution from a cassette, which gets vaporized in the sterilization chamber to a concentration of 6 mg/L
    - The H_2O_2 vapor diffuses through the chamber (50 minutes), exposes all surfaces of the load to the sterilant
    - Low temperature is maintained 37–44°C throughout the cycle.
- **Gas plasma:** In the next step, an **electrical field** is applied to the chamber to create a gas plasma. H_2O_2 breaks into free radicals which initiate microbicidal action, which subsequently interact with essential cell components (e.g. enzymes, nucleic acids)
- **Finally,** the excess gas is removed. The by-products of the cycle (e.g. water vapor, oxygen) are nontoxic and therefore, there is no need of an additional aeration step
- **Cycle duration:** It has a cycle time of 75 min. The newer versions have shorter cycles of 52 min and 24 min
- **Sterilization control:** Spores of *Geobacillus stearothermophilus* is used as a biological indicator. Physical and chemical indicators are the same as discussed for the autoclave.

Uses of Plasma Sterilizer

It is used by CSSD for sterilization of materials and devices that cannot tolerate high temperature and humidity of steam sterilizer, such as some plastics, electrical devices, and corrosion-susceptible metals such as arthroscope, micro and vascular instruments, spine sets and laparoscope.

Precautions/Disadvantages

The following precautions should be followed while using plasma sterilizer:
- Items should be dried before loading
- Linen or paper or cellulose or liquid cannot be processed
- It may not penetrate well, especially in channels or devices designed with long lumens
- It has a small chamber, therefore cannot be used for bulk items
- High cost of equipment and packing materials.

Dry Heat Sterilizer (Hot Air Oven)

This method is used for materials that might be damaged by moist heat or that are impenetrable to the moist heat (e.g. glass wares, powders, petroleum products, sharp instruments).

- **Procedure:** It has a sterilization chamber, which is electrically heated and has a fan or a motor to ensure adequate and even distribution of hot air in the chamber **(Fig. 41.5)**
    - Dry heat acts by oxidation of cell constituents
    - The most common cycles used are 170°C for 60 minutes, 160°C for 120 minutes, and 150°C for 150 minutes.
- **Advantages:** (i) It is non-toxic and does not harm environment, (ii) low operating costs, (iii) penetrates well into materials, (iv) noncorrosive for metals
- **Disadvantages:** The high temperatures are not suitable for most materials

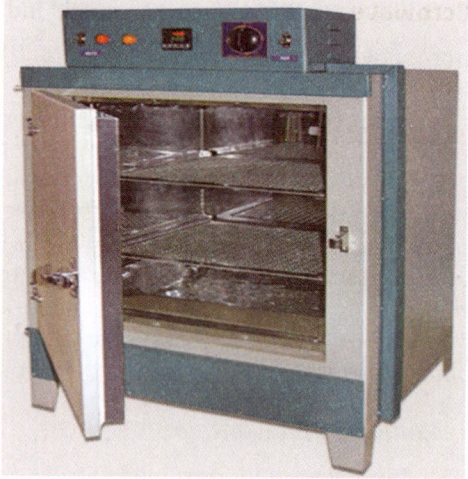

Fig. 41.5: Dry heat sterilizer (hot air oven).

- ❖ **Sterilization control:** Spores of *Bacillus atrophaeus* is used as biological indicator.

Filtration

Filtration acts by removing microorganisms, not by killing. CDC considers filtration as a sterilization method, although some authors arguably disregard this as it does not kill the microorganisms, rather only filters them out. There are two types of filters:
- ❖ **Depth filters:** They retain particles throughout the depth of the filter, rather than just on the surface **(Fig. 41.6A)**. They are used as drinking water purifiers. They do not achieve sterilization and are not suitable for hospital use
- ❖ **Membrane filters:** They are the most widely used filters in hospitals. They retain all the particles on the surface that are larger than their pore size **(Figs. 41.6B and 41.7)**

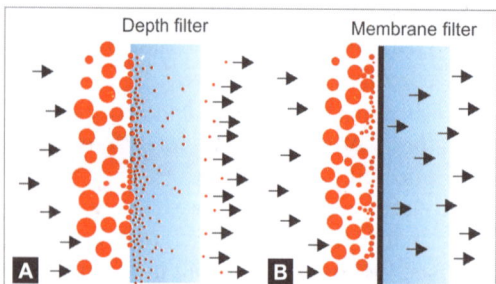

Figs. 41.6A and B: Filtration methods: **A.** Depth filters; **B.** Membrane filters.

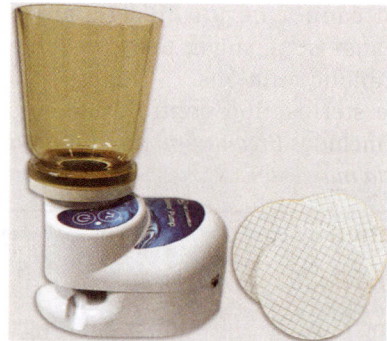

Fig. 41.7: Filter apparatus with membrane filter.
Source: Department of Microbiology, JIPMER, Puducherry.

- Bacterial filters have 0.22 µm pore size which removes most of the bacteria; allowing the viruses to pass-through
- Viral filters have even smaller pore size.
- ❖ Membrane filtration has two wider applications in hospital settings—filtration of air and water.

Filtration of Air

- ❖ **Surgical (3-ply) mask and respirators:** They are simplest examples of filters being used for purification of air. They remove microorganisms based on their pore size. These filters are made up of flat, non-woven fibers
- ❖ **HEPA filters** (high-efficiency particulate air filters):
  - HEPA filter removes 99.97% of particles that have a size of 0.3 µm or more
  - HEPA filters in hospitals are used in biological safety cabinets, airflow system, operation theater, and isolation rooms.
- ❖ **ULPA filters** (ultra-low particulate/penetration air): An ULPA filter can remove from the air at least 99.999% of dust, pollen, mold, bacteria and any airborne particles with a size of 0.12 µm or larger.

Filtration of Liquid

- ❖ Used for bacteriological examination of water in hospital settings, especially dialysis water
- ❖ Also used to remove bacteria from pharmaceutical fluids that are heat labile

and cannot be purified by any other means—sera, sugar, toxin, vaccine and antibiotic solutions.

The sterilization control of membrane filters includes *Brevundimonas diminuta* and *Serratia marcescens*.

Radiation

Ionizing Radiation

Ionizing radiations include cobalt 60 gamma rays or electron accelerators.
- **Use:** It is a low-temperature sterilization method that has been used for a number of medical products (e.g. tissue for transplantation, pharmaceuticals, medical devices)
- **Mechanism:** It causes ionization of the molecules in organisms leading to breakage of DNA
- **Advantages** of ionizing radiation—(1) high penetrating power, (2) rapidity of action, and (3) temperature is not raised (hence this method is also called as **cold sterilization**)
- **Disadvantages:** High sterilization costs and may have deleterious effects on the equipment made up of polyethylene
- **Sterilization control:** Efficacy of ionizing radiation is tested by using *Bacillus pumilus*.

Non-ionizing Radiation

Examples include infrared and ultraviolet radiations.
- **Infrared radiation** technology can be used as an alternate method of sterilization for selected heat-resistant instrument
- **Ultraviolet radiation** does not achieve sterilization, described under intermediate-level disinfectant.

Incineration

Incineration is used for the treatment of biomedical waste materials (for non-plastic infectious waste). It burns (sterilizes) the waste by providing a very high temperature 870–1,200°C and thereby converting the waste into ash, flue gas and heat (Chapter 42).

Microwave

Microwaves are used in hospitals for disinfection of soft contact lenses, dental instruments, dentures, and urinary catheters (for intermittent self-catheterization). It is available in various size from home-type microwave ovens to large-size.
- Large size microwaves are used for disposal of biomedical waste (for plastic infectious waste)
- **Mechanism of action:** Microwaves are radiofrequency waves, which are usually used at a frequency of 2450 MHz. They produce friction of water molecules which generates heat.

HIGH-LEVEL DISINFECTANTS (HLD)

High-level disinfectants (HLD) agents are capable of killing bacterial spores when used in sufficient concentration under suitable conditions. They can kill all the other microorganisms **(Table 41.1)**.

Aldehyde

Formaldehyde, glutaraldehyde and ortho-phthalaldehyde are the commonly used disinfectants. They combine with nucleic acids, proteins and inactivate them, probably by cross-linking and alkylating the molecules.

Glutaraldehyde

- **Semicritical items:** It remains active in the presence of organic matter and is non-corrosive to equipment. Therefore, glutaraldehyde is the most common HLD used for semicritical equipment, such as endoscopes and cystoscopes
  - It is used at 2% or 2.4% concentration (e.g. Cidex). It disinfects objects within 20 minutes but may require longer time to kill spores (10–14 hours)
  - It is available in inactive form; has to be activated by alkalinization before use. Once activated, it remains active only for 14 days.

- ❖ **Aerial disinfection and cleaning:** It is also used for fogging and cleaning of floor and surfaces of critical areas such as operation theatre (e.g. Bacillocid Extra)
- ❖ **Advantages:** It remains active in the presence of organic matter, has excellent material compatibility
- ❖ **Disadvantages:** It has a pungent odor, can produce eye irritation, occupational asthma and contact dermatitis.

Ortho-phthalaldehyde (0.55%)

This can also be used for disinfection of semicritical items, has many advantages over glutaraldehyde—(1) it does not require activation, (2) better odor, (3) less eye irritation, (4) acts faster (5–10 min). However, it does not kill spores effectively and stains skin gray.

Formaldehyde

Although it is an excellent HLD, the healthcare uses of formaldehyde are limited because it produces irritating fumes and pungent odor and also a potential carcinogen. It was used for fumigation of closed areas, such as operation theater, but now this is an obsolete practice.

Peracetic Acid

Peracetic acid is used in automated machines. It is also available for manual immersion; 0.1–0.2%, used for 5–15 min.
- ❖ **Use:** It can be used to sterilize medical (e.g. endoscopes, arthroscopes), surgical, and dental instruments. Peracetic acid in combination with hydrogen peroxide has been used for disinfecting hemodialyzers
- ❖ **Disadvantages:** Expensive, has material compatibility issues, causes chemical irritation and eye damage.

Hydrogen Peroxide (H_2O_2)

H_2O_2 works by producing destructive hydroxyl free radicals that can attack various cell components.
- ❖ **Uses:** H_2O_2 has several usages at various concentrations. It is sporicidal only at >4–5%
  - 3% H_2O_2 is used for environmental surface disinfection, fogging and for wound cleaning
  - 3–6% H_2O_2 is used to disinfect soft contact lens, tonometer biprisms, ventilators, fabrics, and endoscopes, etc.
  - 6–7.5% H_2O_2 is used as chemical sterilant in plasma sterilization
  - Vaporized H_2O_2 is used for industrial sterilization of medical devices and for decontamination of large and small area.
- ❖ **Advantages:** It is rapid in action, nontoxic, has detergent properties with good cleaning ability, and is active in the presence of organic material
- ❖ **Disadvantages** include—expensive, has material compatibility issue (contraindicated for use on copper, brass, zinc, aluminium), can produce chemical irritation and corneal damage. It should be properly stored in dark containers.

INTERMEDIATE-LEVEL DISINFECTANTS

Intermediate-level disinfectants (ILD) destroy all microorganisms, but not bacterial spores **(Table 41.1)**.

Alcohol

Ethyl alcohol and isopropyl alcohol are the most popular alcohols used in hospitals.
- ❖ **Action:** They are rapidly bactericidal to most organisms except spores. The cidal activity drops sharply when diluted below 50% concentration. They act by denaturation of proteins
- ❖ **Uses:** Alcohol (60–80%) is used for various purposes
  - **Alcohol-based handrub** (ABHR), e.g. sterillium, a popular commercial product
  - Disinfecting **smaller non-critical instruments** such as thermometers, which are immersed in alcohol for 10–15 minutes
  - Disinfection of **small medical items/surfaces** such as rubber stoppers of

multiple-dose medication vials or vaccine bottles and hubs of the central line
- **Disinfection of external surfaces of equipment** such as stethoscopes, ventilators, manual ventilation bags, ultrasound machines, etc.
- **Disinfection of non-critical surfaces** such as laboratory bench, medication preparation areas
- **Spirit** (70% alcohol): Used a skin antiseptic.

❖ **Disadvantages:** (i) Flammable and must be stored in a cool, well-ventilated area, (ii) Evaporate rapidly, making exposure time difficult to achieve unless the items are immersed, (iii) May damage tonometer tips and lenses, (iv) Inactivated by organic matter.

Phenolics

Phenol (carbolic acid) was the first widely used antiseptic and disinfectant; was introduced for surgery in 1867 by Joseph Lister (the father of antiseptic surgery). The phenol and its derivatives (called phenolics) are produced by distillation of coal tar.

❖ **Mechanisms:** Phenolics act as protoplasmic poison, disrupt the cell wall and precipitate the cell proteins

❖ **Used as disinfectants:** Cresol, and lysol are the common phenolics used for disinfecting environmental surfaces (e.g. bedside tables, bedrails, and laboratory surfaces) and noncritical medical devices. They are toxic to skin, hence not used as antiseptics. **5% phenol** is mycobactericidal, used for disinfection of sputum specimen

❖ **Used as antiseptics:** Certain phenolics are compatible with skin and are widely used as antiseptics. The classical example is chloroxylenol (the active ingredient of the commercial brand, Dettol)

❖ **Advantages:** Phenolics are the only ILD that retain activity in the presence of organic materials

❖ **Disadvantages:** They can cause hyperbilirubinemia in infants and therefore should not be used in nurseries.

Halogens

Among the halogens, iodine and chlorine have antimicrobial activity. They exist in free state, and form salt with sodium and other metals.

Iodine

Iodine acts by disruption of protein and nucleic acid. Two preparations are available.

❖ **Tincture of iodine:** It used as antiseptic for wound cleaning, but can cause staining and skin allergy

❖ **Iodophor (e.g. povidone iodine):** It is prepared by complexing iodine with carrier (povidone) which helps in sustained-release of iodine. It is nonstaining and free of skin toxicity. Some popular brands available are Wescodyne and Betadine.

Uses: Iodophors are used both as antiseptics and disinfectant at different concentrations
- **Used as antiseptics**
  - 5% topical solution and ointment is used for wound cleaning
  - 7.5% is used for hand scrub
  - 10% is used for surgical skin preparation
  - 1% is used as an oral antiseptic, for mouth wash.
- **Used as disinfectant** for medical equipment, such as hydrotherapy tanks and thermometers.

Chlorine and Hypochlorite

Chlorine is one of the most commonly available disinfectant in hospital.

❖ **Preparations:** Chlorine occurs as—(1) free chlorine, (2) hypochlorite—it is available in two preparations
- Liquid form (sodium hypochlorite or household bleach), or
- Powder form (calcium hypochlorite or bleaching powder)
- Other forms: Include sodium dichloroisocyanurate (NaDCC) available as tablets and chlorine dioxide.

❖ **Mechanisms:** All preparations yield hypochlorous acid (HClO), which causes oxidation of cellular materials and destruction of vegetative bacteria and fungi

- ❖ **Uses (free chlorine):** Chlorine is used for disinfection of municipal water supplies and swimming pool water
- ❖ **Uses (sodium hypochlorite):** It is available at 5.25–6.15%, which is equivalent to 50,000 ppm of available chlorine. It should be used in appropriate dilutions (by adding with water) for disinfection of various hospital supplies. The contact time is about 10–20 minutes
  - Large blood spill: 0.5% (1:10 dilution or 5,000 ppm) is used
  - Small blood spill: 0.05% (1: 100 dilution, or 500 ppm) is used
  - Pre-treatment of liquid waste before disposal: 1% (1:5 dilution, 10,000 ppm) is used
  - Laundry items: 0.1% (1 in 50 dilution 1,000 ppm) is used
  - Surface disinfectant: 0.5% (1:10 dilution or 5,000 ppm) is used
  - *C. difficile* (diarrheal stool): Hypocholorite is sporicidal only >0.5% (5,000 ppm).
- ❖ **Advantages:** Hypochlorites are broad spectrum, rapid in its action, non-flammable, low cost and are widely available
- ❖ **Disadvantages:** (1) Inactivated by organic matter, which can be overcome by adding excess chlorine, (2) Toxic to skin and mucosa, and carcinogenic, (3) It is unstable, evaporates on exposure to sunlight or air. Hence, it has to be prepared daily and stored in opaque container, (4) Corrosive, damages fabrics, carpets, (5) Leaves residue, requires rinsing or neutralization, (6) Offensive odors, (7) Bleaches the fabrics and carpets.

Heat-based Methods

The following heat-based methods can act as ILD, kill all organisms except the spores.

- ❖ **Pasteurization:** Developed by Louis Pasteur and is used for destroying the food-spoiling organisms in milk and fruit juice and thereby extending their shelf-life. In hospitals, pasteurization is used to disinfect respiratory and anesthesia equipment, by immersing in hot water (70°C for 30 min)
- ❖ **Boiling at 100°C:** Boiling of the items in water for 15 minutes may kill most of the vegetative forms but not the spores, hence not suitable for sterilization of surgical instruments
- ❖ **Steaming at 100°C:** When the autoclave is used without closing the pressure valve, the temperature does not rise beyond 100°C. It may be useful for disinfecting those items which cannot withstand the high temperature of autoclave.

Ultraviolet (UV) Radiation

Ultraviolet (UV) radiation is a form of non-ionizing radiation that is emitted by the sun and artificial sources such as mercury vapor bulbs.

- ❖ **Mechanism of action:** Causes destruction of nucleic acid through induction of thymine dimers. Bacteria and viruses are more easily killed by UV light but not spores
- ❖ **Uses:** UV radiation has been employed for:
  - Disinfection of drinking water, titanium implants and contact lenses
  - Disinfection of air and/or surfaces as in operating rooms, isolation rooms, and biologic safety cabinets
  - Sun-rays also contain UV rays, which may disinfect organisms present on environmental surfaces.
- ❖ **Disadvantages:** The effectiveness is influenced by organic matter. In isolation rooms, it may cause skin erythema and keratoconjunctivitis in patients and visitors. Therefore, UV lamps should be placed at least above 2-meters height from the floor level.

LOW-LEVEL DISINFECTANTS

Low-level disinfectants (LLD) destroy vegetative bacteria and enveloped viruses, variable action on nonenveloped viruses, and fungi, but no action on tubercle bacilli and spores (Table 41.1).

Quaternary Ammonium Compound (QAC)

Quaternary ammonium compound (QAC) are commonly used in ordinary environmental sanitation of noncritical surfaces, such as floors, furniture, and walls. Some products are also used for disinfecting non-critical medical equipment that contacts intact skin (e.g. blood pressure cuffs). QAC are also good cleaning agents as they have surfactant like action.

- **Mechanism:** They act by inactivation of energy-producing enzymes, denaturation of essential cell proteins, and disruption of the cell membrane
- **QAC formulations:** Benzyl ammonium chloride is the most popular QAC used in the health care. It does not act in the presence of hard water. The newer generation of QACs (e.g. didecyl dimethyl ammonium bromide) remain active in hard water and are better compatible.

Chlorhexidine Gluconate (CHG)

Chlorhexidine gluconate (CHG) is a biguanide disinfectant, acts by disruption of cytoplasmic membrane.

- **Uses:** CHG is widely used in antiseptic products, at various concentrations
  - **Hand hygiene product:** Hand rub (0.5%), hand wash (4%) (e.g. microshield, a commercial product)
  - **Mouthwash** (0.1–0.2%)
  - **Body wash** solutions (used before surgery)
  - **Skin disinfectant** before surgery (2 %)
  - **Antiseptic** for wound cleaning: Commercially available as **Savlon** which is a combination of CHG 0.3%, cetrimide and isopropyl alcohol.
- **Advantages:** The wide use of CHG is due to its residual activity (prolonged action than alcohol hand rub) and is less irritant
- **Disadvantages:** It is slower in action, activity is pH dependent and is greatly reduced in the presence of organic matter. It produces dermatitis on prolonged use as handrub.

CLEANING AGENTS

Most disinfectants act well only when the instrument or the surface is free from organic matter such as dirt, blood, or other specimens.

- Therefore, cleaning is a very important step which needs to be performed before the disinfectants are applied
- An ideal cleaning agent should have the following properties: easily emulsifiable, saponifiable, water softening, non-toxic and have surfactant like action.

Cleaning Products

Broadly two types of cleaning agents are available.

- **Enzymatic (proteolytic) cleaners:** They contain enzymes such as amylase, lipase, cellulase, protease which break down proteinaceous matter present on equipment. Enzymatic cleaners are not disinfectants; they only remove protein from surfaces
- **Cleaning chemicals (detergents):** These agents act by reducing surface tension and dissolving fat and organic matter. Detergents used for surface and floor cleaning are different than that used for instrument cleaning. Mild alkaline detergents (pH 8.0–10.8) are more efficient cleaning agents for surgical instruments.

Cleaning Methods

The cleaning methods are grouped into:

- **Manual cleaning** by immersion of instruments into the cleaning solution, or by wiping the surfaces with a cloth soaked with the cleaning solution
- **Automatic or mechanical cleaning:** They clean faster with a higher standard of cleaning than manual cleaning. Examples include—ultrasonic washers and washer-disinfector.

ENVIRONMENTAL CLEANING

Environmental cleaning of the floor and surface of hospitals play a vital role in controlling the spread of infections. The general principles of environmental cleaning are as follows:

- **Cleaning followed by disinfections:**
  - **Cleaning:** Always cleaning with a detergent is performed first, before applying disinfectant
  - **Disinfection:** CDC recommends to use low- to intermediate-level disinfectants for environmental cleaning such as QAC, hypochlorite and improved hydrogen peroxide.
- **Cleaning sequence:** Cleaning should be performed in correct sequence to prevent recontamination
  - **Cleaner to dirtier:** The cleaner areas are cleaned first, followed by the dirtier areas; e.g. low-touch surfaces should be cleaned first followed by high-touch surfaces
  - **High to low:** Top area should be cleaned first, then proceed towards bottom (e.g. bedrails → bed legs and table surfaces → floors)
  - **Inward to outwards:** Clean the farthest point from the door first and then proceed towards the door.
- **Frequency of cleaning depends upon:**
  - **Probability of contamination:** Heavily contaminated vs low-contaminated surfaces or instrument
  - **Vulnerability of population to infection:** Immunocompromised vs healthy adults
  - **Frequency of hand contact:** High-touch vs low-touch surfaces.
- **Frequency of cleaning for common situations:**
  - Non-critical surfaces and floors can be cleaned 2–3 times a day
  - Mattress used for patients should be cleaned weekly and after discharge
  - Doors, windows, walls and ceiling should be cleaned once a month and spot-cleaning when soiled
  - **High touch areas** such as doorknobs, elevator buttons, telephones, bedrails, light switches, computer keyboards, monitoring equipment should be cleaned more frequently, every 3–4 hours.

Disinfection of Operation Theater

Environmental cleaning in operation theater (OT) minimizes patients' and HCWs' exposure to potentially infectious microorganisms.

- **Surface disinfection:** Cleaning should be performed first with a cleansing agent, followed by disinfection by using an aldehyde-based disinfectant. Disinfection of OT is carried out in the following situations:
  1. First cleaning of the day (before cases begin)
  2. In between cases (cleaning 3 to 4 feet perimeter around the OT table)
  3. Terminal cleaning of OT after the last case
  4. Detailed wash-down of the OT complex once a week
  5. During renovation or construction of OT or nearby places.
- **Fogging:** Also called aerial disinfection, involves spraying of a disinfectant (e.g. glutaraldehyde, H_2O_2 or QAC based product) with the help of a fogger machine (Fig. 41.8)
  - The procedure takes around 1–2 hours, during which OT should be closed down and personnel need to be vacated
  - Indication: Routine periodic fogging is not recommended, but is indicated only when any outbreak of infection is

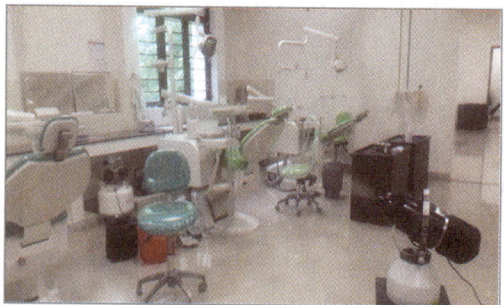

Fig. 41.8: Fogging of dental unit following construction.
Source: Sanitary Department, JIPMER, Puducherry.

suspected or any change in infection control practice implemented or during renovation or construction of OT or nearby places.

METHODS TO TEST EFFICACY OF STERILANT/DISINFECTANT

Tests for Chemical Disinfectants

Chemical disinfectants used in hospitals and laboratories must be tested periodically to ascertain its potency and efficacy. Various methods available are:
- Rideal and Walker test or phenol coefficient test
- Chick Martin test
- Capacity (Kelsey-Sykes) test
- In-use (Kelsey-Maurer) test.

Tests for Sterilizers (Indicators)

The efficacy of sterilizers can be assessed by using physical, chemical and biological indicators.

Physical Indicator

These are the digital displays of the sterilizer equipment showing parameters such as temperature, time and pressure, etc.

Chemical Indicator

They use heat or chemical sensitive materials which undergo a color change if the sterilization parameter (e.g. time, steam quality and temperature) for which it is issued is achieved. Common types used are:
- **Class I:** Also called as exposure indicator or external pack control. They are used on the external surface of each pack, to indicate that the pack has been directly exposed to the sterilant. However, it does not assure sterility **(Fig. 41.9A)**.
- **Class II:** It is called as Bowie-Dick test or as equipment control; i.e. it checks the efficacy of air removal, air leaks and steam penetration and ensures that the steam sterilizer is functioning well

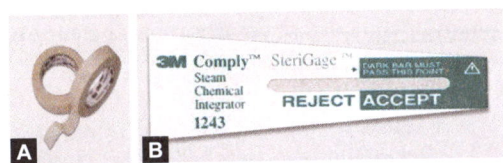

Figs. 41.9A and B: Chemical indicator: **A.** Type I (autoclave tape; **B.** Type V (internal pack control indicator).
Source: Department of CSSD, JIPMER, Puducherry.

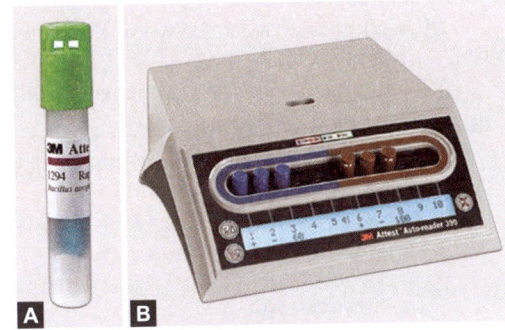

Figs. 41.10A and B: Biological indicator: **A.** Vial; **B.** Incubator.
Source: Department of CSSD, JIPMER, Puducherry.

- **Class IV and V:** Also called as internal pack control indicator. It is placed inside the packs and therefore it verifies whether the critical parameters such as time, steam quality and temperature are attained inside the pack or not **(Fig. 41.9B)**.

Biological Indicator (BI)

It is the most reliable indicator as it uses bacterial spores to check the effectiveness of sterilization. The spores are highly resistant and will be destroyed only when the effective condition is achieved.
- *Geobacillus stearothermophilus* for steam sterilizer and gas plasma (hydrogen peroxide) and liquid acetic acid sterilizer
- *Bacillus atrophaeus* for ethylene oxide sterilizer and dry heat sterilizer (hot air oven)
- Spore containing vials are incubated. Depending upon the incubators used, the result is obtained in 24 min to 48 hours time **(Figs. 41.10A and B)**.

EXPECTED QUESTIONS

I. Write essay on:
1. Define sterilization and disinfection. Describe principle and uses of steam sterilizers.
2. What are chemical sterilants. Discuss their application in healthcare settings.

II. Write short notes on:
1. Membrane filters.
2. Application of glutaraldehyde in healthcare setting.
3. Central Sterile Services Department (CSSD).

III. Multiple Choice Questions (MCQs):

1. Which of the following disinfectant is used in plasma sterilization?
   a. Formaldehyde
   b. Glutaraldehyde
   c. Hydrogen peroxide
   d. Ethylene oxide

2. *Geobacillus stearothermophilus* is used as indicator for efficacy of:
   a. Hot air oven
   b. Autoclave
   c. Filtration
   d. Ultraviolet rays

3. Endoscope is sterilized by:
   a. Glutaraldehyde
   b. Formaldehyde
   c. Autoclaving
   d. Hot air oven

4. Which of the following disinfectant is used for handwash?
   a. Ethylene oxide
   b. Formaldehyde
   c. Chlorhexidine
   d. Povidone iodine

5. Which of the following is used for disinfection of blood spillage area?
   a. Phenol
   b. Hypochlorite
   c. Lysol
   d. Formaldehyde

6. Which of the following is used for disinfection of sputum?
   a. Phenol
   b. Hypochlorite
   c. Lysol
   d. Formaldehyde

7. Which of the following high level disinfectants requires activation before use?
   a. Formaldehyde
   b. Glutaraldehyde
   c. Ortho-phthalaldehyde
   d. Peracetic acid

Answers
1. c   2. b   3. a   4. c   5. b   6. a   7. b

CHAPTER 42: Biomedical Waste Management

CHAPTER PREVIEW
- Biomedical Waste Rule
- Waste Segregation in Hospitals
- Treatment and Disposal Methods
- Blood Spill Management

INTRODUCTION

The waste generated from the hospital carries a higher potential for infections and injuries. Therefore, it is essential to have safe and reliable methods of segregation and disposal of hospital waste.

Definition

Biomedical wastes (BMW) are defined as wastes that are generated during the laboratory diagnosis, treatment or immunization of human beings or animals, or in research activities pertaining thereto, or in the production of biologicals.

Waste Generated in Hospitals

It is estimated that the quantity of solid waste generated in hospitals varies from 1/2 to 2 kg/bed. However, BMW accounts for a minor proportion of the total waste generated in hospitals (~250 gram per bed per day). In developing countries, the waste generated in hospitals falls into two categories:

1. **General (non-hazardous solid waste, 80%):** A large amount of waste falls in the general waste category, which may be disposed of with the usual domestic and urban waste management system. They do not cause any harm to humans. They are not considered as BMW. They should not be mixed with BMW
2. **Biomedical waste:** This includes infectious waste (10%) and chemical/radioactive waste (5%).

Hazards Associated with BMW

Inappropriate and inefficient disposal of BMW can lead to infectious hazards, malignancies, malformations, and environmental (air, land and water) pollution not only to the current generation but also for future generations. The various hazards are:

- ❖ **Hazards from infectious wastes:** This is the component of hospital waste that produces maximum hazards
  - **Pathogens in the infectious waste** may infect HCWs by entering through ingestion, inhalation or direct skin-to-skin contact and can cause various type of infections such as gastrointestinal, respiratory, skin infections, etc.
  - **Hazards from infectious sharps**—leads to transmission of blood borne viruses (hepatitis B, C and HIV).
- ❖ **Hazards from chemical wastes:** They include laboratory reagents, disinfectants, and waste with high content of heavy metals, e.g. mercury from broken thermometers. Most chemicals are toxic, corrosive, explosive and flammable; can cause various physical injuries including chemical burns

- **Pharmaceutical waste:** It includes expired, unused and contaminated drugs, vaccines, sera, etc. Exposure to these agents may cause several adverse effects depending upon the nature of the pharmaceutical waste
- **Hazards from cytotoxic waste:** Cytotoxic drugs used in the treatment of cancers and autoimmune disorders are extremely hazardous to the environment and human health owing to their mutagenic, teratogenic, or carcinogenic properties
- **Hazards from radioactive waste:** They include materials contaminated with radionuclides
  - They are produced as a result of procedures performed by radiology and nuclear medicine departments
  - They are genotoxic, in higher doses can cause severe injuries, including tissue destruction, necessitating the amputation of body parts.

Situation in India

According to the Ministry of Environment and Forests (MoEF), the gross generation of BMW in India is about 484 TPD (tons per day). Unfortunately, only 447 TPD is treated, and 37 TPD (8%) is left untreated. Karnataka tops the chart among all the states in generation of BMW followed by Maharashtra.

Waste Management Hierarchy

The waste management hierarchy is largely based on the concept of the "3Rs", namely reduce, recycle and recover. If none of these methods is available, then the last method opted is disposal.
- **Prevent and reduce:** The most preferable approach, is to prevent or reduce the production of waste as far as possible
- **Reuse and recycle:** The next best option is to reuse the waste as such (if feasible) or after recycling
- **Recover:** Where practicable, recovering waste items for secondary use can be done. It is of two types:
  - *Energy recovery,* whereby waste is converted to fuel for generating electricity or for direct heating
  - *Waste recovery* is a term used for composting of organic waste matter to produce compost or soil conditioner which can be used in agriculture.
- **Treatment:** Wastes that cannot be recycled or recovered, can be subjected to treatment by various methods such as incineration.
  Note: Treatment is also necessary for the biomedical waste before sending for recycling or recovery as these wastes are potentially infectious. This is usually carried out by the autoclave or microwave (explained later)
- **Disposal:** It involves disposal of the waste in landfill or dump yard. This is the least preferable option among all waste management strategies.

BIOMEDICAL WASTE RULE, INDIA

The Ministry of Environment and Forests (MoEF) has formulated biomedical waste rule in 1998; had classified the waste into 10 categories, which used to be segregated into five color-coded containers. There was considerable overlapping between categories which created ambiguity and confusion.

The new BMW guideline was published in 2016 with an amendment added in 2018 and 2019 **(Table 42.1)**.
- It was implemented with a vision of simplifying categorization of BMWs, while improving the ease of segregation, transportation and disposal methods to decrease environmental pollution
- According to this new rule, there are four categories of BMWs, each is segregated by a single color-coded container.

Steps of BMW Management

The management of BMW can overall be summarized into five simple steps.
1. Waste segregation (at the point of generation) into color-coded containers
2. Pre-treatment for laboratory liquid waste
3. Transport of waste from generation site to central storage area of the hospital

Biomedical Waste Management

Table 42.1: Biomedical Waste Management Rule, India, 2016 (including the amendment added in 2018 and 2019).

Category	Type of waste	Type of Bag/container	Treatment/disposal options
Yellow	A. Human anatomical waste	Yellow colored non-chlorinated plastic bags	Incineration/plasma pyrolysis/deep burial
	B. Animal anatomical waste		
	C. Soiled waste		Incineration/plasma pyrolysis/deep burial/autoclaving or hydroclaving + shredding/mutilation
	D. Expired/discarded medicines—pharmaceutical waste, cytotoxic drugs	Yellow colored containers/non-chlorinated plastic bags with cytotoxic label	Sent back to manufacturer/CBMWTF for incineration (cytotoxic drugs at temperature >1,200°C)
	E. Chemical solid waste	Yellow colored containers/nonchlorinated plastic bags	Incineration or plasma pyrolysis or encapsulation
	F. Chemical liquid waste such as discarded disinfectants, infected body fluids and secretions, liquid from house-keeping related activities	To be discharged into separate collection system, which leads to effluent treatment system Not to be discarded into yellow bag	Pre-treated[1] before mixing with other waste water
	G. Discarded linen waste contaminated with blood/body fluids, mask, cap, gown and shoe cover	Non-chlorinated yellow plastic bags/suitable packing material	Non-chlorinated chemical disinfection[2] followed by incineration/plasma pyrolysis
	H. Microbiology, other clinical laboratory waste, blood bags, live attenuated vaccines	Autoclave safe plastic bag/container	Pre-treat to sterilize with non-chlorinated chemicals[2] on-site as per NACO/WHO guidelines (Blue book 2014) + incineration
Red	**Infectious plastic waste** Disposable items such as tubing, bottles, intravenous tubes and sets, catheters, urine bags, syringes (without needles and fixed needle syringes) and vacutainer with their needles cut, gloves, plastic apron and goggles	Red colored non-chlorinated plastic bags or containers	• Autoclaving/microwaving/hydroclaving + shredding • Mutilation/sterilization + shredding Treated waste sent to authorized recyclers or for energy recovery

Contd...

Contd...

Category	Type of waste	Type of Bag/container	Treatment/disposal options
White (Translucent)	**Waste sharps including metal sharps** Needles, syringes with fixed needles, needles from needle tip cutter or burner, scalpels, blades, or any other contaminated sharp (used or discarded)	Puncture-proof, leak-proof, tamper-proof containers	Autoclaving/dry heat sterilization followed by: • Shredding or mutilation or encapsulation in metal container or cement concrete or • Sanitary landfill or • Designated concrete waste sharp pit
Blue	a. **Glasswares:** Broken or discarded and contaminated glass including medicine vials and ampoules except those contaminated with cytotoxic wastes, microscope slides b. **Metallic body implants** Dental implants, other body implants and plates	Puncture proof and leak-proof container	Disinfection can be carried out by: • Soaking the washed glass waste after cleaning with detergent and sodium hypochlorite treatment (1–2%) or • Autoclaving/microwaving/hydroclaving and then it is sent for recycling

Note:
- Biomedical waste rule does not specify any specific color coded bag for general waste segregation in hospital. Depending upon the local policy, hospitals choose any color coded bag for general waste (e.g. JIPMER uses black bag for general waste).
- [1]**Chemical treatment:** Hypochlorite should be used at 1–2% concentration having 30% residual chlorine with contact time of 20 minutes.
- [2]**Non-chlorinated chemicals** include 5% phenol, 5% cresol or 5% lysol.
- The chlorinated plastic bags (except blood bags) and gloves should be phased out and replaced by non-chlorinated bags and gloves.
- Every health care facility should have their own STP (sewage treatment plant).
- Barcoding system should be introduced to monitor the segregation compliance.

Abbreviations: NACO, National AIDS Control Organization; WHO, World Health Organization; CBMWTF, common bio-medical waste treatment facility.

4. Transport of waste from central storage area to common bio-medical waste treatment facility (CBMWTF)
5. Treatment and/or disposal (within 48 hours of generation).

Waste Segregation in Hospitals

Waste segregation refers to the basic separation of different categories of waste generated at source in the hospital and thereby reducing the risks as well as the cost of handling and disposal.

According to BMW Rule (2016), segregation of waste should be done by using containers of four different colors—each is designated for segregation of a particular waste category (*see* **Table 42.1**).

❖ Yellow bag—for infectious non-plastic waste
❖ Red bag—for infectious plastic waste
❖ White or translucent sharp container (puncture-proof box)—for metal sharps
❖ Blue container (puncture-proof box)—for broken glass items and metal implants.

The following general principles need to be followed during segregation, transport and storage of BMW.

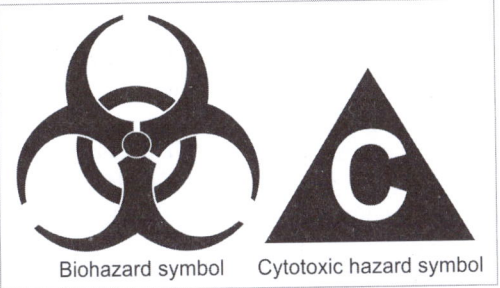

Fig. 42.1: Logos used for segregation of biomedical waste.

- **Waste receptacles:** The waste receptacles should have the following properties
  - **Plastic bags** must be labeled with biohazard logos **(Fig. 42.1)** and should be non-inflammable, autoclave stable and non-chlorinated with a thickness of ≥50 μm
  - **Containers** should have well-fitting lids, either removable by hand or preferably operated by a foot pedal
  - **Sharp box** should be puncture-proof, leak-proof and tamper-proof impermeable container.
- **Importance of segregation:** Segregation is the most crucial step in BMW management. Wrong segregation may lead to serious consequences such as:
  - Needle stick injury transmitting hepatitis B or HIV (if sharp items are segregated in to yellow or red bags)
  - Production of carcinogens (if plastic items are wrongly segregated into yellow bag and subjected to incineration, leads to production of carcinogenic furans).
- **Securement:** All the bags used for waste collection need to be sealed once they are filled to 3/4th of their capacity
- **Labeling:** Bags and containers should be labeled properly with the date and place
- **Pre-treatment:** The laboratory liquid waste should always be pre-treated either with chemical (1–2% hypochlorite) or autoclave before segregating into appropriate containers
- **Transport:** The waste should be transported within 24 hours by **dedicated trolley** to the central BMW storage facility of the hospital. Separate routes should be used for transport to prevent exposure to staff and patients and to minimize the passage of loaded carts through patient care and other clean areas. Interim storage of the waste at ward is strongly discouraged
- **Central storage area:** This is a temporary storage facility present within a hospital where different types of waste should be brought for safe retention until it is treated or collected for transport to CBMWTF
- **Personal protective equipment (PPE):** HCWs handling BMW during transport or in the storage area should wear appropriate PPE such as heavy duty gloves, 3-ply mask, gowns and gumboots.

Treatment and Disposal Methods

As per the mandate of the BMWM rules, 2016, the final disposal and recycling must be performed at common bio-medical waste treatment facility (CBMWTF). Only when there is no CBMWTF within 75 km, the hospital can create its own the disposal facility. The following are the methods used for treatment/disposal of BMW.

Incineration

It has been the method of choice for the disposal of BMW.
- Incineration is a high temperature (800–1,200°C) dry oxidation process that reduces organic and combustible waste into nonorganic incombustible matter, resulting in a very significant reduction of waste volume and weight
- Incineration is usually done for those wastes that cannot be reused, recycled or disposed of in a landfill site, for example human and animal anatomical waste, microbiological waste, and solid non-plastic infectious waste
- Halogenated plastics such as PVC should never be incinerated as it generates furans which are carcinogenic.

Autoclave

Autoclaving is a thermal process where steam is brought into direct contact with waste in a controlled manner and for sufficient duration to sterilize the wastes. It is mainly used for the treatment of infectious plastic and sharp waste.

Chemical Disinfection

A chemical such as hypochlorite 1–2% is mixed to waste which results in disinfection. It is more suitable for liquid waste such as discarded blood and body fluid and also for hospital sewage.

Effluent Treatment Plant

The liquid waste (effluent) generated in the hospital if mixes directly with groundwater it can create significant health risks.
- ❖ Therefore, it is first subjected to chemical treatment and then is drained into effluent treatment plant (ETP)
- ❖ ETP removes the suspended solids and organic matter in wastewater and then disinfects the wastewater (with hypochlorite) and finally drain the water to municipal drainage.

Microwaving

Microwaves are radio-frequency waves, used at a frequency of 2,450 MHz. They produce friction of water molecules which generates heat. Large size microwaves are used for disposal of BMW—mainly infectious plastics and sharp wastes.

Hydroclaving

Hydroclaving is a low-temperature steam sterilizer, involving steam treatment with fragmentation and drying of waste. It breaks up the waste into small pieces of fragmented material; thus obviates postcycle shredding (unlike autoclave).

Shredder

Shredding is a process by which wastes are de-shaped or cut into smaller pieces so as to make the wastes unrecognizable. It helps in prevention of reuse of BMW and also helps to reduce the waste volume.

Deep Burial

Deep burial is a pit dug about two meters deep. It needs to be half-filled with waste, and then covered with lime within 50 cm of the surface, before filling the rest of the pit with soil. The groundwater level should be a minimum of six meters below the lower level of a deep burial pit.

Sharp Pit

A sharp pit constructed within the hospital premises provides an alternative method for disposal of the sharp wastes generated from the facility (**Fig. 42.2**).

Encapsulation

Encapsulation method involves filling the containers with waste, adding immobilizing material and sealing the containers, to prevent the access to unscrupulous activities. The process uses cubic boxes made up of metallic drums which are three quarters filled with sharps or chemicals or pharmaceutical wastes and then filled with a medium such as plastic foam, cement mortar or clay material.

Inertization

The process of inertization involves mixing waste with cement and other substances before disposal to minimize the risk of toxic substances contained in the waste migrating to surface or groundwater. It is especially suitable for pharmaceuticals and for incinerated ashes with a high metal content.

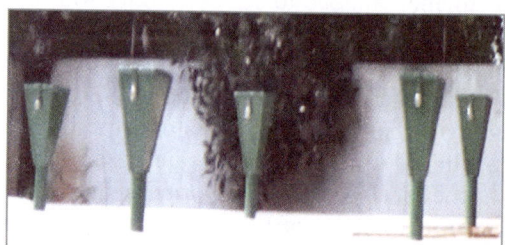

Fig. 42.2: Sharp pit.
Source: Department of Biomedical Waste Management, JIPMER, Puducherry (with permission).

Plasma Pyrolysis

Plasma pyrolysis uses ionized gas in the plasma state to convert electrical energy to temperatures of several thousand degrees using plasma arc torches or electrodes. The system provides high temperatures combined with high UV radiation flux which destroys pathogens completely.

Disposal of Cytotoxic Drug Waste

Expired cytotoxic drugs to be returned back to the manufacturer or supplier or CBMWTF for incineration at >1,200°C or encapsulation or plasma pyrolysis at >1,200°C.

Disposal of General Waste (Solid Waste)

They constitute the large component of hospital waste (80%). They are not biomedical waste; their disposal can be carried out by several strategies.
- **Composting:** It is the decomposition of organic matter by microorganism in warm moist environment
- **Waste-to-energy:** By various methods such as incineration, pelletization, biomethanation, etc.
- Recycling of the waste
- Landfilling in dump yard (least preferred method).

MONITORING OF BMW MANAGEMENT

Monitoring is an essential component of managing biomedical waste in the hospital. BMW management committee should be formed in a healthcare facility, which serves several functions—(1) to oversee the implementation of BMW practices, (2) to educate HCWs about BMWM practices, and (3) to monitor BMW management in a hospital.

BLOOD SPILL MANAGEMENT

Spillage of blood and body fluid poses a substantial risk for the transmission of blood-borne viruses such as hepatitis B, C, and HIV. Therefore, any spillage (small, few drops to large, few mL) should be considered infectious, and need to be cleaned at the earliest.

> **Steps of spill management (CDC protocol, Fig. 42.3)**
> The following steps need to be sequentially followed for the management of blood or body fluid spillage.
> - Any spillage, attend immediately
> - Mark the spill area, place the wet floor signage
> - Wear appropriate PPE (gloves and gown) as mentioned in the spill kit
> - Remove any broken glass pieces with forceps and discard them in the puncture-proof blue waste bin
> - Confine the spill and wipe immediately with an absorbent towel or cloth, which is spread over the spill to solidify the blood or body fluid. Then it is disposed of as infectious waste
> - Clean with hypochlorite (freshly prepared)
>   - For large spills (>10 cm size): Use 1:10 dilution of 5% hypochlorite (5000 ppm) i.e. 0.5%
>   - For small spills (<10 cm size): Use 1:100 dilution of 5% hypochlorite (500 ppm), i.e. 0.05%
> - Allow the disinfectant to remain wet on the surface for at least a contact time of 10 min
> - Rinse the area with clean water to remove the disinfectant residue
> - Discard the PPE and the wastes in appropriate bags
> - Perform hand wash.

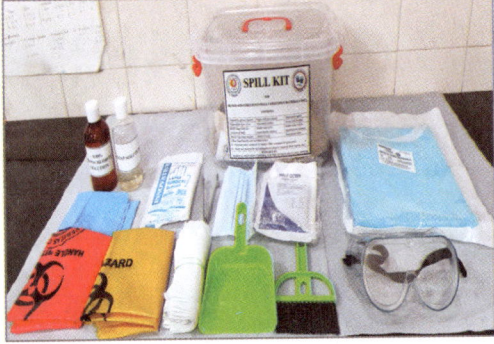

Fig. 42.3: Blood spill kit.

Source: Hospital Infection Control and Prevention Unit, Department of Microbiology, JIPMER, Puducherry *(with permission).*

EXPECTED QUESTIONS

I. Write short notes on:
1. Categories of biomedical waste.
2. Disposal methods available for biomedical waste.
3. Type of containers used for disposal of biomedical waste.

II. Multiple Choice Questions (MCQs):

1. Anatomical waste should be segregated in which color bags?
   a. Yellow b. Red
   c. Blue   d. Black

2. Microbiological waste should be segregated in which color bags?
   a. Yellow b. Red
   c. Blue   d. Black

3. Sharps should be segregated in which color box?
   a. Yellow b. Red
   c. Blue   d. White

4. Solid waste (items contaminated with blood and body fluids including cotton, dressings) belong to which category of biomedical waste?
   a. Yellow b. Red
   c. Blue   d. White

5. Plastic infectious items should be segregated in which color bag?
   a. Yellow b. Red
   c. Blue   d. White

6. Before segregation of microbiological wastes, pre-treatment with what concentration of hypochlorite is recommended?
   a. 1–2%   b. 5%
   c. 10%   d. 15%

7. Blood bag should be segregated in which color bags?
   a. Yellow b. Red
   c. Blue   d. Black

8. N95 respirator should be segregated in which color bags?
   a. Yellow b. Red
   c. Blue   d. Black

9. Gloves should be segregated in which color bags?
   a. Yellow b. Red
   c. Blue   d. Black

10. Treatment and/or disposal should be done within ____ hours of generation:
    a. 24 hr   b. 48 hr
    c. 72 hr   d. 1 week

Answers
1. a   2. a   3. d   4. a   5. b   6. a   7. a   8. a   9. b   10. b

CHAPTER 43

Needle Stick Injury

CHAPTER PREVIEW
- Prevention of Needle Stick Injury
- Post-exposure Management

INTRODUCTION

An occupational exposure is defined as:
- Percutaneous injury, e.g. needle stick injury (NSI) or other sharp injury
- Splash injury:
  - Contact with the mucous membrane (e.g. eye or mouth)
  - Contact with non-intact skin (abraded skin or afflicted with dermatitis)
  - Contact with the intact skin when the duration is prolonged (e.g. several minutes or more).

An occupational injury is often loosely termed as needle stick injury though it includes injury through needle or other sharps and splashes.

Agents transmitted:
Hepatitis B virus (HBV), hepatitis C virus (HCV) and HIV are three major blood-borne viruses (BBVs) that are transmitted through NSI. The risk of transmission is highest for HBV (30%) followed by HCV (3%) and HIV (0.3%).

Infectious specimens for NSI:
- *Potentially infectious body fluids* include blood, genital secretions (semen, vaginal secretions) and all body fluids (CSF, synovial fluid, pleural fluid, peritoneal fluid, pericardial fluid, amniotic fluid)
- *The following are not considered potentially infectious*, unless visibly contaminated with blood: Feces, nasal secretions, saliva, sputum, sweat, tears, urine and vomitus.

Factors that influence the risk of contracting infection following NSI:
The risk of infection following exposure depends on the following factors:
- Type of needle (hollow bore needle has a higher risk than solid needle)
- Device visibly contaminated with blood
- Depth of injury (higher is the depth, more is the risk)
- Volume of blood involved in the exposure
- Viral load present in the blood at the time of exposure
- Timely performing first aid
- Timely start of appropriate post-exposure prophylaxis (PEP) for HBV and HIV.

PREVENTION OF NEEDLE STICK INJURY

Precautions During Handling Needles

The following measures should be taken during handling needles to prevent occupational exposures:
- **Standard precautions** must be followed such as hand hygiene and appropriate use of personal protective equipment (PPE) (e.g. gloves, gowns, masks, and goggles) while handling blood or body fluids
- **Work surfaces** must be disinfected with 0.5% sodium hypochlorite solution
- **HBV vaccination:** Health care workers (HCWs) must be immunized against HBV and protective titer must be documented

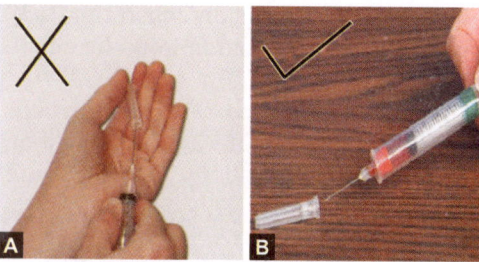

Figs. 43.1A and B: Recapping of needle: **A.** Wrong method; **B.** Correct method (single hand 'scoop' technique).

- **Spill management:** Spillage of blood and other body fluids must be promptly cleaned and surface disinfected with 0.5% sodium hypochlorite solution
- **Disposable needles** should be used. Needles should never be reused
- **Never recap needles:** If unavoidable, single hand-scoop technique may be followed **(Figs. 43.1A and B)**
- **Disposal after use:** Needles must be disposed into the sharp box immediately after use. Needles/sharps should not be left on trolleys and bedside tables
- **Engineering control measures:** Various devices are specially designed with safety features to prevent NSI such as retractable lancets, safety lock syringe with a protective sheath and needleless IV systems.

Precautions During Surgical Procedures

Confine and contain approach should be implemented for every surgical procedure.
- *Passing of sharp instruments* during surgery must be according to the plan decided by the surgeon and his assistant nurse. Sharp instruments should always be passed by non-touch approach, not directly by hands
- *Suturing:* Needles must never be picked up with the fingers while suturing. Forceps or a needle holder is ideal for holding a needle. Where practical, blunt needles should be used to close the abdomen
- Preoperative testing of a patient for BBVs is not mandatory; should be performed only if a clinical indication is present
- **Patient known to have BBV infections** may require the following additional precautions for surgical operation:
  - The lead surgeon should ensure that all members of the team know about infection hazards and appropriate measures should be followed, such as use of *double gloves*
  - The surgical team must be limited to essential members of *trained staff* only
  - It may help theater decontamination if such cases *posted last in the list*, but this is not mandatory.

POST-EXPOSURE MANAGEMENT

Steps of Post-exposure Management

The following are the sequential steps to be followed following an occupational exposure **(Table 43.1)**:
1. **First aid:** First aid has to be started as early as possible **(Table 43.2)**
2. **Report to the designated nodal center:** Every hospital must have a nodal center for the management of NSI. In most hospitals, HICC office acts as a nodal center, other hospitals may designate staff clinic or casualty for the purpose. Nodal centers perform the following functions as mentioned below (steps 3–9)
3. **Take first dose of PEP for HIV:**
   - The first dose of PEP for HIV should be taken as early as possible. Effect is maximum if taken <2 hours and effect is nil if taken after 72 hours of exposure

Table 43.1: Steps of post-exposure management.

1. First aid
2. Report to designated nodal center
3. Take first dose of PEP for HIV
4. Testing for BBVs
5. Decision on PEP for HIV and HBV
6. Documentation and recording of exposure
7. Informed consent and counseling
8. Follow-up testing of HCWs
9. Precautions during the follow-up period

Abbreviations: PEP, post-exposure prophylaxis; HCW, healthcare worker; BBV, blood-borne virus.

Table 43.2: First aid: Management of exposed site.	
Do's	**Don'ts**
Earlier the first aid, lesser is the chance of transmission of BBVs • For splash injury: Irrigate thoroughly the site (e.g. eyes or mouth or other exposed area) vigorously with water at least for 5 minutes • Spit fluid out immediately if gone into mouth and rinse the mouth several times • If wearing contact lenses, leave them in place while irrigating. Once the eye is cleaned, remove the contact lens and clean them in a normal manner	• Do not panic • Do not place the pricked finger into the mouth reflexively • Do not squeeze blood from wound • Do not use antiseptics and detergents

- **NACO recommendation:** The first dose regimen a single tablet, which contains fixed dose combination of Tenofovir (300 mg) + Lamivudine (300 mg) + Dolutegravir (50 mg)
- If the HIV negative status of the source is documented in patient's case record or in the hospital information system, then the first dose of PEP is not required
- If test report is not available, then administer the first dose regimen immediately without waiting for the laboratory result.

4. **Testing for BBVs:** The following tests are done for both source and HCW. The test format should be a rapid method (immunochromatographic test or flow through assay) and result should be available within 1–2 hours
   - Anti-HIV antibody detection
   - HBsAg detection
   - Anti-HCV antibody detection
   - Anti-HBs antibody (done for HCW if previously vaccinated for HBV and titer not tested).

   HCW's baseline status is determined because later it maybe difficult to attribute whether the infection was acquired due to this occupational exposure or any other prior exposure. This may guide while taking a decision, when the HCW claims for compensation from the health authorities

5. **Decision on post-exposure prophylaxis** (PEP) for HIV and HBV is taken based on standard guidelines (NACO for HIV and CDC for HBV) as described in **Tables 43.3 and 43.4** respectively

6. **Informed consent and counseling:** Almost every person feels anxious after exposure. They should be counseled and provided with psychological support
   - They should be informed about the risks and benefits of PEP medications
   - PEP is not mandatory. If the exposed person refuses to take the PEP, it should be documented. However, he should be made to understand about the risk of acquiring infection if PEP is not taken.

7. **Documentation and recording of exposure:**
   - A *structured proforma* should be used to collect the detail information related to exposure such as date, time, and place of exposure, type of procedure done, type of exposure, duration of exposure, source status, volume and type of specimen involved (Refer **Fig. 56.1** of Chapter 56)
   - *Consent form:* For prophylactic treatment, the exposed person must sign a consent form. If the individual refuses to initiate PEP, it should be documented. The designated officer for PEP should keep this document.

8. **Follow-up testing** of HCWs for BBVs should be done if the source status is positive/unknown
   - *HIV testing follow-up is done:* At 6 weeks, 3 months and 6 months after exposure
   - HBV and HCV follow-up testing is done at 6 months after exposure.

9. **Precautions during the follow-up period:** If the source status is positive/unknown, then the following precautions should be adopted by the HCW during the follow-up period, especially the first 6–12 weeks
   - Refraining from blood, semen, organ donation

- Abstinence from sexual intercourse or use of latex condom till both baseline and 3 months HIV tests are found negative
- Women should not breastfeed their infants
- The exposed person is advised to seek medical evaluation for any febrile illness that occurs within 12 weeks of exposure.

Table 43.3: Revised NACO Guidelines for post-exposure prophylaxis (PEP), 2021.

Exposure code (EC)	Source HIV status code (SC)	PEP recommendation
1, 2 or 3	Negative	Not warranted
1	1	Not warranted
1	2	PEP is recommended
2	1	Duration of PEP: 28 days
2	2	**TLD regimen*:** Each tablet contains fixed dose combination of Tenofovir (300 mg) + Lamivudine (300 mg) + Dolutegravir (50 mg); one tablet to be taken daily for 4 weeks.
3	1 or 2	
2 or 3	Unknown (in area with high prevalence)	

Source material: Blood, body fluids or other potentially infectious material (CSF, synovial, pleural, pericardial and amniotic fluid, and pus) or an instrument contaminated with any of these substances

Exposure code:
1. **EC-1 (Mild exposure):** Mucous membrane/non-intact skin exposure with small volumes, or less duration
2. **EC-2 (Moderate exposure):**
   - Mucous membrane/non-intact skin with large volumes/splashes for several minutes or more duration OR
   - Percutaneous superficial exposure with solid needle or superficial scratch
3. **EC-3 (Severe exposure):** Percutaneous exposure with:
   - Large volume transfer
   - By hollow needle, wide bore needle or deep puncture
   - Visible blood on device
   - Needle used in patient's artery or vein

Source HIV Status Code (SC):
1. **SC-1:** HIV positive, asymptomatic or low viral load (<400 copies/mL)
2. **SC-2:** HIV positive, symptomatic (advanced AIDS or primary HIV infection), high viral load
3. **SC unknown:** Status of the patient is unknown and neither the patient nor his/her blood is available for testing
4. **HIV negative:** Tested negative according to NACO strategy

The first dose of PEP
Should be started within 2 hours (for greater impact) and definitely within 72 hours. No need to provide PEP if exposure occurred >72 hours

PEP not required in the following situations:
1. If exposed person is HIV positive: Exposed individuals who are known or discovered to be HIV positive should not receive PEP. They should be referred to ART clinic for counseling and initiation of ART
2. If the exposure is on an intact skin
3. If source is HIV negative
4. Exposure with low-risk specimens like tear, saliva, urine, stool, vomitus, nasal secretion, sweat, etc.
5. For exposures with EC-1 and SC-1
6. Source unknown if HIV prevalence is low
7. In case of delay in reporting the exposure by > 72 hours, PEP initiation becomes optional

Side effects and compliance to PEP:
- Common side effects are:
  - At the initial phase of the course: Nausea, diarrhea, muscular pain, headache or fatigue
  - Later during the course: Anemia, leukopenia or thrombocytopenia
- For most side effects except jaundice or liver tenderness, **PEP should never be discontinued**.
- Compliance of >95% to the PEP schedule is required to maximize the efficacy of PEP. Hence, the person should be counseled to continue the PEP and to take medication to minimize the side effects of PEP.

*Regimen for exposure in pregnant women is essentially same as that of non-pregnant persons.
Abbreviations: NACO, National AIDS Control Organization; ART, antiretroviral therapy.

Table 43.4: Post-exposure prophylaxis (PEP) for hepatitis B.

HCW status	If source is positive or unknown for HBsAg	If source is negative for HBsAg
If the exposed person is completely vaccinated and the antibody titer is protective (≥10 mIU/mL)	No further treatment is required: • Regardless of the HBV status of the source* • Regardless if the titer falls down later*	
If the exposed person is completely vaccinated and the titer is not protective (<10 mIU/mL)	HBIG-1 dose should be started immediately; maximum within 7 days Vaccine: Start the second series (3 doses)	Vaccine: Start the second series (3 doses)
If the exposed person is not vaccinated or partially vaccinated	HBIG-1 dose should be started immediately; maximum within 7 days Vaccine: Complete the vaccine series from the last dose given (do not restart)	Vaccine: Complete the vaccine series from the last dose given (do not restart)
Nonresponders (If the exposed person is vaccinated for 2 series, i.e. 6 doses and the titer is not protective)	HBIG-2 doses at 1 month apart (0.06 mL/kg or 10–12 IU/kg)	Nothing is required

Note:
- HCW is said to be protected when titer rises (anti-HBs ≥10 mIU/mL), after three or more doses of vaccination. Rise of titer after one or two doses of vaccine should not be considered as protective.
- HCWs who are not protected must be checked for their HBsAg status at baseline and follow-up testing 6 months later, regardless of their vaccination status.
- Anti-HBs antibody titer should be checked only after 2 months of last dose of vaccine and 6 months after HBIG administration; otherwise, it will give erratic results.
- HBIG and HBV vaccine can be administered simultaneously but at different sites.
- HBIG provides a temporary protection for 3–6 months.
- Previous report of Anti-HBs titer is acceptable only if it is documented. Verbal reports should not be considered.

*In a previously protected person, the memory B cells will start producing antibodies soon after the antigenic challenge, hence revaccination by booster doses is not recommended even if the titer falls down later.
Adapted from CDC Guidelines, 2013.
Abbreviations: HBIG, hepatitis B immunoglobulin; HCW, health-care worker; HBsAg, hepatitis B surface antigen.

EXPECTED QUESTIONS

I. **Write short notes on:**
   1. Sequential steps to be followed after a needle stick injury.
   2. Post-exposure prophylaxis for HIV.
   3. Post-exposure prophylaxis for hepatitis B.

II. **Multiple Choice Questions (MCQs):**
   1. **The decreasing order of risk of transmission following occupational exposure:**
      a. HIV>HBV>HCV
      b. HBV>HIV>HCV
      c. HBV>HCV>HIV
      d. HCV>HBV>HIV
   2. **All are potentially highly infectious specimen for occupational injury, *except*:**
      a. Blood
      b. Semen
      c. CSF
      d. Saliva
   3. **The sequence of steps to be followed after accidental exposure to blood/fluid:**
      a. First aid Reach to nodal center and try to get report of source status Take first dose of PEP for HIV → Testing of source and HCW status for BBVs → Prophylactic treatment for HIV and HBV
      b. Reach to nodal center and try to get report of source status → First aid → Take first dose of PEP for HIV → Testing of source and HCW status for BBVs → Prophylactic treatment for HIV and HBV
      c. Take first dose of PEP for HIV → Testing of source and HCW status for BBVs → First aid → Reach to nodal center and try to get report of source status → Prophylactic treatment for HIV and HBV
      d. Prophylactic treatment for HIV and HBV → Take first dose of PEP for HIV → Testing of source and HCW status for BBVs → First aid → Reach to nodal center and try to get report of source status

Answers
1. c   2. d   3. a

CHAPTER 44: Environmental Surveillance

CHAPTER PREVIEW
- Water Surveillance
- Air Surveillance
- Surface Surveillance

The environment in the hospital plays an important role in the occurrence of healthcare-associated infections. The various environmental sources from which microorganisms can be transmitted to patients and healthcare workers include water, air and environmental surfaces. Therefore, monitoring of microbiological quality of water, air and surfaces are of paramount importance for safe hospital environment.

WATER SURVEILLANCE

Waterborne Pathogens

Hospital water and water-containing devices may serve as a reservoir of healthcare associated waterborne pathogens. Microbial contamination of water in healthcare settings is broadly of two types.

Category 1 (Enteric Pathogens)

This results from fecal contamination of drinking water supplies. This group of waterborne pathogens are common in community settings than in hospitals. These agents are transmitted by ingestion of contaminated water. Most of them cause diarrheal outbreaks, while few agents cause extraintestinal illness. Examples include:
- **Bacteria:** Gram-negative bacilli such as *Salmonella, Shigella, Vibrio cholerae*
- **Viruses:** Rotavirus, norovirus, hepatitis A and E viruses
- **Parasites:** *Entamoeba histolytica, Giardia lamblia, Cryptosporidium, Cyclospora*, etc.

Category 2 (Common Hospital Pathogens)

These include multidrug resistant gram-negative bacilli (MDR-GNB), legionellae, etc.
- This group of waterborne pathogens are more important in hospital-setting, than community
- They are commonly present in hospital environment and can contaminate various hospital water reservoirs such as potable water, sinks, dialysis water, ice and ice machines, etc.
- They are transmitted by various routes such as ingestion, contact, aspiration, etc.
- Waterborne outbreaks caused by these pathogens and their reservoirs in healthcare settings have been a serious threat to high-risk patients who are critically ill or immunocompromised.

Test of Drinking Water Contaminated with Enteric Pathogens

Hospital drinking water should be free of enteric pathogens and safe for drinking. Therefore, water supplies should be regularly tested to confirm that they are free from such contamination.

- However, it is impracticable to attempt directly to detect the presence of all types of enteric pathogen in water because they are usually present in minute quantity; such as *Shigella, Salmonella*, etc.
- Instead, it is wise to test the water supplies for those microorganisms which indicate that fecal contamination has taken place. These organisms are called as indicator organisms.

Indicator Organisms

Indicator organisms are usually the commensal bacteria of intestine. Their presence in water supplies indicates that there may be a contamination of sewage with enteric pathogens and the water supplies needs to be disinfected.

There are a number of intestinal commensals, used as indicator organisms, of which important ones are as follows.
- Fecal (thermotolerant) *Escherichia coli*: It is the most sensitive indicator, confirms recent fecal contamination of water
- Coliform (other than *Escherichia coli*): Indicates remote contamination—either by fecal (presumptive) or soil and vegetation.

Collection and Transport of Water Sample

Water specimen should be collected in a screw-capped wide sterile container.
- **Volume:** At least 150–200 mL of water should be collected
- **Neutralizer:** Sodium thiosulfate is added to neutralize the bactericidal effect of residual chlorine present in water if any
- **Sampling points** in hospitals must represent different sources from which water is obtained such as portable water from pipelines, endoscopy rinse water, dialysis water, dental chair unit waterline, etc.
- **Sampling method from the tap:** Care should be taken while collecting water to minimize extraneous contamination. Hand washing should be performed and gloves should be worn before collection **(Fig. 44.1)**

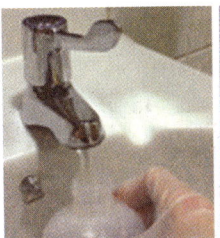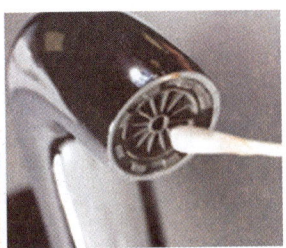

Fig. 44.1: Water sampling methods.

- **Tap swabs:** Sterile swab is inserted into the nozzle of the tap carefully, without touching the outer tap surface. The swab is then rubbed around–that is, moved backwards and forwards and up and down, as much as possible, on the inside surface of the tap outlet or flow straightener **(Fig. 44.1)**
- There are two methods employed for detection of microbial contamination of water—(1) Multiple-tube method and (2) membrane filtration method.

Multiple-tube Method

It is the most common method used for water surveillance. It is so named as it involves mixing of specific volume (100 mL) of water samples, divided into multiple tubes containing a special culture medium—MacConkey purple broth.
- **Positive result:** After being incubated for 24–48 hours, the medium turns to yellow from purple, along with turbidity and production of gas **(Fig. 44.2)**. This indicates presence of coliform bacteria. However, it cannot differentiate between fecal *E. coli* and other coliform bacteria
- **Differential coliform count (Eijkman test):** Subsequently fecal *E. coli* can be differentiated from other coliform bacteria by its ability to grow at 44°C
- **Determination of MPN:** The number of tubes giving positive reaction is compared with specialized statistical table (called McCrady table) to determine the most probable number (MPN) of coliform count present per 100 mL of water. This is called as presumptive coliform count
- **Quality of water supply:** Depending upon the MPN/100 mL, the quality of the water

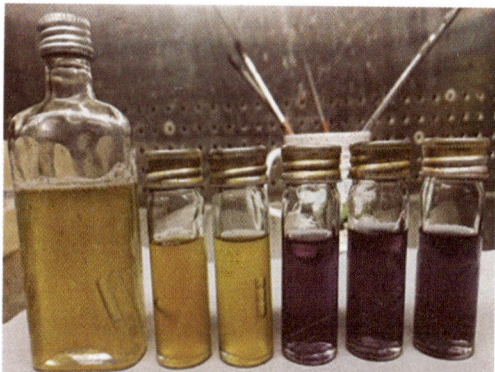

Fig. 44.2: MacConkey purple broth for multiple tube method (one 50 mL and five 10 mL tubes are needed for testing unpolluted water); if negative, media appears purple; if positive, media turn yellow.

Source: Department of Microbiology, JIPMER, Puducherry (with permission).

Table 44.1: Classification of quality of drinking water supply.

Quality of drinking water supply	Most probable number (MPN)/100 mL of water	
	Coliform count/100 mL	Thermotolerant E. coli count/100 mL
Excellent	0	0
Satisfactory	1–3	0
Intermediate	4–9	0
Unsatisfactory	≥10	≥1

specimen can be interpreted as excellent, satisfactory, intermediate or unsatisfactory **(Table 44.1)**.

Membrane Filtration Method

This method is based on the filtration of a known volume (e.g. 100 mL) of water through a cellulose membrane of pore size 0.2 or 0.45 μm.
- **Advantages:** Membrane filtration is the recommended method for—(1) testing dialysis water, (2) for testing clean water, where the bacterial count in water is expected to be low and (3) for testing a large volume of water
- **Disadvantages:** It is not suitable for turbid water. Expensive than multiple tube method.

Test of Water Contaminated with Healthcare Associated Pathogens

Most of the healthcare associated pathogens are recovered by membrane filtration method, followed by plating on to a suitable culture medium.

Endotoxin Detection

Endotoxins are the component of the cell wall of gram-negative bacteria. Dialysis water, devices, etc. contaminated with endotoxin can elicit a variety of inflammatory responses in our body and thereby cause serious toxic effects. Therefore, apart from bacteriological testing, the dialysis water used for hemodialysis is also tested for presence of endotoxin.
- **Methods:** Three methods are available—(i) gel clot assay (Limulus amebocyte lysate assay), (ii) turbidimetric method, and (iii) chromogenic technique
- **Permissive level:** Water used to prepare dialysate and to reprocess hemodialyzers should contain endotoxin unit <0.25 EU/mL.

AIR SURVEILLANCE

Air is an important vehicle of transmission of many pathogenic organisms. Therefore, the examination of air to detect the number of bacteria carrying particles is important particularly in critical areas such as operation theatres (OTs), bone marrow transplant units, etc.

Indication (CDC Recommendations)

Routine air sampling (i.e. random or periodic sampling) is not recommended because (i) HAI rates are not related with levels of general microbial contamination of air or environmental surfaces, (ii) there is no standard guideline mentioning for permissible levels of microbial contamination of environmental surfaces or air.

CDC recommends targeted air surveillance, which should be carried out for the following indications:
- Investigation of an outbreak

- For research purpose
- After reconstruction or newly constructed buildings
- After fogging (to monitor the quality)
- For short-term evaluation of a change in infection control practice.

Evaluation of the Quality of Air in OT

Evaluation of the quality of air includes both microbiological and non-microbiological (physical) parameters.

Microbiological Parameters

There are two principle means of monitoring the microbiological parameters present in the air, passive monitoring and active sampling.

Passive Monitoring (Settle Plate) Method

Standard Petri dishes containing culture media (e.g. blood agar) are exposed to the air for a given time and then the plates are incubated at 37°C for 24 hours aerobically.
- **1, 1, 1 method:** The ideal recommendation is the 1, 1, 1 method where the plates are placed at different locations in the OT one meter away from the side walls, one meter above the floor and for a duration of 1 hour
- **Disadvantages:** (1) It cannot detect smaller particles or droplets suspended in the air, (2) This method cannot quantify the volume of air sampled, (3) This method is not recommended when sampling air for fungal spores, because single spores can remain suspended in air indefinitely.

Active Monitoring (Slit Sampler Method)

In active monitoring, a microbiological air sampler (e.g. sieve impactor) is used. It has a vacuum pump, and a perforated lid **(Fig. 44.3B)**, in which an agar plate can be placed.
- The vacuum pump physically draws a known volume of air through the perforated lid and allows it to impact on the agar plate (e.g. blood agar)
- Following incubation, the quantity of microorganisms present in the culture plate is measured in terms of CFU/m^3 of air **(Fig. 44.3A)**

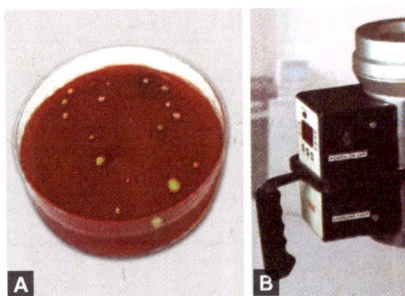

Figs. 44.3A and B: A. Air sampler method showing blood agar with bacterial colonies; **B.** Air sampler (HiMedia).
Source: Department of Microbiology, JIPMER, Puducherry *(with permission)*.

- Active monitoring is applicable when the concentration of microorganisms is not very high, such as in an operating theatre, bone marrow transplant unit, etc.

Air Particle Counters

Air particle counters have been developed recently, that are capable of detecting airborne particles containing microorganisms in real time.

The particle count of an OT is considered acceptable only when it falls in the acceptable range of clean room standard, according to the international standards system ISO 14644-1
- Most of the HEPA filtered OT should satisfy ISO 6 level of clean room standard, which refers that the room should maintain <35,200 particles of 0.5 µm in size per cubic meter
- Ultra-clean OT (e.g. orthopedics) should have clean room standard ISO 5; which refers that the room should maintain <3,520 particles of 0.5 µm size per cubic meter.

Non-microbiological Parameters

The number of bacteria in air at any given point of time depends upon various non-microbiological parameters such as air changes per hour, air velocity, positive pressure environment, temperature and relative humidity inside OT, etc. Therefore, there should be periodic monitoring of these parameters.

SURFACE SURVEILLANCE

Environmental surface sampling has been used to determine (a) reservoirs of potential environmental pathogens, and (b) the sources of the environmental contamination.

❖ **Locations:** It is required for high-risk locations such as operation theatres and ICU settings
❖ **Sites for sampling (high touch areas):** Surface sampling is taken from sites where there is high-risk of contaminations
❖ **Indications (CDC recommendation):**
  ▪ Surface sampling is currently indicated for research, as a part of an epidemiologic investigation, or during an outbreak investigation
  ▪ Routine periodic surface surveillance is not recommended.
❖ **Method:** Moistened sterile swabs (soaked in sterile saline) are used to collect the samples from high-risk areas and then inoculated on to blood agar for the recovery of aerobic bacteria
❖ **Reporting:** Only pathogenic organisms isolated are reported. A semi-quantitative report (as heavy, moderate or light growth) should be provided. Contaminants such as aerobic spore bearers are not reported
❖ **Newer techniques** such as luminometer (expresses bacterial contamination as CFU/mL) and glow gel techniques are available which are easy to perform though expensive.

EXPECTED QUESTIONS

I. Write short notes on:
1. Water surveillance.
2. Air surveillance.

II. Multiple Choice Questions (MCQs):
1. Which is the best indicator organism of fecal contamination of water?
   a. Fecal *E. coli*
   b. Fecal streptococci
   c. *Pseudomonas*
   d. *Vibrio cholerae*
2. Evaluation of the quality of air in OTs can be performed by all the following methods, *except*:
   a. Settle plate
   b. Slit sampler
   c. Particle count
   d. Multiple tube method
3. Eijkman test is performed to detect:
   a. Thermotolerant *Escherichia coli*
   b. Coliform bacteria
   c. *Clostridium perfringens*
   d. Fecal streptococci
4. Which of the following method is used for detection of endotoxin in water?
   a. Multiple tube method
   b. Membrane filtration method
   c. Limulus amebocyte lysate assay
   d. Slit sampler method

Answers
1. a   2. d   3. a   4. c

CHAPTER 45

Laundry Management

CHAPTER PREVIEW
- Collection and Transport of Linens
- Laundry Process
- Post-laundry Process

Laundry' in a healthcare facility (HCF) is a process by which various hospital linens are cleaned and disinfected.

- ❖ **Purpose:** The purpose of the laundry is to protect the health care workers (HCWs) from exposure to potentially infectious materials during the collection, handling, and sorting of contaminated linens
- ❖ **Linens:** The reusable linens in a HCF includes bed linens, curtains, towels, patient clothing, and HCWs' clothing (uniforms, coats, scrub suits, etc.).

Used or Contaminated Linen

For laundry purposes, the contaminated (i.e. used) linen generated in the HCF is classified into two categories:

- ❖ **Dirty linen:** They are used linen, but not visibly soiled with blood or blood-tinged body secretions
- ❖ **Soiled linen:** They are contaminated with excreta, blood, or body fluids. These also include the dirty used linen received from known cases of infected patients. These linen have a higher risk of transmitting infections.

Route of transmission: There are several routes by which these infections can be transmitted from the contaminated linens, which include:

- ❖ Direct contact with contaminated linen
- ❖ Aerosols generated from sorting and handling of contaminated linen.

Infection control measures: Adherence to standard precautions (such as hand hygiene and wearing appropriate PPE) when handling contaminated laundry is adequate to reduce the risk of disease transmission to patients and staff. Other important infection control measures include:

- ❖ Processing of linens in isolation areas
- ❖ Minimizing agitation of the linens to prevent the dispersal of aerosols
- ❖ Effective cleaning and disinfection of linens.

COLLECTION AND TRANSPORT

The used linen is collected at the point of generation such as in wards, ICUs, OTs, laboratories, etc., and are transported to the laundry facility.

- ❖ Used linen should be handled with **minimum agitation**, to prevent the generation of potentially contaminated lint aerosols in patient-care areas
- ❖ Linen needs to be **collected immediately** in bags and should not be placed on the floor or any other surfaces for a long time
- ❖ **Segregation:** All the linen generated from patient care areas should be segregated into dirty and soiled linen and preferably need to be collected in different color-coded trolleys

- To minimize aerosolization of any organisms contaminating linen, linen **should not be** rinsed, shaken, or sorted in the clinical area
- The personnel should keep his/her **hands away from the face** while handling linen
- **Storage:** The collected linen needs to be stored at a designated place, i.e. in dirty utility of the area of the ward
- **Packing:** Linens are packaged in bags, which are securely tied to prevent leakage if the laundry is wet. Bags must be clearly labelled, or color-coded so that HCWs handling these items are aware of the nature of the contaminated linen **(Fig. 45.1)**
- **Labelling:** Proper labelling of the linen helps in identification, traceability, and inventory management
- **Inventory:** The inventory should be maintained by the sister-in-charge of the area while giving and receiving the linens
- **Transport:** Clean and used linen should be transported in a separate dedicated closed system such as a trolley, cart, or chute. The trolleys should be cleaned and disinfected after transport **(Fig. 45.1)**.

LAUNDRY PROCESS

The laundry staff must wear appropriate PPE such as heavy-duty gloves, masks, and gowns, depending on the risk of work involved.

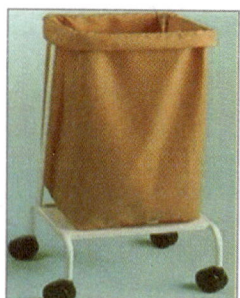 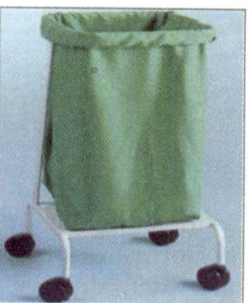

Fig. 45.1: Dirty linen in green and soiled linen in yellow-colored trolleys.

The laundering cycle consists of flush, main wash, bleaching, rinsing, and souring.
- **Flush:** The first step is to wet the linen with warm water (37–44°C) for 1 to 3 minutes to remove water-soluble soils
- **Wash:** This involves washing the linen with soaps or detergents in low-level hot water (57–62°C) for 5–8 minutes. Washing removes major stains and dirt and also sets the pH to 11–12, which is needed for the bleach step
- **Bleach:** This involves the treatment of linen with hypochlorite (50–200 ppm) in hot water 60–70°C for about 5 to 8 minutes. The bleaching step is for stain removal and disinfection of linen
- **Rinse:** This involves rinsing the linen in warm water (37–48°C) for 2–3 minutes, which helps to remove the residuals of stain and soiling, and also to neutralize the chlorine
- **Souring cycle:** It is the final rinse cycle, where a low level of warm water mixed with products such as softeners, etc. is used for 3–5 minutes, which makes the fabrics soft.

POST LAUNDRY PROCESS

The post laundry activities must be carried out in a well-separated clean area in the laundry, which involves the following steps:
- **Sorting of linen** into specific product types is carried out in a designated area. Sorting can also be performed before putting the linen for the laundry process
- **Drying of processed linen:** Can be carried out either by the mechanical dryer or manual drying (sunlight)
- **Packing of dried linen:** The linen is ironed (i.e. calendered) and folded by either manually or using specialized equipment
- **Storage:** Then the linen are kept in storage in a clean well-separated area which ensures their cleanliness until use.

EXPECTED QUESTIONS

I. **Write short notes on:**
   1. Collection and transport of linens.
   2. Steps of laundry process.

CHAPTER 46: Immunization of Healthcare Workers

CHAPTER PREVIEW
- Hepatitis B Vaccine
- Other Vaccines for HCWs

INTRODUCTION

Healthcare workers (HCWs) are at increased risk of exposure to infectious pathogens in their workplace and in turn, may act as a source of that infection and pose a risk of transmission to patients, other HCWs, members of their household, or other community contacts. Therefore, it is important that the HCWs should receive certain vaccines to protect them from the potential risk of acquiring healthcare-associated infections.

❖ The hospital administration must take the sole responsibility to provide a safe working environment and appropriate immunization to all the HCWs including the contractual, temporary, and outsourced HCWs.

❖ To achieve the above-said aim, hospitals should have staff clinics or staff health services. In many healthcare facilities, the hospital infection control committee (HICC) plays an active role in providing support to staff clinics to achieve its objectives.

IMMUNIZATION PROGRAM FOR HCW

Ensuring that HCWs are immune to vaccine-preventable diseases is an essential part of a successful staff health program **(Table 46.1)**.

Table 46.1: Vaccines that are recommended for all HCWs (adapted from CDC and WHO).

Vaccine	Recommendations	Schedule/dosage
Vaccines that are strongly recommended for all HCWs		
Hepatitis B	All HCWs at risk for exposure to blood or body fluids; vaccinate unless laboratory evidence of immunity	Three doses, at 0, 1, 6 months, IM route*
Influenza	• All HCWs are at high risk for contact with patients with influenza • Both trivalent and quadrivalent vaccines are available, in inactivated and live-attenuated forms	• Single-dose, yearly once • Inactivated vaccine is given IM route • Live attenuated vaccine given intranasally
COVID-19 vaccine	All HCWs must receive two doses of COVID-19 vaccine and thereafter the annual precautionary dose every year • **Covaxin:** Two doses (4–6 weeks apart) by IM route • **Covishield:** Two doses (12–16 weeks apart) by IM route	Precautionary dose every year
Measles, mumps and rubella	Vaccinate if there is no laboratory evidence of immunity	Single-dose, SC route
Varicella	Consider vaccinating unless there is a history of physician-diagnosed disease or laboratory evidence of immunity	Single-dose, SC route

Contd...

Contd...

Vaccines recommended for HCWs working in high-risk areas		
Td (tetanus toxoid, diphtheria toxoid, adult dose)	• **HCW (>18 year age) completed primary vaccination:** Td booster dose is indicated every 10 years till 65 years • **HCW (>18 year age) not completed primary vaccination:** 3 doses of Td are given at 0, 1 month, and 1 year • **Pregnant HCWs** need to get two doses of Td at 4 weeks interval during early pregnancy and a single dose of Td booster is recommended in a pregnancy, if received two doses of Td in a previous pregnancy within last 3 years	IM route, deltoid
Meningococcal polysaccharide vaccine	Give both MenACWY and MenB to microbiologists who are routinely exposed to isolates of *Neisseria meningitidis*	• Single-dose, IM route • Booster every 5 years if risk continues
Rabies	Persons working in a research laboratory setting	IM or ID single dose on days 0, 7, and 28 days
Typhoid (Vi capsular vaccIne)	HCWs with moderate to high-risk exposure	• Single-dose SC/IM route • Booster every 3 years
Hepatitis A	Persons working with HAV in a research laboratory setting	2-dose schedule: 0 and 6–12 months

Abbreviations: IM, intramuscular; ID, intradermal; SC, subcutaneous
Protective titer: Anti-HBs titer of ≥10 mIU/mL after three doses of hepatitis B vaccination is considered as protective.

- Optimal use of vaccines can prevent the transmission of vaccine-preventable diseases and eliminate unnecessary work restrictions.
- Prevention of illness through a comprehensive staff immunization program is far more cost-effective than case management and outbreak control.
- A mandatory immunization program that includes both newly recruited and currently employed HCWs is more effective than voluntary immunization program in ensuring that HCWs are vaccinated.

Decision about which vaccines to include in the staff immunization program has been made by considering the following aspects:

- The likelihood of HCWs' exposure to vaccine-preventable diseases and the potential consequences of not vaccinating
- The nature of employment (type of contact with patients and their environment)
- The characteristics of the patient population within the healthcare organization.

EXPECTED QUESTIONS

I. **Write short notes on:**
   1. Discuss the vaccines that are recommended for healthcare workers.

II. **Multiple Choice Questions (MCQs):**
   1. All the following vaccines are recommended for healthcare workers, *except*?
      a. COVID
      b. Hepatitis B
      c. Hepatitis A
      d. Tetanus

2. Which of the following vaccines is given to healthcare workers, as a precautionary dose?
   a. Influenza
   b. Varicella
   c. Hepatitis B
   d. COVID

Answers
1. c   2. d

CHAPTER 47

Antimicrobial Stewardship

CHAPTER PREVIEW

- Introduction
- Implementation of Antimicrobial Stewardship Program
- Monitoring the Compliance to Antimicrobial Stewardship Program
- Rational Use of Antimicrobial Agents
- Hospital Antibiogram

INTRODUCTION

Antimicrobial stewardship program (AMSP) provides strategies for rationalizing the use of antimicrobials in the hospital.

Definition

Centers for disease control and prevention (CDC) has defined antimicrobial stewardship as use of the right antimicrobial agent, for the right patient, at the right time, with the right dose, route and frequency, causing the least harm to the patient and future patients.

Why AMSP is Needed?

Antimicrobial stewardship program in a hospital is required for the following reasons.

Antimicrobial Resistance (AMR)

AMR is a rising threat across the globe. The multidrug resistant organisms (MDROs) are prevalent in every country though the extent and the severity of the problem varies. Extensive use of antimicrobials is the single most important factor for the bacteria to undergo mutation, which leads bacteria to become resistant to antimicrobials and then the resistant strain flourish exponentially in the presence of selective pressure of antimicrobials.

Misuse and Over-use of Antimicrobials

The last eight decades since the discovery of penicillin witnessed the saving of millions of lives due to use of antimicrobials in treating infections. However, at the same time, this has also led to their misuse through various ways—(1) use without a prescription, (2) overuse for self-limiting infections, non-bacterial infections, and (3) treatment of colonizer/contaminant.

Widespread Use of Antimicrobials in Other Sectors

World's largest antimicrobial use occurs for animal non-therapeutic purpose (70%), followed by animal therapeutic purpose (15%). Human use accounts only 15% of total antimicrobial consumption, out of which only 9% is being used for human therapeutic purpose. This data explains that just bringing in stewardship program in health care facility would not bring down antimicrobial use dramatically. A robust plan should also be in place for control of antimicrobial use in animals.

Poor Antimicrobial Research

Research in the development of new antimicrobial is a huge investment for the pharmaceutical industry. More so, soon after the discovery of an antimicrobial, the bacteria develop resistance mechanisms to tackle the antimicrobial. As a result, investment goes waste. It is also hypothesized that there could be a return to the pre-antibiotic era, where many people could suffer or die from untreatable bacterial infections.

IMPLEMENTATION OF AMSP

The key steps of implementation of antimicrobial stewardship program (AMSP) in a hospital is as follows.

Administrative Support (Leadership)

The most important prerequisite for implementing AMSP is a strong administrative support. They should be publicly committed to the program and provide necessary funding and infrastructure support.

Formulating AMS Team

Antimicrobial stewardship team (AMS team) is a multidisciplinary committee which is responsible for framing, implementing and monitoring the compliance to antimicrobial policy of the hospital.
- AMS team is led by the antimicrobial steward who may be an infectious disease physician or infection control officer or clinical microbiologist
- **Antimicrobial steward** is the central driving force behind this program. A larger hospital may require more than one antimicrobial steward
- Other members of AMS team include stewardship nurses, clinical pharmacists and officer in-charge of pharmacy.

Infrastructure Support

Infrastructure support is essential to initiate appropriate pathogen-directed antimicrobial agent at the earliest.
- **Support from the microbiology laboratory**
    - *Automations:* Facility for automated culture (e.g. BACTEC, BacT/ALERT or Virtuo), identification (MALDI-TOF) and sensitivity (e.g. VITEK) should be available. This reduces the turn-around time to 24–48 hours; compared to conventional cultures which takes 2–5 days
    - *Biomarkers:* Facility for testing biomarkers such as procalcitonin and C-reactive protein (CRP) must be available (discussed subsequently)
    - *Molecular tests:* Facility to perform rapid molecular tests must be available; e.g. Biofire FilmArray multiplex PCR
    - *Emergency laboratory:* Emergency lab functioning round the clock is a marker of a quality microbiology laboratory.
- **Hospital information system (HIS):** Fully functional HIS including laboratory information system will augment the stewardship program by many folds
- Supporting manpower availability.

Framing Antimicrobial Policy

Every hospital should frame their own hospital antimicrobial policy which is usually a pocket handbook, comprising of system/syndrome wise indications for antimicrobial choice and their dosage.
- It should be prepared by AMS team after discussing with all the clinicians, microbiologists and administrators
- The policy must be compliant to the standard national and international antimicrobial guidelines and local antibiogram pattern
- Common consensus between all clinicians must be arrived, before framing the policy; which facilitates better adherence to policy.

Implementing AMS Strategies

Two types of strategies are available for implementing AMSP.
- Front end strategies (formulary restriction)
- Back end strategies (prospective audit and feedback).

Front End Strategy (Formulary Restriction)

This involves classifying antimicrobial agents into restricted, semi-restricted and non-

Table 47.1: Proposed formulary restriction.		
Restricted antimicrobials	**Semi-restricted antimicrobials**	**Unrestricted antimicrobials**
Pharmacy supply of >1 days requires prior approval by AMS team	Pharmacy supply of >3 days requires prior approval by AMS team	Pharmacy supply does not require AMS team approval
Colistin Carbapenem Tigecycline	Teicoplanin, Vancomycin, Daptomycin, Linezolid, Third and fourth generation cephalosporins	First and second generation cephalosporins, Cotrimoxazole, Azithromycin, Clarithromycin, Fluoroquinolones

restricted antimicrobials with indications for their use combined with an approval system regulated by the AMS team **(Table 47.1)**.

❖ This strategy sounds more attractive, impact is immediate and appears to be the most ideal way to achieve antimicrobial stewardship, but practically implementing formulary restrictions is challenging and a difficult task
❖ It creates a lot of confusion as it directly compromises the clinician's freedom to choose antimicrobials
❖ More so availability of the AMSP consultants to give approval all the time further complicates the problem, especially in emergency situations.

Back End Strategy

This is carried out by **prospective audit and feedback**. Though difficult to perform, but it is the most effective strategy to implement AMSP.

❖ The AMS team goes for stewardship round during which they discuss with the clinical team in detail about the compliance to the antimicrobial policy in terms of appropriateness of the antimicrobials used, dosage with renal adjustment, compliance to susceptibility report, etc. The clinical team gives justification about the non-compliance occurred, if any
❖ The prospective audit and feedback is a mutually agreed upon constructive discussion between AMS team and the clinical team on the cases with daily follow up
❖ Although the back end strategy is more labor-intensive, it has several advantages:
 ▪ It is more widely practiced
 ▪ It is more easily accepted by clinicians
 ▪ It provides a higher opportunity for educating and training health care professionals
 ▪ Impact is delayed but sustainable improving the overall quality of antimicrobial prescribing practice.

Education and Training

Similar to any other health care program, AMSP also needs continuous education, training, motivation and assessment of the health care providers. Developing antimicrobial stewardship is a behavioral change within the person. Hence, adequate motivational education is a must to bring in such change.

MONITORING THE COMPLIANCE TO AMSP

It is said that "If you cannot measure it, you cannot improve it". Measurement of the compliance to AMSP is achieved by looking at both process and outcome indicators.

1. **Policy adherence indicator** (process indicator): This is achieved by conducting antimicrobial stewardship audit as described under backward strategy. Both prescription and administrative compliance can be calculated

Indicators of Prescription Compliance

Examples of prescription compliance indicators include:
- Percentage of time the empirical antibiotic given, is according to the infective syndrome suspected
- Percentage of time the empirical antibiotic is modified according to antimicrobial susceptibility report.
- Percentage of time cultures are taken before the start of antibiotics
- Percentage of time the choice of surgical antimicrobial prophylaxis given is according to the policy

Indicators of administrative compliance

Examples of administrative compliance indicators include:
- Percentage of time the antibiotic is administrated in correct dose, correct frequency, correct route (IV, oral or infusion)
- Percentage of time the surgical antimicrobial prophylaxis is administered in correct dose, correct time and correct frequency

2. **Antimicrobial usage outcome indicators** such as defined daily dosage (DDD) and days of therapy (DOT). These indicators are used to estimate the antibiotic consumption. They are discussed below
3. **AMR outcome indicator**: The change in AMR pattern is analyzed by conducting periodic AMR surveillance
4. **Clinical outcome indicators** such as morbidity (e.g. length of stay) and mortality (e.g. infection-related deaths) indicators
5. **Financial outcome indicators** such as antimicrobial cost per patient day or per year or per admission.

DDD (Defined Daily Dosage)

Defined Daily Dose (DDD) is the average maintenance dose per day for a drug used for its main indication in adults.
- ❖ Therapeutic dose should not be used for calculating antibiotic usage because it varies between the persons depending upon the weight, disease type, associated factors such as renal adjustment, etc. Therefore, DDD is a better indicator to calculate the antimicrobial consumption
- ❖ WHO assigned DDD are available in website, which should be used while calculating the number of DDDs consumed
- ❖ DDD cannot be used for estimating antibiotic consumption in patients with renal failure and pediatric patients, because the daily dose actually prescribed is typically lower than the average dose defining the DDD.

Calculation of DDDs

No. of DDDs =

$$\frac{\text{Therapeutic dose (No. of tablets/vials used} \times \text{gm per tablet/vial)}}{\text{WHO defined DDD of the antimicrobial agent}}$$

Contd...

Contd...

Example

Levofloxacin is administered as 750 mg PO daily for 7 days. The WHO assigned DDD for levofloxacin is 0.5 g.
Therefore the number of DDD is calculated as:
= (0.75 g dose × 7 days/0.5 g DDD) = 10.5 DDDs

Days of Therapy (DOT)

DOT of an antibiotic is the number of days that patient receives at least one dose of that antibiotic. It can be used for estimating antibiotic consumption in patients with renal failure, pediatric patients and therefore is preferred over DDDs.

Examples include:
- A patient has received meropenem 1 g, twice daily for 3 days; the DOT is 3
- A patient has received meropenem 0.5 g, thrice daily for 3 days; the DOT is 3
- A patient has received meropenem 1 g, twice daily and vancomycin 1g thrice daily for 3 days; the DOT is 3+3=6

RATIONAL USE OF ANTIMICROBIAL AGENTS

When prescribing antimicrobial agents, the clinicians should consider the following advice.

Prescribe Only when Indicated

Prescribe antibiotics only when it is indicated. There are various conditions where antibiotics are not required.
- ❖ **Diarrhea:** Oral rehydration solution is the mainstay of treatment, not antibiotics. More so, the most common cause of diarrhea is of viral etiology
- ❖ **Upper respiratory tract infections** such as common cold and sore throat, where the primary cause is viral infections (except when bacterial infections such as streptococcal sore throat or diphtheria are strongly suspected)
- ❖ When an **alternative diagnosis** is suspected/confirmed such as dengue, chikungunya, malaria, etc.
- ❖ **Prophylaxis:** Routine antibiotic prophylaxis should not be given to prevent

infection, except for particular situations such as cotrimoxazole prophylaxis in HIV-infected individuals.

Culture of Cultures

Antibiotics should always be started only after site-specific specimens are collected for culture. If specimens are collected after antibiotic start, then cultures become false-negative and thus it will not help in targeted therapy.

Empirical vs Targeted Therapy

Empirical therapy: Empirical antibiotic should not be given randomly, but based on three important elements.
- The infective syndrome likely to be present
- The common etiological bacterial agents for that infective syndrome
- The local antibiogram for those organisms, indicating the antimicrobial resistance pattern.

Targeted or pathogen-directed therapy: The empirical therapy should be modified subsequently, based on antimicrobial susceptibility test (AST) report. The modifications may be of two types—escalation or de-escalation.

Escalation vs De-escalation Approach

There are two approaches by which antimicrobial agents are prescribed—escalation and de-escalation.
- The approach needs to be chosen based on local antimicrobial resistance pattern and the spectrum of activity of the antibiotic
- Antibiotics prescribed for an organism can be ranked based on their spectrum of activity and local antimicrobial resistance pattern
- For example; In hospital X, the antibiotics given for gram-negative organisms such as *E. coli* are ranked according to decreasing order of susceptibility: colistin (rank-1) → tigecycline → carbapenems → piperacillin-tazobactam → cefoperazone sulbactam → amikacin → cefepime → ceftazidime → cotrimoxazole → ceftazidime → ciprofloxacin → ceftriaxone (lowest rank).

Escalation Approach

This approach is chosen if local antimicrobial resistance pattern is unlikely and/or the patient is clinically stable. The empirical therapy is started with a narrow spectrum antibiotics (e.g. ceftriaxone for *E.coli*). If AST report shows resistance, then can be escalated to a higher rank antibiotic subsequently (e.g. meropenem for *E.coli*).

De-escalation Approach

This approach is chosen if local antimicrobial resistance pattern is expected to be high and/or patient is critically ill. Empirical therapy is started with broad spectrum antibiotics (e.g. meropenem for *E.coli*). If AST report shows susceptible, it can be de-escalated to a narrow spectrum antibiotic subsequently (e.g. ceftriaxone for *E.coli)*.

However, the reserved/restricted antimicrobials such as colistin and tigecycline should not be given as empirical therapy even under de-escalation strategy. They should be prescribed only when AST report is available and shows resistant results to all other antimicrobials tested.

Site-specific Antimicrobials

Only those antimicrobials should be prescribed which are active at the infection site. The following antimicrobials are not active at the respective sites and therefore should be excluded from treatment.
- **Lungs:** Daptomycin is not active at respiratory site as it gets inactivated by pulmonary surfactants
- **CSF:** Any oral antibiotic, 1st and second generation cephalosporins, tetracyclines, macrolides, quinolones and clindamycin are not active in CSF
- **Urine:** Antibiotics such as chloramphenicol, macrolide and clindamycin should be avoided in UTI; as they do not achieve adequate urinary concentrations.

Avoid Administration Errors

Antimicrobials must be administrated at the correct dose (as per the age/body weight), and frequency and duration of therapy.

- **Loading dose:** Certain concentration dependent antimicrobials such as aminoglycoside, vancomycin and colistin should be administered with a loading dose
- **Infusion:** The efficacy of certain antimicrobials such as vancomycin is better when mixed with saline and given as an IV infusion over 2–3 hours
- **Renal adjustment:** The dosage of the nephrotoxic drugs (such as aminoglycoside, vancomycin, and colistin) should be adjusted according to the creatinine clearance.

MIC-guided Therapy

The AST can be performed by disk diffusion or by MIC (minimum inhibitory concentration)-based method; the latter being more accurate and reliable. There are certain situations, where the antibiotic treatment is MIC-guided.
- Clinical conditions such as endocarditis, pneumococcal meningitis/pneumonia, etc.
- Vancomycin for *S. aureus*: Vancomycin should be avoided if MIC is >1 µg/mL.

Timely Stoppage of Antimicrobial

Antimicrobial agent must be stopped at appropriate time, which may be determined by clinical improvement or after obtaining negative culture or by use of biomarkers.

Biomarkers-guided Therapy

Biomarkers such as procalcitonin (PCT) or C-reactive protein (CRP) may be used for predicting bacterial infection. PCT is more reliable marker than CRP. It is raised in bacterial infections, but not in viral infections.

Misuse of Antimicrobials

The following are the common examples of misuse of antimicrobials which should be avoided.
- **Avoid overlapping spectra:** Meropenem and piperacillin–tazobactam combination therapy for double gram-negative coverage should be avoided as both these drugs belong to beta-lactam group of antimicrobials and therefore share similar antibacterial spectra
- **Redundant antibiotic:** Meropenem and metronidazole combination therapy for suspected gram-negative/ anaerobic sepsis should be avoided as meropenem is active against anaerobes in addition to gram-negative bacteria. Therefore, metronidazole can be withdrawn from therapy
- **Ineffective antibiotic:** Cloxacillin in MRSA (methicillin resistant *S. aureus*) infection is ineffective and therefore should be avoided. Vancomycin is the drug of choice for MRSA
- **Inferior antibiotic:** Vancomycin is an inferior cell wall acting agent compared to cloxacillin for MSSA (methicillin susceptible *S. aureus*) infection.

HOSPITAL ANTIBIOGRAM

An **antibiogram** is an overall profile of antimicrobial susceptibility testing results of a specific microorganism to a battery of antimicrobial agents **(Table 47.2)**. It is the responsibility of the department of Microbiology to construct a hospital antibiogram and share it with clinicians. It has the following uses.
- Antibiogram guides the clinicians in selecting the best empirical antimicrobial treatment in the event of pending culture and susceptibility results
- It is also an useful tool for detecting and monitoring trends in antimicrobial resistance within the hospital
- Antibiogram can also be used to compare susceptibility rates across institutions and track resistance trends and thereby contributing to national AMR surveillance database.

Table 47.2: Hospital antibiogram of gram-negative bacteria for the year 2020, expressed in terms of susceptibility rate.

	Ciprofloxacin	Amikacin	Ceftazidime	Piperacillin-tazobactam	Meropenem	Colistin
E. coli	25	85	55	75	82	99
Klebsiella	15	75	35	65	70	85
Pseudomonas	32	80	60	80	80	99
Acinetobacter	29	70	10	18	20	99

EXPECTED QUESTIONS

I. Write short notes on:
1. Strategies of antimicrobial stewardship program.
2. Monitoring of antimicrobial stewardship program.

II. Multiple Choice Questions (MCQs):
1. **Antimicrobial stewardship program in a hospital is required for the following reasons, *except*:**
   a. Rapid development of antimicrobial resistance
   b. Misuse and over-use of antimicrobials
   c. Widespread use of antimicrobials in humans compared to animal industry
   d. Poor antimicrobial research
2. **Who can act as antimicrobial steward?**
   a. Infectious disease physician
   b. Clinical microbiologists
   c. Medicine consultant
   d. Any of the above
3. **Which is not a Back End Strategy of Antimicrobial stewardship program?**
   a. Prospective audit and feedback is an example
   b. Formulary restriction is an example
   c. It is labor intensive than front-end strategy
   d. Sustainable than front-end strategy
4. **Maximum consumption of antibiotics occurs for:**
   a. Human therapeutic use
   b. Human non-therapeutic use
   c. Animal therapeutic use
   d. Animal non-therapeutic use

Answer
1. c   2. d   3. b   4. d

SAY NO TO HANGING MASK SYNDROME

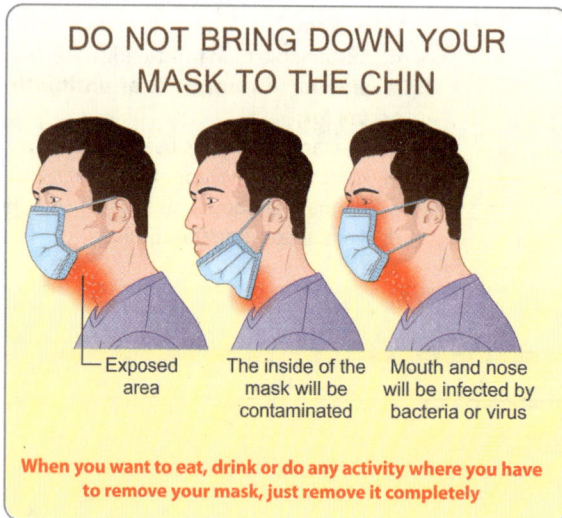

DO NOT BRING DOWN YOUR MASK TO THE CHIN

- Exposed area
- The inside of the mask will be contaminated
- Mouth and nose will be infected by bacteria or virus

When you want to eat, drink or do any activity where you have to remove your mask, just remove it completely

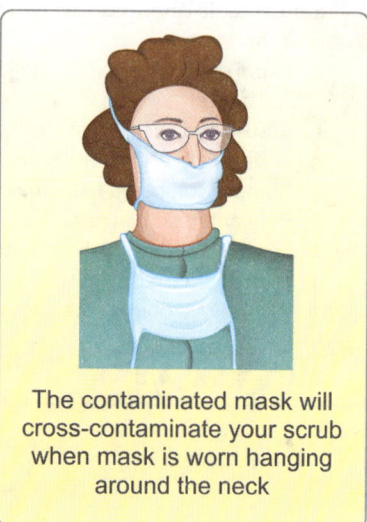

The contaminated mask will cross-contaminate your scrub when mask is worn hanging around the neck

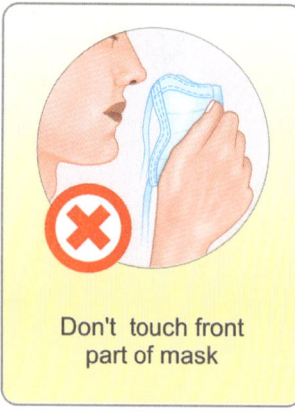

Don't touch front part of mask

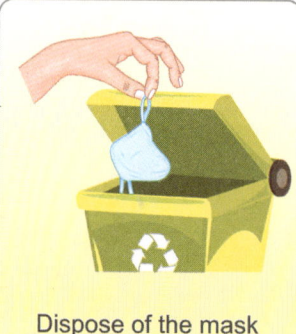

Dispose of the mask into the waste bin

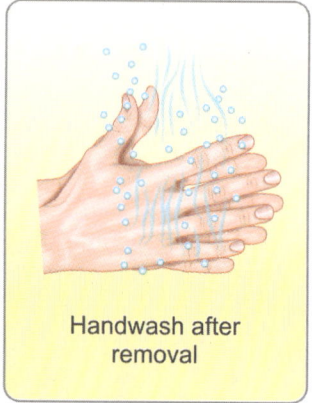

Handwash after removal

Mask is meant to protect you from infection, Do not make it as a mean to acquire infection

SECTION 8: Applied Microbiology and Miscellaneous

SECTION OUTLINE

48. Bloodstream Infections
49. Meningitis
50. Urinary Tract Infection (UTI)
51. Diarrheal Diseases
52. Respiratory Tract Infections
53. Miscellaneous Infectious Syndromes
54. Specimen Collection and Transport
55. Practical Microbiology
56. Patient Safety
57. Safety Protocol for Healthcare Personnel

Prevention of
Sexually Transmitted Infections
is in your hands

S

- Safe sex: Use Condoms

- Avoid Multiple Partners

T

- Talk to Your Partner

- Test Appropriately

- Treat Both Partners

I

- Abstinence Till Recovery

- Get Vaccinated

(e.g. HBV, HPV)

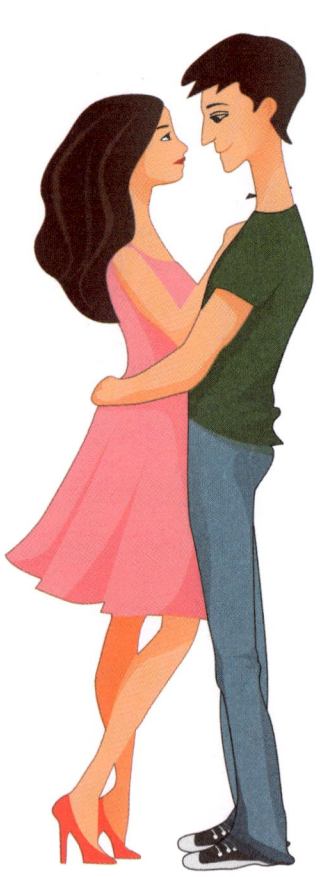

CHAPTER 48

Bloodstream Infections

CHAPTER PREVIEW

- Introduction
- Etiological Agents of BSI
- Types of Bloodstream Infections
- Clinical Manifestations
- Laboratory Diagnosis
- Fever of Unknown Origin (FUO)

INTRODUCTION

Bloodstream infections (BSI) refer to the presence of microorganisms in blood, which constitute one of the most serious situations among infectious diseases; as they are a threat to every organ in the body. Therefore, timely detection of the causative agent is one of the most important goals of the microbiology laboratory.

Terminologies

- Bacteremia refers to the presence of bacteria in blood without any multiplication
- Septicemia is a condition in which bacteria circulate and actively multiply in the bloodstream and may produce their products (e.g. toxins) that cause harm to the host
- Similarly, the presence of viruses, parasites, and fungi in the blood can be described as 'viremia', 'parasitemia', and 'fungemia' respectively.

Types of Bacteremia

Bacteremia may be transient, continuous, or intermittent.

1. **Transient bacteremia**: It may occur spontaneously or with minor events such as brushing teeth or chewing food, instrumentation of contaminated mucosal site, and surgery involving a non-sterile site. These bacteria are normally cleared from the blood by the host immune system
2. **Continuous bacteremia**: Here, the organisms are released into the bloodstream at a fairly constant rate. It occurs in conditions such as endocarditis
3. **Intermittent bacteremia**: In most other infections, bacteria are released into blood intermittently; e.g. undrained abscess (bacteria are released approximately 45 minutes before a febrile episode).

ETIOLOGICAL AGENTS OF BSI

Pathogens of all four major groups of microbes—bacteria, viruses, fungi, and parasites can cause bloodstream infections.

Bacterial Etiology

Bacterial agents account for the majority of BSIs. The common agents causing **primary BSI** include typhoidal salmonellae, brucellae, or spirochetes (*Leptospira*, *Borrelia*), HACEK group of pathogens, viridans streptococci, and Rickettsiae.

However, there are various other bacterial agents which can primarily infect other sites and subsequently spill over to the bloodstream to cause **secondary BSI**. These include:

- Gram-positive cocci—staphylococci, beta-hemolytic streptococci, enterococci, and pneumococci
- Gram-negative cocci—meningococci
- Gram-positive bacilli—*Bacillus anthracis* and *Listeria*
- Gram-negative bacilli—*E. coli, Klebsiella, Enterobacter*, non-fermenters (e.g. *Pseudomonas, Acinetobacter, Burkholderia, Stenotrophomonas*), *Haemophilus, Aeromonas*, etc.
- Anaerobes—*Bacteroides*.

Viral Etiology

Although many viruses do circulate in the peripheral blood at some stage of the disease and have a viremic phase, the primary infection usually occurs in the target organs. There are a few viruses that preferentially infect blood cells, which can be considered as **primary viral agents of BSI** such as HIV, agents of hemorrhagic fever such as dengue, chikungunya, Ebola, Marburg, Lassa, yellow fever, etc.

Parasitic Etiology

The parasites causing bloodstream infections are:
- Parasites that directly infect blood cells such as *Plasmodium* and *Babesia* infecting RBCs
- Parasites that may be found in the bloodstream before they migrate to other tissues or organs; e.g. include tachyzoites of *Toxoplasma gondii*, amastigote forms of *Leishmania*, and trypomastigote forms of *Trypanosoma*
- Parasites that may be present in the lymphatics and come to the bloodstream transiently; e.g. microfilariae of filarial parasites.

Fungal Etiology

Fungemia occurs primarily in immunosuppressed patients, patients with malignancies, patients on chemotherapy, and in those with serious or terminal illness—*Candida* species, agents of systemic mycoses (*Histoplasma, Blastomyces, Coccidioides,* and *Paracoccidioides*) and *Cryptococcus*.

As bacterial agents are the most common group to cause bloodstream infections, therefore the rest of the discussion in this chapter is largely limited to bacterial agents.

TYPES OF BLOODSTREAM INFECTIONS

There are two major categories of bloodstream infections (BSIs): Intravascular and extravascular.

Intravascular Bloodstream Infections

They originate within the cardiovascular system which includes infection of the heart (endocarditis, myocarditis, and pericarditis) and catheter-related BSI (CRBSI).

Extravascular Bloodstream Infections

Most cases of clinically significant bacteremia are of extravascular origin.
- The organisms multiply at the primary site such as the urinary tract, lungs and then invade to reach the bloodstream
- The organisms are either removed by the cells of the reticuloendothelial system or they multiply more widely and thereby causing septicemia
- **Portal of entry:** The most common portals of entry for bacteremia are the genitourinary tract (25%), followed by respiratory tract (20%), abscesses (10%), surgical site wound infections (5%), and biliary tract (5%). In up to 25% of cases, the portal of entry remains uncertain.

CLINICAL MANIFESTATIONS

Bloodstream infections have a bacteremia stage followed by a septicemic stage. The clinical manifestations are evident only in the septicemic stage. In this stage, the bacteria multiply and release their products (e.g. toxins) which travel to various organs affecting their functions. Based on the severity and the extent of organ failure; bloodstream infection can be divided into two stages: sepsis and septic shock.

- ❖ **Sepsis:** The common signs and symptoms include:
  - Fever or hypothermia with/without chills and rigors
  - Hyperventilation leads to excess loss of CO_2 and subsequent respiratory alkalosis
  - Skin lesions, change of mental status, and diarrhea.
- ❖ **Septic shock:** This is the gravest late-stage complication of septicemia and is manifested as—hypotension, multi-organ failure, etc.

In sepsis, the severity and degree of organ failure can be determined by an assessment score called SOFA (Sepsis-related Organ Failure Assessment) score or Quick SOFA criteria.

LABORATORY DIAGNOSIS

Diagnosis of bloodstream infection depends on the isolation of the causative agent from the blood by performing a blood culture.

Specimen Collection for Blood Culture

Extreme care should be taken while collecting blood for culture, as there is a high risk of contamination with skin flora.

- ❖ **Site:** Blood for culture should always be collected in pairs; from two separate venipuncture and 2 separate skin decontamination process. If a central line is present, then one sample from the central line and one from the venipuncture should be collected
- ❖ **Preparation of the site:** To avoid contamination with skin flora, blood should be collected under strict aseptic conditions using sterile disposable syringe (Fig. 48.1)
- ❖ **Skin decontamination:** Skin should be disinfected by two-step procedure—first, treated with 70% isopropyl alcohol, and then a second antiseptic solution such as povidone-iodine or chlorhexidine should be applied
  - The disinfectants should be applied in a circular motion, starting from the center to the periphery
  - The area should be allowed to air dry before venipuncture.
- ❖ **Timing of collection:** Blood should be collected before starting antimicrobial therapy. If the antimicrobial agent is already started, then the best time for collection is just before the next dose of the antimicrobial agent
- ❖ **Blood volume:** A blood specimen is drawn using a sterile syringe and needle. At least **8–10 mL** of blood per bottle for an adult and **1–3 mL** per pediatric bottle is recommended
- ❖ **Number of blood cultures:** At least 2–3 blood culture sets (each set consists of two bottles: 1 aerobic and 1 anaerobic) are required to have a good isolation rate. Multiple blood cultures should be collected for endocarditis cases

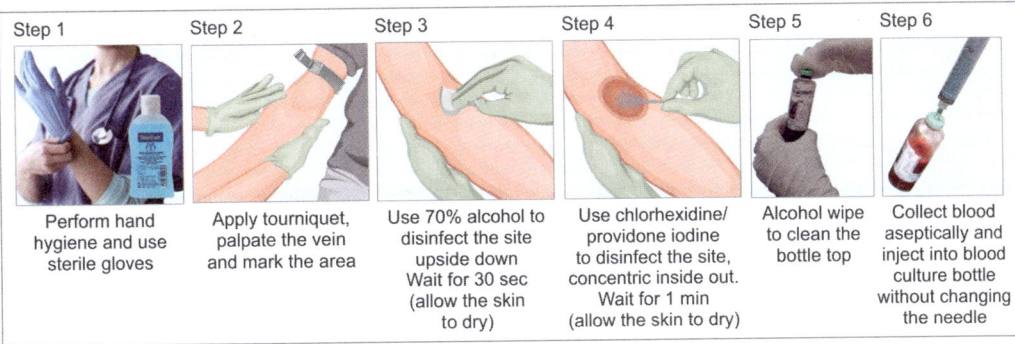

Fig. 48.1: Steps of collection of blood for culture.

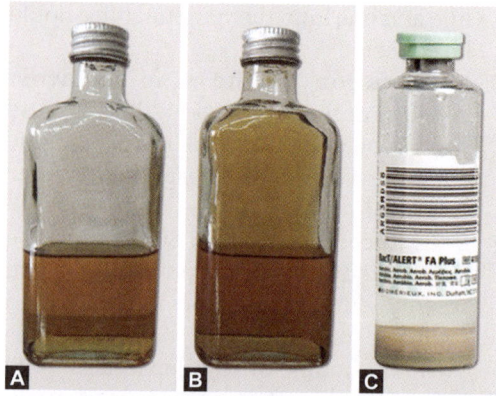

Figs. 48.2A to C: Blood culture bottles: **A.** Monophasic medium (BHI broth); **B.** Biphasic medium (Castaneda's), containing BHI broth and BHI agar slant; **C.** BacT/ALERT bottle.

Source: **A to C.** Department of Microbiology, JIPMER, Puducherry (*with permission*).

- **Dispensing:** Collected blood is then directly dispensed into a blood culture bottle at the bedside—either a conventional or automated blood culture **(Figs. 48.2A to C)**. Change of needle between collection and dispensing, an old practice is no longer recommended
- **Transport of blood specimen:** The collected blood is gently mixed with the broth and then transported immediately to the laboratory. In case of delay, the blood culture bottle **should never be refrigerated**. It can be kept at 35°C in an incubator (if available) or left at room temperature.

FEVER OF UNKNOWN ORIGIN (FUO)

Fever of unknown origin (FUO) is a very common term used by clinicians to refer to any febrile illness without an initial obvious etiology.

- Most febrile illnesses either resolve before a diagnosis can be made or eventually show typical clinical features or positive for specific investigations that lead to arriving at a correct diagnosis. This group of febrile illnesses is not called as FUO
- The term FUO is reserved only for prolonged febrile illnesses without an established etiology despite of intensive evaluation and diagnostic testing.

Definition of FUO

The definition of FUO is as follows:
- Fever ≥38.3°C (≥101°F) on at least two occasions
- Duration of illness of ≥3 weeks
- No known immunocompromised state
- The diagnosis that remains uncertain after a thorough history-taking, physical examination, and a set of laboratory investigations.

Etiology of FUO

FUO has both infectious and non-infectious etiology.
- **Infections (36%):** This accounts for the majority of FUO cases. All groups of microbial infections (both localized and systemic) can cause FUO such as mycobacterial infections, typhoid fever, rickettsial infections, etc.
- **Neoplasms (19%):** For example, lymphoma, leukemia, myeloma, renal, colon, and liver cancers, etc.
- **Non-infectious inflammatory diseases (19%):** For example, connective tissue disorders like rheumatoid arthritis, SLE (systemic lupus erythematosus), etc.
- Miscellaneous and undiagnosed causes (26%).

EXPECTED QUESTIONS

I. Write short notes on:
1. List the etiological agents of bloodstream infection.
2. List the etiological agents of FUO.
3. Write in detail about steps involved in blood collection for culture.

CHAPTER 49

Meningitis

CHAPTER PREVIEW

- Acute Bacterial Meningitis
- Acute Viral Meningitis
- Chronic Meningitis

Meningitis is a life-threatening infection of the leptomeninges (arachnoid and pia mater) surrounding the brain and spinal cord, with involvement of the subarachnoid space.

Based on the onset, meningitis can be classified into:

- ❖ **Acute meningitis:** Presents as an acute fulminant illness that progresses rapidly in a few hours. It is further divided into acute bacterial (or pyogenic) and acute viral meningitis
- ❖ **Chronic meningitis:** Progressively worsens over weeks (>4 weeks).

ACUTE BACTERIAL MENINGITIS

Acute bacterial meningitis (also called as pyogenic meningitis), is an acute purulent infection within the subarachnoid space. It is characterized by elevated polymorphonuclear cells in CSF.

The agents implicated in pyogenic meningitis may vary according to age.

- ❖ **Overall:** *Streptococcus pneumoniae* is the most common cause of pyogenic meningitis (~50%). Other agents include meningococcus (~25%), *Streptococcus agalactiae* (~15%), *Listeria* (~10%), and *Haemophilus influenzae* (<10%)
- ❖ **Neonates:** The common agents of neonatal meningitis include *Streptococcus agalactiae*, gram-negative bacilli such as *Escherichia coli* and *Klebsiella,* and *Listeria monocytogenes*
- ❖ **Elderly (>60 years):** Common agents are *Streptococcus agalactiae* and *Listeria monocytogenes.*

Pathogenesis

The bacteria that cause acute meningitis are transmitted from person-to-person through droplets of respiratory secretions from cases or nasopharyngeal carriers. Organisms may gain access to the meninges by several routes:

- ❖ **Hematogenous spread** (most common route)
- ❖ **Direct spread from an infected site** present close to meninges—e.g. otitis media, sinusitis, etc.
- ❖ **Anatomical defects in the CNS** as a result of surgery, trauma, and congenital defects, can allow organisms for ready and easy access to the CNS.

Clinical Manifestations

The average incubation period is 4 days but can range between 2 and 10 days. Patients with meningitis develop various manifestations such as:

- ❖ **Important symptoms** include fever, vomiting, intense headache, altered consciousness, etc.

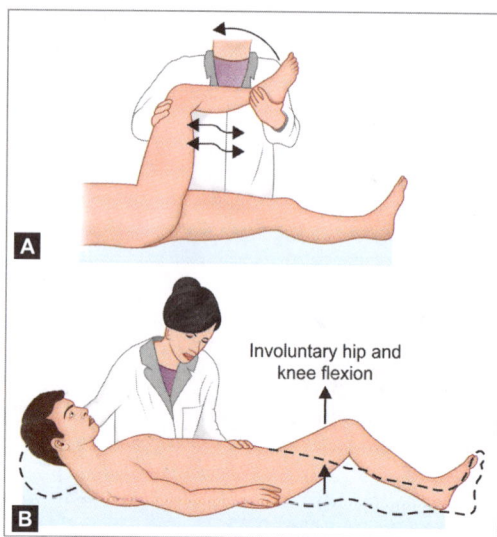

Figs. 49.1A and B: Signs seen in meningitis: **A.** Kernig's sign; **B.** Brudzinski's sign.

- **Signs of meningism** (meningeal irritation) such as:
  - *Nuchal rigidity* (stiff neck): The neck becomes stiff and resists passive flexion
  - *Kernig's sign:* Severe stiffness of the hamstrings causes an inability to straighten the leg when the hip is flexed to 90° **(Fig. 49.1A)**
  - *Brudzinski's sign:* When the neck is passively flexed, results in spontaneous flexion of the hips and knees **(Fig. 49.1B)**.
- **In infants:** Babies usually present with fever, irritability, and bulging fontanelle.

Laboratory Diagnosis

CSF is the most ideal specimen for bacterial meningitis. Blood culture is also collected in addition.

- **CSF collection:** CSF is obtained by lumbar puncture under strict aseptic conditions. It is divided into three sterile containers; one each for cell count, biochemical analysis, and bacteriological examination
- **CSF transport:** CSF being the most precious specimen should be examined immediately, and should never be refrigerated as delicate pathogens such as *H. influenzae* may die.

Cytological and Biochemical Analysis

Biochemical analysis and cell count of CSF give a preliminary clue about the type of meningitis **(Table 49.1)**.

In acute bacterial (pyogenic) meningitis:
- CSF usually contains >1,000 leukocytes/μL and predominantly neutrophils (90–95%)
- The total protein content is elevated and the glucose level is diminished or even absent
- CSF pressure is highly elevated.

CSF Microscopy (Gram Staining)

Gram staining of CSF may give a preliminary clue about the etiological agent, based on the morphology of the bacteria **(Table 49.2)**. This

Table 49.1: Cytological and biochemical parameters in CSF of normal individuals and in different types of meningitis.

Characteristics	Normal individual	Pyogenic meningitis	Tuberculous meningitis	Viral meningitis
CSF pressure (mm of water)	Normal (50–150)	Highly elevated (>180)	Moderately elevated	Slightly elevated/normal
Total leukocyte count (per mm^3)	0–5	100–10,000	10–500	25–500
Predominant cell type	Lymphocytes	Neutrophils	Lymphocytes	Lymphocytes
Glucose (mg%)	40–70	<40 mg/dL (decreased to absent)	20–40 mg/dL (slightly decreased)	Normal
Total proteins (mg%)	15–45	>45 mg/dL (usually >250; markedly increased)	100–500 mg/dL (moderate to markedly increased)	20–80 mg/dL (normal or slightly elevated)

Table 49.2: Preliminary clue about the etiological agents of pyogenic meningitis based on CSF Gram stain.

Appearance in CSF Gram stain	Suggestive of
Gram-positive diplococci, flame or lanceolate-shaped with clear halo (capsulated) (**Fig. 12.7**, Chapter 12)	Streptococcus pneumoniae
Gram-negative diplococci, capsulated, with adjacent sides flattened (lens or half-moon shaped) (**Fig. 12.9**, Chapter 12)	Neisseria meningitidis
Pleomorphic gram-negative coccobacilli, capsulated	Haemophilus influenzae
Gram-negative bacilli, arranged singly	Escherichia coli or others
Gram-positive cocci in short chain	Streptococcus agalactiae
Gram-positive short bacilli, often confused with diphtheroids	Listeria monocytogenes

helps in the early initiation of appropriate empirical antimicrobial therapy.

Direct Antigen Detection

After centrifugation of CSF, the supernatant can be used for antigen detection by latex agglutination test.
- It is available for the detection of capsular antigens of common agents of meningitis such as *S. pneumoniae, N. meningitidis, H. influenzae*, etc.
- Detection of capsular antigens in CSF is more sensitive than CSF microscopy.

Culture

Ideal media for CSF culture are chocolate agar, blood agar, and MacConkey agar.
- **Culture plates** are incubated at 37°C for 48 hours
- **Identification:** Colonies grown on solid media are processed for identification of the organism either by an automated identification system such as MALDI-TOF or VITEK or by conventional biochemical tests
- **Antimicrobial susceptibility test** should be done to initiate definitive antimicrobial therapy. It is carried out by disk diffusion test or preferably by automated MIC-based methods such as VITEK.

Molecular Methods

Molecular tests are highly sensitive and provide faster results.
- **Formats:** Multiplex PCR and multiplex real-time PCR can be used for simultaneous detection of common agents of pyogenic meningitis
- **BioFire FilmArray** is an automated nested multiplex PCR commercially available, which can detect common agents of meningitis in CSF, with a turnaround time of 1 hour.

> **TREATMENT** — **Pyogenic meningitis**
>
> The mortality of pyogenic meningitis is very high and the survivors may develop complications. Therefore, treatment should be initiated as early as possible.
> The **empirical therapy** comprises of:
> - *Adult:* IV ceftriaxone and vancomycin
> - *For neonates:* IV ampicillin plus gentamicin
> - *IV dexamethasone* is added to the regimen to reduce intra-cranial pressure.
>
> **Definitive therapy:** After the culture report is available, the empirical therapy is modified based on the organism isolated and its antimicrobial susceptibility pattern.

ACUTE VIRAL MENINGITIS

It is caused by a number of viruses, among which enteroviruses account for the majority of cases (>85%). Others include herpesviruses, arboviruses (encephalitis group), HIV, mumps virus, etc.
- The CSF is predominantly lymphocytic
- Although they usually develop meningitis in few days after the infection; many of these viruses progress slower and can also occasionally cause chronic meningitis.

CHRONIC MENINGITIS

Chronic meningitis is defined as the persistence of meningitis that exists for >4 weeks; associated with a persistent inflammatory response in CSF (white blood cell count >5/μL)

- **Etiology:** Caused by both infective etiology (Table 49.3) and non-infectious causes such as malignancy, autoimmune diseases, etc.
- **CSF findings:** In chronic meningitis, the CSF is predominantly lymphocytic.

Note: The term 'aseptic meningitis' was traditionally used to describe the agents of chronic meningitis which are not able to be grown in culture (aseptic meaning lack of infection). However, with molecular methods, it is now possible to detect most of these agents. Therefore, the term 'aseptic meningitis' is no longer correct, although in clinical practice it may still be used widely by clinicians.

Table 49.3: Agents of chronic meningitis.

Bacterial agents
- Partially treated suppurative meningitis
- *Mycobacterium tuberculosis*
- *Treponema pallidum* (tertiary syphilis)
- *Borrelia burgdorferi* (Lyme disease)

Viral agents
Agents of acute viral meningitis may also present as chronic meningitis, e.g. enteroviruses, herpesviruses, HIV, mumps, etc.

Parasitic agents: *Toxoplasma gondii*, free-living amoebae

Fungal agents: *Cryptococcus neoformans* and *Candida*

Note: Some of these agents may present as a subacute form of meningitis, that progresses over several days to <4 weeks.

 EXPECTED QUESTIONS

I. Write essays on:
1. Discuss the etiological agents, pathogenesis and clinical manifestations, and laboratory diagnosis of acute pyogenic meningitis?

II. Write short notes on:
1. Acute viral meningitis
2. Chronic meningitis.

III. Multiple Choice Questions (MCQs):
1. **Neonatal meningitis acquired through an infected birth canal is due to:**
    a. *S. pyogenes*
    b. Viridans streptococci
    c. *S. agalactiae*
    d. *S. pneumoniae*
2. **Biochemical analysis of pyogenic meningitis reveals all, *except*:**
    a. CSF pressure: highly elevated
    b. Total leukocyte count: Highly elevated, neutrophilic
    c. Glucose: highly elevated
    d. Total proteins: markedly increased
3. **All are the bacterial agents causing meningitis, *except*:**
    a. Meningococcus
    b. Cryptococcus
    c. *H. influenzae*
    d. Pneumococcus
4. **All of the following bacterial agents can cause chronic meningitis, *except*:**
    a. *Listeria monocytogenes*
    b. *Mycobacterium tuberculosis*
    c. *Borrelia burgdorferi*
    d. *Treponema pallidum*

Answers
1. c   2. c   3. b   4. a

CHAPTER 50

Urinary Tract Infection (UTI)

CHAPTER PREVIEW

- Classification
- Predisposing Factors
- Etiology and Pathogenesis
- Clinical Manifestations
- Laboratory Diagnosis
- Treatment

URINARY TRACT INFECTION

Urinary tract infection (UTI) is defined as a disease caused by microbial invasion of the urinary tract (i.e. kidney, bladder, or urethra). UTI is one of the most common infective syndrome encountered.

Classification

- UTIs may be broadly classified into two types—lower UTI and upper UTI **(Table 50.1)** depending on the anatomical sites involved
- Depending upon the source of infection, UTI can be of two types: healthcare-associated (e.g. CAUTI, Chapter 39 for detail) and community-acquired.

Table 50.1: Comparison between lower and upper UTIs.

	Lower UTI	Upper UTI
Sites involved	Urethra and bladder	Kidney and ureter
Symptoms	Local manifestations: dysuria, urgency, frequency	Local and systemic manifestations (fever, vomiting, abdominal pain)
Route of spread	Ascending route	Both ascending (common) and descending route
Occurrence	More common	Less common

Predisposing Factors

There are a number of factors that predispose to the pathogenesis of UTI.

- **Gender:** UTI more commonly affects females, which is due to—(i) short urethra, and (ii) close proximity of urethral meatus to anus; so that there is more chance of migration of bacteria present in perineum into the urinary tract
- **Age:** For females, the incidence of UTI increases with age (10–20% incidence in adult life). Whereas males have a higher risk during infancy and in old age (due to prostate enlargement)
- **Pregnancy:** Anatomical and hormonal changes in pregnancy favor the development of UTIs. Most pregnant women develop asymptomatic bacteriuria
- **Structural and functional abnormality** of the urinary tract may obstruct the urine flow, which can lead to urinary stasis; which predisposes to infection
  - *Structural obstruction:* Renal and ureteric stones, prostate enlargement, etc.
  - *Functional obstruction:* Neurogenic bladder due to spinal cord injury.
- **Catheter:** The presence of an indwelling urinary catheter is the single most important risk factor to develop UTI in hospitalized patients

❖ **Bacterial virulence** such as the expression of pili helps in bacterial adhesion to uroepithelium.

Etiology

Escherichia coli (uropathogenic *E. coli*) is by far the most common cause of UTIs, accounting for 70% of total cases.
❖ The endogenous flora such as *E. coli*, *Klebsiella*, *Proteus* and enterococci are the important agents
❖ In healthcare-associated UTIs, in addition to the above agents, multidrug-resistant *Pseudomonas*, and *Acinetobacter* can also cause UTI.
❖ In general, viruses, parasites and fungi infrequently infect the urinary tract.

Bacterial pathogens are the major cause of UTI; their pathogenesis, clinical features, laboratory diagnosis and treatment have been discussed in detail in this chapter.

Refer **Table 50.2** for the list of common microorganisms causing UTIs.

Table 50.2: Common microorganisms causing UTIs.

Bacterial agents	Other agents
Gram-negative bacilli: Enterobacteriaceae • *Escherichia coli*: Most common (70%) • *Klebsiella pneumoniae* • *Enterobacter* species • *Proteus* species • *Serratia* species **Non-fermenters** • *Pseudomonas aeruginosa* • *Acinetobacter* species	**Fungus:** *Candida albicans* **Parasites:** • *Schistosoma haematobium* • *Trichomonas vaginalis* • *Dioctophyme renale*
Gram-positive cocci: • *Enterococcus* species • *Staphylococcus saprophyticus** • *Staphylococcus aureus* • *Staphylococcus epidermidis* • *Streptococcus agalactiae*	**Viruses:** • BK virus • Adenovirus types–11 and 21

Abbreviation: UTI, Urinary tract infection.
*Common in sexually active females.

Pathogenesis

Bacteria invade the urinary tract mainly by two routes—ascending and descending routes **(Fig. 50.1)**.

Ascending Route

It is the most common route; the enteric endogenous bacteria enter the urinary tract which is facilitated by sexual intercourse, catheterization, etc.
❖ **Colonization:** Adhesion to the urethral epithelium is the first and the most important step in pathogenesis. A number of virulence factors (e.g. fimbriae) help in adhesion
❖ **Ascension:** Following colonization, the pathogen ascends through the urethra upwards towards the bladder to cause cystitis
❖ **Further ascension** through the ureter may occasionally occur if there is vesicoureteral reflux leading to pyelonephritis (infection of renal parenchyma)
❖ **Acute tubular injury:** If the inflammatory cascade continues, tubular obstruction and damage occurs which may lead to interstitial nephritis.

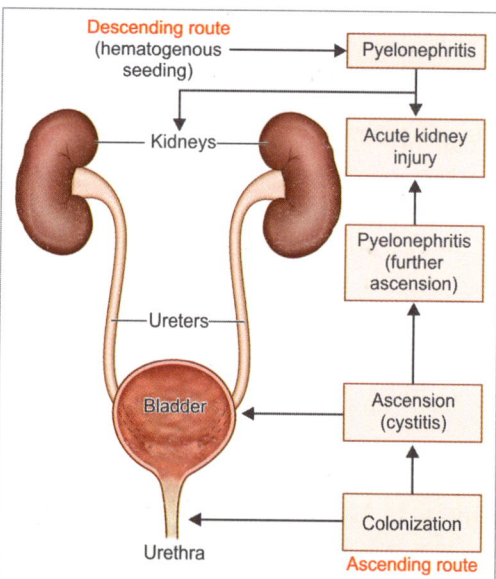

Fig. 50.1: Pathogenesis of urinary tract infection.

Descending Route

This refers to the invasion of organisms to renal parenchyma from other organs through the hematogenous route, causing pyelonephritis. This accounts for 5% of total UTIs. Common agents include—*S. aureus*, *Salmonella*, *M. tuberculosis*, and *Leptospira*.

Clinical Manifestations

UTIs may be presented in various forms:
- **Lower UTI:** Asymptomatic bacteriuria, cystitis, urethritis, acute urethral syndrome
- **Upper UTI:** Pyelonephritis.

Lower UTI

Asymptomatic Bacteriuria

It refers to the isolation of a significant count of bacteria in an appropriately collected urine specimen, obtained from a person without symptoms of UTI. It is more common in females and its incidence increases with age.
- **Asymptomatic UTI** is clinically significant in a certain group of people such as pregnant women (as chances of complication in mother and fetus are more), people undergoing prostatic surgery, or any urologic procedure where bleeding is anticipated. Therefore, in this group, routine screening and treatment for asymptomatic UTI is highly recommended
- In contrast, **asymptomatic UTI** is not clinically significant in non-pregnant, pre-menopausal women, old age, catheterized patients, or patients with spinal injury. In such cases, neither screening nor treatment of asymptomatic UTI is needed.

Cystitis (Infection of the Bladder)

It is characterized by localized symptoms such as:
- Dysuria (pain while micturition), frequency, urgency, and suprapubic tenderness (over the bladder area)
- Urine becomes cloudy, with a bad odor, and in some cases grossly bloody (hematuria)
- There is no associated systemic manifestation.

Acute Urethral Syndrome

This is another form of lower UTI seen in young sexually active females, characterized by:
- Presence of classical symptoms of lower UTI as described for cystitis
- Bacterial count is often low (10^2 to 10^5 CFU/mL)
- Pyuria (pus in urine) is present
- **Agents:** Mostly due to the usual agents of UTI, a few cases may be caused by gonococcus, *Chlamydia*, herpes simplex virus, etc.

Upper UTI (Pyelonephritis)

Pyelonephritis refers to inflammation of kidney parenchyma, calyces, and the renal pelvis, i.e. the part of the ureter present inside the kidney **(Fig. 50.1)**.
- Associated with systemic manifestations such as—fever, flank pain, vomiting **(Table 50.1)**
- Lower urinary tract symptoms such as frequency, urgency, and dysuria may also be present.

Laboratory Diagnosis

Specimen Collection

Urine should be collected in a wide mouth screw-capped sterile container by various methods.
- **Clean-voided midstream urine:** It is the most common specimen for UTI; collected after properly cleaning the urethral meatus or glans
- **Suprapubic aspiration** of urine from the bladder: It is the most ideal specimen. It is recommended for patients in coma or infants
- **In catheterized patients,** urine should be collected from the catheter tube (after clamping distally and disinfecting); but not from the urobag.

Transport

The urine sample should be processed immediately. If a delay is expected for more than 1–2 hours, then it can be stored in the refrigerator.

Direct Examination

The screening tests done are as follows:
- **Wet mount examination:** It is done to demonstrate the pus cells in urine. Pyuria of >8 pus cells/mm³ is taken as significant
- **Leukocyte esterase test:** It is a rapid and cheaper method that detects leukocyte esterases secreted by pus cells present in urine.

Culture

- ❖ **Culture media:** Urine sample should be inoculated onto CLED agar (cysteine lactose electrolyte deficient agar) or a combination of MacConkey agar and blood agar. CLED agar is preferred in laboratories with higher sample load
- ❖ **Kass concept of significant bacteriuria:** This is based on the fact that, though the normal urine is sterile it may get contaminated during voiding, with normal urethral flora. However, the bacterial count in contaminated urine would be lower than that caused by an infection

> **Significant bacteriuria**
> - A count of $\geq 10^5$ **colony forming units (CFU)/mL** of urine is considered as significant—indicates infection (referred to as 'significant bacteriuria')
> - **Count between 10^4 to 10^5 CFU/mL** indicates doubtful significance; should be clinically correlated
> - **Low count of $<10^4$** CFU/mL is due to the presence of commensal bacteria (due to contamination during voiding) and is of no significance. However, low counts can be significant in the following conditions:
>   ➢ Patient on antibiotic treatment
>   ➢ Pyelonephritis and acute urethral syndrome
>   ➢ Sample taken by suprapubic aspiration.

- ❖ **Quantitative culture:** This is done to count the number of colonies. Each colony on the plate corresponds to one bacterium in the urine sample. Quantitation is done by:
  - A semi-quantitative method such as a standardized loop technique
  - A quantitative method such as the pour plate method.
- ❖ **Colony appearance:** It depends upon the organism grown. For example, lactose fermenters such as *E. coli* and *Klebsiella* produce pink colonies on MacConkey agar and yellow colonies on CLED agar; whereas non-lactose fermenters such as *Proteus, Pseudomonas* and *Acinetobacter* produce pale colonies
- ❖ **Identification:** The colonies grown are identified either by conventional biochemical tests or automated identification systems such as MALDI-TOF or VITEK
- ❖ **AST:** Antimicrobial susceptibility test is essential to guide the appropriate treatment. It is performed conventionally by disk diffusion test (on Mueller-Hinton agar) or by automated MIC-based methods such as VITEK.

TREATMENT Urinary tract infections

Treatment should be based on the AST report. Quinolones (e.g. norfloxacin), nitrofurantoin, cephalosporins, and aminoglycosides are among the preferred drugs.

Higher antibiotics such as carbapenem (e.g. meropenem), β-lactam/β-lactamase inhibitor combinations (e.g. piperacillin-tazobactam), or fosfomycin are used for the treatment of healthcare-associated UTIs caused by multidrug-resistant gram-negative bacilli.

EXPECTED QUESTIONS

I. **Write an essay on:**
   1. Discuss the etiological agents, pathogenesis, clinical manifestations, and laboratory diagnosis of UTI.

II. **Write short notes on:**
   1. Significant bacteriuria.
   2. Asymptomatic bacteriuria.

III. **Multiple Choice Questions (MCQs):**
   1. Which culture medium is preferred for processing of urine specimens?
      a. TCBS agar   b. CLED agar
      c. Chocolate agar d. XLD agar
   2. Which of the following is the most common etiological agent of UTI?
      a. *Escherichia coli*   b. *Klebsiella*
      c. *Proteus*   d. *Enterobacter*

Answers
1. b   2. a

CHAPTER 51: Diarrheal Diseases

CHAPTER PREVIEW
- Types of Diarrheal Diseases
- Pathogenesis
- Laboratory Diagnosis

DIARRHEAL DISEASES

The diarrheal diseases are one of the leading cause of illness globally; cause significant morbidity and mortality. It is more common in developing countries, where young children get diarrhea on an average three times a year.

There are various clinical types of diarrheal diseases; caused by a wide variety of infectious agents including bacteria, viruses, and parasites **(Table 51.1)**.

Diarrhea

Diarrhea is defined as passage of three or more loose or liquid stools per day, in excess than the usual habit for that person.

❖ Acute diarrhea usually lasts for <14 days; most often caused by viral agents, followed by bacterial or parasitic agents

Table 51.1: Infectious agents of acute diarrhea and the underlying mechanism.

Mechanism	Examples of pathogens involved	

Non-inflammatory	**Bacteria** (mostly enterotoxin mediated):
	• *Vibrio cholerae*
	• Diarrheagenic *Escherichia coli*:
	  ➢ Enteropathogenic *E. coli*
	  ➢ Enterotoxigenic *E. coli*
	  ➢ Enteroaggregative *E. coli*
	• *Clostridium perfringens*
	• *Bacillus cereus*
	• *Staphylococcus aureus*
	Viruses: Rotavirus, norovirus, adenoviruses—40, 41, caliciviruses and astrovirus
		Parasites (protozoa):
		• *Giardia duodenalis*
		• *Cryptosporidium parvum*
		• *Cyclospora cayetanensis*
		• *Cystoisospora belli*
		Parasites (helminths):
		• *Ascaris*, hookworm
		• *Strongyloides*, *Trichinella*
		• *Taenia saginata*, *T. solium*
		• *Hymenolepis nana*
		• *Fasciolopsis buski*

Inflammatory	**Predominantly dysentery:**
	• *Shigella* species
	• *Campylobacter jejuni*
	• Diarrheagenic *Escherichia coli*:
	  ➢ Enterohemorrhagic *E. coli*
	  ➢ Enteroinvasive *E. coli*
	• *Vibrio parahaemolyticus*
	Predominantly inflammatory diarrhea:
	• Non-typhoidal salmonellae
	• *Yersinia enterocolitica*
		Parasite (predominantly dysentery):
		• *Entamoeba histolytica*
		• *Balantidium coli*
		• *Trichuris trichiura*
		• *Schistosoma mansoni*
		• *Schistosoma japonicum*

Penetrating	*Salmonella typhi* (enteric fever)	

❖ Common microbial agents causing diarrhea and the mechanisms involved are summarized in **Table 51.1**.

Dysentery

Dysentery is characterized by diarrhea with increased blood and mucus, often associated with fever, abdominal pain, and tenesmus (feeling of constant need to pass stools, despite an empty colon) **(Table 51.1)**.

Traveler's Diarrhea

Traveler's diarrhea is the most common travel-related infectious illness.
 ❖ **Epidemiology:** Occurs in about 20–50% of people traveling from temperate industrialized countries to tropical regions of Asia, Africa, etc.
 ❖ **Microbial agents:** Overall, enterotoxigenic *Escherichia coli* is the most common agent, followed by enteroaggregative *E. coli*, *Campylobacter* and *Shigella*
 ❖ **Clinical presentation:** Most cases begin within the first 3–5 days; characterized by a sudden onset of abdominal cramps, anorexia, and watery diarrhea.

Persistent and Chronic Diarrhea

Diarrhea that lasts for ≥14 days (usually 2–4 weeks) is considered persistent. Chronic diarrhea usually lasts for >4 weeks. May result from infections due to various organisms.
 ❖ Parasites such as *Cryptosporidium*, *Cyclospora*, *Entamoeba histolytica*, *Giardia*
 ❖ Bacteria: *Campylobacter*, *Clostridioides difficile*.

Gastroenteritis

Gastroenteritis or infectious diarrhea may be defined as inflammation of the mucous membrane of the stomach and intestine resulting in combination of diarrhea, vomiting and pain abdomen with or without mucus or blood in stool, fever or dehydration.

Food Poisoning

Food poisoning refers to an illness acquired through consumption of food or drink contaminated either with microorganisms, or their toxins. The agents of food poisoning have different incubation periods.

> **Microbial agents of food poisoning**
> **1–6 h incubation period:** Food contaminated with preformed toxins, which directly act following intake:
> - *Staphylococcus aureus* (enterotoxin)
> - *Bacillus cereus* (emetic toxin)
>
> **8–16 h incubation period:** Food contaminated with organisms which release toxin in the intestine:
> - *Clostridium perfringens*
> - *Bacillus cereus* (diarrheal toxin)
>
> **>16 h incubation period:** Food contaminated with organisms which release toxin in the intestine or by other mechanisms:
> - *Vibrio cholerae*
> - Enterotoxigenic *E. coli*
> - Enterohemorrhagic *E. coli*
> - Non-typhoidal salmonellae and *Shigella* species

Pathogenic Mechanisms of Diarrhea

Enteric pathogens have developed a variety of strategies to overcome host defenses.

Inoculum Size

Enteric pathogens differ from each other in their infective dose to initiate the infection. For example:
 ❖ *Shigella*: 10–100 bacilli
 ❖ *Vibrio cholerae*: 10^5–10^8 bacilli
 ❖ *Salmonella*: 10^3–10^5 bacilli.

Adherence

Adherence to intestinal mucosa helps the organism to compete with the normal bowel flora and there by colonizing the intestinal mucosa.

Toxin Production

Enteric organisms can produce variety of toxins, which are implicated in pathogenesis of diarrhea. These include:
 ❖ *Vibrio cholerae:* Cholera toxin
 ❖ *Diarrheagenic E. coli:* Heat labile, heat stable and verocytotoxin
 ❖ *Shigella:* Shiga toxin, enterotoxin

- *Clostridioides difficile:* Toxin A and B
- Neurotoxins: *S. aureus* enterotoxin, *Bacillus cereus* toxin, *Clostridium botulinum* toxin.

Invasion

In addition to production of toxins, bacterial invasion is another mechanism by which destruction of intestinal mucosal cells takes place resulting in dysentery.

Predisposing Factors

Alterations of the host defense mechanisms can promote the diarrheal diseases.
- **Suppression of the normal flora:** Leads to loss of protective effect of intestinal normal flora
- **Neutralization of gastric acidity:** Promote the acid labile pathogens (e.g. *V. cholerae*)
- **Inhibition of intestinal motility:** Interfere with the clearance of bacteria from the small intestine
- **Age:** Children (<5 years) are more likely to contract most of the diarrheal diseases (e.g. rotavirus) than adults
- **Location:** Closed and semi-closed communities, including day-care centers, schools, residential facilities, and cruise ships are among the important settings for outbreaks of diarrheal diseases
- **Antibiotic-associated:** Patients on prolonged antibiotic course are more likely to develop *C. difficile* infection leading to diarrhea (Chapter 14)
- **Impaired host immunity:** Immunocompromised hosts (e.g. AIDS) are at a higher risk of developing diarrhea.

Laboratory Diagnosis of Diarrheal Diseases

Specimen Collection

Fecal specimen (containing mucus flakes) is collected in a sterile screw capped wide mouthed container. In carriers, a rectal swab may be collected.
- Specimens should be transported to the laboratory within 1 hour
- If a delay of longer than 1 hour is anticipated, the fecal specimen should be collected in transport media like Cary-Blair medium, or alkaline peptone water (if cholera is suspected).

Macroscopy

The following macroscopic appearances are noted:
- Color of the specimen
- Consistency—formed, semi-formed or liquid
- Presence of blood (suggestive of dysentery), mucus or pus (suggestive of inflammatory diarrhea)
- Presence of adult parasitic forms, e.g. *Enterobius*, *Ascaris*, or *Taenia* segments.

Microscopy

- **Wet mount preparation** in saline or iodine is done for detection of pus cells, RBCs and detection of parasitic cysts, trophozoites, eggs or larvae
- **Hanging drop preparation:** To demonstrate darting motility of *Vibrio cholerae*
- **Gram-stained smear:** Not routinely done because of presence of normal flora
- **Modified acid-fast staining** can be carried out for the detection of oocysts of *Cryptosporidium*, *Cyclospora* and *Cystoisospora*
- **Electron microscopy** of stool specimen: For the detection of viruses, e.g. rotavirus, astrovirus, etc.

Bacterial Culture

- **Culture media:** Fecal specimen should be inoculated onto the following media:
  - *Enrichment broth:* Selenite F broth and alkaline peptone water
  - *Selective medium:* MacConkey agar, DCA (deoxycholate citrate agar), XLD (xylose lysine deoxycholate) agar and TCBS (thiosulfate citrate bile salt sucrose) agar.
- **Identification** of the enteric pathogens is made by performing either conventional biochemical tests or automated identification systems. Then serotyping is performed with specific group or type specific antisera

❖ **Antimicrobial susceptibility test:** It is done to choose appropriate drug for treatment.

Tissue Culture

This is carried out for the detection of enteric viruses and also for some diarrheagenic *E. coli*.

Antigen Detection

Various test formats are available to detect microbial antigens in stool.
❖ ELISA is available for detection of rotavirus antigen in stool
❖ Immunochromatographic test (e.g. **triage parasite panel**) is available for simultaneous detection of *E. histolytica*, *Giardia* and *Cryptosporidium* in stool
❖ Rapid test is available to detect *C. difficile* antigens (glutamate dehydrogenase and toxin A/B) in stool.

TREATMENT — Diarrhea

Treatment depends up on the severity.
- Fluid therapy is the main stay of treatment
- Anti-motility agents and adsorbents may be considered in moderate-to-severe diarrhea
- Antibiotic therapy is required only for severe diarrhea:
  ➢ Ciprofloxacin or levofloxacin
  ➢ Azithromycin for *Campylobacter*
  ➢ Metronidazole or vancomycin (for *C. difficile*).

EXPECTED QUESTIONS

I. Write essay on:
1. Discuss the etiological agents, pathogenesis, clinical manifestations and laboratory diagnosis of diarrhea.

II. Write short notes on:
1. Dysentery
2. Traveler's diarrhea
3. Food poisoning

III. Multiple Choice Questions (MCQs):
1. Which is most common cause of Traveler's diarrhea?
   a. *Shigella*   b. ETEC
   c. *V. cholerae*   d. EHEC

2. Which of the following is the most common etiological agent of acute diarrhea?
   a. Rotavirus
   b. *Shigella*
   c. *V. cholerae*
   d. *Salmonella*

3. All of the following are predisposing factors for developing diarrhea, *except*:
   a. Suppression of the normal flora
   b. Neutralization of gastric acidity
   c. Inhibition of intestinal motility
   d. Common in adults

Answers
1. b   2. a   3. d

CHAPTER 52: Respiratory Tract Infections

CHAPTER PREVIEW
- Upper Respiratory Tract Infections
- Lower Respiratory Tract Infections

INTRODUCTION

The respiratory tract is divided into two segments, the upper and the lower respiratory tract.
- The upper respiratory tract (URT) includes the nasal cavity, paranasal sinuses, pharynx (throat), epiglottis, and larynx
- The lower respiratory tract (LRT) comprises of trachea, and bronchi, which are divided into bronchioles and lungs, with the surrounding pleura.

Defense Mechanisms of Respiratory Tract

The respiratory tract provides several defense mechanisms which prevent the entry of respiratory pathogens:
- **Normal respiratory flora** compete with the pathogens and prevent their colonization in the pharynx
- **Mucociliary clearance:** Cilia and mucus lining of the trachea helps in clearing the pathogens
- **Nasal cavity:** Nasal hairs, convoluted passages, etc.
- **Secretory products**: Secretory IgA and lysozyme, etc. in respiratory secretion
- **Tracheobronchial tree:** The branching architecture traps particles on the airway lining.

UPPER RESPIRATORY TRACT INFECTIONS

The various URT infections (URTI) are pharyngitis and tonsillitis, laryngitis, acute laryngotracheobronchitis (croup), epiglottitis, parapharyngeal infections, infections of the nasal cavity and sinuses.

Pharyngitis and Tonsillitis

Pharyngitis (or sore throat) refers to the inflammation of the pharynx. It commonly affects children, where it presents along with tonsillitis (inflamed tonsils) **(Figs. 52.1A and B)**.
- **Agents:** Viral agents are the most common cause, followed by bacterial agents

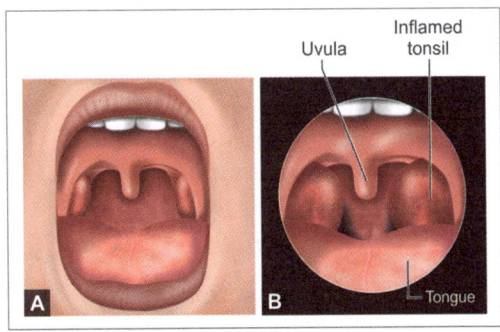

Figs. 52.1A and B: A. Healthy throat; **B.** Sore throat, showing inflamed pharynx with enlarged and inflamed tonsils and uvula.

- Viral agents: Influenza, parainfluenza viruses, coronaviruses (e.g. COVID-19), adenoviruses, etc.
- Bacterial agents: *Streptococcus pyogenes, Corynebacterium diphtheriae*, etc.

❖ **Clinical manifestations** include throat pain, difficulty in swallowing, erythematous (red) and swollen pharynx/tonsil, inflammatory exudate over the pharynx, and rarely membrane over the tonsils (e.g. diphtheria).

Laryngitis

Laryngitis (inflammation of the larynx) has an abrupt onset and is usually self-limited.
- ❖ **Clinical manifestations:** The patient presents with hoarseness and lowering or deepening of the voice
- ❖ **Agents:** Viruses like influenza and parainfluenza viruses, adenoviruses, coronaviruses, etc.

Acute Laryngotracheobronchitis (Croup)

Croup is a potentially more serious disease as the infection extends downward from the larynx to involve the trachea or even the bronchi.
- ❖ **Agent:** Parainfluenza viruses are the most common cause of croup
- ❖ **Manifestation:** Illness is characterized by fever, inspiratory stridor, hoarseness, and dry cough.

Epiglottitis

Epiglottitis is an infection of the epiglottis and other soft tissues above the vocal cords. It can lead to significant edema and inflammation, causing respiratory obstruction.
- ❖ **Agents:** *Haemophilus influenzae* type b is the primary cause of epiglottitis
- ❖ **Age:** Children are commonly infected.

Parapharyngeal Infections

- ❖ **Peritonsillar abscess (or quinsy):** It is a deep neck infection that occurs as a complication of tonsillitis. It usually affects children. The common organisms implicated are *S. pyogenes, S. aureus*, etc.
- ❖ **Ludwig's angina:** It is a form of diffuse cellulitis of the mandibular space on the floor of the mouth
  - *Source:* This infection most commonly arises from an adjacent dental infection
  - *Etiology:* Often polymicrobial and anaerobic
  - *Manifestations:* It is aggressive, rapidly spreading cellulitis, without lymphadenopathy, with potential for airway obstruction.

Infections of Nasal Cavity and Sinuses

- ❖ **Rhinitis (or common cold)** is an inflammation of the nasal mucous membrane. It clinically presents as a running nose, sneezing, watery eyes, etc. Rhinoviruses are the most common cause
- ❖ **Atrophic rhinitis:** It is caused by *Klebsiella ozaenae*, characterized by chronic foul-smelling mucopurulent nasal discharge; affecting elderly people
- ❖ **Rhinoscleroma:** It is chronic, granulomatous hypertrophy of the nose, caused by *Klebsiella rhinoscleromatis*
- ❖ **Sinusitis** (i.e. inflammation of the paranasal sinuses):
  - *Agents:* The common agents are *S. pneumoniae, H. influenzae,* and *Moraxella catarrhalis*. Viral and fungal sinusitis is rare
  - *Clinical features:* Presents with facial pressure, frontal headache, loss of smell, nasal congestion, and postnasal drip
  - *Diagnosis* is often made clinically, in adjunction with radiological features.

Laboratory Diagnosis of URTI

Specimen Collection and Transport

- ❖ **A throat swab** (oropharyngeal swab) containing fibrous exudates is the ideal specimen for pharyngitis. It should be collected by vigorous rubbing of a sterile swab over the posterior pharynx and both the tonsillar pillars. Two swabs may be collected, one for direct smear and the other for culture

- **Specimens** other than throat swabs include:
  - In suspected diphtheria, a portion of the pseudomembrane may be obtained
  - The nasopharyngeal swab is preferred for *B. pertussis* or viruses like influenza or coronavirus. It is collected by inserting a flexible swab through the nose into the posterior nasopharynx and then rotating for 5 seconds.
- **Types of swabs:** Dacron or Rayon swabs are suitable for collecting most URT microorganisms. Flocked swabs are preferable. Cotton swabs can be used for *S. pyogenes*, but are not suitable for viruses
- **Transport:** For isolation of most URT bacterial pathogens, swabs should be processed within 4 hours. However, for molecular diagnosis (bacteria or viruses), the specimens can be stored at 4°C and can be processed late.

Diagnostic Methods

- **Direct smear:** Gram staining is not useful for most of the URTI. Albert stain may be performed when diphtheria is suspected
- **Culture:** Specimens may be inoculated onto blood agar and chocolate agar
- **Molecular methods** such as real-time PCR is the gold standard method for the detection of respiratory viruses such as influenza or coronaviruses and others
- **Antigen detection tests** may be useful for the detection of certain URT pathogens such as SARS CoV-2 from nasopharyngeal swabs.

ORAL CAVITY INFECTIONS

Common infections of the oral cavity include:
- **Stomatitis:** It is an inflammation of the mucous membranes of the oral cavity. It is caused by the herpes simplex virus (HSV); characterized by multiple painful tiny vesicular lesions on the oral mucosa and in the oropharynx
- **Oral thrush:** It is characterized by whitish patches of exudate on the buccal mucosa. It is caused by *Candida* spp., especially in HIV-infected individuals
- **Dental infections**: Common infections include: root canal infections, dental abscesses, periodontal abscesses, etc. These infections are most commonly caused by anaerobic bacteria and viridans streptococci present in the oral cavity
- **Salivary gland infections** such as parotitis (inflammation is most often caused by mumps) and bacteria (acute suppurative parotitis, due to *Staphylococcus aureus*)
- **Vincent's angina:** It is an acute necrotizing ulcerative gingivitis, caused by *Borrelia vincentii* and an anaerobe *Fusobacterium fusiformis*. They are found as normal flora in the mouth.

LOWER RESPIRATORY TRACT INFECTIONS

Various lower respiratory tract infections (LRTI) include the infections affecting the bronchus, bronchioles, lungs, and pleura.
- **Bronchitis and bronchiolitis:** Refer to inflammation of the bronchial tree and bronchioles respectively:
  - Most commonly caused by respiratory viruses such as a respiratory syncytial virus (RSV), influenza, and coronavirus and rarely by bacterial agents like *Mycoplasma pneumoniae*
  - Characterized by respiratory distress with expiratory wheeze, tachypnea, nasal flaring, retractions, and irritability.
- **Whooping cough:** Caused by *Bordetella pertussis*, characterized by paroxysmal cough—repetitive violent spasmodic coughs, within a single expiration which ends with an audible sound or whoop
- **Pneumonia:** Refers to inflammation of lungs, i.e. either alveoli or interstitium space (discussed below)
- **Tuberculosis:** Caused by *Mycobacterium tuberculosis* (discussed in Chapter 15)
- **Fungal lung disease:** It is most often caused by *Pneumocystis jirovecii* and agents causing systemic mycoses like *Histoplasma*
- **Parasitic lung disease:** Agents include *Paragonimus westermani* or larvae of nematodes like *Ascaris*

- **Lung abscess:** Abscess formation in the lung parenchyma, either primary (due to anaerobic bacteria) or secondary to low immunity
- **Pleural effusion:** Presence of an excess quantity of fluid in the pleural space. It could be due to secondary to bacterial pneumonia or tuberculous pleuritic or viral pleural effusion. When fluid collection in the pleural cavity is pyogenic in nature, called as empyema.

Pneumonia

Pneumonia refers to inflammation of the lungs. Based on the area of lungs involved, and the type of cough produced, pneumonia is traditionally classified into two groups.

- **Lobar or typical pneumonia:** It involves infection of the lung parenchyma and its alveoli. It is characterized by consolidation (gives a dull note on percussion) and productive cough with purulent sputum. It is mostly caused by pyogenic organisms such as:
    - *Streptococcus pneumoniae*
    - *Haemophilus influenzae*
    - *Staphylococcus aureus*
    - Gram-negative bacilli such as *E. coli, Klebsiella, Pseudomonas, Acinetobacter,* etc.
- **Interstitial or atypical pneumonia** occurs in the interstitial space of the lungs. Cough is characteristically non-productive. It is caused by:
    - Bacteria such as *Mycoplasma, Chlamydia, Legionella* species, etc.
    - Viruses such as influenza, coronaviruses (including COVID-19), respiratory syncytial virus, parainfluenza, adenoviruses, etc.
    - Fungal agents causing pneumonia.

In lieu of epidemiological point of view, pneumonia can also be classified into:

Community-acquired: Patients acquire the infection in the community.
- Pneumococcus followed by *Mycoplasma pneumoniae* are the most common agents
- Others: *H. influenzae, Chlamydia pneumoniae,* and viral pneumonia.

Healthcare-associated: Patients acquire the infection in the hospital setting.
- This is more frequently observed in patients on mechanical ventilation, called as **ventilator-associated pneumonia (VAP)**
- It is most often caused by the **multidrug-resistant** pathogens found in the hospital environment such as *Pseudomonas, Acinetobacter, Escherichia coli, Klebsiella pneumoniae, and* MRSA (methicillin-resistant *S. aureus*).

Clinical Features

Common clinical features of pneumonia include:
- Fever, with chills and/or sweats, tachycardia
- Increased respiratory rate (tachypnea), with increased use of accessory muscles of respiration
- Dyspnea (shortness of breath)
- If the pleura is involved, the patient may experience pleuritic chest pain
- Cough: Productive cough in lobar and dry cough in atypical pneumonia.

Pathogenesis

Pathogenesis of pneumonia involves the following steps:
- Organisms gain access to the lower respiratory tract:
    - By aspiration from the oropharynx (most common): It occurs frequently during sleep (in the elderly), or when consciousness is lowered or in ventilated patients
    - Inhalation of pathogens through infected droplets
    - Via hematogenous spread
    - Spread from pleural or mediastinal space.
- Organisms escape the defense mechanisms of the host's respiratory tract
- Inability of the host immune response to clear the pathogen. Organisms in the lungs are normally phagocytosed by the alveolar macrophages.

Laboratory Diagnosis of LRTI

Specimen Collection

Important specimens for LRTI include sputum, induced sputum, tracheal aspirate, bronchoalveolar lavage (BAL), protected specimen brush (PSB), lung aspirate, and pleural fluid.

Microscopy

- **Gram staining** of the sputum specimens is done to determine the specimen quality (pus cells are >25 and epithelial cells are <10 per low power field) and also to detect organisms:
    - Gram-positive cocci, pair, lanceolate shaped—suggestive of pneumococcus
    - Pleomorphic gram-negative coccobacilli—suggestive of *Haemophilus influenzae*.
- **Acid-fast staining** of sputum by Ziehl-Neelsen technique is performed to demonstrate the acid-fast bacilli, e.g. *M. tuberculosis*
- **GMS stain** (Gomori methenamine silver stain) is used to demonstrate *Pneumocystis jirovecii*.

Culture

Specimens should be collected before antibiotic therapy for better yield of organisms.
- **Bacterial culture** is performed by using media such as blood agar, chocolate agar, and MacConkey agar
- **For *M. tuberculosis*:** Lowenstein Jensen medium or automated MGIT (mycobacteria growth indicator tube) may be used
- **For fungal pathogen isolation:** Sabouraud dextrose agar is used.

Serology (Antibody Detection)

Antibody detection tests by methods such as ELISA can be used for the diagnosis of atypical pneumonia pathogens such as *Mycoplasma*, *Chlamydia*, and viruses.

Antigen Detection Tests

Various antigen detection methods available for lower respiratory tract pathogens include:
- **Enzyme immunoassay** is available to detect *Legionella pneumophila* specific soluble antigens in urine
- **Direct fluorescent antibody tests** are available for influenza virus and respiratory syncytial virus, and *B. pertussis*, but are poorly sensitive and technically challenging.

Molecular Test

Molecular methods such as multiplex PCR assays are available targeting the genes specific for the common suspected agents of LRTI.
- **Real-time PCR** is the gold standard diagnostic method for detection of the agents of viral pneumonia such as influenza and SARS-CoV-2
- **Automated real-time PCR** such as GeneXpert and Truenat can be used for the identification of *M. tuberculosis* in sputum. They can be also used for detection of agents of viral pneumonia such as influenza and SARS-CoV-2.

EXPECTED QUESTIONS

I. **Write short notes on:**
   1. Pharyngitis.
   2. Laboratory diagnosis of pneumonia.

II. **Multiple Choice Questions (MCQs):**
   1. **All are upper respiratory tract infections, except:**
      a. Pharyngitis
      b. Acute laryngotracheobronchitis
      c. Bronchiolitis
      d. Peritonsillar abscess
   2. **Interstitial pneumonia is caused by all, except:**
      a. *Mycoplasma*
      b. *Chlamydia*
      c. *Legionella*
      d. Pneumococci

Answers
1. c   2. d

CHAPTER 53

Miscellaneous Infectious Syndromes

CHAPTER PREVIEW
- Skin and Soft Tissue Infections (SSTI)
- Sexually Transmitted Infections (STI)
- Congenital Infections
- Eye Infections
- Ear Infections

SKIN AND SOFT TISSUE INFECTIONS (SSTI)

Skin and soft tissue infections (SSTIs) can arise from invasion of organism through skin or from organisms that reach the skin from blood as a part of systemic infection.

- Skin comprises of epidermis, dermis and subcutaneous tissues. Hair follicles and sweat glands originate in the subcutaneous tissues
- Infection can involve any of these layers of skin **(Table 53.1)**.

Clinical Types of SSTIs

Skin infections can be subdivided into primary and secondary lesions:
- **Primary lesion:** An area of tissue with impaired structure/function due to damage by trauma or disease
- **Secondary lesion:** A lesion arising as a consequence of any primary infection.

Agents implicated in surgical site infections and burn wound infections are listed in **Tables 53.2 and 53.3** respectively.

Laboratory Diagnosis

Specimen Collection

Appropriate specimens include:
- Pus from the wound collected by sterile swab
- Pus from abscess collected by incision and drainage, or needle aspiration
- Vesicle or bulla fluid, collected by needle aspiration or sterile swab
- Subcutaneous infections: Sample collected from the base of the lesion or biopsy of the deep tissues
- Skin scrapings, plucked hair or nail clippings in suspected fungal infections.

Microscopy

- Gram staining of the specimen may demonstrate the morphology of the causative organisms
- KOH mount is done for suspected fungal infections (e.g. dermatophyte)
- Tzanck smear of the vesicle fluid suspected of herpes simplex or varicella virus infections.

Culture

- For the culture of aerobic bacteria, specimens are inoculated onto blood agar and MacConkey agar and incubated overnight at 37°C
- **For culture of atypical *Mycobacterium*:** Lowenstein Jensen medium may be used
- **For dermatophytes:** Sabouraud's dextrose agar is used
- **For anaerobic organisms:** Robertson's cooked meat broth and BHIS (brain heart

Table 53.1: Infective skin manifestations and their common causative agents.

Skin lesions	Description	Common etiological agents
Macule	Flat, non-palpable discoloration of skin (≤5 mm size) If size exceeds 5 mm, is called as patch	Dermatophytes Viral rashes (e.g. enterovirus)
Papule	Elevated palpable solid lesion, usually ≤5 mm in size	Molluscum contagiosum Scabies (*Sarcoptes scabiei*) Warts (Human Papilloma virus)
Nodule	Elevated palpable solid lesion, usually >5 mm in size	*Corynebacterium diphtheriae*, Post kala-azar dermal leishmaniasis, *Nocardia* species, etc.
Vesicle	Fluid-filled lesions with a diameter ≤5 mm	Herpes simplex virus, varicella-zoster virus
Bulla	Fluid-filled lesions with a diameter >5 mm	Herpes simplex virus, *Staphylococcus aureus*
Pustule	A fluid-filled vesicle containing pus and is ≤5 mm	*Staphylococcus aureus*
Abscess	A fluid-filled lesion containing pus and is >5 mm	*Streptococcus pyogenes*
Secondary lesions		
Scale	Excess dead epidermal layer	Dermatophytes
Ulcer	A lesion with loss of epidermis and dermis	*Mycobacterium leprae* (leprosy), *Mycobacterium ulcerans* (Buruli ulcer), *T. pallidum* (hard chancre)
Impetigo	Erythematous lesions which may be bullous or non-bullous with exudates and golden-yellow crusts	Non-bullous: *Streptococcus pyogenes* Bullous: *Staphylococcus aureus*
Cellulitis	Diffuse spreading infection involving deep layers of dermis Ill-defined flat red, painful lesions	*Streptococcus pyogenes* *Staphylococcus aureus*
Hair follicle infections		
Folliculitis	Superficial infection of single hair follicle, presents as pustule	
Furuncle	Deeper infections of the hair follicles, presents as abscess, spread deeply into dermis and subcutaneous tissues	*Staphylococcus aureus*
Carbuncle	Represents the coalescence of a number of furuncles	
Infection of fascia and muscles		
Necrotizing fasciitis	Rapidly spreading infection of fascia	*Streptococcus pyogenes* *Staphylococcus aureus*
Pyomyositis	Pus formation in the muscle layer	*Staphylococcus aureus* *Streptococcus pyogenes*
Myonecrosis	Extensive necrosis of the muscle layer with gangrene formation	Clostridial myonecrosis Other anaerobic infections

infusion agar with supplements) should be used. The plates should be incubated anaerobically.

Quantitative Culture

As the degree of bacterial contamination of the wound, is directly related to the chance of development of wound sepsis, hence quantitative culture may be performed to determine the number of colony forming units/gram of the tissue collected from the wound.

Identification

Accurate identification of the causative agent is done based on colony morphology,

Table 53.2: Agents causing surgical site wound infection.

Bacterial agents	Fungi
For most clean wounds: • Staphylococcus aureus • Coagulase-negative staphylococci • Enterococcus	Candida albicans
If bowel integrity is compromised: • Gram-negative flora like E. coli and • Anaerobic organisms like Bacteroides, Prevotella, etc.	

Table 53.3: Agents causing burn wound infections.

Bacteria	Fungi
Staphylococcus aureus (may be MRSA) Pseudomonas aeruginosa Coagulase-negative staphylococci (e.g. S. epidermidis)	Candida albicans

Abbreviation: MRSA, methicillin resistant *staphylococcus aureus*.

culture smear, and biochemical reactions or automated identification systems.

Antimicrobial Susceptibility Test

It helps in initiation of appropriate therapy.

> **TREATMENT** — SSTIs
>
> Skin and soft tissue infections are treated by both surgically (incision and drainage or surgical debridement) and medically (antibiotics).

SEXUALLY TRANSMITTED INFECTIONS

The sexually transmitted infections (STIs) are a group of communicable diseases which are transmitted by sexual contact.

Causative agents of STIs may be classified into two groups:
1. Agents causing local manifestations such as:
   - Genital ulcers
   - Urethral discharge
   - Vaginal discharge
   - Genital warts
   - Pelvic inflammatory diseases.
2. Agents transmitted by sexual route, producing only systemic manifestations and do not cause local manifestations (e.g. HIV).

The microorganisms causing STIs are listed in **Table 53.4** and the important features of STIs producing genital ulcers are compared in **Table 53.5**.

Table 53.4: Causative agents of sexually transmitted infections (STIs).

Agents causing local manifestations	
Genital ulcers	
Syphilis	Treponema pallidum
Herpes genitalis	Herpes simplex viruses
Chancroid	Haemophilus ducreyi
Lymphogranuloma venereum	Chlamydia trachomatis
Donovanosis	Klebsiella granulomatis
Urethral discharge	
Gonorrhea	Neisseria gonorrhoeae
Non-gonococcal urethritis (NGU)	• Chlamydia trachomatis (D-K) • Ureaplasma urealyticum • Mycoplasma genitalium • Mycoplasma hominis • Herpes simplex virus • Candida albicans • Trichomonas vaginalis
Vaginal discharge	
Vulvovaginal candidiasis	Candida albicans Non-albicans Candida species
Bacterial vaginosis	Gardnerella vaginalis
Trichomonal vaginitis	Trichomonas vaginalis
Genital warts	
Condyloma acuminata	Human papilloma viruses
Agents causing systemic manifestations	
Pelvic inflammatory diseases (PID)	Neisseria gonorrhoeae Chlamydia trachomatis
No genital lesions but only systemic manifestations	HIV Hepatitis B virus (HBV) Hepatitis C virus (HCV)

Table 53.5: Comparison of sexually transmitted infections (STIs) producing genital ulcer.

Feature	Syphilis	Herpes	Chancroid	LGV	Donovanosis
Incubation period	9–90 days	2–7 days	1–14 days	3 days–6 weeks	1–4 weeks (up to 6 months)
Genital ulcer	Painless, indurated, single	Multiple, painful	Painful, soft usually multiple	Painless, firm single lesion	Painless, single/multiple, beefy-red ulcer
Lymphadenopathy	Painless, firm, bilateral	Painful, firm, often bilateral	Painful, soft, marked swelling leads to bubo formation	Painful and soft, unilateral	Absent (pseudobubo may be present due to subcutaneous swelling)

Abbreviation: LGV, lymphogranuloma venereum.

Laboratory Diagnosis of STIs

Specimen Collection

- Discharge from the infected area such as vaginal or urethral discharge are collected in a sterile container
- **Sterile swabs may be used to collect the discharge** (if scanty): Charcoal impregnated swabs are used for suspected gonococcal infection
- Fluid from the vesicles (genital herpes).

Microscopy

- **Wet mount examination:** It is carried out for the vaginal discharge:
  - In trichomoniasis: Pus cells along with motile trophozoites are seen
  - In candidiasis: Yeast cells along with pseudohyphae are seen.
- **Gram-stained smear** of the discharge or the swab is useful for:
  - Bacterial vaginosis—clue cells are seen, which are vaginal epithelial cells studded with gram variable pleomorphic coccobacilli: suggestive of *Gardnerella vaginalis*
  - In gonorrhea—intracellular kidney-shaped diplococci are seen
  - In candidiasis—gram-positive budding yeast cells along with pseudohyphae are seen.
- **Giemsa stain** is done for:
  - *Klebsiella granulomatis* to detect the presence of Donovan's bodies (macrophage filled with bipolar stained bacilli)
  - *Chlamydia trachomatis* inclusion bodies.
- **Dark field microscopy** and silver impregnation methods—in syphilis, reveals characteristic spirally coiled bacilli.

Culture

Specimens are inoculated onto the appropriate culture media or cell line for the isolation of the causative organism.
- Thayer-Martin medium—for *N. gonorrhoeae*
- McCoy cell line—for *Chlamydia trachomatis*
- Sabouraud's dextrose agar (SDA)—for *Candida* species
- Cell lines such as Vero cells, monkey kidney cell line for herpes simplex virus.

Serology

Serological tests such as venereal disease research laboratory (VDRL) or rapid plasma reagin (RPR) test can be performed for the diagnosis of syphilis.

Molecular Test

Multiplex PCR and real-time PCR have been developed for simultaneous detection of pathogens causing STIs.

> **TREATMENT** — Urethritis
>
> Combination of ceftriaxone + azithromycin is the recommended regimen. Ceftriaxone will act against gonococcus and azithromycin will treat *C. trachomatis*; as these are the common causative agents of urethritis. Treatment to both the sexual partners is needed.

CONGENITAL INFECTIONS

Vertical transmission refers to the spread of infections from mother-to-baby. These infections may occur by transplacental route (congenital infection), during delivery, or after delivery.

Congenital Infection

A congenital infection is an infection that crosses the placenta to infect the fetus. They often lead to defects in fetal development or even death.

TORCH is an acronym used for some common congenital infections. These are:
* **T**oxoplasmosis
* **O**ther infections (congenital syphilis, hepatitis B, Coxsackie virus, Epstein-Barr virus, varicella-zoster virus, *Plasmodium falciparum* and human parvovirus)
* **R**ubella
* **C**ytomegalovirus (CMV)
* **H**erpes simplex virus.

Perinatal Infections (During Delivery)

Perinatal infections occur while the baby moves through an infected birth canal. These infections are usually caused by the agents of STIs. These also include the infections transmitted through contamination with fecal matter during delivery. Common examples of agents causing perinatal infections include:
* Cytomegalovirus
* *Neisseria gonorrhoeae*
* *Chlamydia* species
* Herpes simplex virus
* Human papilloma virus (genital warts)
* Group B streptococci.

Postnatal Infections (After Delivery)

These infections spread from mother to baby following delivery, usually during breastfeeding. Some examples of postnatal infections are: CMV, HIV and group B streptococci.

EYE INFECTIONS

In general, ocular infections are grouped into:
* **Infections involving external structures of the eyes:** such as eyelid (blepharitis), conjunctiva (conjunctivitis), cornea (keratitis) and sclera (scleritis).
* **Infections involving internal structures:** Retina (retinitis), uvea (uveitis) and aqueous humor or vitreous humor (endophthalmitis).

The list of the organisms causing various ocular infections is given in **Table 53.6**.

EAR INFECTIONS

Common ear infections are **(Table 53.7)**.

Table 53.6: Ocular infections and their causative agents.

Infections	Organisms
Blepharitis (Infection of eyelids)	Staphylococcus aureus
Conjunctivitis (Infection of conjunctiva)	• Haemophilus influenzae • Staphylococcus aureus • Chlamydia trachomatis • Neisseria gonorrhoeae • Adenovirus, Herpes simplex virus
Keratitis (Infection of cornea)	• Staphylococcus aureus • Streptococcus pneumoniae • Fusarium, Candida • Acanthamoeba
Scleritis (Infection of sclera)	Staphylococcus aureus
Chorioretinitis and uveitis (Infection of choroid, retina, and uvea)	• Mycobacterium tuberculosis • Treponema pallidum • Cytomegalovirus • Toxoplasma gondii
Endophthalmitis (Infection of aqueous humor or vitreous humor)	• Staphylococcus aureus • Streptococcus pneumoniae • Pseudomonas aeruginosa • Other gram-negative bacilli • Herpes simplex virus, Candida

Table 53.7: Organisms causing ear infections.

Otitis externa: Infection of external ears	Otitis media: (middle ear infections)
Acute otitis externa • *Staphylococcus aureus* (most common) • *Streptococcus pyogenes* • *Pseudomonas* (malignant otitis externa) • Other gram-negative bacilli • *Aspergillus* species • *Candida* species	**Acute otitis media** • *Streptococcus pneumoniae*: Most common (33%, in children) • *Haemophilus influenzae* type b (second most common) • *Moraxella catarrhalis* • *Streptococcus pyogenes* • Respiratory syncytial virus • Influenza virus
Chronic otitis externa • Anaerobes (most common) • *Pseudomonas*	**Chronic otitis media** Anaerobes (most common)

❖ **Otitis externa:** Inflammation, irritation, or infection of the outer ear and ear canal
  ■ Also called as swimmer's ear—swimming in contaminated water is one of the reasons of contracting swimmer's ear
  ■ Symptoms—itchy ear canal, Inflammation of ear canal's skin and pus formation in ear canal and earache that is aggravated when the ear lobe is pulled.

❖ **Otitis media:** Infections of middle ear; characterized by earache and ear discharge
  ■ It often begins with an infection that causes a sore throat, cold or respiratory problem and eventually spread to the middle ear
  ■ Symptoms include: Intense earache, headache, fever and nausea and leaking of discharge from ear following rupture of the tympanic membrane.

EXPECTED QUESTIONS

I. Write short notes on:
1. TORCH infections.
2. Skin and soft tissue infections.
3. Sexually transmitted infections.

II. Multiple Choice Questions (MCQs):
1. Which of the following sexually transmitted infection produces painful genital ulcers and painful lymph nodes?
   a. Syphilis
   b. Chancroid
   c. LGV
   d. Donovanosis

2. The agent of malignant otitis externa is:
   a. *Staphylococcus aureus*
   b. *Pseudomonas* species
   c. *Streptococcus pyogenes*
   d. *Candida* species

3. Not a common cause of surgical site infection is____:
   a. *Staphylococcus epidermidis*
   b. *Pseudomonas aeruginosa*
   c. *Acinetobacter* species
   d. *Burkholderia pseudomallei*

Answers
1. b   2. b   3. d

CHAPTER 54: Specimen Collection and Transport

CHAPTER PREVIEW
- Specimen Collection
- Specimen Transport

SPECIMEN COLLECTION

Specimen Collection

A young patient with history of high grade fever with chills for two days, presents to the out patient department. Upon detailed clinical examination, clinician decides to admit him and requests for his blood and urine culture and susceptibility testing. After two days of hospitalization he develops diarrhea with two episodes of vomiting. His stool specimen was collected and sent for culture. Discuss the method of collection of the following specimens for culture.
- Blood for blood culture
- Urine specimen for microscopy and culture
- Stool specimen for microscopy and culture

Explanation

The specimen collection has been explained in the following Chapters
- Blood collection for culture: Refer Chapter 48
- Urine specimen collection for microscopy and culture: Explained subsequently in this chapter
- Stool specimen collection for microscopy and culture: Explained subsequently in this chapter

Specimen collection depends upon the type of underlying infections **(Table 54.1)**.

General Principles

The following general principles should be followed while collecting the specimen:

- ❖ **Standard precautions** should be followed for collecting and handling all specimens (Chapter 37 for details)
- ❖ **Before antibiotics start:** Whenever possible, culture specimens should be collected prior to administration of any antimicrobial agents
- ❖ **Contamination** with indigenous flora should be avoided, especially when collecting urine and blood culture specimens
- ❖ **Swabs** are though convenient but considered inferior to tissue, aspirate and body fluids
- ❖ **Container:** Specimens should be collected in sterile, tightly sealed, leak proof, wide-mouth, screw-capped containers
- ❖ **Labeling:** All specimens must be appropriately labeled with name, age, gender, name of the treating physician, clinical diagnosis, antibiotic history, type of specimen, and desired investigation name
- ❖ **Rejection:** Specimens grossly contaminated or compromised or improperly labeled may be rejected (see highlight box below)
- ❖ If **anaerobic culture** is requested, proper anaerobic collection containers with media should be used
- ❖ Specimen should not be sent in container containing **formalin** for microbiological culture analysis.

Specimen Rejection Criteria

Microbiology samples that do not meet the *appropriate sample* and the *test request requirements* need to be rejected, so as to prevent

Contd...

Table 54.1: Types of infections and various specimens collected.

Type of infections	Specimens collected
Bloodstream infection, sepsis, endocarditis	Paired blood culture specimens • Collected aseptically by two-step disinfection of skin; first with alcohol followed by chlorhexidine • 8–10 mL of blood (for adults) collected in blood culture bottles
Infectious diseases requiring serology	• Blood (2 mL/investigation) • Collected by minimal asepsis (one-step skin disinfection with alcohol) • Collected in vacutainer
Diarrheal diseases	Stool (mucus flakes), rectal swab
Meningitis	Cerebrospinal fluid (CSF)
Infections of other sterile body area	Sterile body fluids, e.g., pleural fluid, synovial fluid, peritoneal fluid
Skin and soft tissue infections	Pus or exudate, wound swabs, aspirates from abscess and tissue bits
Anaerobic infections	Aspirates, tissue specimens, blood and sterile body fluids, bone marrow (swabs, sputum not satisfactory)
Upper respiratory tract infections	Throat swab with membrane over the tonsil, nasopharyngeal swab, pernasal swab
Lower respiratory tract infections	Sputum, endotracheal aspirate, bronchoalveolar lavage (BAL), protected specimen brush (PSB) and lung biopsy
Pulmonary tuberculosis	• Sputum—early morning and spot • Collected in well-ventilated area • Gastric aspirate for infants
Urinary tract infections	• Midstream urine • Suprapubic aspirated urine • Catheterized patient—collected from the catheter tube, after clamping distally and disinfecting; not from urobag
Genital infections	• Urethral swab, cervical swab—for urethritis • Exudate from genital ulcers
Eye infections	• Conjunctival swabs • Corneal scrapings • Aqueous or vitreous fluid
Ear infections	• Swabs from outer ear • Aspirate from inner ear

Contd...

inaccurate data and to ensure the safety of patients and laboratory personnel. Reasons for sample rejection may include the following:
- Improperly labeled or unlabeled sample
- Incomplete specimen-related or clinical information on the sample and/or on the requisition form
- Sub-optimal sample, i.e., leaking urine and/or stool containers, insufficient quantity or inappropriate sample for the test requested
- Duplicate microbiology samples received on the same day, i.e., multiple stool, sputum samples
- Sample delayed in transit more than the accepted limit.

SPECIMEN COLLECTION FOR BACTERIAL INFECTIONS

Blood Specimen

In clinical microbiology laboratories, blood collection is indicated either for blood culture or for serological tests.

Collection of Blood Specimen for Culture

Blood culture is regarded as one of the most important culture investigation performed by clinical microbiology laboratory. As there is a high risk of contamination with skin flora, sterile aseptic precautions must be taken for collection and skin is disinfected with two agents—70% alcohol followed by chlorhexidine. It is discussed in detail in Chapter 48.

Collection of Blood Specimen for Serology

Collection of blood specimen for serological (e.g., virology or immunology) diagnostic tests is similar to as done for culture; except that skin disinfection is performed by only one agent i.e., 70% isopropyl alcohol. This is because contamination with skin flora is not an issue while performing these investigations.

- The blood sample is collected in clean sterile tubes (Vacutainers, **Fig. 54.1B**)
- Tube is filled 3/4th full and then allowed to stand at room temperature for a few hours to allow a solid clot to form and retract
- Then the tube is centrifuged, serum is separated, placed in another clean tube, which can be used for further diagnostic testing.

CSF and Other Sterile Body Fluids

CSF and other sterile body fluids should be collected before the starting of antimicrobial therapy, in sterile screw capped container, under adequate aseptic precautions.

- **CSF:** It is collected by lumbar puncture at interspace L3-L4, or L4-L5. The site is first disinfected with antiseptics similar to that used for blood culture. After collection, CSF is then divided into three sterile tubes (2 mL each) for three diagnostic laboratories
  - Biochemistry (for total protein and glucose)
  - Bacteriology (culture and susceptibility, Gram staining, antigen detection)
  - Cytology (for cell count).
- **Body fluids from other sterile sites** such as ascitic fluid, pleural fluid, peritoneal fluid, and synovial fluid specimens are collected by percutaneous aspiration under aseptic precautions with syringe and needle
- **Body fluid specimens** can also be inoculated at bedside directly on to BacT/ALERT bottles for culture. In these case, a portion of the specimen should be aliquoted separately for Gram stain

- **Transport:** Specimens should be transported immediately (within 15 min) to the laboratory; If any delay is expected, body fluid specimens can be stored at 37°C (in incubator) or at room temperature; **but never refrigerated**, as delicate pathogens such as *H. influenzae*, pneumococci or meningococci may die.

> **Sterile Universal Specimen Container (Fig. 54.1A)**
>
> These are designed for collecting biological specimens, including urine, stool, sputum, peritoneal exudate, joint fluid, biopsy specimen, sterile body fluids and aspirates for microbiological culture and susceptibility testing. It is very convenient for sample collection at the bed side. These containers should have the following specifications:
> - They should be sterile, leak-proof, wide mouthed and screw capped
> - Each container should bear the name of the patient, from whom the specimen was collected and his hospital register number
> - Specimen type and date and time of collection
> - A completely filled investigation requisition form should always accompany the specimen indicating the investigation requested along with the probable clinical diagnosis and current antibiotic therapy

Fecal Specimens

A small quantity of semisolid/solid stool or one third of the container in case of liquid

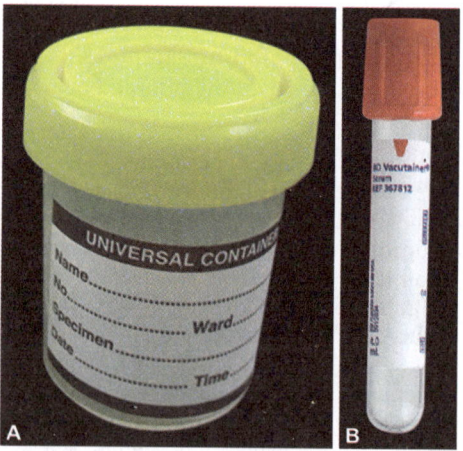

Figs. 54.1A and B: A. Sterile universal container; **B.** Blood collection Vacutainer tube.

stool specimen is collected in a wide mouthed, sterile screw capped, leak proof container **(Fig. 54.1A)**; preferably prior to initiation of antibiotics.
- ❖ **Rectal swabs** may be collected in case of asymptomatic carriers
- ❖ **Transport:** Sample should be immediately transported to the laboratory. In case of delay, suitable transport media may be employed such as Cary Blair medium or Venkatraman Ramakrishnan (VR) medium.

Respiratory Specimens

Respiratory specimens are categorized into two groups.
- ❖ Upper respiratory tract specimens such as throat swab, nasopharyngeal swabs, bits of membrane from tonsil
- ❖ Lower respiratory tract specimens such as sputum, endotracheal aspirate (ETA) and bronchoalveolar lavage (BAL), protected specimen brush (PSB) and lung biopsy.

Sputum

Sputum cultures are indicated to identify the pathogens causing pneumonia.
- ❖ Sputum specimen that results following a deep cough is preferable and is collected in a sterile screw capped, wide-mouthed, leak proof container **(Fig. 54.1A)**. Patient should be instructed to place the rim of the container under the lower lip to catch entire expectorated mucopurulent sputum
- ❖ **Early morning sputum** samples should be obtained as they contain pooled overnight secretions, as they may contain increased concentration of pathogens
- ❖ **For suspected tuberculosis**
  - ▪ **Two sputum** specimens are collected- spot and early morning. Sputum collection booths should be located away from other people, outside in an open well ventilated space
  - ▪ **Gastric aspirate** may be collected for infants in suspected case of tuberculosis. Early morning specimen is ideal before eating/getting up. Transport time should be < 15 minutes.

- ❖ Collected specimen has to be transported to the laboratory as soon as possible (within two hours); as delicate pathogens may otherwise die, if there is a delay.

ETA, BAL, PSB and Lung Biopsy Specimens

Collection of endotracheal aspirate (ETA), bronchoalveolar lavage (BAL), protected specimen brush (PSB) and lung biopsy specimens is technically demanding and requires specialized techniques. These specimens should be transported immediately to the laboratory and cultured within one hour of collection.

Throat Swab

Throat swab samples for bacterial culture is collected by depressing the tongue with a tongue depressor. The oropharyngeal swab is rubbed on the back of the throat, over the tonsils, and in any other area where there is redness or pus. Whenever possible, a portion of pseudomembrane may be collected.

Nasopharyngeal Secretions

Nasopharyngeal specimens are the best specimens which may be obtained by:
- ❖ **Nasopharyngeal aspiration** (best method): Collected by inserting flexible swab through nose into posterior nasopharynx and rotating for 5 seconds; specimen of choice for *Bordetella pertussis*
- ❖ **Per-nasal swab**: Collected by using a sterile swab on a flexible wire.

Note: For culture in a suspected case of pertussis, alginate swabs are the best followed by dacron swabs. Cotton swabs are not satisfactory. It is recommended to collect six swabs, at 1–2 days intervals to achieve maximum yield.

Exudate Specimens

Wound swabs (sterile cotton swab, **Fig. 54.2**) are recommended to identify the

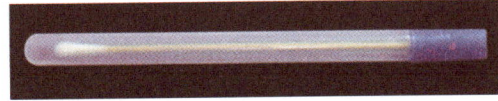

Fig. 54.2: Sterile cotton swab.

etiological agents causing deep-seated wound infection.
- ❖ Wound swabs are ideally collected prior to starting of antibiotic therapy and only for clinically infected wounds or that fail to heal even after a long period
- ❖ **For closed wounds** disinfect with 70% alcohol or 2% chlorhexidine followed by 10% povidone-iodine. Remove iodine with alcohol just prior to specimen collection
- ❖ **Open wounds** are first debrided and then thoroughly rinsed with sterile saline prior to collection
- ❖ Preferably sample the **viable tissue** and not the superficial debris
- ❖ A portion of the sample also must be placed in Robertson's Cooked Meat (RCM) medium, if anaerobic culture is indicated
- ❖ For collection of pus in the form of **abscess**, aspirate the deepest portion of the lesion with a syringe and needle
- ❖ **For burn wound** swab collection, consider sampling different areas of the burn, as organisms may not be evenly distributed in a burn wound
- ❖ **Aspirates and tissue specimens** should be delivered to the laboratory for further processing within 30 minutes of collection for best recovery. Tissue specimens must be kept moist to preserve viability of organisms
- ❖ **For anaerobic culture,** aspirates or tissue specimens are recommended. Specimen which are not suitable include swab, urine, sputum etc.
- ❖ **Discharging sinus:** In case of actinomycetoma, **granules** present in the discharge are collected in sterile gauze or loop by pressing the sinuses from the periphery to express them out.

Urine Specimen

It is extremely important to collect the urine specimens carefully to avoid the contamination with normal urethral flora. The various type of collection of urine specimen for culture has been described below.
- ❖ **Midstream clean catch urine:** It is the most common type of urine specimen collected for culture. After properly cleaning the urethral meatus or glans with soap and water, urine specimen is collected in a sterile, wide mouthed, screw capped, leak proof container by voiding the first portion (which is likely to be contaminated with normal urethral flora) **(Fig. 54.1A)**
- ❖ **Indwelling catheter:** Urine specimen should be collected from the catheter tubing (after clamping and disinfecting a portion of the catheter tubing with alcohol), by inserting a sterile syringe and needle directly into the catheter tubing. Urine *must not be* collected from the drainage bag
- ❖ **Suprapubic aspiration:** It is the **most ideal** urine specimen, as it avoids the risk of contamination with urethral flora
  - However it is invasive and therefore is recommended only for patients in coma or infants
  - The skin above the bladder is disinfected and then urine is collected needle aspiration above the symphysis pubis through the abdominal wall into the full bladder.
- ❖ **Transport:** Urine specimen must be transported to the microbiology laboratory as soon as possible and should be processed immediately. If delay is expected for more than two hours, then it can be stored in refrigerator or stored by adding boric acid or glycerol for maximum 24 hours before plating.

Genital Specimens

Common genital specimens include urethral discharge for urethritis and exudate from genital ulcers

Urethral Discharge

Urethral swab in men and cervical swab in women are the preferred specimens. Vaginal swab is not satisfactory.
- ❖ **Method:** The urethral meatus is cleaned with gauze soaked in saline. The purulent discharge is expressed out by pressing at the base of the penis and collected directly on to slides or swabs

- **Swab:** Dacron or rayon swabs are preferred, as cotton and alginate swabs are inhibitory to many urethral pathogens such as gonococci
- **In chronic urethritis:** As discharge is minimal, prostatic massage is done to collect the secretion; alternatively, the morning drop of secretion may also be collected
- **Transport Media:** Specimens should be transported immediately. If not possible, then charcoal containing Stuart's or Amies transport medium can be used.

Exudate from Genital Ulcers

Surface of the genital ulcer is cleaned with saline, gentle pressure is applied at the base of the lesion, and a drop of exudate is collected on a slide.

Endometrial specimens: Collected by surgical biopsy or trans-cervical aspirate via sheathed catheter.

Other Specimens

- **Ocular specimens:** They are precious specimens, should be transported to laboratory within 15 min. Bedside inoculation onto blood agar may be considered if delay is unavoidable
  - **Conjunctival swab:** Swabs should be pre-moistened with sterile saline and samples should be collected from both the eyes
  - **Corneal scrapings:** Clinicians should instill local anesthetics before collection
  - **Aqueous or vitreous fluid** for endophthalmitis cases.
- **Ear specimens:**
  - **External ear:** Specimen is collected by firmly rotating the swab into the outer ear **(Fig. 54.2)**
  - **Inner ear specimens:** If ear drum is intact, material behind the drum is aspirated with syringe; if ear drum is ruptured, swab is used to collect material from the inner ear. Ear canal should be cleaned with mild soap solution before aspiration.

SPECIMEN TRANSPORT AND STORAGE BEFORE PROCESSING

Specimen Transport

The specimens should reach the laboratory for further processing as soon as possible after the collection. If required appropriate transport media should be used.

For most of the specimens, transport time should not exceed **two hours**. However, there are some exceptions.

- Specimens such as CSF and body fluids, ocular specimens, tissue specimens, suprapubic aspirate and bone specimen should be **transported immediately** (<15 minutes)
- **Urine (midstream)** added with preservative (boric acid) is acceptable up to 24 hours, otherwise should be transported within 2 hours
- **Stool culture:** Stool specimen should be transported within 1 hour, but with transport media such as Cary-Blair medium or Venkatraman Ramakrishnan (VR) medium, is acceptable up to 24 hours
- **Rectal swabs**—up to 24 hours is acceptable
- **For anaerobic culture:** Specimens should be put into Robertson's cooked meat broth or any specialized anaerobic transport system and transported immediately to the laboratory.

Specimen Storage before Processing

Most specimens can be stored **at room temperature** immediately after receipt, for **up to 24 hours**. However, there are some exceptions.

- **Blood cultures**—should be incubated at 37°C immediately upon receipt
- Sterile body fluids, bone, vitreous fluid, suprapubic aspirate—should be immediately plated upon receipt and incubated at 37°C
- **Corneal scraping**—should be immediately plated at bed-side on to blood agar and chocolate agar
- **Stool culture**—stool specimen for culture can be stored up to 72 hours at 4°C
- **Urine** (mid-stream and from the catheter), **lower respiratory** tract specimen, **gastric**

biopsy (for *Helicobacter pylori*)—can be stored up to 24 hours at 4°C.

Prioritizing the Specimen for Processing

Certain precious specimens such as CSF and sterile body fluids, ocular specimens, tissue specimens, suprapubic aspirate and bone specimen should be processed immediately as soon as received, not more than 15 min delay. Similarly, blood culture bottles should be immediately incubated upon receipt.

SPECIMEN COLLECTION FOR VIRAL INFECTIONS

Specimen collection has to be done early in the patient's illness as possible, as viruses can be recovered only for a few days after the onset of illness. The following steps should be kept in mind during specimen collection:

Appropriate time: Specimens should be collected as soon as possible, preferably within 3 days after onset of symptoms.
* From the correct site **(Table 54.2)**
* In the correct method of collection
* In adequate volume **(Fig. 54.3)**

Table 54.2: Various types of viral infections and specimen of choice.

Systemic infections	Specimens to be collected
Respiratory infections	• Swabs (nasal, throat, nasopharyngeal) • Bronchoalveolar lavage, nasal washings • Aspirates (nasal or sinus), serum
Viral encephalitis	• Cerebrospinal fluid • Throat washings • Tissue by brain biopsy (postmortem) • Stool and serum
Viral gastroenteritis	Stool and serum
Exanthematous infections	• Vesicle aspirate • Skin scrapping • Skin biopsy
Poliomyelitis	• Stool and rectal swabs • Serum
Sexually-transmitted infections	Serum
Teratogenic viruses	Serum
Conjunctivitis	Conjunctival swab
Vector-borne diseases	Serum

* In suitable containers (sterile and chemical free)—e.g., viral transport media
* Transport in correct temperature: Specimen to be kept at 4°C for 3–5 days, after which the sample should be kept at –70°C **(Fig. 54.3)**
* Correctly labeled (patient details and specimen details).

Specimen Collection for COVID-19

Combined oropharyngeal and nasopharyngeal swab is recommended (NP/OP swab) for the diagnosis of COVID-19. Refer highlight box below for details.

> **Specimen collection for COVID-19**
> Combined oropharyngeal and nasopharyngeal swab is recommended (NP/OP swab)—first take the oropharyngeal sample; then using the same swab take nasopharyngeal sample.
> * Dacron or polyester flocked swabs are used, dipped in viral transport media (VTM) after collection **(Fig. 54.4)**
> * Explain the procedure to the patient
>
> *Contd...*

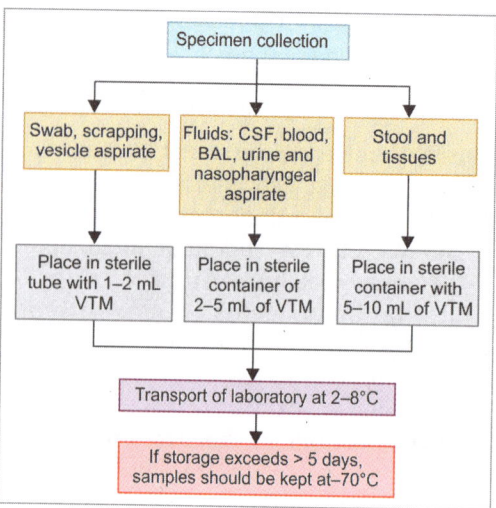

Fig. 54.3: Process of specimen collection and transport for viral infections.
Abbreviations: VTM, viral transport medium; CSF, cerebrospinal fluid; BAL, bronchoalveolar lavage.

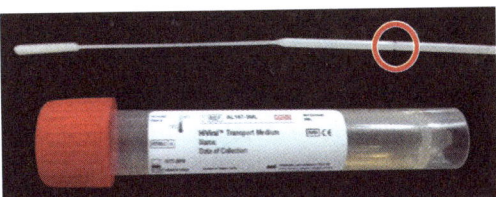

Fig. 54.4: Viral transport medium and swab.
Source: Department of Microbiology, JIPMER, Puducherry (*with permission*).

Contd...

Oropharyngeal swab (e.g., throat swab)
- Tilt patient's head back slightly to improve the view of the throat. Ask the patient to say Ah
- Place a tongue depressor over the anterior 1/3 to anterior 1/2 of the tongue and depress the tongue gently
- Do not press the tongue depressor firmly
- Collect specimen by gently swiping the tip of the swab over tonsillar pillars and posterior pharyngeal wall

Nasopharyngeal swab
- Tilt the patient's head back slightly, so that the nasal passages become more accessible
- Ask the patient to close his eyes to lessen the mild discomfort of the procedure
- Insert the swab into the nostril, and direct it posteriorly. The swab should be passed keeping it close to the nasal septum
- Keep the swab just above the floor of the nasal passage and parallel to the palate. It should not be directed laterally away from the septum or superiorly away from the floor
- You will feel resistance when you reach the nasopharynx
- Once you reach the nasopharynx, leave the swab in place for several seconds to absorb secretions; then rotate the swab several times before removing it

Break of the stem of both the swabs (oropharyngeal and nasopharyngeal) at the groove as shown below (red circle, **Fig. 54.4**),

Contd...

Contd...

and place the swab into the tube containing the VTM **without touching the outer surface of the tube**.

SPECIMEN COLLECTION FOR PARASITIC INFECTIONS

The proper and timely collection of specimen is of paramount importance for diagnosis of parasitic infections.
- As many parasites inhabit in the intestinal tract, stool examination is the most common diagnostic technique used for the diagnosis of parasitic infections. Refer Chapter 4 for details on stool specimen collection for stool microscopy and for other diagnostic techniques
- Blood examination is useful in the diagnosis of infection caused by blood parasites, such as *Plasmodium, Leishmania* and *Wuchereria bancrofti*. Blood collection technique has been already discussed under specimen collection for bacterial infections.

SPECIMEN COLLECTION FOR FUNGAL INFECTIONS

Specimen collection for diagnosis of fungal infection depends on the site of infection such as skin scraping, hair, nail, sputum, etc.
- Skin, hair and nail are collected for superficial fungal infections
- For systemic mycoses, blood sample is collected
- Cerebrospinal fluid (CSF) is collected for cryptococcal meningitis.

Details on specimen collection for various fungal infections are discussed in Chapter 35.

EXPECTED QUESTIONS

I. Write short notes on:
1. Sterile universal specimen container.
2. Specimen transport for bacterial infections.
3. Specimen collection and transport for viral infections.

CHAPTER 55: Practical Microbiology

The practical exercises conducted for the nursing students perusing BSc Nursing course vary among the universities in India. In general, the following are the practical exercises that are important for BSc Nursing students.

GRAM STAIN: EXERCISE-1

Case Scenario 1: A smear is provided, made from a sputum specimen of a 5-year-old child with acute onset of fever, productive cough and dyspnea for the past two days. Physical examination revealed dull note on percussion.

Case Scenario 2: A smear is provided, made from a CSF specimen of a 2-year-old baby presented with high-grade fever, vomiting and excessive crying for past three days.

Case Scenario 3: A smear is provided, made from a pus discharge of a postoperative wound infection of a 65-year-old man who has undergone an abdominal surgery.

Case Scenario 4: A smear is provided, made from a wound swab specimen of a foot ulcer of a diabetic patient.

Questions (common to all case scenarios):
1. Perform Gram stain of the smear provided.
2. Draw your observations with the help of a neat labeled diagram and give your interpretation.
3. Suggest which antibiotic can be started empirically for the treatment of this case?
4. What are various theories of Gram staining?
5. What are the various uses of Gram staining?

Explanation

The above clinical presentations are suggestive of a case of:
- Lobar pneumonia (case scenario 1)
- Pyogenic meningitis (case scenario 2)
- Surgical site infection (case scenario 3)
- Diabetic foot ulcer (case scenario 4).

The answers to the above questions have been explained in Chapter 2.2.

ACID-FAST STAINING: EXERCISE-2

A smear is provided, made from a sputum specimen of a 15-year-old boy who presented with fever, productive cough, and hemoptysis for the past two weeks.
1. Perform acid-fast staining of the smear provided.
2. Draw your observations with the help of a neat labeled diagram and give your interpretation.
3. Suggest the treatment regimen given in this case.
4. What is RNTCP grading and its implications?
5. Which is the conventional culture medium used and describe the colonies grown?
6. What is the recommended molecular method available for rapid and accurate identification? Mention its advantages?

Explanation

The above clinical presentation is suggestive of a case of pulmonary tuberculosis. The answers to the above questions have been explained in this chapter and also in Chapters 2.2 and 15.

HAND HYGIENE: EXERCISE-3

A nurse in an ICU records the pulse of a patient, records it in the case sheet and then goes back to nursing station. Then she draws the blood of another patient. While transporting the specimen, a drop of blood fell on her palm. Then she enters the operation theater to assist for a surgery.

1. How many times she has to perform hand hygiene?
2. What are the hand hygiene methods she has to perform and for how much duration?
3. What are the hand hygiene products to be used?
4. Preform handwash by following the WHO steps (Objective Structured Practical Examination).

Explanation

The nurse has to perform totally seven times hand hygiene: Five times hand rub, once handwash and hand scrub each (**Figs. 37.1 to 37.3**).

Hand rub: Nurse has to perform hand rub five times, 20–30 seconds in each time with 70–80% alcohol hand rub.
- Before recording pulse (WHO Moment 1)
- After recording pulse (WHO Moment 4)
- Before drawing blood (WHO Moment 2)
- After drawing blood (WHO Moment 3)
- After recording in the case sheet (WHO Moment 5).

Handwash: She has to perform handwash once (after blood drop fell on her palm), with 2–4% chlorhexidine handwash for 40–60 seconds.

Hand scrub: She has to perform hand scrub once (before assisting for surgery), with 4% chlorhexidine handwash for 3–5 minutes.

Refer Chapter 37 for further details.

	Handwash (OSPE checklist)		Scores (Attempt)		
Step	Student's performance	Total	First	Second	Third
1	Removes all hand accessories (finger ring, wrist watch, etc.) (0.5) and applies sufficient amount of soap/handwash/hand rub (0.5)	1.0			
2	Rubs palm to palm	0.5			
3	Rubs back of palm on both sides (0.5 + 0.5)	1.0			
4	Interlaces fingers in the web spaces	1.0			
5	Rubs back of fingers on palm on both sides (0.5 + 0.5)	1.0			
6	Follows rotational rubbing of thumb on both sides (0.5 + 0.5)	1.0			
7	Rubs nails on palms on both sides (0.5 + 0.5)	1.0			
8	Rinses hands with water	0.5			
9	Dries hands with paper with single use towel (0.5) and closes the tap with same paper towel/elbow (0.5)	1.0			
10	Disposes the paper towel appropriately	1.0			
	Completes the steps 2–8 in 40–60 seconds time	1.0			
	Total score	10			

Faculty Remarks/Feedback:

Faculty Signature
Date

GLOVES (DONNING AND DOFFING): EXERCISE-4

A nurse performs phlebotomy to collect blood specimen for culture. Before starting the procedure, she performs hand hygiene and wears a pair of hand gloves. Perform donning and doffing of hand gloves (Objective Structured Practical Examination).

Explanation

Donning (wearing) and doffing (removal) of hand gloves (OSPE checklist)				Scores (Attempt)		
Step	Student's performance		Total	First	Second	Third
Donning	Glove: 1	Wears by touching and pulling only the edge of the cuff	1.0			
	Glove: 2	a. Wears by pulling the external surface of second glove by the finger of gloved hand (0.5) and b. Avoids touching the forearm skin (0.5)	1.0			
Doffing	Glove: 1	Removes first glove by using the other gloved hand, grasps the palm area of the first glove and peels it off	1.0			
	Glove: 2	a. Holds the removed glove in the other gloved hand (0.5) and b. Slides fingers of the ungloved hand under the other glove at wrist and peels off second glove over first glove (0.5)	1.0			
		a. Disposes the gloves appropriately (0.5) and b. Performs hand hygiene after gloves removal (0.5)	1.0			
		Total score	5.0			

Faculty Remarks/Feedback:

Faculty Signature
Date

PERSONAL PROTECTIVE EQUIPMENT: EXERCISE-5

In COVID-19 healthcare setup, what are the personal protective equipment (PPE), the nurse should wear while giving care to the patient? Perform donning and doffing of PPE in a sequential manner (Objective Structured Practical Examination).

Explanation

The PPE needed for giving care to the COVID-19 patient are a pair of gloves, 3-ply mask (surgical mask), gown and goggle or face shield. If aerosol-generating procedure is to be performed, N95 respirator needs to be worn in place of a 3-ply mask.

Sequential donning (wearing) of PPE (OSPE checklist)		Scores (Attempt)		
Student's performance	Total	First	Second	Third
Performs proper hand hygiene	1.0			
Wears the gown first in sequence	0.25			
Wears the gown by fully covering torso from neck to knees, arms to end of wrists, and wraps around the back and fasten it at the waist and back of neck	0.5			
Wears the mask second in sequence	0.25			

Contd...

Contd...

Sequential donning (wearing) of PPE (OSPE checklist)		Scores (Attempt)		
Student's performance	Total	First	Second	Third
Pulls the straps tight and pulls the mask to below chin and then applies knots	0.5			
Presses on the nasal bridge part of the mask to seal tightly and for N95 respirator, performs fit check	0.5			
Wears the goggles/face shield third in sequence	0.25			
Wears the goggles/face shield by touching the front part only	0.5			
Wears the gloves last in sequence	0.25			
Glove: 1 Wears by touching and pulling only the edge of the cuff	0.5			
Glove: 2 a. Wears by pulling the external surface of second glove by the finger of gloved hand (0.25)				
b. Avoids touching the forearm skin (0.25)	0.5			
Total score	5.0			

Faculty Remarks/Feedback:

Faculty Signature
Date

Sequential doffing (removal) of PPE (OSPE checklist)		Scores (Attempt)		
Student's performance	Total	First	Second	Third
Removes the gloves first	0.5			
Does not touch outside of the gloves (contaminated)	0.5			
Glove: 1 Removes first glove by using the other gloved hand, grasps the palm area of the first glove and peels it off	0.5			
Glove: 2 a. Holds the removed glove in the other gloved hand (0.25) and b. Slides fingers of the ungloved hand under the other glove at wrist and peels off second glove over first glove (0.25)	0.5			
Discards the gloves into red bin	0.5			
Performs hand hygiene after gloves removal	0.5			
Removes gown second in sequence: Does not touch the front part of the gown while removing	0.5			
Unfastens the gown ties, taking care that sleeves do not touch the body while reaching for ties	0.5			
Pulls the gown away from neck and shoulders, by touching inside of gown only	0.5			
Turn the gown inside out and rolls it into a bundle and discards	0.5			
Discards the gown into yellow bin	0.5			
Performs hand hygiene after removal	0.5			
Removes face shield/goggles third in sequence	0.5			
Removes face shield/goggles by touching the sides only and bending forward	0.5			

Contd...

Contd...

Sequential doffing (removal) of PPE (OSPE checklist)		Scores (Attempt)		
Student's performance	Total	First	Second	Third
Discards face shield/goggles into red bin	0.5			
Performs hand hygiene after removal	0.5			
Takes off mask fourth in sequence	0.5			
Does not touch front part of the mask	0.5			
Unties the lower knot first, then the upper knot and removes the mask by holding its straps, without touching the front				
Discards the mask into yellow bin	0.5			
Performs hand hygiene at the last after removal of all PPE	0.5			
Total score	10			
Faculty Remarks/Feedback				
	Faculty Signature Date			

CONTACT PRECAUTIONS: EXERCISE-6

A 70-year-old woman after surgery for total knee replacement, is transferred to the postoperative ward. Four days later, the patient develops erythema and pus discharge at the wound site. The wound swab sent for culture shows growth of MRSA (methicillin-resistant *S. aureus*); sensitive only to vancomycin and linezolid. Total of 10 patients are housed in the same ward and only two nurses are posted. Hand rub is available only at the entrance and at the nursing station. There is only one stethoscope, blood pressure (BP) apparatus and thermometer in the ward. It is a practice in the ward to use the same gloves continuously, due to shortage of supply. After 2 days, another patient following appendectomy develops discharge from the wound site and MRSA grows on culture with the same antimicrobial sensitivity pattern. Identify the risks for transmission and the type of transmission-based precaution applicable?

Explanation

A cluster of cases of surgical site infection occurred with MRSA infection which resulted from the lack of standard and contact precautions of the index case.

- **Inadequate staffing:** Ten patients are there in the ward and only two nurses are posted there for their care
- **Inaccessibility to hand rub:** Hand rubs are available only at the entrance and nursing station but not at the bedside
- **No patient dedicated equipment:** There was only one stethoscope, BP apparatus and thermometer, etc. in the ward
- **Inappropriate use of gloves:** HCWs are using the same gloves in multiple occasions, without changing them when indicated
- **Patient placement is not followed:** Patient isolation or cohorting are not followed.

Refer Chapter 38 for further details.

DROPLET PRECAUTIONS: EXERCISE-7

A cluster of cases of upper respiratory tract infection (URTI) occurred in a long-term care facility, following a group activity held in a common food area of the hospital. All cases who attended the group activity had food, sitting close to each other at the dining table. One of the individual who attended the group activity was already suffering from URTI for four days. Due to the lack of waste bins in the dining room, used tissues were placed on the dining room tables.

The shared bathrooms were far from the dining area, therefore hand hygiene was not performed during the event. Eight individuals reported symptoms consistent with COVID-19, which was later confirmed by molecular test.
❖ Discuss the infection control breach that occurred
❖ What type of transmission-based precautions are needed for these cases when they are admitted in the ward?

Explanation

A cluster of COVID-19 (URTI) cases occurred in a long-term care facility following a group activity where one of the individual was already suffering from URTI. The factor which promoted the spread of infection include:
❖ **Overcrowding:** Group activity held in a common food area and individuals had food, sitting close to each other at the dining tables
❖ **Lack of droplet precaution by the index case:** The index case did not follow any measures of droplet precaution, such as wearing a surgical mask, hand hygiene, etc. He should not have attended any group activity when suffering from URTI
❖ **Inappropriate respiratory hygiene:** Due to the lack of waste bins in the dining room, used tissues were placed on the dining room tables
❖ **Inadequate hand hygiene** as hand hygiene facility was far away from the dining area.
Refer Chapter 38 for further details.

AIRBORNE PRECAUTIONS: EXERCISE-8

An intern is posted in tuberculosis isolation ward, which comprises of individual isolation rooms. His nature of job is to draw blood specimen, give injections, measure blood pressure, etc.
1. What type of transmission-based precaution is needed in a tuberculosis isolation ward? Discuss its components.
2. What are the recommended personal protective equipment (PPE) to be worn before he enters an isolation room?
3. Demonstrate the method of donning and doffing of each PPE with the correct sequence.
4. What are the precautions to be followed while donning and doffing of each PPE?

Explanation

M. tuberculosis is transmitted through aerosol. Therefore, aerosol precaution is needed. The recommended PPE to be worn before entering an isolation room are gloves, gown, N95 respirator and goggles/face shield. Refer Chapter 38 for further details.

STERILIZATION AND DISINFECTION PRACTICES: EXERCISE-9

What are the recommended methods for sterilization/disinfection of the following items in a healthcare facility—endoscope, culture media, ventilator tubes, operation theater disinfection, cleaning of the surgical instrument, stethoscope, wound disinfection?

Explanation

The recommended methods for sterilization/disinfection of following items in a healthcare facility are:
❖ **Endoscope:** 2% glutaraldehyde or 0.55% orthophthalaldehyde
❖ **Culture media:** Should be sterilized by autoclave (121°C for 15 min)
❖ **Ventilator tubes:** Can be sterilized at CSSD by ethylene oxide sterilizer, plasma sterilizer
❖ **Operation theater disinfection:** Cleaning with a detergent, followed by disinfection with a high level disinfectant, such as glutaraldehyde or hydrogen peroxide
❖ **Cleaning of surgical instruments:** The surgical instruments should be cleaned first with enzymatic (proteolytic) cleaners before sending to CSSD for sterilization

- **Stethoscope:** The external surfaces of stethoscope should be disinfected with alcohol 60–80% (isopropyl alcohol) after each use
- **Wound disinfection:** Povidone-iodine (5% topical solution and ointment) is recommended for wound disinfection. Refer Chapter 41 for further details.

BIOMEDICAL WASTE SEGREGATION AUDIT: EXERCISE-10

While examining the biomedical waste receptacles at the common collection point in a hospital, the following items were found. Find out how many items are segregated appropriately according to biomedical waste rule 2016.

Yellow bag	Red bag	White box	Blue box
1. N95 mask 2. Cyclophosphamide vial 3. Nitrile gloves 4. Central venous catheter 5. Coverall	1. Syringe 2. IV set 3. Blood bag 4. Nasogastric tube 5. Syringe with fixed needle	1. Microscopy slide 2. Metallic implant 3. Needle 4. Scalpel 5. Broken glass ampoule	1. Cytotoxic drug bottle 2. Glass ampoule (amikacin) 3. Stained cloth 4. Stained cotton 5. BacT/ALERT bottle

Explanation

The following are the correct items segregated in the biomedical waste receptacles.

Yellow bag	Red bag	White box	Blue box
Correctly segregated 1. N95 mask 2. Cyclophosphamide vial 3. Coverall **Not segregated correctly** 1. Nitrile gloves (red) 2. Central venous catheter (red)	**Correctly segregated** 1. Syringe 2. IV set 3. Nasogastric tube **Not segregated correctly** 1. Blood bag (yellow) 2. Syringe with fixed needle (white)	**Correctly segregated** 1. Needle 2. Scalpel **Not segregated correctly** 1. Microscopy slide (blue) 2. Metallic implant (blue) 3. Broken glass ampoule (blue)	**Correctly segregated** 1. Glass ampoule (amikacin) **Not segregated correctly** 1. Cytotoxic drug bottle (yellow) 2. Stained cloth (yellow) 3. Stained cotton (yellow) 4. BacT/ALERT bottle (red)

Refer Chapter 42 for further details.

NEEDLE STICK INJURY: EXERCISE-11 (CASE SCENARIO-1)

A 32-year-old staff working in the biomedical waste department reported to HICC with complaints of needle stick injury while segregating a yellow bag. The incident happened 18 hours back. He did not perform any first aid measures at the time of injury. He has not received any hepatitis B vaccination before. Discuss the post-exposure prophylaxis measures that should be undertaken.

Explanation

The source is unknown as the prick happened while segregating a yellow bag. Therefore, the following post-exposure prophylaxis measures need to be taken.
- **For HIV:** First dose of ART has to be given immediately (within 2 hr of exposure); followed by full course of ART for 28 days (Refer Chapter 43 for the drugs given in ART and the dosage)
- **For hepatitis B:** He should receive hepatitis B immunoglobulin plus hepatitis B vaccine series (three doses); 1st dose

to be taken now, followed by 2nd and 3rd dose after 1 month and 6 months respectively (Refer Chapter 43 for further details).

NEEDLE STICK INJURY: EXERCISE-12 (CASE SCENARIO-2)

A 28-year-old medicine resident reported to HICC with complaints of needle stick injury on his left thumb while recapping the needle. The incident happened 1 hr back. On enquiry, he mentioned that he had immediately washed his finger with running tap water for 2 minutes. The source sample was tested and was found to be positive for hepatitis B surface antigen and reactive for HIV antibodies. The resident had received a complete course (one series) of hepatitis B vaccine 10 years back, following which he had an anti-HBs titer of 550 mIU/mL. Discuss the post-exposure prophylaxis measures that should be undertaken.

Explanation

The source sample was found to be positive for hepatitis B surface antigen and reactive for HIV antibodies. Therefore, the following post-exposure prophylaxis measures need to be taken.

- **For HIV:** First dose of ART has to be given immediately (within 2 hr of exposure); followed by full course of ART for 28 days (Refer Chapter 43 for the drugs given in ART and the dosage)
- **For hepatitis B:** As he was vaccinated and protected with anti-HBs titer of 550 mIU/mL; therefore no further action (post-exposure prophylaxis) is necessary.

NEEDLE STICK INJURY: EXERCISE-13 (CASE SCENARIO-3)

A 41-year-old surgeon reported to HICC with complaints of surgical blade injury on his left thumb, 3 hr back. The source sample was tested positive for hepatitis B surface antigen, but negative for HIV antibodies and HCV antibodies. The surgeon had received two doses of hepatitis B vaccine 2 years back. Discuss the post-exposure prophylaxis measures that should be undertaken.

Explanation

The source sample was found to be positive for hepatitis B surface antigen but non-reactive for HIV. Therefore, the following post-exposure prophylaxis measures need to be taken.

- **For HIV:** No further action (post-exposure prophylaxis) is necessary
- **For hepatitis B:** He was partially vaccinated for hepatitis B, therefore, he should be given hepatitis B immunoglobulin plus the third dose hepatitis B vaccine (Refer Chapter 43 for further details).

CHAPTER 56: Patient Safety

CHAPTER PREVIEW
- What is Patient Safety?
- Patient Safety Indicators
- Incidents and Adverse Events
- International Patient Safety Goals

WHAT IS PATIENT SAFETY?

Patient safety is a healthcare discipline that has emerged with the evolving complexity in healthcare systems as a result of the rise in patient harm in healthcare facilities.
- ❖ It aims to prevent and reduce errors, risks, and harm that occur to patients while providing healthcare
- ❖ This discipline relies on continuous improvement based on learning from errors and adverse events
- ❖ Patient safety is fundamental to delivering quality essential health services. Quality health services across the world should be effective, safe, and patient-centered
- ❖ To ensure successful implementation of patient safety strategies, skilled health care professionals, effective involvement of patients in their care, and data to drive safety improvements are all needed
- ❖ It is essential to gather information on potentially avoidable safety events which can improve the delivery of care to patients and this can be achieved by:
  - Monitoring a certain set of indicators named—patient safety indicators (PSIs)
  - Capturing incidents and adverse events and their root cause analysis (RCA).

PATIENT SAFETY INDICATORS

The patient safety indicators (PSIs) are a set of measures that can be used with hospital inpatient discharge data in turn to provide a correct perspective on patient safety. More specifically, they focus on potential in-hospital complications and iatrogenic adverse events following surgeries, procedures, and childbirth.

The examples of commonly used patient safety indicators in the healthcare setting are:
- ❖ Care for vulnerable patients
- ❖ Prevention of iatrogenic injury
- ❖ Care of lines, drains, and tubing's
- ❖ Restrain policy and care—physical and chemical
- ❖ Blood and blood transfusion policy
- ❖ Prevention of IV complication
- ❖ Prevention of fall
- ❖ Prevention of DVT
- ❖ Shifting and transporting of patients
- ❖ Surgical safety
- ❖ Care coordination events related to medication reconciliation and administration
- ❖ Prevention of communication errors
- ❖ **Prevention of HAI:** This component has been discussed in detail in Chapters 36 to 40 of this book
- ❖ Documentation.

A brief explanation of some of the important safety indicators has given below.

Care for Vulnerable Patients

Vulnerable patient: A patient may be for any reason unable to protect and take care of themselves, against significant harm or exploitation. Five important strategies to manage vulnerable patients:
1. Understand their needs
2. Partner with other community resources
3. Match needs to services
4. Execute safe transitions
5. Determine post-discharge steps for care.

Prevention of Iatrogenic Injury

Iatrogenic injury refers to tissue or organ damage caused by needed medical treatment, pharmacotherapy, or the use of medical devices. The steps that can prevent iatrogenic injury include— restriction of self-medication, increased knowledge of contraindications, and lowering the number of simultaneous drugs.

Care of Lines, Drains, and Tubings

Safety considerations to be followed are as follows:
- The drain or all tubings should be below the patient's chest level to facilitate drainage
- Tubing should have no obstructions
- Ensure all connections between chest tubes and drainage unit are tight and secure.

Restrain Policy and Care

Restrain policy must be followed, if any patient's behavior has the potential to cause harm to the individual, others, or serious property damage. Nurses assess and reassess the patients regularly to ensure the safety of that patient as well as of others.

Blood and Blood Transfusion Policy

This policy aims to ensure an easily accessible and adequate supply of safe blood and blood products procured from a voluntary blood donor, which is free from transfusion-transmitted infections and is stored under optimum conditions.

Prevention of Fall

Falls can take a serious impact on the quality of life and independence. Steps to be taken to prevent patient falls in hospitals are:
- Secure locks on beds, stretchers, and wheelchairs. Keep floors obstacle-free
- Place call light and frequently needed objects within patient reach.

Surgical Safety

Surgical safety is a very important patient safety indicator. WHO has developed a surgical safety checklist to ensure patient safety for those undergoing the surgery. These checklists should be filled by a nurse, anesthesiologist, and a surgeon. Important components of this checklist are:
- Before induction of anesthesia
- Before skin incision
- Before a patient leaves the operating room.

Prevention of Communication Errors

Patient safety can be ensured by effective communication among physicians, staff, and patients. The use of universal precautions for health literacy, appropriate medical interpretations, and shared decision-making are evidence-based tools that improve communication and increase patient safety.

Documentation

Good documentation is important to protect patients. It promotes patient safety and quality of care. Complete and accurate medical recordkeeping can help to ensure that patients get the right care at the right time.

INCIDENTS AND ADVERSE EVENTS

An incident or adverse event is an event that causes or could have caused damage to the patient, and which is not due to the patient's underlying condition.

- Examples of adverse drug events include— dosage errors, incorrect administration of the medicine, or mix-ups of product names or packaging
- The approach that can be followed by most healthcare organizations to detect adverse events and incidents includes the following sequential steps.

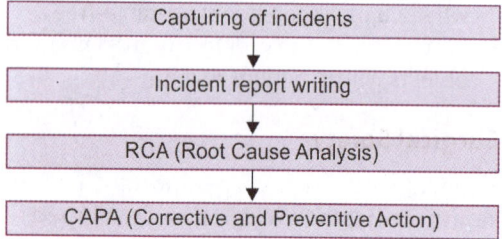

Capturing of Incidents

Identifying an incident and subsequent analysis to determine its characteristics is a crucial step in patient safety improvement. This is because it enables subsequent development and implementation of preventative measures. A certain set of indicators or checklists are used to capture the incident and the adverse events in a healthcare setting. An incident is usually presented via an incident report.

Incident Report Writing

An incident report is a form to document all workplace injuries, illnesses, near misses, and accidents. An incident report should be completed at the time the incident occurs, no matter how minor the injury is.

- Completing an incident report form when an incident occurrence has happened and following it up with an additional investigation, corrective action, hazard report, and sign-off
- These follow-on forms ensure that the causes of incident occurrence are investigated to prevent the same from happening again
- An incident report form might be completed by the staff involved in the incident that occurred or it might be completed by a safety manager on their behalf
- An illustration of the incident report form has been depicted in **Figure 56.1**— Needlestick injury reporting proforma.

Root Cause Analysis

Root cause analysis (RCA) is the investigation process following an incident. The incident may or may not have caused harm to a person or property. Incidents may not have occurred at all, but instead, someone reported a dangerous situation. In both the above situation, a root cause analysis should be conducted.

- An RCA is conducted by following 6 steps, beginning with the incident report and ending with a comprehensive root cause analysis
- Understanding each stage of the root cause analysis is vital for successful preventive action plans and implementation
- Various steps of RCA are depicted in **Figure 56.2**.

Corrective and Preventive Actions

The purpose of the corrective and preventive action (CAPA) subsystem is to collect information, analyze information, identify, investigate and take appropriate and effective corrective and/or preventive action to prevent their recurrence. The following steps are followed in a CAPA:

- Verifying or validating corrective and preventive actions
- Communicating corrective and preventive action activities to responsible people
- Providing relevant information for management review and documenting these activities.

The above steps are essential in dealing effectively with product and quality problems, preventing their recurrence, and preventing or minimizing device failures.

INTERNATIONAL PATIENT SAFETY GOALS

The International Patient Safety Goals (IPSG) were developed in 2006 by the Joint

Employment ID:	**Date of exposure:**		**Time:**	**Date of reporting:**	**Time:**

Name: **Age:** **Sex:** **Hospital no:**

Mobile no: **Intercom no:**

Job category: Doctor ☐ Nurse ☐ Technician ☐ Attender ☐ Housekeeping staff ☐
Student ☐ Others: ....

Place of the incident:

Source/Patient: Known ☐ Unknown ☐ **Name:** **Hospital number:**

Type of contact: Needle-stick ☐ Sharp ☐ (OR) Mucocutaneous exposure ☐

If the exposure involved needle stick and sharp object
1. Were you the original user of the sharp item?   Yes ☐   No ☐
2. Was there blood on the device?   Yes ☐   No ☐   Unknown ☐

3. Source patient status for blood borne viruses (BBVs) at the time of exposure/reporting:
 - Test for BBVs done in last six months and report available ☐
   – HIV: Positive ☐/Negative ☐ Date_____
   – HBV: Positive ☐/Negative ☐ Date_____
   – HCV: Positive ☐/Negative ☐ Date_____
 -Test for BBVs is either not done in last six months, or done but report not available ☐

4. For what purpose was the sharp item originally used?
    a. Unknown ☐
    b. Injection -- intra-muscular ☐ subcutaneous ☐ intradermal ☐
    C. To draw blood sample ---   arterial ☐   venous ☐   subcutaneous ☐
    d. To place IV line --   arterial ☐   central line ☐
    e. To obtain a body fluid or tissue sample --   urine ☐ CSF ☐ Amniotic fluid ☐ Other fluid.........
    f. Suturing ☐   Biopsy ☐   During operation ☐
    g. Other: Specify......................

5. Did the injury occur?   ☐ Before use of item (item broke/slipped, assembling device, etc.)   ☐ During use of item *(item slipped, patient jarred item, etc.)*   ☐ While recapping the used needle   ☐ Device left on floor, table, bed or other inappropriate place   ☐ While cleaning the item   ☐ From item left on or near disposal container   ☐ While putting item into disposal container   ☐ After disposal, stuck by item protruding from opening of disposal container   ☐ Other: Specify: ....
6. Type of device caused the injury: Needle   Hollow-bore ☐ Plain ☐ Instrument ☐ Glass ☐ Unknown ☐
7. Specify the instrument that caused the injury:
8. What was the site of the injury?
9. Was the injury?   ☐ Superficial *(little of no bleeding)*   ☐ Moderate *(skin puncture, some bleeding)*   ☐ Severe *(deep stick/cut, or profuse bleeding)*
10. Gloves used   Single pair ☐   Double pair ☐   No gloves ☐   Not applicable ☐
Describe the incidence in own words

Contd...

Contd...

The exposure (splashes) involved blood and body fluid:
1. Type of body fluid which was involved in the exposure?
2. Was the body fluid visibly contaminated with blood? Yes ☐ No ☐ Unknown ☐
3. What was the exposed part? (Check all that apply)   Intact skin ☐ Non-intact skin ☐ Nose (mucosa) ☐ Mouth ☐ Conjunctiva ☐ Others ....
4. What were all barrier garment(s) worn at the time of exposure?   Gloves ☐ Surgical mask ☐ Plastic apron ☐ Goggle ☐ Surgical gown ☐   Eyeglasses (Not a protective item) ☐ Lab coat ☐ Other ....

5. Was the exposure the result of?
    a. Direct patient contact
    b. Specimen container leaked/spilled/broke
    C. Touched contaminated drapes/sheets/gowns, etc.

6. If equipment failure (device malfunction), Specify: Equipment type and manufacturer
7. For how long was the blood or body fluid in contact with your skin or mucous membranes?   < 5 minutes ☐   5-14 minutes ☐   15 min-1 hour ☐   >1 hour ☐

8. How much blood/body fluid came in contact with your skin or mucous membranes?
    a. Small amount - Few drops
    b. Large amount - Several drops or splashes

9. Do you have an opinion that any other engineering control, administrative or work practice could have prevented the injury? Yes ☐ No ☐ Unknown ☐ If yes then specify-   ....

POST EXPOSURE FOLLOW-UP

SOURCE INFORMATION:
1. Source known and tested:
2. Source known but not tested, reason:
3. Source not known

If the source patient was believed to be high-risk group for blood borne pathogens:
Blood product recipient ☐ Injection drug use ☐ Sex worker ☐ Hemophilia ☐ Dialysis ☐ Others ....

INFORMATION OF THE HEALTHCARE WORKER:

First aid:

First dose of ART taken:	Yes ☐ No ☐	If Yes, Date:	Time:

Vaccination status of HCW
1. Complete vaccination with anti HBs titer tested   Date.......... Protective ☐ Not protective ☐
2. Complete vaccination with no titer testing   Date of last dose: ....
3. Incomplete vaccination   Date of last dose: .... No. of doses ....
4. No vaccination

Whether HCW is pregnant: Yes ☐ No ☐ Not applicable ☐ If yes, trimester: First ☐ second ☐ third ☐

RESULTS OF BASELINE TESTS:

Test	SOURCE		HEALTHCARE WORKER	
HIV antibody	Positive ☐	Negative ☐	Positive ☐	Negative ☐
HBsAg	Positive ☐	Negative ☐	Positive ☐	Negative ☐
HCV antibody	Positive ☐	Negative ☐	Positive ☐	Negative ☐
Anti-HBs antibody	Not applicable		Protective ☐	Not protective ☐

Follow-up advice given-
1. Tests for HIV, HBV, HCV are scheduled on.............
2. Referred to ART clinic Yes/No
3. HBV vaccine taken on next dose scheduled on.............
4. Hepatitis B immunoglobulin taken on ....

INFECTION CONTROL NURSE (SIGNATURE)

Fig. 56.1: Needlestick injury reporting proforma.

Source: Form adapted and modified from Hospital Infection Control Committee (HICC), JIPMER, Puducherry *(with permission).*
Courtesy: Medical Superintendent, JIPMER, Puducherry.

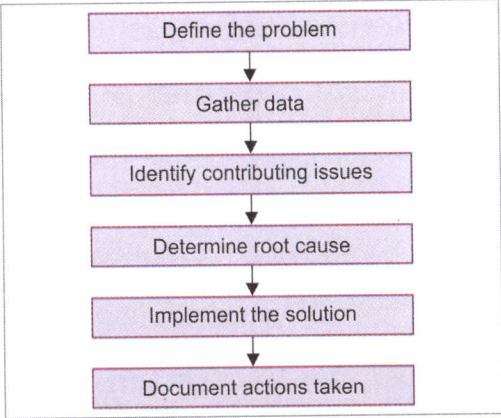

Fig. 56.2: Steps of root cause analysis (RCA).

Commission International (JCI). Compliance with IPSG has been monitored in JCI-accredited hospitals since January 2006. The JCI recommends targeted solution tools to help the hospital to meet IPSG standards. The Joint Commission has updated the IPSGs over time: The current version has the following goals:

- Goal 1: Identify patients correctly
- Goal 2: Improve effective communication
- Goal 3: Improve the safety of high-alert medications
- Goal 4: Ensure safe surgery
- Goal 5: Reduce the risk of healthcare-associated infections. This component has been discussed in detail in Chapters 36 to 40 of this book
- Goal 6: Reduce the risk of patient harm resulting from falls.

The above components of patient safety goals have been already explained under patient safety indicators.

CHAPTER 57: Safety Protocol for Healthcare Personnel

CHAPTER PREVIEW
- Safety Protocol
- Role of Nurse in Disaster Management
- Employee Safety Indicators

SAFETY PROTOCOL

Hospitals always strive to ensure their patients' safety but ignore the fact that even healthcare staff also face work-related hazards and need protection from both physical as well as psychological harm.

- ❖ A healthcare facility usually involves working with various physical, chemical, and biological hazards and handling equipment of different nature
- ❖ Healthcare staff needs to be aware of the various hazards specific to their workspace
- ❖ Standard precautions and transmission-based precautions are followed to reduce the risk of transmission of infection from both recognized and unrecognized sources (refer to Chapters 37 and 38 for details)
- ❖ To ensure workplace safety for all healthcare workers safety protocol should be in place and should be followed by all healthcare workers.

Various components of the safety protocol are listed in **Table 57.1**.

Table 57.1: Various components of safety protocol to be followed in a healthcare facility.
- Five S's (Sort, Set in order, Shine, Standardize, Sustain)
- Radiation safety
- Laser safety
- Fire safety
  - Types and classification of fire
  - Fire alarms
  - Firefighting equipment
- HAZMAT (Hazardous Materials) safety
- Types of spill and spillage management
- MSDS (Material Safety Data Sheets)
- Environmental safety
- Risk assessment
- Maintenance of temperature and humidity
- Audits
- Emergency codes

Five S's (Sort, Set in order, Shine, Standardize, Sustain)

It provides a methodology for organizing, cleaning, developing, and sustaining a productive work environment. Various steps of 5 S's are:
1. **Sort:** Remove unnecessary items from each area
2. **Set in order:** Organize and identify storage for effective use
3. **Shine:** Clean and inspect each area regularly
4. **Standardize:** Setting up procedures for performing these tasks
5. **Sustain:** Perform these tasks on regular basis.

Radiation Safety

The radiation safety principle includes—"**ALARA**". ALARA stands for "as low as reasonably achievable". It means that even if it is a small dose, if there is no benefit to receiving the dose, then better try to avoid it. Three basic protective measures involved are: time, distance, and shielding.

- **Time:** Minimize the time near a radiation source to only as long as it takes to complete a task
- **Distance:** Maximize your distance from a radioactive source as much as possible to minimize the exposure
- **Shielding:** In a radiation emergency, to shield yourself from a radiation source, put something between you and the source.

Laser Safety

Five important laser safety measures are:
1. Wear laser safety glasses: As lasers can cause significant damage to the eyes, wearing laser safety glasses is a must
2. Ensure proper storage
3. Follow standards and regulations
4. Work with trained personnel
5. Use warning signs boards.

Fire Safety

Personnel working in the hospitals should be familiar with the location and operation of all safety equipment like fire extinguishers and other facilities available like electrical mains, electrical fuses, and gas connections. Keep exits and passageways clear at all times for easy evacuation in case of fire accidents.

Types and Classification of Fire

Various types of fire are:
- Class A—fires involving solid materials such as wood, paper, etc.
- Class B—fires involving flammable liquids such as petrol, or oils
- Class C—fires involving gases
- Class D—fires involving metals
- Electrical fires: Any fire involving electrical equipment.

Firefighting Equipment

Fire detection and alarm systems include—smoke or spark detectors, and automatic or manual fire alarm systems. Other accessories include—water and sand bucket, hammer, fire axe, fire blanket, emergency lights, etc.

- **A fire alarm system** warns people when smoke, fire, carbon monoxide, or other fire-related emergencies are detected
- These alarms may be activated automatically from smoke detectors and heat detectors.

HAZMAT (Hazardous Materials) Safety

A hazardous material is any waste that poses a substantial or potential threat to human health or the environment. Classifications of hazardous materials:
- Class 1: Explosives
- Class 2: Gases
- Class 3: Flammable liquids
- Class 4: Flammable solids
- Class 5: Organic peroxides
- Class 6: Toxic and infectious substances
- Class 7: Radioactive material
- Class 8: Corrosives.

This waste, if not managed properly, increases the risk of infection, injuries, and exposure to harmful toxins. The process of dealing with healthcare waste consists of the following steps:
- Waste minimization by re-use and recycling
- Waste segregation
- Waste collection
- Waste storage
- Waste transportation
- Waste treatment
- Waste disposal.

Types of Spill and Spillage Management

Two types of spills are minor and major spills.

A minor chemical spill is one that the healthcare staff is capable of handling safely without the assistance of safety and emergency personnel. All other chemical spills are considered major.

Safety During Spills

Steps involved in the management of various spillages have been described below:

- Reagent spills should be washed with copious amounts of water
- Spillages of non-hazardous materials, such as water or saline, onto the floor can make the floor slippery and thus a potential danger of causing injury due to falling. Clean up such spills immediately
- If an inflammable spill is large, contact Maintenance Department. Arrange to isolate the electrical supply. Do not use switches in the immediate area as a spark from the switch may ignite a spill. Provide adequate ventilation and open the doors/windows wherever possible. Do not cross the spill or move further into the room
- In case of urine spill, do not use a chlorine releasing agent directly on a urine spill, as it promotes the release of free chlorine from the treated area
  - Place a mop cloth/gauze pad over the spill area, to allow urine and debris to get absorbed
  - Clean the surface thoroughly using detergent and water and dry thoroughly
  - Decontaminate the area with a solution of 1,000 ppm available chlorine solution.
- Blood spills management is described in detail in Chapter 42.

Material Safety Data Sheets (MSDS)

It is a technical document that provides comprehensive information on a controlled product related to:
- Health effects of exposure to the product
- Hazard evaluation related to the product's handling, storage, or use
- Measure to protect workers at risk of exposure
- Emergency procedures.

The data sheet may be written, or printed and must meet the availability, design, and content requirements of Workplace Hazardous Materials Information System (WHMIS) legislation.

Environmental Safety

Environmental safety is the guidance, policies, and practices enforced to ensure that the surrounding environment is free from hazards that will warrant the safety and well-being of healthcare staff and residents near the healthcare facility.

The best ways to ensure environmental and workplace safety are:
- Train thoroughly
- Review past mistakes
- Ensure proper communication
- Check your equipment
- Focus on risk management
- Coordinate with professionals.

Risk Assessment

It is a process to identify potential hazards and to analyze what could happen if a hazard occurs. There are numerous hazards to consider. In healthcare premises, hazards can range from slips, trips, and fire, the chemicals used, electrical equipment, and even microbiological hazards.

Recording the findings on a datasheet
- Every datasheet requires the date of the assessment and documented copies should be kept for five years
- Each assessment should be shared with the relevant staff members, who should also date and sign it
- This helps improve procedures and is key to training staff and enhancing service levels.

Maintenance of Temperature and Humidity

The Centers for Disease Control and Prevention (CDC) recommends the following temperature ranges for healthcare facilities based on zone:
- **Cool temperature standards (20–23°C)** are typically associated with operating rooms, endoscopy, and clean workrooms
- **Warmer temperatures (24°C)** are recommended in hospital patient rooms
- **A standard temperature range of (21–24°C)** can be used in most other healthcare zones.

Relative humidity should be maintained between 20% and 60% in a healthcare facility.

Audits

Audits are about accountability.
- ❖ Audits assure that effective programs are in place for identifying, eliminating, or controlling hazards that could adversely impact a hospital's physical and human assets
- ❖ The best time to conduct an audit is during a time when work practices can be observed as they are normally conducted and when there will be the least number of distractions to the normal work procedures.

Emergency Codes

Hospitals often use code names to alert their staff to an emergency. These codes can be communicated through an intercom in the hospital or directly to staff using communication devices.

Codes allow trained hospital personnel to respond quickly and appropriately to various events. The use of codes can also help prevent concern or panic by visitors and people being treated at the hospital.

Examples of some of the emergency codes used in the hospitals are:
- ❖ Code blue: Cardiac arrest
- ❖ Code red: Fire or smoke
- ❖ Code orange: Hazardous material or spill incident
- ❖ Code yellow: Disaster
- ❖ Code white: Evacuation
- ❖ Code green: Emergency activation.

ROLE OF NURSE IN TIMES OF DISASTER

During the disaster, nurses activate the disaster plan in their hospitals, triage cases, provide emergency treatment for injured people, and coordinate evacuations and the transportation of patients to other medical facilities. A nurse may be assigned a variety of tasks during a disaster such as delivering first aid and medication, assessing the state of victims, and monitoring mental health needs.

EMPLOYEE SAFETY INDICATORS

Employee safety indicators are as followed:
- ❖ **Vaccination:** The immunization indicated for healthcare workers has been described in Chapter 46
- ❖ **Needlestick injuries (NSI):** It has been discussed in Chapter 43
- ❖ **Fall prevention:** Work-related slip, trip, and fall incidents can frequently result in serious disabling injuries that impact a healthcare employee's ability to do his or her job and diminished ability to care for patients. Fall can be prevented by:
  - Keep floors clean and dry
  - Wear slip-resistant shoes
  - Prevent entry into areas that are wet by keeping caution boards
  - Clear walkways and work areas to allow employees to move more freely and safely
  - Incorporate slip, trip, and fall awareness and prevention into routine safety training.
- ❖ **Radiation safety:** It has been already discussed under the safety protocol
- ❖ **Annual health check:** An annual health checkup or periodic health check is useful as it can help detect and identify diseases or the warning signs of an impending disease very early. Hospitals can develop their own policies for the list of investigations to be included in annual health checkups for their healthcare workers.

For Multidrug Resistant Organisms (MDROs) in Hospital

CONTACT PRECAUTIONS
EVERYONE MUST:

Clean their hands, including before entering and when leaving the room.

PROVIDERS AND STAFF MUST ALSO:

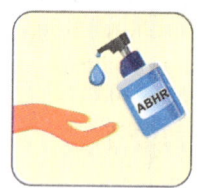

Put on gloves before room entry. Discard gloves before room exit.

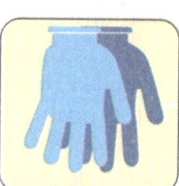

Put on gown before room entry. Discard gown before room exit.

Do not wear the same gown and gloves for the care of more than one person.

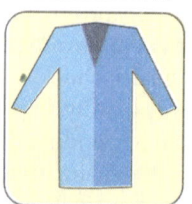

Use dedicated of disposable equipment. Clean and disinfect reusable equipment before use on another person.

Material is developed by CDC

Index

Page numbers followed by *f* refer to figure and *t* refer to table.

A

Abscess 376
  amoebic liver 198
Acid-fast bacilli 21*f*, 121*f*
Acid-fast staining 22, 124, 365, 380
Acinetobacter 35, 274, 281, 287, 354, 356
Acquired immunity 68, 68*t*
Acquired immunodeficiency syndrome 176, 178, 193
Actinomycetes 115
Actinomycetoma 247, 248
Active immunity 69, 70, 70*t*
Active immunoprophylaxis 93
Adaptive immunity 68
Adenovirus 44, 62, 153, 275
Adult respiratory distress syndrome 285
Aedes
  aegypti 165, 168
  albopictus 165
Aerosol generating procedures 276, 277
African sleeping sickness 207
Agglutination reaction 76, 81
Air surveillance 328
Airborne precautions 276, 385
Albert's stain 22, 113, 113*f*
Alcohol 306
Aldehyde 305
Algid malaria 210
Amoeba 51, 197
  free-living 7*f*, 197, 201
Anaerobic culture 19, 20, 376
Anaphylactic reactions 223
Anchovy sauce pus 198
Ancylostoma 233
Antibiogram 340
Antibody 74, 75, 91, 186
Antibody-mediated immune response 72
Antigen 74, 130
Antigen-antibody reactions, types of 81
Antigenic drift 156, 156*t*
Antigenic shift 156
Antimicrobial agent 34, 35*t*, 338
Antimicrobial resistance 34, 335
Antimicrobial stewardship program 294, 335
Anti-rabies prophylaxis 172*t*
Antiretroviral therapy 324
Arbovirus 165
Ascaris lumbricoides 231
Aspergillosis 250, 252-254
Automated antimicrobial susceptibility tests 28
Automated blood culture systems 25, 129
Automated identification systems 105

B

B lymphocytes 71
Babesia 214, 346
Bacillus
  anthracis 12, 13, 42, 114
Bacteremia 103, 136, 345
Bacterial endotoxins 42*t*
Bacterial genetics 31
Bacterial growth 15
  curve 15, 16*f*, 16*t*
Bacterial meningitis, acute 349, 350
Bacterial pathogenesis 39
Bacteriophages 154, 154*f*
Bacteroides fragilis 39, 119
Balamuthia mandrillaris 201
Balantidium coli 218
Bartonella 144
Biofire film array 351
Biomedical waste 262, 270, 313, 317*f*
Biphasic medium 24*f*, 25, 348*f*
BK virus 153
Blackwater fever 210
Blastocystis hominis 218
Blastomyces 346
Blood 262
  collection of 347*f*
  spill management 319
Blood culture 20, 129
  bottles 348*f*
  specimen collection for 347
Bloodstream infection 345, 346, 373
Bordetella pertussis 138, 363, 375
Borrelia 345
  vincentii 363
Botulism, infant 118
Brugia malayi 53, 229, 237, 239, 239*f*, 240

C

Calabar swelling 240
Candida albicans 250, 251*f*, 260
Capsule, demonstration of 12
Castleman's disease 193
Catheter-associated urinary tract infection 135, 280, 282, 292*t*, 294
Catheter-related bloodstream infection 282
Central sterile services department 298, 299*f*
Chagas' disease 207
Chemiluminescence immunoassay 86, 186
Chickenpox 62, 151
Chlamydia 35, 144, 274, 355, 364, 365
Cholera 134
Christie-Atkins-Munch-Peterson test 104
Chronic meningitis 349, 351
  agents of 352*t*
Clonorchis sinensis 227
Clostridium
  botulinum 42, 116, 118, 359
  difficile 118
  perfringens 35, 116, 117*f*
  tetani 16, 42, 61, 94, 116, 117, 118*f*
Clue cells 139
Coagulase test 105*f*
Coagulase-negative staphylococci 104, 106

Index

Coccidioidomycosis 249
Complement pathways 68, 78f
Condylomata lata 141
Congenital rubella syndrome 160
Coronavirus disease 2019 (COVID-19) 62, 63, 95, 161, 163, 382
Corynebacterium diphtheriae 22, 35, 42, 94, 112, 113f, 362
Cough etiquette 262, 276, 279
Coxiella burnetii 144
Creutzfeldt-Jakob disease 194
Cryptococcus neoformans 56, 251, 252f
Cryptosporidium 217, 218f, 326, 358
Cutaneous anthrax 114
Cutaneous larva migrans 235, 241
Cyclospora 217, 218f, 358
  cayetanensis 217
Cysticercosis 220-222
Cystoisospora 217, 218f
  belli 217
Cytomegalovirus 152
  infections 152

D

Dendritic cells 68, 72
Dengue 165, 166
Dermatophytoses 246, 246t, 247
Diarrheal diseases 357, 373
  laboratory diagnosis of 359
Dimorphic fungi 56, 249
Diphtheria 70, 112, 113, 275, 362
  toxin 112
Diphyllobothrium latum 224
Direct fluorescent antibody 171
  tests 365
Dracunculiasis 241
Droplet transmission 62
Dry heat sterilizer 303, 304f
Dysentery 218

E

Ear infections 136, 370, 371, 373
Echinococcus granulosus 219, 222
Eijkman test 327
Elek's gel precipitation test 81
Endotoxins 42
Entamoeba coli 197
Entamoeba histolytica 197, 199f, 326, 358
Enteric fever 128, 131
Enterobacterales 35, 126
Enterobiasis 231
Enterococcus 35, 109, 287

Entero-test 201
Enzyme-linked fluorescence assay 47, 85
Enzyme-linked immunosorbent assay 47, 83, 167, 200
Epidermodysplasia verruciformis 153
Epstein-Barr virus 152, 193, 370
Escherichia coli 13, 15, 16, 24, 35, 39, 126, 327, 349, 354
ESKAPE pathogens 260
Eumycetoma 247, 248

F

Fasciola hepatica 227, 227f
Fasciolopsis buski 226, 227, 227f
Fatty diarrhea 201
Filarial dance sign 239
Filarial nematodes 7, 237
Fimbriae 13, 41
Flagella 13
Flash sterilization 302
Floppy child syndrome 118
Fluorescence microscope 7, 8f, 46
Food poisoning 104, 358
Food-borne botulism 118
Fusobacterium fusiformis 363

G

Gardnerella vaginalis 135, 139, 369
Gas gangrene 116, 117
GeneXpert 122
German measles 159
Giant-cell pneumonitis 158
Giardia 197, 358
  duodenalis 201, 202, 202f
Gloves 264, 265, 382
  donning, steps of 266f
Gonococcus 111f
Gown donning, steps of 269f
Gown removal, steps of 269f
Gram stain 9, 10t, 15, 20, 21f, 56, 110, 113, 114, 117, 286, 351t, 380
Griffith experiment 32
Guinea worm disease 229, 241

H

H1N1 flu 156
HACEK group 138
Haemophilus
  ducreyi 138
  influenzae 12, 13, 15, 23, 36, 95, 114, 137, 138f, 275, 349, 362, 364, 365

Halophilic vibrio 134
Hand hygiene 262, 263, 263f, 264, 265, 270, 274, 275, 381
Hand wash 263, 264, 381
  steps of 263, 264f
Healthcare-associated infection 59, 104, 135, 259, 260, 280, 292, 294t
Helicobacter pylori 40, 135, 139
Helminths 51, 51t, 357
Hemorrhagic cystitis 153
Hepatitis viruses 183, 183t
Hepatitis A virus 183
Hepatitis B 184, 184, 184f, 187, 193, 260, 295, 325t, 333, 386, 387
Hepatitis C 183, 188, 189, 193, 260
Herd immunity 70
Herpes simplex virus 149
Hide Porter's disease 114
Histoplasmosis 249
Hospital antibiogram 340
Hospital infection control 3, 257
Human immunodeficiency virus 176
Human oncogenic viruses 193t
Hydatid disease 224
Hymenolepis nana 219, 224

I

Immunity 11, 67
Immunochromatographic test 47, 53, 87, 200
Immunoglobulin 49, 96
Infection control 262, 296
  measures 106, 113, 123, 151, 274, 275, 331
Infectious mononucleosis 82, 152
Infective endocarditis 103, 136
Influenza 62, 157, 295, 333
Innate immunity 67, 68, 68t
Interferon 48
Intestinal amoebae 197
Intestinal flagellates 201
Intestinal flukes 226, 227
Intestinal nematodes infections 51, 229
Intestinal taeniasis 220, 220f, 221
Intrinsic resistance 34
Invasive aspergillosis 254
Ionizing radiation 305

J

Japanese B encephalitis 168
JC virus 153

Index

K

Kala-azar elimination 207
Kaposi's sarcoma 193
Katayama fever 226
Kirby-Bauer's disk diffusion 28
Klebsiella 35, 281, 354
Koch's postulates 4
Koplik's spots 157, 158*f*
Kyasanur forest disease virus 167

L

Lancefield grouping 106, 107
Larva 219, 232
    currens 235
    migrans 241
Legionnaires disease 139
Leishmaniasis 205*f*
Lepromatous leprosy 124, 124*t*
Leprosy 125
Leptospirosis 144
Listeria 35, 115
Loa loa 229, 237, 240
Loeffler's syndrome 231
Ludwig's angina 362
Lymphatic filariasis 237, 240

M

Madura foot 247
Malaria 208, 213
Malassezia furfur 245
Malignant pustule 114*f*
Maltese cross forms 214
McFadyean's reaction 114
McIntosh and Filde's anaerobic jar 26, 26*f*
Measles 63, 158
Megaloblastic anemia 224
Methicillin-resistant *Staphylococcus aureus* 38, 105
Microscopic agglutination test 82, 144
Molluscum contagiosum virus 153
Monkeypox virus 153
Monoclonal antibody 77
Montenegro test 206
Moraxella catarrhalis 362
Morganella 281
Mucormycosis 252
Mueller-Hinton agar 28, 356
Multiple tube method 327, 328*f*
Mumps 62, 275
Mycetoma 247, 248
Mycobacteria infections 120
Mycoplasma 35, 36, 146, 364, 365
Mycotoxicosis 253
Myxoviruses 155

N

Naegleria fowleri 201
Natural killer cells 68, 71
Needle stick injury 321, 386, 387, 397
Neisseria
    gonorrhoeae 63, 109, 110, 370
    meningitidis 41, 109
Neurocysticercosis 221, 222*f*
Nipah virus 159
Nocardia 115, 248
    species 247
Nonfermenter gram-negative bacilli 135
Non-sporing anaerobes 119
Nontuberculous mycobacteria 120, 125
Non-typhoidal salmonellae 128
Nonvenereal treponema species 143

O

Omicron detection 163
Onchocerca volvulus 229, 237, 240
Oncogenic viruses 193
Opisthorchis viverrini 227
Oral live attenuated vaccines 134
Oral polio vaccine 70, 174, 174*t*, 175
Oriental sore 207
Orientia tsutsugamushi 144
Orthomyxoviruses 155
Otitis externa 371
Otitis media 371

P

P24 antigen detection 179, 181
Papillomaviruses 153
Paracoccidioides 346
    brasiliensis 56, 249
Paracoccidioidomycosis 249
Paragonimus westermani 226, 227, 227*f*, 363
Parainfluenza viruses 157
Paramyxoviruses 155
Parvovirus B19 62, 153, 275
Paul Bunnell test 82
Penicillium marneffei 56, 254
Pernicious malaria 210
Personal protective equipment 157, 193, 262, 263, 266*f*, 270, 274, 275, 277, 317, 382, 385
Pertussis 275
Piedra 245
Plasmodium 7, 208, 346, 379
Pneumococcus 108
Polyomaviruses 153
Post-kala-azar dermal leishmaniasis 206
Pour plate technique 25
Prozone phenomenon 81
Pseudomonas 35, 42, 274, 281, 287, 354, 356
Pulmonary anthrax 114
Pulmonary aspergillosis 253
Pulmonary tuberculosis 120, 373
Pulse polio immunization 175
Pyogenic meningitis 350, 351, 351*t*

Q

Quantitative buffy coat examination 212, 239
Quellung reaction 13

R

Rabies 170, 172, 334
Rapid diagnostic test 213
Rat-bite fever 139
Real-time polymerase chain reaction 29, 30, 47, 163, 189, 200
Reye's syndrome 151
Rhinoscleroma 362
Rhinosporidiosis 248
Rhinovirus 62, 275
Rhizopus 253*f*
Rice-water stool 133
Rickettsia 35, 144
Ringworm 246
Rose Gardner's disease 248
Rotavirus 44, 192*f*
Roundworm 231
Rubella 62, 63, 159, 275

S

Salmonella 128, 326, 327, 354
Schistosoma 226
Seasonal flu 156
Serratia marcescens 132, 305
Serum, sickness 92
Shigella 131, 326, 327, 358
Sleeping sickness 207

Slow virus 194*t*
Smallpox virus 62, 153
Spaulding's classification 300*t*
Spill management 322
Sporotrichosis 248
Staphylococcus 35, 103
Streptobacillus moniliformis 135, 139
Streptococcus 36, 106
Strongyloidiasis 235
Surgical mask 266
    and respirators 265
Surgical site infection 135, 286, 287*t*, 288, 293*t*
Swimmer's ear 136
Swimming pool granuloma 125
Syphilis 141, 143

T

Taenia saginata 219, 220
Taenia solium 219-221
Tinea 246
Toxic shock syndrome 104
Toxoplasmosis 217
Trematode infections 226
Treponema pallidum 17, 35, 141
Trichinella spiralis 229, 237, 241

Trichomonas infections 197
Trichuris 229
Trypanosoma 204, 207, 346
    brucei complex 207
Tuberculosis 122, 123, 363
Typhoidal salmonella 128
Typhus fever 82

U

Ureaplasma urealyticum 146
Urinary tract infection 103, 126, 250, 292, 353, 354, 356, 373

V

Vaccination 93, 213
Varicella-zoster virus 151, 370
Ventilator-associated pneumonia 135, 261, 280, 284, 286, 286*t*, 364
Vibrio cholerae 13, 17, 23, 35, 41, 42, 61, 132, 134*f*, 326, 358
Vincent's angina 363
Viral gastroenteritis 191, 192, 378
Viral hemorrhagic fever 62, 275

Viral hepatitis 183
Visceral larva migrans 241

W

Warthin-Finkeldey cells 158
Weil Felix test 144
Weil's disease 143
West Nile virus 168
Western blot 86
Whooping cough 138, 275, 363
Widal test 82, 130, 130*f*
Wool sorter's disease 114
Wuchereria bancrofti 53, 229, 237, 239, 240*f*, 379

Y

Yeasts 21
Yellow fever 168
    17D vaccine 168
Yersinia pestis 132

Z

Ziehl-Neelsen staining 15, 121
Zika virus disease 169
Zoster 62, 151
Zygomycoses 250, 252